Differential Diagnosis
in
RADIOLOGY

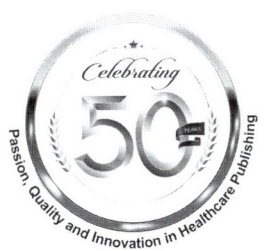

Differential Diagnosis in
RADIOLOGY

Third Edition

Sumeet Bhargava
MBBS DNB (Radiodiagnosis) FCGP FIAMS FICRI FIMSA MNAMS

Formerly Associate Professor
Department of Radiodiagnosis and Imaging
Rama Medical College and Superspecialty Hospital
Ghaziabad, Uttar Pradesh, India

Satish K Bhargava
MD (Radiodiagnosis) MD (Radiotherapy) DMRD FICRI FIAMS FCCP FUSI FIMSA FAMS

Formerly Professor and Head
Department of Radiology and Imaging
School of Medical Sciences and Research
Sharda Hospital, Sharda University
Greater Noida

Professor and Head
Department of Radiology and Imaging
University College of Medical Sciences (University of Delhi)
and Guru Teg Bahadur Hospital
New Delhi

Head, Department of Radiology and Imaging
JN Medical College, Aligarh Muslim University
Aligarh, Uttar Pradesh, India

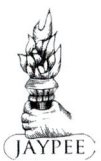

JAYPEE BROTHERS MEDICAL PUBLISHERS
The Health Sciences Publisher
New Delhi | London | Panama

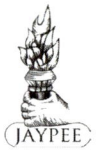 **Jaypee Brothers Medical Publishers (P) Ltd**

Headquarters
Jaypee Brothers Medical Publishers (P) Ltd
4838/24, Ansari Road, Daryaganj
New Delhi 110 002, India
Phone: +91-11-43574357
Fax: +91-11-43574314
Email: jaypee@jaypeebrothers.com

Overseas Offices

J.P. Medical Ltd
83 Victoria Street, London
SW1H 0HW (UK)
Phone: +44 20 3170 8910
Fax: +44 (0)20 3008 6180
Email: info@jpmedpub.com

Jaypee-Highlights Medical Publishers Inc
City of Knowledge, Bld. 235, 2nd Floor
Clayton, Panama City, Panama
Phone: +1 507-301-0496
Fax: +1 507-301-0499
Email: cservice@jphmedical.com

Jaypee Brothers Medical Publishers (P) Ltd
Bhotahity, Kathmandu, Nepal
Phone: +977-9741283608
Email: kathmandu@jaypeebrothers.com

Website: www.jaypeebrothers.com
Website: www.jaypeedigital.com

© 2019, Jaypee Brothers Medical Publishers

The views and opinions expressed in this book are solely those of the original contributor(s)/author(s) and do not necessarily represent those of editor(s) of the book.

All rights reserved. No part of this publication may be reproduced, stored or transmitted in any form or by any means, electronic, mechanical, photocopying, recording or otherwise, without the prior permission in writing of the publishers.

All brand names and product names used in this book are trade names, service marks, trademarks or registered trademarks of their respective owners. The publisher is not associated with any product or vendor mentioned in this book.

Medical knowledge and practice change constantly. This book is designed to provide accurate, authoritative information about the subject matter in question. However, readers are advised to check the most current information available on procedures included and check information from the manufacturer of each product to be administered, to verify the recommended dose, formula, method and duration of administration, adverse effects and contraindications. It is the responsibility of the practitioner to take all appropriate safety precautions. Neither the publisher nor the author(s)/editor(s) assume any liability for any injury and/or damage to persons or property arising from or related to use of material in this book.

This book is sold on the understanding that the publisher is not engaged in providing professional medical services. If such advice or services are required, the services of a competent medical professional should be sought.

Every effort has been made where necessary to contact holders of copyright to obtain permission to reproduce copyright material. If any have been inadvertently overlooked, the publisher will be pleased to make the necessary arrangements at the first opportunity. The **CD/DVD-ROM** (if any) provided in the sealed envelope with this book is complimentary and free of cost. **Not meant for sale.**

Inquiries for bulk sales may be solicited at: jaypee@jaypeebrothers.com

Differential Diagnosis in Radiology

First Edition: 2005

Second Edition: 2014

Third Edition: **2019**

ISBN: 978-93-5270-290-9

Printed at: Ajanta Offset & Packagings Ltd., Faridabad, Haryana

Dedicated to

*My loving late wife Kalpana
whose inspiration and sacrifice have made it
possible to bring out this book*

Satish K Bhargava

Contributors

Amit Sahu
Senior Consultant Radiology
Max Superspecialty Hospital
Saket, New Delhi, India

Anubhav Sarikwal
Ex-Senior Resident
Department of Radiology and Imaging
University College of Medical Sciences
(University of Delhi)
and Guru Teg Bahadur Hospital
New Delhi, India

Ashish Verma
Associate Professor
Department of Radiodiagnosis and Imaging
Institute of Medical Sciences
Banaras Hindu University
Varanasi, Uttar Pradesh, India

HM Kansal
Ex-Professor
Department of Pulmonary Medicine
School of Medical Sciences and Research
Sharda Hospital, Sharda University
Greater Noida, Uttar Pradesh, India

Mamta Motla
Ex-Senior Resident
Department of Radiology and Imaging
University College of Medical Sciences
(University of Delhi)
and Guru Teg Bahadur Hospital
New Delhi, India

Nidhi Bhargava
Ex-Senior Resident
Department of Radiology and Imaging
University College of Medical Sciences
(University of Delhi)
and Guru Teg Bahadur Hospital
New Delhi, India

OP Sharma
Ex-Professor
Department of Radiodiagnosis
Institute of Medical Sciences
Banaras Hindu University
Varanasi, Uttar Pradesh, India

Pardeep Kumar
Ex-Resident
Department of Radiology and Imaging
University College of Medical Sciences (University of Delhi) and Guru Teg Bahadur Hospital
New Delhi, India

Pushpender Gupta
Department of Radiology
Wake Forest Baptist Medical Center
Winston-Salem, North Carolina, USA

Rajeev Chaturvedi
Ex-Senior Resident
Department of Radiology and Imaging
University College of Medical Sciences (University of Delhi) and Guru Teg Bahadur Hospital
New Delhi, India

Rajul Rastogi
Associate Professor
Department of Radiology and Imaging
Teerthanker Mahaveer University
Moradabad, Uttar Pradesh, India

Satish K Bhargava
Formerly Professor and Head
Department of Radiology and Imaging
School of Medical Sciences and Research
Sharda Hospital, Sharda University
Greater Noida
Professor and Head
Department of Radiology and Imaging
University College of Medical Sciences (University of Delhi) and Guru Teg Bahadur Hospital
New Delhi

Head
Department of Radiology and Imaging
JN Medical College
Aligarh Muslim University
Aligarh, Uttar Pradesh, India

Shuchi Bhatt
Associate Professor
Department of Radiology and Imaging
University College of Medical Sciences (University of Delhi)
and Guru Teg Bahadur Hospital
New Delhi, India

Sumeet Bhargava
Formerly Associate Professor
Department of Radiodiagnosis and Imaging
Rama Medical College and Superspecialty Hospital
Ghaziabad, Uttar Pradesh, India

Vinita Rathi
Professor
Department of Radiology and Imaging
University College of Medical Sciences (University of Delhi) and Guru Teg Bahadur Hospital
New Delhi, India

Preface to the Third Edition

In the era of imaging, interpretation of plain radiograph and to arrive a proper diagnosis for proper management is very crucial for a radiologists, physicians and orthopedic surgeons. Keeping in view of this and enormous demand of the book from the residents of various specialties and radiologists from all over the country and abroad. It was thought proper to add more illustrations for better understanding of various diseases.

We are sure that this third edition will be more beneficial to the residents and practicing consulting physicians in solving day- to-day problems so as to arrive at a correct diagnosis and help in proper management.

Sumeet Bhargava
Satish K Bhargava

Preface to the First Edition

The advancement in Radiology and subspecialties over a period of two decades has tremendously enhanced this course and indepth knowledge of image interpretation. This is particularly true in a developing country like ours, where still majority of radiologists practice in broader specialty and it is not always feasible to update the knowledge because of paucity of time and availability of literature/newer books at all places. However, an interpretation of any radiograph is extremely essential for a radiologist to arrive at a correct diagnosis, keeping in view various salient features of disease entity on various imaging modalities and to exclude other similar looking pictures. Thus, it is more important for a trainee radiologist and a radiologist in practice to have a book, which should be a valuable primer and also the concise and handy reference to use in day-to-day practice. An attempt has been made to list out as many important conditions as possible, enumerated their salient features and important differential diagnoses so as to arrive at a particular diagnosis.

Sumeet Bhargava
Satish K Bhargava

Acknowledgments

We are grateful to our colleagues and friends, who gave timely support and stood solidly behind us in our joint endeavor of bringing out this book, which was required keeping in view the wide acceptability of the ultrasound technique.

We are thankful to Shri Jitendar P Vij (Group Chairman), Mr Ankit Vij (Managing Director), Ms Chetna Malhotra Vohra (Associate Director—Content Strategy) and Ms Madhuri Aggarwal (Development Editor) of M/s Jaypee Brothers Medical Publishers (P) Ltd, New Delhi, India, and all the contributors, who have always been in keen desire to work with smiling faces and with polite voices, as a result of which this book has seen the light of the day.

Contents

1. **Chest** 1
    - Lesions of Thoracic Inlet 1
      Satish K Bhargava, Rajeev Chaturvedi, Amit Sahu
    - Cystic Lymphangioma 6
      Sumeet Bhargava, Satish K Bhargava
    - Solid with Fat Density 6
      Sumeet Bhargava, Satish K Bhargava
    - Solid without Fat Density 6
      Sumeet Bhargava, Satish K Bhargava
    - Mediastinal Masses 7
      Satish K Bhargava, Nidhi Bhargava
    - Pleuropericardial Cyst 8
      Sumeet Bhargava, Satish K Bhargava
    - Differential Diagnosis of Soft Tissue Lesions in
      Right Anterior Cardiophrenic Angle 8
      Sumeet Bhargava, Satish K Bhargava
    - Middle Mediastinal Masses 9
      Sumeet Bhargava, Satish K Bhargava
    - Posterior Mediastinal Masses 10
      Sumeet Bhargava, Satish K Bhargava
    - Hiatus Hernia 10
      Sumeet Bhargava, Satish K Bhargava
    - Esophageal Lesions 10
      Sumeet Bhargava, Satish K Bhargava
    - Paravertebral Lesions 10
      Sumeet Bhargava, Satish K Bhargava
    - Differential Diagnosis of Superior Mediastinal Masses 11
      Sumeet Bhargava, Satish K Bhargava
    - Differential Diagnosis of Anterior Mediastinal Masses 14
      Shuchi Bhatt, Rajul Rastogi, Sumeet Bhargava
    - Anterior Mediastinal Mass 16
      Satish K Bhargava, Pardeep Kumar
    - Middle Mediastinal Mass 16
      Sumeet Bhargava, Satish K Bhargava
    - Lymph Nodes 17
      Sumeet Bhargava, Satish K Bhargava
    - Differential Diagnosis of Posterior Mediastinal Masses 19
      Pushpender Gupta, Satish K Bhargava

- Chest Wall Abnormalities 21
  Rajul Rastogi, Vinita Rathi
- Superior Rib Notching 22
  Shuchi Bhatt, Pardeep Kumar
- Inferior Rib Notching 24
  Satish K Bhargava, Nidhi Bhargava
- Elevation of Diaphragm 25
  Amit Sahu, Nidhi Bhargava, Shuchi Bhatt
- Pneumomediastinum 27
  Nidhi Bhargava, Satish K Bhargava
- Lung Tumors 27
  Satish K Bhargava, Nidhi Bhargava
- Hilar Enlargement 29
  HM Kansal, Nidhi Bhargava, Satish K Bhargava
- Apical Shadows 29
  Sumeet Bhargava, Satish K Bhargava
- Calcification on Chest Radiograph 29
  Satish K Bhargava, Nidhi Bhargava
- Air-Fluid Levels on Chest X-ray 31
  Satish K Bhargava, Nidhi Bhargava
- Cavitating Pulmonary Lesions 32
  Amit Sahu, Nidhi Bhargava, Satish K Bhargava
- Mass within Cavity 32
  Nidhi Bhargava, Satish K Bhargava
- Cavitating Pulmonary Lesions 32
  Pardeep Kumar, Rajul Rastogi, Satish K Bhargava
- Trauma 35
  Sumeet Bhargava, Satish K Bhargava
- Lucent Lung Lesions 35
  Nidhi Bhargava, Satish K Bhargava
- Solitary Pulmonary Nodule 36
  Nidhi Bhargava, Shuchi Bhatt
- Solitary Pulmonary Nodule 37
  Satish K Bhargava, HM Kansal, Sumeet Bhargava
- Pulmonary Edema on the Opposite Side to a Pre-existing Abnormality 42
  Nidhi Bhargava, Rajul Rastogi
- Miliary Shadowing 44
  HM Kansal, Satish K Bhargava, Sumeet Bhargava
- Miliary Shadowing (0.5–2 mm) 46
  Satish K Bhargava, Nidhi Bhargava, Sumeet Bhargava
- Multiple Opacities 47
  Sumeet Bhargava, Nidhi Bhargava, Shuchi Bhatt
- Complete Opaque Hemithorax 48
  Sumeet Bhargava, Nidhi Bhargava, Vinita Rathi

- Opaque Hemithorax 48
  Satish K Bhargava, Pushpender Gupta, HM Kansal
- Hypertransradiant Lung Field 50
  Sumeet Bhargava, Satish K Bhargava, Anubhav Sarikwal
- Hypertranslucent Lung Field 53
  Nidhi Bhargava, Sumeet Bhargava
- Honeycomb Lung 54
  Sumeet Bhargava, Nidhi Bhargava, Satish K Bhargava
- Honeycomb Pattern 55
  Satish K Bhargava, Vinita Rathi, Sumeet Bhargava
- Asbestosis 56
  Sumeet Bhargava, Satish K Bhargava
- Pleural Diseases or Lesions 57
  Rajul Rastogi, Sumeet Bhargava
- Pleural Fluid 61
  Shuchi Bhatt, Nidhi Bhargava
- Pleural Tumors 62
  Nidhi Bhargava, Sumeet Bhargava, Amit Sahu, Satish K Bhargava
- Pleural Calcification 62
  Sumeet Bhargava, HM Kansal, Rajeev Chaturvedi, Satish K Bhargava
- High Resolution CT-Pattern of Parenchymal Disease 63
  Rajul Rastogi, Nidhi Bhargava, Satish K Bhargava
- Cardiophrenic Angle Mass 63
  Sumeet Bhargava, Satish K Bhargava, HM Kansal

2. Breast: Mammographic Differential Diagnosis 66
  Sumeet Bhargava, Rajul Rastogi, Satish K Bhargava, Pushpender Gupta
- Density of Lesion on Mammogram 66
  Sumeet Bhargava, Satish K Bhargava
- Margins of Lesion 66
  Sumeet Bhargava, Satish K Bhargava
- Circumscribed Radiolucent Lesion 66
  Sumeet Bhargava, Satish K Bhargava
- Mixed Density Lesions 66
  Sumeet Bhargava, Satish K Bhargava
- Radiopaque (Soft Tissue Density Lesion) 68
  Sumeet Bhargava, Satish K Bhargava
- Circumscribed Malignant Lesions (Circumscribed Carcinoma) 70
  Sumeet Bhargava, Satish K Bhargava
- Breast Calcification Types 72
  Sumeet Bhargava, Satish K Bhargava
- Carcinoma 76
  Sumeet Bhargava, Satish K Bhargava

3. Cardiovascular System 77

- Differential Diagnosis of Cardiovascular Disorders 77
  Sumeet Bhargava, Satish K Bhargava, Rajul Rastogi
- Invisible Main Pulmonary Artery 77
  Sumeet Bhargava, Satish K Bhargava
- Pulmonary Arterial Hypertension 78
  Sumeet Bhargava, Satish K Bhargava
- Enlarged Left Ventricle 79
  Sumeet Bhargava, Satish K Bhargava
- Enlarged Left Atrium 80
  Rajul Rastogi, Satish K Bhargava, Sumeet Bhargava
- Dilatation of Pulmonary Trunk 82
  Rajul Rastogi, Satish K Bhargava, Sumeet Bhargava
- Enlargement Aorta 82
  Sumeet Bhargava, Satish K Bhargava
- Small Aorta 83
  Sumeet Bhargava, Satish K Bhargava
- Enlarged Right Atrium 83
  Sumeet Bhargava, Satish K Bhargava
- Enlarged Right Ventricle 85
  Sumeet Bhargava, Satish K Bhargava
- Right Aortic Arch 85
  Rajul Rastogi, Satish K Bhargava, Sumeet Bhargava
- Pulmonary Venous Hypertension 87
  Rajul Rastogi, Satish K Bhargava, Sumeet Bhargava
- Enlarged Superior Vena Cava 87
  Sumeet Bhargava, Satish K Bhargava
- Cardiac Calcifications 88
  Sumeet Bhargava, Satish K Bhargava
- Cardiac Valve Calcifications 88
  Amit Sahu, Sumeet Bhargava, Satish K Bhargava
- Situs 89
  Sumeet Bhargava, Satish K Bhargava
- Cyanotic Heart Disease 89
  Sumeet Bhargava, Satish K Bhargava

4. Soft Tissue Lesions 91

Sumeet Bhargava, Satish K Bhargava, Shuchi Bhatt
- Differential Diagnosis of Soft Tissue Lesions 91
- Soft Tissue Ossification 92
- Linear Calcification of Soft Tissues 93
- Parasitic Calcification 94
- Areas of Decreased Density 94

- Periarticular Soft Tissue Calcification 96
- Generalized Calcinosis 97
- Sheet-like Calcification in Soft Tissue 97

5. Abdomen and Gastrointestinal Tract and Hepatobiliary System 98

- Dilated Esophagus 98
  Rajul Rastogi, Satish K Bhargava, Rajeev Chaturvedi
- Esophageal Carcinoma 100
  Rajul Rastogi, Rajeev Chaturvedi, Satish K Bhargava
- Thickened Mucosal Folds Esophagus and Stomach 103
  Ashish Verma, Shuchi Bhatt, Sumeet Bhargava
- Thickened Gastric Folds 104
  Sumeet Bhargava, Satish K Bhargava
- Thickened Small Bowel 108
  Sumeet Bhargava, Satish K Bhargava
- Thickened Gastric Folds 110
  Rajul Rastogi, Satish K Bhargava, Sumeet Bhargava
- Thickened Duodenal Folds 111
  Amit Sahu, Rajul Rastogi, Satish K Bhargava, Sumeet Bhargava
- Massively Dilated Stomach 112
  Satish K Bhargava, Rajul Rastogi, Sumeet Bhargava
- Target Lesions in Stomach on Barium Study 112
  Sumeet Bhargava, Satish K Bhargava, Rajul Rastogi
- Gas in Gastric Wall 113
  Satish K Bhargava, Rajul Rastogi, Sumeet Bhargava
- Cobblestone Duodenal Cap on Barium Study 113
  Satish K Bhargava, Rajul Rastogi, Sumeet Bhargava
- Dilated Duodenum/Obstruction of Duodenum 113
  Rajul Rastogi, Sumeet Bhargava, Satish K Bhargava
- Dilated Small Bowel/Jejunal and Ileal Obstruction 114
  Sumeet Bhargava, Rajul Rastogi, Shuchi Bhatt
- Strictures Small Bowel 114
  Rajul Rastogi, Satish K Bhargava
- Small Intestinal Stricture 115
  Anubhav Sarikwal, Sumeet Bhargava
- Thickened Folds in Small Bowel 118
  Rajul Rastogi, Shuchi Bhatt, Sumeet Bhargava
- Thickened Small Bowel Folds with Gastric Abnormality 119
  Rajul Rastogi, Sumeet Bhargava, Satish K Bhargava
- Nodular Appearance of Small Bowel 119
  Rajul Rastogi, Sumeet Bhargava, Satish K Bhargava
- Malabsorption 119
  Satish K Bhargava, Rajul Rastogi, Sumeet Bhargava
- Protein Losing Enteropathy 124
  Satish K Bhargava, Rajul Rastogi, Sumeet Bhargava

- Pathologic Lesions in Terminal Ileum ... 124
  Satish K Bhargava, Rajul Rastogi, Sumeet Bhargava
- Colonic Polyps ... 125
  Satish K Bhargava, Rajul Rastogi, Sumeet Bhargava
- Colonic Polyps ... 126
  Sumeet Bhargava, Satish K Bhargava
- Colonic Strictures/Narrowing ... 127
  Rajul Rastogi, Sumeet Bhargava, Satish K Bhargava
- Pneumatosis Intestinalis ... 128
  Rajul Rastogi, Sumeet Bhargava, Satish K Bhargava
- Megacolon in Adults ... 129
  Rajul Rastogi, Satish K Bhargava
- Thumbprinting in Colon ... 129
  Rajul Rastogi, Sumeet Bhargava, Satish K Bhargava
- Aphthous Ulcers ... 129
  Rajul Rastogi, Sumeet Bhargava, Satish K Bhargava
- Anterior Indentation of Rectosigmoid Junction ... 130
  Rajul Rastogi, Sumeet Bhargava, Satish K Bhargava
- Widening/Enlargement of Presacral/Retrorectal Space ... 130
  Sumeet Bhargava, Rajul Rastogi, Satish K Bhargava
- Cystic Mesenteric Masses ... 131
  Sumeet Bhargava, Rajul Rastogi, Satish K Bhargava
- Nonvisualization of Gallbladder on Ultrasound ... 131
  Rajul Rastogi, Sumeet Bhargava
- Gas in Biliary Tree ... 131
  Rajul Rastogi, Sumeet Bhargava, Satish K Bhargava
- Gas in Portal Venous ... 131
  Rajul Rastogi, Sumeet Bhargava, Satish K Bhargava
- Diffuse Hepatomegaly ... 132
  Rajul Rastogi, Sumeet Bhargava, Satish K Bhargava
- Hepatic Calcification ... 132
  Amit Sahu, Rajul Rastogi, Sumeet Bhargava, Satish K Bhargava
- Primary Hepatic Masses ... 133
  Rajul Rastogi, Sumeet Bhargava, Satish K Bhargava
- Neonatal Obstructive Jaundice ... 134
  Rajul Rastogi, Sumeet Bhargava, Satish K Bhargava
- Fetal/Neonatal Hepatic Calcification ... 134
  Rajul Rastogi, Sumeet Bhargava, Satish K Bhargava
- Diffusely Hypoechoic Liver ... 135
  Rajul Rastogi, Sumeet Bhargava, Satish K Bhargava
- Diffusely Hyperechoic Liver (Bright Liver) ... 135
  Rajul Rastogi, Sumeet Bhargava, Satish K Bhargava
- Focal and Hyperechoic Hepatic Lesions ... 135
  Rajul Rastogi, Satish K Bhargava

- Focal, Hypoechoic and Hepatic Lesions 135
  Sumeet Bhargava, Satish K Bhargava, Rajul Rastogi
- Periportal Hyperechogenicity 135
  Sumeet Bhargava, Satish K Bhargava, Rajul Rastogi
- Thickened Gallbladder Wall 136
  Sumeet Bhargava, Satish K Bhargava, Rajul Rastogi
- Focal Hypodense Lesions on NECT Liver 136
  Satish K Bhargava, Sumeet Bhargava, Rajul Rastogi
- Hyperperfusion Abnormalities of Liver 137
  Satish K Bhargava, Rajul Rastogi, Sumeet Bhargava
- Hepatic Tumors with Vascular "Scar" 137
  Satish K Bhargava, Rajul Rastogi, Sumeet Bhargava
- Diffusely Hypodense Liver on NECT 137
  Satish K Bhargava, Rajul Rastogi, Sumeet Bhargava
- Splenomegaly 137
  Sumeet Bhargava
- Splenic Calcification 138
  Rajul Rastogi, Sumeet Bhargava, Satish K Bhargava
- Hyperechoic Splenic Lesion 138
  Rajul Rastogi, Sumeet Bhargava, Satish K Bhargava
- Focal Hypoattenuating Lesions in Spleen 138
  Rajul Rastogi, Sumeet Bhargava, Satish K Bhargava
- Pancreatic Calcification 138
  Rajul Rastogi, Sumeet Bhargava, Satish K Bhargava
- Pancreatic Masses 139
  Satish K Bhargava, Pushpender Gupta, Pardeep Kumar
- Focal Pancreatic Masses 141
  Rajul Rastogi, Sumeet Bhargava, Satish K Bhargava
- Adrenal Mass 142
  Rajul Rastogi, Sumeet Bhargava, Satish K Bhargava
- Adrenal Calcification 142
  Rajul Rastogi, Sumeet Bhargava, Satish K Bhargava
- Extraluminal Intra-abdominal Gas 142
  Rajul Rastogi, Sumeet Bhargava, Satish K Bhargava
- Pneumoperitoneum 143
  Sumeet Bhargava, Anubhav Sarikwal, Shuchi Bhatt
- Pneumoperitoneum 145
  Rajul Rastogi, Sumeet Bhargava, Satish K Bhargava
- Gasless Abdomen 146
  Rajul Rastogi, Sumeet Bhargava, Satish K Bhargava
- Ascites 146
  Rajul Rastogi, Sumeet Bhargava, Satish K Bhargava
- Abdominal Mass in Neonate 147
  Rajul Rastogi, Sumeet Bhargava

- Abdominal Mass in Child 148
  Sumeet Bhargava, Satish K Bhargava, Rajul Rastogi
- Intestinal Obstruction in Neonate 149
  Sumeet Bhargava, Rajul Rastogi, Satish K Bhargava
- Abnormalities of Bowel Rotation 150
  Sumeet Bhargava, Rajul Rastogi, Satish K Bhargava
- Intra-abdominal Calcification in Neonate 150
  Sumeet Bhargava, Rajul Rastogi, Satish K Bhargava
- Hematemesis 151
  Sumeet Bhargava, Satish K Bhargava, Rajul Rastogi
- Dysphagia in Adults 151
  Sumeet Bhargava, Satish K Bhargava, Rajul Rastogi
- Neonatal Dysphagia 152
  Sumeet Bhargava, Satish K Bhargava, Rajul Rastogi
- Pharyngeal/Esophageal Diverticula 152
  Sumeet Bhargava, Satish K Bhargava, Rajul Rastogi
- Esophagitis/Esophageal Ulcers 153
  Rajul Rastogi, Sumeet Bhargava, Satish K Bhargava
- Esophageal Strictures 155
  Satish K Bhargava, Rajul Rastogi
- Tertiary Contractions in Esophagus 155
  Rajul Rastogi, Sumeet Bhargava, Satish K Bhargava
- Gastric Masses and Filling Defects 156
  Sumeet Bhargava, Satish K Bhargava, Rajul Rastogi
- Linitis Plastica 157
  Rajul Rastogi, Shuchi Bhatt, Sumeet Bhargava
- Gastrocolic Fistula 159
  Rajul Rastogi, Satish K Bhargava
- Retroperitoneal Fibrosis 159
  Sumeet Bhargava, Shuchi Bhatt, Satish K Bhargava
- Mass of Iliopsoas Compartment 160
  Satish K Bhargava, Sumeet Bhargava, Ashish Verma
- Anatomy of Liver, Bile Ducts and Pancreas 161
  Sumeet Bhargava
- Congenital Gallbladder Anomalies 164
  Sumeet Bhargava, Satish K Bhargava
- Inflammatory Bowel Disease 166
  Satish K Bhargava, Pushpender Gupta, Shuchi Bhatt, Pardeep Kumar

6. Skeletal System and Joints 172

- Abnormal Skeletal Maturation 172
  Sumeet Bhargava, Satish K Bhargava, Rajul Rastogi
- Short Limb Skeletal Dysplasia 173
  Satish K Bhargava, Rajul Rastogi, Sumeet Bhargava

Contents

- Short Spine Skeletal Dysplasia 174
  Sumeet Bhargava, Satish K Bhargava, Rajul Rastogi
- Lethal Neonatal Dysplasia 175
  Satish K Bhargava, Rajul Rastogi
- Dumbbell-Shaped Long Bones 175
  Satish K Bhargava, Rajul Rastogi
- Mucopolysaccharidoses and Mucolipidosis 175
  Satish K Bhargava, Rajul Rastogi
- Mucolipidoses 176
  Sumeet Bhargava, Satish K Bhargava, Rajul Rastogi
- Generalized Osteosclerosis 176
  Satish K Bhargava, Rajul Rastogi
- Sclerotic Bone Lesions 176
  Satish K Bhargava, Rajul Rastogi, Sumeet Bhargava
- Bone Sclerosis Associated with Periosteal Reaction 179
  Satish K Bhargava, Rajul Rastogi
- Solitary Sclerotic Lesion with Lucent Center 180
  Satish K Bhargava, Rajul Rastogi
- Coarse Trabecular Pattern of Bone 180
  Satish K Bhargava, Rajul Rastogi
- Characteristics of Metastatic Lesions to the Primary Tumors 180
  Sumeet Bhargava, Satish K Bhargava
- Childhood Tumors Metastasizing to Bone 180
  Satish K Bhargava, Rajul Rastogi
- Bubbly Bone Lesions 180
  Satish K Bhargava, Rajul Rastogi
- Primary Bone Tumors: Clinical Features, Site of Predilection, and
  Radiologic Presentation 182
  Satish K Bhargava, Rajul Rastogi, Sumeet Bhargava
- Radiologic Characteristics of Benign and Malignant Bone Lesions 182
  Satish K Bhargava, Rajul Rastogi
- Subarticular Lytic Bone Lesion 183
  Satish K Bhargava, Rajul Rastogi, Sumeet Bhargava
- Osteolytic Defects in the Medulla 184
  Satish K Bhargava, Rajul Rastogi
- Lucent Bone Lesion Containing Bone/Calcium 187
  Satish K Bhargava, Rajul Rastogi
- Common Lytic Bone Lesions 188
  Satish K Bhargava, Rajul Rastogi
- Location of Some Common Neoplasms/Lesions 188
  Satish K Bhargava, Rajul Rastogi
- Septated Bone Lesions 189
  Satish K Bhargava, Rajul Rastogi
- Moth-Eaten Bone 189
  Satish K Bhargava, Rajul Rastogi

- Osteopenia 190
  Satish K Bhargava, Rajul Rastogi
- Periosteal Reactions: Types and Conditions 192
  Sumeet Bhargava, Satish K Bhargava, Rajul Rastogi
- Types of Periosteal Reactions 193
  Satish K Bhargava, Rajul Rastogi
- Periosteal Reaction in Childhood 194
  Satish K Bhargava, Rajul Rastogi
- Hypertrophic Osteoarthropathy 195
  Satish K Bhargava, Rajul Rastogi
- Bone Dysplasias: Associated with Multiple Fractures 196
  Sumeet Bhargava, Satish K Bhargava, Rajul Rastogi
- Excessive Callus Formation 196
  Rajul Rastogi, Sumeet Bhargava, Satish K Bhargava
- Bone within Bone Appearance 196
  Rajul Rastogi, Sumeet Bhargava, Satish K Bhargava
- Fatigue Fractures 196
  Rajul Rastogi, Sumeet Bhargava, Satish K Bhargava
- Pseudoarthrosis 197
  Rajul Rastogi, Sumeet Bhargava, Satish K Bhargava
- Irregular/Stippled Epiphysis 197
  Amit Sahu, Rajul Rastogi, Sumeet Bhargava, Satish K Bhargava
- Avascular Necrosis/Osteonecrosis/Aseptic Necrosis 198
  Rajul Rastogi, Sumeet Bhargava, Satish K Bhargava
- Solitary Radiolucent Metaphyseal Bands 199
  Sumeet Bhargava, Rajul Rastogi, Satish K Bhargava
- Solitary Dense Metaphyseal Band 200
  Rajul Rastogi, Satish K Bhargava
- Alternating Radiolucent/Dense Metaphyseal Bands 200
  Sumeet Bhargava, Rajul Rastogi, Satish K Bhargava
- Dense Vertical Metaphyseal Lines 200
  Rajul Rastogi, Satish K Bhargava
- Frayed Metaphysis 200
  Rajul Rastogi
- Cupping of Metaphysis 200
  Rajul Rastogi, Satish K Bhargava
- Erlenmeyer Flask Deformity 200
  Rajul Rastogi, Sumeet Bhargava, Satish K Bhargava
- Erosion of Medial Metaphyses of Proximal Humerus 201
  Rajul Rastogi, Satish K Bhargava
- Abnormality Related to Clavicles 201
  Rajul Rastogi, Sumeet Bhargava, Satish K Bhargava
- Rib Lesions 201
  Rajul Rastogi, Satish K Bhargava

- Rib Notching 202
  Rajul Rastogi, Sumeet Bhargava, Satish K Bhargava
- Abnormal Shape, Size, and Density of Ribs 202
  Rajul Rastogi, Sumeet Bhargava, Satish K Bhargava
- Madelung Deformity 202
  Rajul Rastogi, Sumeet Bhargava, Satish K Bhargava
- Carpal Fusion 203
  Rajul Rastogi, Satish K Bhargava
- Abnormal Digits 203
  Rajul Rastogi, Satish K Bhargava
- Abnormal Thumb 204
  Rajul Rastogi, Satish K Bhargava
- Lytic Lesion in Digits 204
  Rajul Rastogi, Satish K Bhargava
- Acro-Osteal Changes 204
  Rajul Rastogi, Sumeet Bhargava, Satish K Bhargava
- Monoarthritis 205
  Rajul Rastogi, Satish K Bhargava
- Arthritis with Periostitis 206
  Rajul Rastogi, Satish K Bhargava
- Arthritis with Demineralization 206
  Rajul Rastogi, Sumeet Bhargava, Satish K Bhargava
- Arthritis without Demineralization 207
  Rajul Rastogi, Sumeet Bhargava, Satish K Bhargava
- Arthritis with Preserved/Widened Joint Space 207
  Rajul Rastogi, Sumeet Bhargava, Satish K Bhargava
- Enlarged Femoral Intercondylar Notch 208
  Rajul Rastogi, Sumeet Bhargava, Satish K Bhargava
- Plantar Calcaneal Spur 208
  Sumeet Bhargava, Rajul Rastogi, Satish K Bhargava
- Chondrocalcinosis 208
  Sumeet Bhargava, Rajul Rastogi, Satish K Bhargava
- Ankylosis of Interphalangeal Joints 208
  Rajul Rastogi, Sumeet Bhargava, Satish K Bhargava
- Enthesiopathy 208
  Rajul Rastogi, Sumeet Bhargava, Satish K Bhargava
- Sacroiliitis 208
  Rajul Rastogi, Satish K Bhargava
- Protrusio Acetabuli 209
  Sumeet Bhargava, Rajul Rastogi, Satish K Bhargava
- Widening of Symphysis Pubis (Diastasis) 210
  Rajul Rastogi, Sumeet Bhargava, Satish K Bhargava
- Fusion of Symphysis Pubis 210
  Rajul Rastogi, Sumeet Bhargava, Satish K Bhargava

- Radiographic Findings in Degenerative, Inflammatory, and Neuropathic Arthritis 210
  Rajul Rastogi, Satish K Bhargava
- Comparative Features of Seronegative Spondyloarthritides D/D of Dwarfism 210
  Rajul Rastogi, Satish K Bhargava
- Dysplasias 212
  Sumeet Bhargava, Satish K Bhargava
- Thanatophoric Dwarfism 213
  Sumeet Bhargava, Satish K Bhargava
- Mesomelic Dwarfism 213
  Sumeet Bhargava, Satish K Bhargava
- Acromesomelic Dwarfism 213
  Sumeet Bhargava, Satish K Bhargava
- Acromelic Dwarfism 213
  Sumeet Bhargava, Satish K Bhargava
- Sclerotic Lesions of Bone 214
  Ashish Verma, Sumeet Bhargava
- Lytic Lesions in Bone 217
  Satish K Bhargava, Shuchi Bhatt
- Differential Diagnosis of Generalized Osteoporosis 222
  Sumeet Bhargava, Satish K Bhargava
- Solitary Dense Vertebra 225
  Pushpender Gupta, Satish K Bhargava
- Acro-Osteolysis 226
  Vinita Rathi, Sumeet Bhargava
- Sacroiliitis 227
  Satish K Bhargava
- Arthritis Involving Spinal Column 228
  Sumeet Bhargava, Satish K Bhargava
- Bone Cyst 230
  Satish K Bhargava, Anubhav Sarikwal

7. Urogenital System 235

- Adult and Neonatal Kidney: Differences 235
  Sumeet Bhargava, Satish K Bhargava
- Smooth and Small Kidneys 235
  Rajul Rastogi, Satish K Bhargava
- Small, Smooth, and Unilateral Kidneys 235
  Sumeet Bhargava, Satish K Bhargava
- Small, Smooth, and Bilateral Kidneys 237
  Sumeet Bhargava, Satish K Bhargava
- Small and Smooth Kidneys 237
  Shuchi Bhatt, Ashish Verma

- Small and Smooth Kidneys 239
  Sumeet Bhargava, Satish K Bhargava
- Small and Irregular Kidneys 239
  Satish K Bhargava, Rajul Rastogi
- Large and Smooth Kidneys 241
  Sumeet Bhargava, Rajul Rastogi, Satish K Bhargava
- Bilateral Large Smooth Kidneys 243
  Sumeet Bhargava, Satish K Bhargava
- Extraskeletal Features 244
  Sumeet Bhargava, Satish K Bhargava
- Leukemia 245
  Sumeet Bhargava, Satish K Bhargava
- Acute Interstitial Nephritis 245
  Sumeet Bhargava, Satish K Bhargava
- Autosomal Recessive (Infantile) Polycystic Kidney Disease 245
  Sumeet Bhargava, Satish K Bhargava
- Nephromegaly Associated with Cirrhosis, Hyperalimentation, and Diabetes Mellitus 246
  Sumeet Bhargava, Satish K Bhargava
- Nonvisualization of a Kidney during Excretion Urography 246
  Satish K Bhargava
- Dilated Calyx and Dilated Ureter 249
  Amit Sahu, Pardeep Kumar, Shuchi Bhatt
- Dilated Ureter and Calyces 249
  Sumeet Bhargava, Satish K Bhargava
- Dilated Calyx 250
  Sumeet Bhargava, Satish K Bhargava
- Gas in Urinary Tract 252
  Satish K Bhargava, Sumeet Bhargava
- Loss of Renal Outline on Plain Film 252
  Sumeet Bhargava, Satish K Bhargava
- Renovascular Hypertension 254
  Sumeet Bhargava
- Renal Calcification 255
  Sumeet Bhargava, Satish K Bhargava
- Renal Mass 257
  Sumeet Bhargava, Satish K Bhargava, Pushpender Gupta
- Abscess Typical Imaging Features 262
  Sumeet Bhargava, Satish K Bhargava
- Cystic Disease of Kidneys 262
  Sumeet Bhargava, Satish K Bhargava
- Carcinoma of the Bladder 266
  Rajul Rastogi, Sumeet Bhargava, Satish K Bhargava

- Bladder Outflow Obstruction 267
  Rajul Rastogi, Shuchi Bhatt
- Testicular Tumors 271
  Rajul Rastogi, Shuchi Bhatt
- Seminal Vesicle Calcification 273
  Anubhav Sarikwal, Satish K Bhargava
- Differential Diagnosis of Abnormal Nephrograms 274
  Sumeet Bhargava, Mamta Motla, Shuchi Bhatt
- Filling Defect in the Bladder 274
  Mamta Motla, Satish K Bhargava
- Carcinoma Prostate 274
  Satish K Bhargava, Anubhav Sarikwal
- The Prostate 279
  Sumeet Bhargava, Shuchi Bhatt
- Differential Diagnosis of Adrenal Mass 282
  Sumeet Bhargava, Satish K Bhargava
- Painless Hematuria 284
  Satish K Bhargava, Ashish Verma

8. Head, Neck, and Spine 287

- Lucency in the Skull Vault: Without Sclerosis 287
  Sumeet Bhargava, Satish K Bhargava
- Lucency in the Skull Vault: With Surrounding Sclerosis 288
  Sumeet Bhargava, Satish K Bhargava
- Thickening of the Skull Vault 289
  Vinita Rathi, Sumeet Bhargava
- Generalized Increase in Density of Skull Vault 290
  Sumeet Bhargava, Satish K Bhargava
- Metabolic 291
  Sumeet Bhargava, Satish K Bhargava
- Localized Increase in Density of the Skull Vault 292
  Sumeet Bhargava, Satish K Bhargava
- Destruction of Petrous Bone (Apex) 293
  Sumeet Bhargava, Satish K Bhargava
- Basilar Invagination 294
  Sumeet Bhargava, Satish K Bhargava
- Hair on End Skull Vault 295
  Rajul Rastogi, Satish K Bhargava
- Multiple Wormian Bones 296
  Sumeet Bhargava, Satish K Bhargava
- Posterior Fossa Cysts and Cysts-like Masses 297
  Sumeet Bhargava, Satish K Bhargava
- Enlarged Sylvian Fissure/Midline Cranial Fossa of CSF Density 297
  Sumeet Bhargava, Amit Sahu, Satish K Bhargava

- Skull Base and Cavernous Sinus 298
  Sumeet Bhargava, Satish K Bhargava
- Central Skull Base Lesions 300
  Sumeet Bhargava, Satish K Bhargava
- Cerebellopontine Angle Masses 301
  Sumeet Bhargava, Amit Sahu, Satish K Bhargava
- Suprasellar Mass 303
  Sumeet Bhargava, Satish K Bhargava
- Sellar and Suprasellar Masses 305
  Sumeet Bhargava, Satish K Bhargava
- Pituitary Apoplexy 306
  Sumeet Bhargava, Satish K Bhargava
- Aneurysm 307
  Sumeet Bhargava, Satish K Bhargava
- Rathke's Cleft Cyst 307
  Sumeet Bhargava, Satish K Bhargava
- Arachnoid Cyst 307
  Sumeet Bhargava, Satish K Bhargava
- Epidermoid and Dermoid 307
  Sumeet Bhargava, Satish K Bhargava
- Teratoma 308
  Sumeet Bhargava, Satish K Bhargava
- Germinoma (Atypical Teratoma) 308
  Sumeet Bhargava, Satish K Bhargava
- Visual Pathway Glioma 308
  Sumeet Bhargava, Satish K Bhargava
- Chordoma 308
  Sumeet Bhargava, Satish K Bhargava
- Neurosurgeon's Queries 308
  Sumeet Bhargava, Satish K Bhargava
- Expanded Pituitary Fossa 308
  Sumeet Bhargava, Satish K Bhargava
- Ring Enhancing Lesions on Contrast-enhanced Computed Tomography 310
  Sumeet Bhargava, Satish K Bhargava
- Superior Orbital Fissure Enlargement 311
  Sumeet Bhargava, Satish K Bhargava
- Neoplasm 313
  Sumeet Bhargava, Satish K Bhargava
- Temporal Bone Sclerosis 314
  Sumeet Bhargava, Satish K Bhargava
- Intervertebral Disk Space Calcification 316
  Satish K Bhargava, Sumeet Bhargava
- Ivory Vertebral Body 317
  Sumeet Bhargava, Satish K Bhargava

- Atlantoaxial Subluxation 318
  Sumeet Bhargava, Satish K Bhargava
- Posterior Scalloping of Vertebral Body 318
  Sumeet Bhargava, Satish K Bhargava
- Anterior Scalloping of Vertebral Bodies 319
  Sumeet Bhargava, Satish K Bhargava
- Anterior Vertebral Body Beaks 320
  Sumeet Bhargava, Satish K Bhargava
- Block Vertebra 321
  Sumeet Bhargava, Satish K Bhargava
- Enlarged Vertebral Body 322
  Sumeet Bhargava, Satish K Bhargava
- Solitary Collapsed Vertebra 322
  Sumeet Bhargava, Satish K Bhargava
- Multiple Collapsed Vertebrae 323
  Sumeet Bhargava, Satish K Bhargava
- Intraspinal Masses 325
  Sumeet Bhargava, Satish K Bhargava
- Differential Diagnosis of Posterior Fossa Cysts 327
  Sumeet Bhargava, Satish K Bhargava
- Enlarged Optic Foramen 328
  Pardeep Kumar, Satish K Bhargava, Rajul Rastogi
- Bare Orbit/Hypoplasia of Greater Wing of Sphenoid 329
  Rajul Rastogi, Shuchi Bhatt
- Orbital Hyperostosis 331
  Rajul Rastogi, Sumeet Bhargava
- Cephaloceles 332
  Sumeet Bhargava, Satish K Bhargava
- Pathological Intracranial Calcification 333
  Rajul Rastogi, Shuchi Bhatt
- Vascular Lesions 335
  Sumeet Bhargava, Satish K Bhargava
- J-Shaped Sella 336
  Sumeet Bhargava
- Cerebellar Malformations 338
  Pardeep Kumar, Satish K Bhargava
- Demyelinating Disorders 339
  Amit Sahu, Anubhav Sarikwal, Satish K Bhargava
- Demyelination 339
  Sumeet Bhargava, Satish K Bhargava
- Infectious 340
  Sumeet Bhargava, Satish K Bhargava
- Human Immunodeficiency Virus Encephalopathy 341
  Sumeet Bhargava, Satish K Bhargava

Contents

- Dysmyelination (Leukodystrophies) 342
  Sumeet Bhargava, Satish K Bhargava
- MELAS Syndrome 344
  Sumeet Bhargava, Satish K Bhargava
- MERRF Syndrome 344
  Sumeet Bhargava, Satish K Bhargava
- Leukodystrophies: Distinctive Features 344
  Sumeet Bhargava, Satish K Bhargava
- Prevertebral Soft Tissue Thickening 344
  Sumeet Bhargava, Satish K Bhargava
- Nasopharyngeal Masses 346
  Sumeet Bhargava, Satish K Bhargava
- Laryngeal Masses 348
  Satish K Bhargava, Anubhav Sarikwal
- Orbital Masses 349
  Rajul Rastogi, Satish K Bhargava
- Cavernous Hemangioma (Encapsulated Venous Malformation) 351
  Sumeet Bhargava, Satish K Bhargava
- Metastatic Tumors 351
  Sumeet Bhargava, Satish K Bhargava
- Miscellaneous 351
  Sumeet Bhargava, Satish K Bhargava
- Orbital Pseudotumor (Idiopathic Orbital Inflammation) 352
  Sumeet Bhargava, Satish K Bhargava
- Ocular Masses 353
  Sumeet Bhargava, Satish K Bhargava
- Intraorbital Calcification 353
  Sumeet Bhargava, Satish K Bhargava
- Inner Ear Masses 355
  Sumeet Bhargava, Satish K Bhargava
- Methods of Imaging 356
  Sumeet Bhargava, Satish K Bhargava
- Middle Ear Masses 357
  Sumeet Bhargava, Satish K Bhargava
- External Acoustic Masses 359
  Rajul Rastogi, Sumeet Bhargava, Satish K Bhargava
- Intramedullary Lesions 361
  Sumeet Bhargava, Amit Sahu, Rajeev Chaturvedi, Satish K Bhargava
- Intradural Extramedullary Masses 363
  Satish K Bhargava, Pushpender Gupta
- Extradural Extramedullary Lesion 366
  Rajul Rastogi, Shuchi Bhatt
- Differential Diagnosis of Floating Tooth 369
  Sumeet Bhargava, Satish K Bhargava

- Cysts of Jaw 371
  Sumeet Bhargava, Ashish Verma, Satish K Bhargava
- Loss of Lamina Dura of Teeth 372
  Rajul Rastogi, Vinita Rathi
- Opaque Maxillary Antrum 375
  Rajul Rastogi, Satish K Bhargava
- Thyroid Lesions.. 376
  Rajul Rastogi, Shuchi Bhatt
- Decreased or No Uptake of Radiotracer 380
  Sumeet Bhargava, Satish K Bhargava

9. Obstetrics and Gynecology 383

- Ultrasound Characteristics of Abnormal Gestation Sac... 383
  Sumeet Bhargava, Satish K Bhargava
- Differential Diagnosis between Blighted Ovum and
  Pseudogestation of Ectopic Pregnancy 383
  OP Sharma
- Differential Diagnosis between Ectopic Pregnancy, Abortion in
  Progress (Early Gestation) and Nabothian Cysts 383
  OP Sharma
- Differential Diagnosis between Partial Mole, Intrauterine Fetal Death
  with Hydropic Placental Degeneration, and Twin Pregnancy
  (Mole and Fetus)... 384
  OP Sharma
- Differential Diagnosis between Pelvic Masses, Extruded Fetal Parts
  with Uterine Perforation and Ectopic Pregnancy
  (Postpartum/Intervention) 384
  OP Sharma, Rajul Rastogi
- Differential Diagnosis of a Presacral Fetal Mass 384
  OP Sharma, Rajul Rastogi
- Fetal Neck Masses.. 386
  OP Sharma, Rajul Rastogi
- Differential Diagnosis of Fetal Renal Cystic Diseases 386
  OP Sharma, Rajul Rastogi
- Differential Diagnosis of various Fetal Anterior Abdominal Wall Defects 386
  OP Sharma
- Differential Diagnosis between Renal Cysts and Hydronephrosis....................................... 386
  OP Sharma, Rajul Rastogi
- Differential Diagnosis of Cystic Adnexal Masses 386
  OP Sharma, Rajul Rastogi
- Differential Diagnosis of Ovarian Masses.. 388
  Ashish Verma, Sumeet Bhargava, Satish K Bhargava
- Differential Diagnosis of Benign and Malignant Ovarian Masses 388
  OP Sharma

- Differential Diagnosis of Cystic Abdominal Masses 388
  OP Sharma
- Differential Diagnosis of Non-gynecological Pelvic Lesions 389
  Ashish Verma, Sumeet Bhargava, Satish K Bhargava
- Differential Diagnosis of Postoperative Pelvic Mass 389
  Sumeet Bhargava, Satish K Bhargava
- Differential Diagnosis of Ovarian Adnexal Mass 390
  Sumeet Bhargava, Satish K Bhargava
- Differential Diagnosis of Ovarian Adnexal Mass of Ovarian Masses 390
  Sumeet Bhargava, Satish K Bhargava
- Sonographic Classification of Adnexal Masses 391
  Ashish Verma, Sumeet Bhargava, Satish K Bhargava
- Absent Intrauterine Pregnancy with Positive Pregnancy Test 392
  Ashish Verma, Sumeet Bhargava, Satish K Bhargava, Rajul Rastogi
- Differential Diagnosis of Thickened Placenta 393
  Ashish Verma, Sumeet Bhargava, Satish K Bhargava, Rajul Rastogi
- Ultrasound Signs of Chromosomal Abnormality 394
  Ashish Verma, Sumeet Bhargava, Satish K Bhargava, Rajul Rastogi
- Differential Diagnosis of Enlarged Uterus 396
  Ashish Verma, Sumeet Bhargava, Satish K Bhargava, Rajul Rastogi
- Cystic Structures in Fetal Abdomen 396
  Satish K Bhargava, Sumeet Bhargava, Ashish Verma, Rajul Rastogi
- Differential Diagnosis of Fetal Hydrops 397
  Satish K Bhargava, Sumeet Bhargava, Ashish Verma, Rajul Rastogi
- Differential Diagnosis of Fetal Brain and Head Abnormalities 398
  Satish K Bhargava, Ashish Verma, Rajul Rastogi, Sumeet Bhargava
- Differential Diagnosis of Brain and Head Abnormality 399
  Satish K Bhargava, Ashish Verma, Rajul Rastogi, Sumeet Bhargava
- Differential Diagnosis of Thickened Endometrium 400
  Sumeet Bhargava, Satish K Bhargava, Ashish Verma
- USG Signs in Abortions/Miscarriage 401
  Satish K Bhargava, Ashish Verma
- Differential Diagnosis of Fetal Causes of Abnormality in Liquor Volume 402
  Satish K Bhargava, Ashish Verma
- Differential Diagnosis of Gas in the Genital Tract 404
  Satish K Bhargava, Ashish Verma
- Differential Diagnosis of Fetal Intra-abdominal Calcification 405
  Satish K Bhargava, Ashish Verma
- Differential Diagnosis of Fetal Thoracic Abnormalities 406
  Satish K Bhargava, Ashish Verma

Index *409*

Chapter 1

Chest

LESIONS OF THORACIC INLET

Anatomy of Thoracic Inlet (Fig. 1.1)
- Thoracic inlet/root of neck is a narrow space that serves as a junction between the neck and the thorax.
- Boundaries are:
  - *Anteriorly*: Manubrium
  - *Posteriorly*: First thoracic vertebra
  - *Laterally*: First ribs.
- This area is further delineated by Sibson's fascia which extends from the transverse process of C7 vertebra to the medial border of first rib.
- Plane of the thoracic inlet is tilted downward anteriorly and laterally on either side being highest medially and posteriorly.

Differential Diagnosis of Lesions at Thoracic Inlet (Flowchart 1.1)

Congenital Lesions
- Lymphangioma
- Hemangioma
- Cervical extension of mediastinal thymus

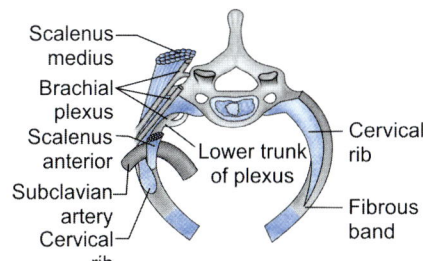

Fig. 1.1: Thoracic inlet.

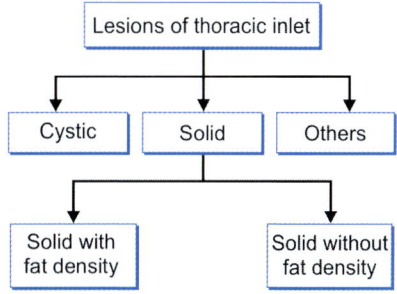

Flowchart 1.1: Lesions of thoracic inlet.

- Thymic cyst
- *Vascular anomalies*: Aneurysm of aberrant subclavian artery, asymmetric dilatation of jugular veins (refer to Navigating thoracic inlet; Radiographics).

Inflammatory Lesions
- Inflammatory adenopathy—tuberculosis, infectious mononucleosis, HIV infection, etc.
- Cervical abscess
- Tubercular spondylitis with abscess
- Retropharyngeal abscess with mediastinal extension.

Benign Lesions
- Thyroid lesions: Nodule, cysts, and adenomas (extending downward)
- Esophageal lesions: Upper esophagus duplication, malignancies
- Lipoma
- Lipoblastoma
- Schwannomas and neurofibromas

- Fibromatosis
- Desmoid tumor.

Malignant Tumors

- Lymphoma
- Neuroblastoma
- Thyroid carcinoma
- Tracheal malignancies
- Pancoast's tumor
- Lymph node metastasis
- Liposarcoma
- Metastasis to thoracic vertebra and ribs.

Traumatic Lesions

- Pneumomediastinum
- Esophageal foreign body
- Cervicothoracic hematoma.

Miscellaneous

- Cervical rib (Fig. 1.2)
  - Thoracic outlet syndrome
  - Intrathoracic goiter (Fig. 1.3).

Lymphangioma

- Develops from congenital obstruction of lymphatic drainage.

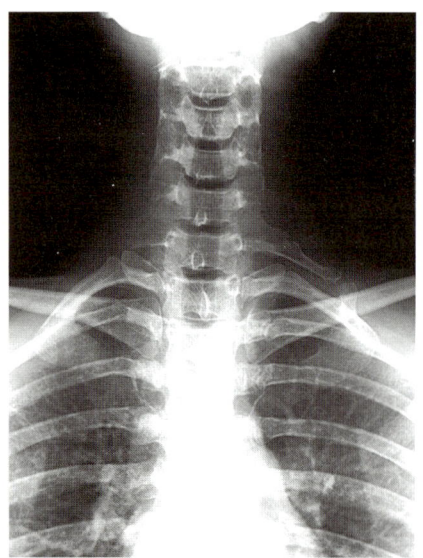

Fig. 1.2: Anteroposterior radiograph of cervical spine shows cervical rib arising from C7 on the left side forming pseudarthrosis with left first rib.

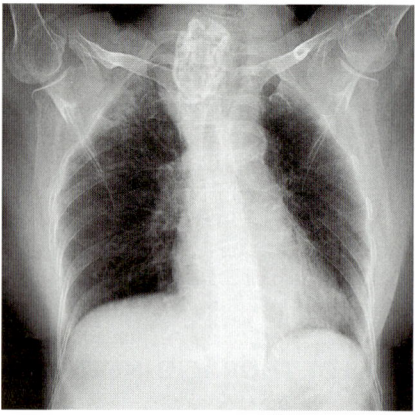

Fig. 1.3: Anteroposterior radiograph of chest shows superior mediastinal widening caused by enlarged thyroid gland with a large calcification in its right lobe.

- Tends to surround and invade normal anatomical structures. Five percent occur in neck (posterior triangle); 3–10% extends into mediastinum, asymptomatic and painless masses, 90% detected by 2 years of age.

Imaging: Multilocular trans-septal masses of fluid attenuation, walls of septa-enhance (if history of surgery/infection). Occasionally hemorrhagic areas and fluid-fluid levels are present.

Hemangiomas

Benign masses composed of proliferating endothelial cells characteristically increase in size and gradually involute. It most commonly occurs in the first year of life.

Imaging: Calcified phleboliths within the mass may be present. Enhance with adjacent vascular structure and fill with contrast over a short time.

Magnetic resonance imaging (MRI): Intermediate signal intensity (SI) on T1WI and high SI on T2WI, fatty replacement may be present.

Cervical Extension of Mediastinal Thymus

- Due to incomplete mediastinal descent and manifests as solid midline thymus at thoracic inlet.

- Diagnosis is made on the basis of homogeneous SI similar to that of the thymus with all magnetic resonance (MR) imaging sequences or connection to the normally located thymus.

Thymic Cyst
- Caused by persistence or degeneration of the thymopharyngeal ducts.
- 50% of cervical thymic cysts are continuous with mediastinal masses. Most commonly seen on the left side.

Computed tomography (CT): Well-marginated, unilocular/multilocular, attenuation is close to water.

MR: Decrease SI on T1WI and intermediate/high SI on T2WI.
- SI on T1WI may increase if cyst contains blood/protein.
- Then septa may be present.
- When these cysts occur in the neck, they are located partially within the carotid sheath.
- Most thymic cysts are congenital but they have also been reported with infection, neoplasms, radiation therapy, trauma, and thoracotomy.

Vascular Anomalies
- Venous malformations and arteriovenous malformation (AVM) are rarely seen in the neck.
- Jugular vein thrombosis occurs after placement of a central catheter or in association with compressive lesion and is seen as luminal obstruction with thin rim of enhancement of the vasa vasorum.
- Cervical aortic arch—high-positioned, usually right-sided aortic arch. Occasionally associated with other cardiac and vascular anomalies, patient presents with respiratory problems/dysphagia.
- A pulsatile mass is found in the neck.

Cervical Abscess
- Cervical abscesses seldom cross the thoracic inlet into the mediastinum.
- Infection in the visceral space may extend into the anterior mediastinum, whereas infection in the retropharyngeal and prevertebral spaces may extend into the posterior mediastinum.

Imaging is required to distinguish cellulitis and suppuration adenopathy from the abscesses which require surgical treatment.

In suppuration—focal hypoattenuating mass with an enhancing rim on contrast-enhanced computed tomography (CECT) and a complete hypoechoic to anechoic mass with a variable thick rim of solid tissue is seen on ultrasound scans. In fluid collection—SI on MR varies according to protein content, skin thickening and reticulated fat planes may be seen adjacent to the abscess margins in CT and MR.

Tuberculous Spondylitis with Abscess Formation
- Infection usually starts anteriorly in the vertebral body
- In 90% cases, at least two vertebrae are affected
- Skip lesions occur in 4% cases
- Paraspinal abscesses are present in 55–90% cases
- *Imaging features*:
  - Vertebral body destruction
  - Loss of disk space
  - Paraspinal abscess
  - Prevertebral and epidural collections
  - Paraspinal calcification.
- In the neck—dysphagia, hoarseness, and lymphadenopathy are the accompanying features.

Retropharyngeal Abscess with Mediastinal Extension

Causes of Retropharyngeal Abscess
- Tonsillar infection
- Iatrogenic/traumatic
- Perforation of pharynx.

X-ray neck soft tissue: Retropharyngeal soft tissue thickening, forward displacement of airway.

CT/MR: Retropharyngeal collection continuing into the post-mediastinum through the thoracic inlet.

Lipoma

- Most common cervical neoplasms of mesenchymal origin.
- Typically present as painless slowly-growing masses, most commonly occurring in posterior triangle.

CT: Homogeneous non-enhancing mass, isodense with subcutaneous fat, usually well-encapsulated lesions (–10 to –100 HU).

MRI: Signal intensity similar to subcutaneous fat (increase on T1WI, intermediate SI on T2WI and loss of SI on fat suppressed MR images).

Lipoblastoma

Rare, usually encapsulated benign neoplasm of the embryonal fat. Composed of mature and immature fat and found almost exclusively in infants (90% <3 years) and children.
Most common site—extremities → trunk → head → neck.
CT: Fat separated by septa of soft tissue which does not enhance.
MR: Heterogeneous and have intermediate to high SI on T1WI according to the amount of immature fat. On fat suppressed images—area of high SI is suggestive lipoblastoma.

Schwannomas and Neurofibromas

- Common sites are—vagus nerve, ventral and cervical nerve roots, cervical sympathetic chains, and brachial plexus.
- Plexiform neurofibromas are pathognomonic of type I neurofibromatosis.

CT: Hypo- to isoattenuating at CT. Contrast enhancement is more often seen with schwannomas.

MR: Low to intermediate SI on T1WI and intermediate to high SI on T2WI. They show non-uniform enhancement. Plexiform neurofibromas usually involve cartilaginous soft tissue.

- Malignant degeneration is seen in 15–30% cases.
- Tumors arising in vagus nerve displace the common carotid and internal carotid arteries. Anteromedially and the internal jugular vein posterolaterally.
- Sympathetic chain tumors demonstrate a constant relationship with the longus colli muscle.
- Brachial plexus tumors displace the anterior scalene muscle anteriorly.

Aggressive Fibromatosis

- Characterized by proliferation of fibrous tissue with locally aggressive behavior and a tendency toward recurrence after resection.
- Etiology is unknown.
- Appearance on MR is often infiltrative and can suggest malignancy. Usually has decreased SI on T1 and T2WI that permits diagnosis.

Lymphoma

- Hodgkin's disease accounts for majority of lymphomatous anterior mediastinal masses and the neoplastic cells typically infiltrate the thymus.
- Thymic involvement is always accompanied by involvement of mediastinal lymph node.
- Lymphoma of neck involves cervical lymph node chain, Waldeyer's tonsillar ring and lymphoid tissue at the base of tongue. Such lymphoma is most often of the non-Hodgkin's type.
- Calcification and necrosis can be seen if lymphoma was treated previously.

Thyroid Carcinoma

- Papillary carcinoma accounts for 75–90% of all the cases and is especially prevalent in younger patients.
- Medullary, follicular, and anaplastic carcinoma account for 10–25%.
- Usually evaluated by ultrasound or scintigraphy. CT/MR is required to evaluate tumoral extent when malignant tumors are suspected.
- Difficult to distinguish benign from malignant nodule because the findings are

nonspecific. However, thyroid masses with infiltrating margins that obscure soft tissue plane and associated with adenopathy are suggestive of carcinoma.
- Cold nodules on scintigraphy have a higher frequency of malignancy.
- MR is preferred as compared to CT because iodine administered during CT scan cause iodine 131 therapy to be postponed for up to 6 months after the removal of maximum tumor volume.

Neuroblastoma

- 10–15% neuroblastomas are located in posterior mediastinum. More than 5% neuroblastomas arise in the neck.
- Arise from the renal cell rest blasts located in the adrenal gland or sympathetic chain.
- Osteochondritis and ipsilateral Horner's syndrome are related to lesion of cervical sympathetic nerve.
- 50% neuroblastoma shows calcification on X-ray.
- 90% shows calcification on CT.
- MR imaging is the modality of choice for demonstrating the full extent of mass, chest wall invasion, and extra-adrenal intraspinal involvement.
- Lymph nodes involved are deep cervical lymph nodes along the internal jugular vein, supraclavicular lymph node, scalene nodes, and highest lymph node in superior mediastinum.

Pancoast's Tumor

- Pancoast's syndrome consists of a constellation of signs and symptoms that include shoulder and arm pain in the distribution of C8, T1 and T2 nerve roots, Horner's syndrome, and atrophy of hand muscle.
- This is caused by tumor in lung apex (squamous cell carcinoma) which is causing invasion of the chest wall, and prevertebral sympathetic chain or the inferior or stellate ganglion.
- This tumor should be ruled out if unilateral pleural thickening or asymmetric thickening more than 5 mm is noted on chest X-ray (CXR).

Metastases: (To rib and thoracic vertebra).
- *Usually has a mixed pattern*: Breast/lung
- Blastic—prostate
- Lytic—thyroid and kidney
- Vertebra—pedicles and vertebral body are involved.
- Ribs—lesions are recognized early when the rib is expanded.

Pneumomediastinum

Air can travel from the mediastinum along the fascial planes to the neck; subcutaneous tissue and chest wall.

Most common causes in children are asthma, aspiration of foreign body and trauma.

Esophageal—foreign body granuloma.
- Most commonly seen in infants and children.
- Most common site of retention is the upper esophagus at the thoracic inlet.
- Long-standing foreign body produces a granulomatous tissue reaction that manifests as a mass.
- Mediastinitis and abscess can be seen in this region as a complication of foreign body perforation.

Cervicothoracic Hematoma

Causes
- Trauma
- Faulty placement of central catheter
- Hematomas are usually trans-spatial lesions.

Computed Tomography
- Hyperdense in acute phase.
- Hypodense in chronic phase and on MR SI varies depending on the phase.

Cervical Rib

- Seen in 1% of population
- Symptomatic in 10%
- Unilateral in 50–80%
- Cervical ribs vary in length and may be connected to the first rib by a fibrous band
- Cervical rib may affect the brachial plexus in any one of the following two ways:
    1. May narrow the space between the posterior aspect of first rib and anterior scalene muscle through which the nerve and subclavian artery passes.
      Or
    2. Cervical rib may be situated such that a portion of the brachial plexus must pass over it, thereby stretching the lower trunks.
- Results in cervical rib syndrome—sensory symptoms usually antedate motor involvement and occur along the ulnar border of forearm and hand
- Muscle wasting of thenar eminence.

Thoracic Outlet Syndrome

Because of compression of the subclavian artery and C8/T1 nerve.

Usual Causes

- Cervical rib
- Elongated transverse process of C7
- Fibrous band extending from transverse process of C7 to the first rib
- Low set shoulder girdle
- Pancoast's tumor.

Intrathoracic Goiter

Characterized by:
- Continuity with cervical thyroid gland
- Marked enhancement on CECT
- Well-defined margins
- Inhomogeneity
- Focal calcification.

CYSTIC LYMPHANGIOMA

Detected by 2 years of age and seen to extend from posterior triangle multilocular cystic mass.

Thymic Cyst

Unilocular/multilocular cystic mass seen in continuation with thymus.

Cervical Abscess

Hypodense collection with enhancing rim with adjacent reticulated fat plane.

Pott's Spine with Abscess

Vertebral body destruction with loss of IVD space with adjacent collection and calcification.

SOLID WITH FAT DENSITY

Lipoma

Painless progressive mass, well-encapsulated isointense to fat.

Liposarcoma

- Fast growing; adults
- Soft tissue admixed with fat.

Lipoblastoma

- 90% less than 3 years
- Areas of increase SI on T2WI
- Fat separated by septa.

SOLID WITHOUT FAT DENSITY

- Schwannoma and neurofibroma
- Plexiform neurofibroma associated with neurofibroma.

Neuroblastoma

- Arises from sympathetic chain
- Children
- Calcification present in 90%
- Horner's syndrome.

Thyroid Carcinoma

Mass is contiguous with thyroid and has infiltrating margins and obscures soft tissue plane.

Pancoast's Tumor

Mass lesion in lung apex with destruction of first rib.
- Patient presents with Pancoast's syndrome.

Chest

Metastatic Lymph Node Mass
Primary lesion can be localized.

Others
Hemangioma
- Compressible mass lesion, multiple small cystic spaces, phlebolith is present, and vascular enhancement is present.

Cervical Rib
- Extra rib is seen to arise from transverse process of C7.
- May cause symptoms due to compression of subclavian vessels or brachial plexus.

MEDIASTINAL MASSES (TABLE 1.1 AND FIG. 1.4)

Mediastinum
Felson's method of mediastinal division has been shown in Figure 1.4.

Anterior Mediastinal Masses

Thyroid Tumor (Table 1.2)
- Nontoxic enlargement of the gland
- Thyrotoxicosis
- Carcinoma thyroid
- Hashimoto's disease.

Thymic Tumors
- *Normal thymic shadow*: Triangular soft tissue mass that projects to one side of the mediastinum.
- *Prominent*:
  - On expiratory film
  - Slightly rotated film
- *Disappears*:
  - Severe neonatal infection
  - After major surgery
  - Use of steroids.

Most Common Tumors of Mediastinum (Table 1.1)
- Thymoma
  - Benign
  - Malignant 30%

Table 1.1: Tumors of mediastinum (both common and rare).

Common	Rare
Anterior	
• Tortuous innominate artery • Lymph node • Retrosternal goiter • Fat deposition	• Innominate artery aneurysm • Parathyroid adenoma • Lymphangioma
• Lymph node enlargement • Aneurysm of ascending aorta • Thymoma • Teratoma	• Sternal mass • Lipoma • Hemangioma
• Epicardial fat pad • Diaphragmatic hump • Pleuropericardial cyst	• Morgagni hernia
Middle	
• Lymph node enlargement • Aortic arch aneurysm • Enlarged pulmonary artery • Dilatation of superior vena cava (SVC) • Bronchogenic cyst	• Tracheal lesion • Cardiac tumor
Posterior	
• Neurogenic tumor • Pharyngoesophageal pouch	
• Aneurysm of descending aorta • Esophageal dilation • Azygos diltation • Hiatus hernia	• Neurenteric cyst • Pancreatic pseudocyst • Sequestrated lung
• Neurogenic tumor • Paravertebral mass	• Bochdalek hernia • Extramedullary hematopoiesis

- Hyperplasia of the gland
- Thymic cyst
- Thymolipoma
- Lymphoma
- Germ cell tumor
- Carcinoids.

Teratodermoid Tumors

- Dermoid cyst
- Teratoma
  - Benign
  - Malignant
- All arise from the primitive germ cell nests in the urogenital ridge
- Dermoid cyst contains mainly ectodermal tissues

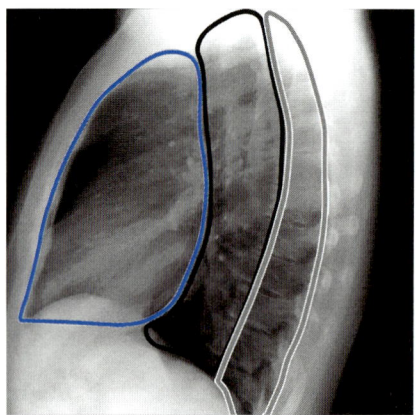

Fig. 1.4: Felson's method of mediastinal division: the anterior, middle, and posterior compartments of the mediastinum are easy to identify on the lateral chest X-ray (CXR).

- Solid teratoma contains tissues of ectodermal, mesodermal and endodermal origins.

Dermoid cyst appears as a round or oval soft tissue mass, which may show peripheral rim or central nodular calcification. A fat-fluid level or a rudimentary tooth is diagnostic radiological sign. Teratoma appears as a lobulated soft tissue mass which on CT shows a mass of mixed attenuation containing soft tissue, cyst fluid, fat, and calcification of bone.

PLEUROPERICARDIAL CYST

- Anterior mediastinal mass
- 75% occur in right anterior cardiophrenic angle
- Cysts have thin walls, which contain clear fluid
- These change shape with respiration.

DIFFERENTIAL DIAGNOSIS OF SOFT TISSUE LESIONS IN RIGHT ANTERIOR CARDIOPHRENIC ANGLE (TABLE 1.3)

Morgagni Hernia

- Persistent developmental defect in the diaphragm anteriorly.
- Anterior mediastinal mass.
- May contain omentum or transverse colon.
- Appears as a soft tissue mass.
- Containing either gas or air-fluid level or fat.
- Diagnosis is confirmed by barium meal and follow through or barium enema.

Table 1.2: Differential diagnosis of retrosternal goiter.

	Nontoxic enlargement of thyroid	Thyrotoxicosis	Carcinoma (CA) thyroid	Hashimoto's disease
Vocal cord involvement	–	–	+	–
Superior vena cava (SVC) compression	–	–	+	–
Calcification	±	–	±	–
Rapid increase in size	Hemorrhage cyst	-do-	++	–
Symptom severity	±	Clinical manifestation	+	–
Orbital lesion	–	+	–	–

Chest

Table 1.3: Differential diagnosis of soft tissue lesions in right anterior cardiophrenic angle.

	Change shape with respiration	Density	Content	Separate from pericardium	Silhouette sign
Pleuropericardial cyst	+	Soft tissue	Fluid	+	+
Epicardial fat pad	–	Fatty	Fat	+	+
Partial eventration of right hemidiaphragm	+	Soft tissue	Diaphragm contour	+	–
Right middle lobe pathology	–	Soft tissue	Lung	+	+
Morgagni hernia	–	Fat if omentum +	Omentum	+	+
Right atrial tumor	–	Soft tissue	Soft tissue	+	–
Pericardial lesion	–	-do-	Soft tissue fluid	–	+

MIDDLE MEDIASTINAL MASSES

Lymph Node Enlargement

Metastatic (Table 1.4)

- *Intrathoracic*:
  - Bronchial carcinoma
  - Esophageal carcinoma
- *Extrathoracic*:
  - Breast and renal
  - Adrenal and testicular
  - Tumors of pharynx and larynx.
- Lymphoma leukemia.
- *Sarcoidosis*: Bilateral hilar masses with well-defined outline. These show egg shell calcification.
- Primary tuberculous infection produces an area of consolidation in one of the lobes with unilateral hilar mass and an associated pleural effusion.
- Low attenuation areas due to cyst formation or necrosis are seen in lymph nodes involved with Hodgkin's disease and metastatic testicular or squamous cell tumors, particularly after treatment with radiotherapy or chemotherapy.

Aortic Aneurysm (Fig. 1.5)

This produces either widening of the mediastinum or a round or oval soft tissue mass in any part of the mediastinum with a well-defined outline. Curvilinear or peripheral calcification may be due to syphilitic aortitis or

Table 1.4: Metastatic lymph nodes.

Head and neck squamous cell carcinoma	Renal cell carcinoma
Breast carcinoma	Seminoma
Melanomas	Mucinous adenocarcinoma of gastrointestinal tract (GIT)
Neuroblastomas	Nasopharyngeal carcinoma
Rhabdomyosarcomas	Thyroid carcinoma
Small cell carcinoma of lung	Ovarian and prostate carcinoma

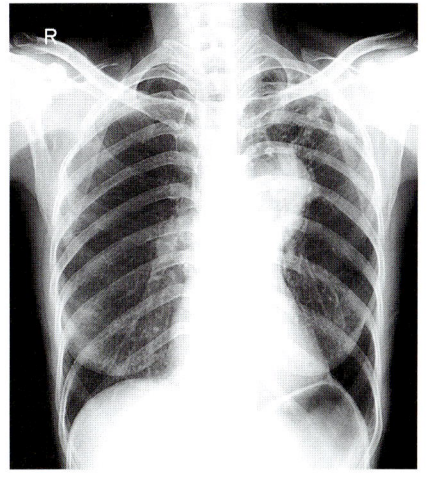

Fig. 1.5: Posteroanterior radiograph of chest shows aneurysm of arch of aorta. Incidental note is made of the fibrotic changes in the left upper lobe.

atherosclerosis. It may cause pressure erosion defect of the sternum or anterior scalloping of one or two vertebral bodies. The subintimal flap and false lumen of a dissecting aneurysm can be demonstrated by CT.

Tortuous Innominate Artery

It occurs in 20% of the elderly patients with hypertension and produces widening of the superior part of the mediastinum on the right without displacement of the trachea to the left.

Bronchogenic Cyst

- Middle or posterior mediastinal mass
- Majority occur around the carina in the paratracheal, tracheobronchial or subcarinal region
- Can alter in shape on respiration
- Pericardial defect may occur in association.

Tracheal Tumors

Tracheal tumors include carcinoma, plasmacytoma. They narrow the tracheal lumen and appear as soft tissue mass.

POSTERIOR MEDIASTINAL MASSES

Neurogenic Tumors (Table 1.5)

Adults

- Neurofibroma
- Neurilemmoma.

Children

Neuroblastoma.
- These may be asymptomatic or may produce back pain and may even extend through an intervertebral foramen into the spinal canal (dumb-bell tumors) to produce spinal cord compressions.
- Involvement of the posterior ribs or adjacent thoracic vertebrae—produce ribs splaying, localized pressure erosion defect of one or two vertebral bodies and ribs notching.

HIATUS HERNIA

- Most common cause of a mediastinal mass on a chest radiograph in an elderly patient. It appears as a soft tissue mass with an air-fluid level.
- Lies to the left of the midline.
- Contents could be liver, omentum, and small intestine.

ESOPHAGEAL LESIONS

Present with dysphagia.

Pharyngoesophageal pouch: Soft tissue mass with an air-fluid level, lies in the midline, displaces trachea forward.

Carcinoma/leiomyoma: Soft tissue mass with an air-fluid level, behind the heart.

Achalasia: Large soft tissue mass with air-fluid level with barium flowing in spurts. Pulmonary consolidation/bronchiectasis may be present.

PARAVERTEBRAL LESIONS

Involves the thoracic vertebrae or intervertebral disk space. They appear as an elongated or lobulated soft tissue mass with a well-defined outline.

Differential diagnosis would be:
- Hematoma
- Pyogenic abscess
- Tubercular abscess
- Multiple myeloma
- Lymphoma
- Metastasis
- Extramedullary hematopoiesis.

Bochdalek Hernia

- Its persistency develops mental defect in the diaphragm posteriorly.
- Occurs in the left hemidiaphragm.

Table 1.5: Neurogenic tumors.

	Shape	Calcification	Dumb-bell
Neurofibroma	Rounded	±	+
Neurilemmoma	-do-	-	-
Neuroblastoma	Elongated	Central spicules or peripheral rim	+

- Small hernias usually contain retroperitoneal fat, kidney or spleen, that appear as a soft tissue mass in the posterior costophrenic angle.
- Larger hernias may contain jejunum, ileum, and colon.

Neurenteric Cysts

Result due to partial or complete persistence of the neurenteric canal or its incomplete resorption includes gastrointestinal duplication, enteric cyst, neurenteric cyst, anterior meningocele and cysts of the canal.

Pancreatic Pseudocyst

- Posterior mediastinal mass
- Round/oval soft tissue mass behind the heart
- A left basal pleural effusion or atelectasis in the lower lobes may result
- Extramedullary hematopoiesis
- Appears as lobulated paravertebral soft tissue mass behind the heart.

DIFFERENTIAL DIAGNOSIS OF SUPERIOR MEDIASTINAL MASSES

Contents

1. Trachea and esophagus.
2. Muscles—sternohyoid, sternothyroid, and lower ends of longus colli.
3. Anterior arch of aorta, brachiocephalic artery, ICC, and left subclavian artery.
4. Veins—right and left brachiocephalic vein and upper-half of superior vena cava (SVC).
5. Nerves—vagus, phrenic, cardiac nerve, and right laryngeal nerve.
6. Thymus.
7. Thoracic duct.
8. Lymph nodes (LNs)—paratracheal, brachiocephalic, and tuberculosis.

Criteria for Superior Mediastinum Widening

More than 8 cm in the transverse diameter.
   More than 25% of the thoracic diameter at that level.

- *Retrosternal goiter*: Less than 5% of enlarged thyroid in the neck. Extend into mediastinum due to nontoxic enlargement, thyrotoxicosis, carcinoma, and Hashimoto's disease (see Table 1.2).
   – Soft tissue swelling that moves on swallowing
   – Dysphagia, stridor if benign, vocal cord paralysis or SVC compression-malignancy
   – Patients present soft tissue mass in anterior part; extend down from the neck
   – Outline well-defined in mediastinum but fades off into the neck
   – Displacement and compression of trachea to the left, 20% are retrotracheal
   – Ca^{++} nodules, linear or crescent pattern
   – CT mass of mixed attenuation extending from one of the lower poles of thyroid
   – Radionuclide scan 99 Tc pertechnetate on 123I-NaI
   – MRI—diagnostic.
- Thymus—normal thymus—most common in infants.
   – Most common in adult benign and malignant thymoma
   – Associated with myasthenia gravis, red cells aplasia or decreased granulocytes
   – Plain X-ray chest –ve
   – CT:
      ◆ Grossly asymmetrical lobular configuration
      ◆ Homogeneous with mild contrast enhancement
      ◆ Less commonly decreased attenuation areas—hemorrhage/necrosis/cyst Ca^{++} occasionally.
   – MRI = T1 = Med. SI, T2 $\Rightarrow$ fat
   Thymic hyperplasia:
   – Seen in two-thirds of myasthenia gravis
   – CT = symmetric diffuse enlargement
   – MR = same signal as normal gland
   – Enlargement of thymus may also be seen in thymic cyst, thymolipoma, lymphoma, germ cell tumor, and carcinoid.
- Teratodermoid tumors/germ cell tumor—extragonadal germ cell tumor located within or adjacent to thymus
   – Most common germ cell tumor in superior mediastinum is dermoid cyst

and benign and malignant teratoma. Chest radiograph (CXR) may show round or oval soft mass with well-defined border and may contain peripheral rim or central nodules of Ca^{++}.
– III on CT, fat-fluid level, Ca^{++} calcifications, well-defined border and soft tissue attenuation mass is highly suggestive of germ cell tumor.
– *Malignancy*—more solid component and aggressive features.
- Lymph node enlargement (Figs. 1.6 and 1.7)
  – Widened mediastinum may have lobulated margins in case of LN enlargement
  – Hodgkin/non-Hodgkin disease—paratracheal and tracheobronchial, asymmetrical widening of middle part of superior mediastinum
    - Associated feature—parenchymal lung disease
    - Ca^{++} in LN seen after irradiation
  – Tuberculosis—unilateral paratracheal lymphadenopathy without obvious mediastinum or pleural involvement seen in immunocompromised patients
  – In an adult/children area of consolidation/caseation
  – Fungal disease histoplasmosis, coccidioidomycosis, and blastomycosis
    - Enlargement of hila or paratracheal LN
    - Ca^{++} in healing histoplasmosis Sarcoidosis—bilateral lobulated hilar mass.

Metastasis:
– Primary tumor is usually intrathoracic—esophagus/bronchus.
– Benign—in adult
  - Papilloma
  - Chordoma Ca^{++} smooth, well-defined and fibroma less than 2 cm in diameter
  - Hemangioma.
– Mucus plug—decreased alternation, mixed with air and will change in position and resolve after coughing.
– Malignant—squamous cell carcinoma and adenoid cystic Ca_2—most commonly a smooth or irregular intraluminal mass with asymmetry. Narrowing of tracheal lumen is seen.
- *Aneurysm and dissection of arch of aorta*—true, pseudo, post-traumatic atherosclerotic, post-traumatic elderly, and fusiform.
  – Younger, contained by adventitia only, saccular
  – Clinical presentation → asymptomatic
  – Symptoms—enlarged compresses adjacent structure

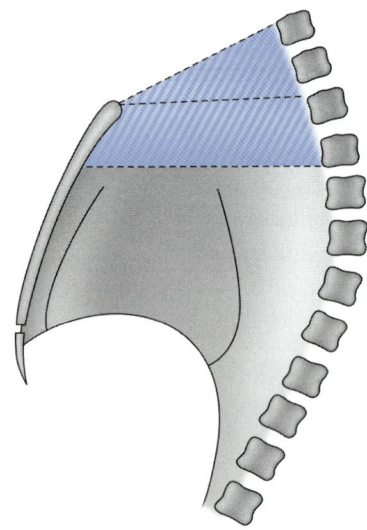

Fig. 1.6: Boundaries of superior mediastinum.

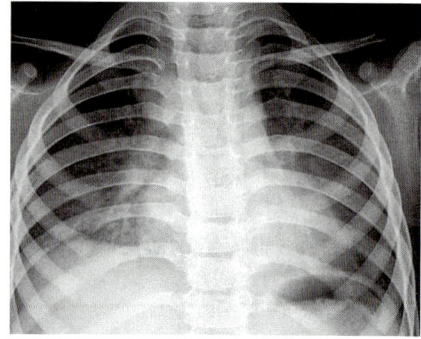

Fig. 1.7: Posteroanterior (PA) radiograph of chest shows superior mediastinal widening caused by right paratracheal adenopathy in a case of Koch's chest.

- C × R = Widening with or without Ca^{++}
- CT = Saccular and fusiform dilatation of segment of aorta
- >4 cm; use short-axis diameter
- Ca^{++} in aortic wall, peripheral
- Intraluminal thrombus—crescentic/circumferential
- Displacement of adjacent structure = Trachea, bronchus and pulmonary artery, SVC, esophagus, bony erosion, growth rate 5.6 cm/year.

Aortic dissection emergency situation:
- Peak 7th–8th decade
- Most common predisposing condition is hypertension—congenital heart disease, coarctation, bicuspid aortic valve (AV)
- Intimal tear—blood enters into the aortic wall and creates a false and true lumen
- CXR wide mediastinum aortic contour displaced, intimal Ca^{++}
- CT = Internal displacement or intimal Ca^{++}
- Visible internal flap increased in attenuation
- High density thrombus in false lumen if acute hemorrhage
- CECT—contrast-filled true and false lumen separated by intimal flap
- Delayed enhancement of false lumen because of slow flow
- MR—very well-demonstrate the intimal flap
- Aortography—highly accurate.

- *Dilatation of SVC and other veins*:
  - Dilatation of SVC seen in raised CVP
  - CCF
  - Tricuspid valve disease
  - Mediastinal mass
  - Constrictive pericarditis
  - Total anomalous pulmonary venous drainage (TAPVD)—supracardiac variety. All the pulmonary veins open into large ascending vein on the left side which is a remnant of embryonic. Left SVC. This connects into the left brachiocephalic vein which then passes into the right-sided SVC and into the RA.

- *A pharyngoesophageal pouch/Zenker's diverticulum*:
  - CXR = Soft tissue mass in posterior part of superior mediastinum which contains an air-fluid level.
  - Soft tissue mass lies in the midline and displaces the trachea forward.
  - Barium-esophagogram—confirm the diagnoses.

- Fat deposition—superior mediastinum widening and epicardial fat pad seen in obese adult patients, Cushing's disease, and steroid therapy
  - CT = Shows an excessive amount of mediastinal fat.

- Tracheal mass—positive with nonspecific symptoms like cough, dyspnea, stridor, and wheezing
  - CXR = Not very helpful
  - Benign—in adult
  - Papilloma
  - Chordoma Ca^{++}: Smooth well-defined and less than 2 cm in diameter
  - Fibroma
  - Hemangioma
  - Mucus plug—decrease attenuation, mixed with air and will change in position and resolve after coughing
  - Malignant—squamous cell carcinoma and adenoid cystic carcinoma are most common
  - A smooth or irregular intraluminal mass with asymmetric narrowing of tracheae lumen is seen.

- *Neurogenic tumor*:
  - Adult—NF and schwannoma—peripheral intercostal nerve children—ganglioneuroma and neuroblastoma—which arise is thoracic sympathetic ganglia.
  - CXR: A round or oval soft tissue mass in paravertebral gutter which usually project to one side of mediastinum.

- Neuroblastoma—central spicules or peripheral rim Ca^{++} splaying of posterior ribs.
- Pressure erosion and defect of vertebral bodies.
- Rib notching.
- Enlargement of an intervertebral foramen.
- CT = Solid mass of soft tissue attenuation, may contain Ca^{++} and involve the adjacent bone.
- MRI = Intraspinal extension.
- MRI = Transaxial SE.
- GRF/phase velocity mapping.

DIFFERENTIAL DIAGNOSIS OF ANTERIOR MEDIASTINAL MASSES

Anterior mediastinum lies anterior to anterior pericardium and trachea. For ease of differential diagnosis, it can be divided into three areas (Table 1.6).

Salient Features

Region 1 (Fig. 1.8)

- *Thyroid tumor (retrosternal goiter)*:
  - Less than 5% goiters extend into the mediastinum.
  - Mostly females presenting with soft tissue swelling, dysphagia, and stridor.
  - Chest X-ray shows oval soft tissue mass in superior part of anterior mediastinum fading off into the neck.
  - Well-defined smooth or lobulated.
  - Central nodular and linear calcification.
  - Displacement and compression of trachea.
  - CT shows mass of mixed attenuation with cysts and calcifications, contiguous with one of the poles of thyroid.
- *Lymph node enlargement*:
  May be due to lymphoma, metastasis or infection.
  - Widening of mediastinum on CXR.
  - Lobulated soft tissue mass due to indentation by ribs.
  - Calcification may be present.
  - Lymphadenopathy elsewhere in the body.
  - CT shows discrete round or slightly irregular densities of various sizes ± enhancement and necrosis.
- *Fat deposition*:
  - Cushing's disease, corticosteroid therapy
  - Widening of superior mediastinum on CXR
  - CT shows excessive amount of mediastinal fat with density—50–100 HU.
- *Tortuous innominate artery or aneurysm*:
  - Common in elderly
  - Widening of superior mediastinum
  - CT shows dilatation of innominate artery.
- *Lymphangioma/cystic hygroma*:
  - Mainly in children.
  - Transilluminating soft tissue swelling in the root of the neck.
  - Chest X-ray shows: Oval soft tissue mass extending into the neck.
  - Alters shape on respiration but does not displace trachea
  - Ultrasound and CT shows cystic septated mass.

Table 1.6: Differential diagnosis of anterior mediastinal lesion.

Region 1	Region 2	Region 3
Tortuous innominate artery	Lymph node (LN) enlargement	Epicardial fat pad
Lymph nodes	Aneurysm of aorta	Diaphragmatic hump
Retrosternal goiter	Thymoma tumors	Pleuropericardial cyst
Fat deposition	Teratodermoid	Morgagni's hernia
Aneurysm of innominate artery	Sternal mass lipoma	
Parathyroid adenoma	Hemangioma	
Cystic hygroma or lymphangioma		

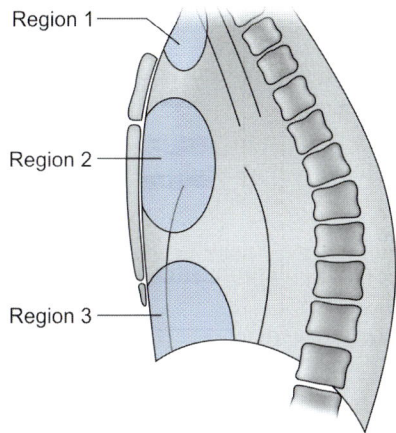

Fig. 1.8: Anterior mediastinal masses.

- *Parathyroid adenoma*:
  – Hypercalcemia with hyperparathyroidism.
  – Usually small with normal CXR.
  – Confirmed by radionuclide scan with 201Tl chloride with increased activity.

Region 2
- *Thymoma*: Usually adults.
  – Can present with myasthenia gravis (10–15%)
  – Round oval and smooth or lobulated
  – May have nodular or rim calcification
  – CT shows mixed attenuation mass with calcification and cysts.
- *Teratodermoid tumor*: Commonly dermoid cysts and benign and malignant teratomas.
  – Anterior mediastinal mass in young adult patient, dyspnea, cough, and chest pain.
  – Round or oval soft tissue mass, projects to one side.
  – Calcification, especially rim, fragments of bone and teeth are diagnostic.
  – Fat with fat-fluid level.
- *Lymph node enlargement*.
- *Aneurysm of ascending aorta*:
  – Widening of mediastinum or mediastinal mass
  – Well-defined outline
  – Peripheral rim of calcification
  – Pulsatile mass on fluoroscopy
  – Pressure erosion of sternum
  – CT shows dilated aorta with blood of higher attenuation.
- *Sternal mass*: Metastasis, plasmacytoma, chondrosarcoma, and osteomyelitis.
  – Soft tissue mass with sternal destruction.
  – Tumor new bone formation or lytic expansion of sternum.
  – Collection in anterior mediastinum with sternal destruction in osteomyelitis.
- *Lipomas*:
  – Round or oval soft tissue density mass with low density
  – Alters shape on respiration
  – CT shows solid mass of fatty attenuation.
- *Hemangioma*: Widening of mediastinum, round or oval soft tissue mass, pheboliths are diagnostic.

Region 3
- *Epicardial fat pad*:
  – Especially in obesity
  – Triangular opacity in cardiophrenic angle
  – Less dense due to fat
  – CT shows fat density and is diagnostic.
- *Diaphragmatic hump*:
  – Localized eventration
  – Common on anteromedial portion of right dome
  – Portion of liver extends into it
  – Can be confirmed by ultrasound.
- *Pleuropericardial cyst*:
  – Spring water cyst or pericardial diverticulum
  – 75% in right anterior cardiophrenic angle
  – Round/oval/triangular soft tissue mass
  – Alters shape on respiration
  – Ultrasound or CT shows trans-sonic or cystic mass adjacent to pericardium with density 0–20 HU.

- *Morgagni's hernia*:
  - 90% in right anterior cardiophrenic angle
  - Round or oval soft tissue mass
  - Lower radiographic density than expected for its size
  - Larger hernias contain transverse colon which appears as soft tissue mass with air-fluid level
  - Diagnosis by ultrasound, confirmed by barium meal examination or CT.

ANTERIOR MEDIASTINAL MASS
Children
Congenital

- *Normal thymus*:
  - Sail sign +ve
  - Wave sign +ve
  - Notch sign +ve
- *Cystic hygroma*:
  - Cystic septated mass in neck and mediastinum
- *Morgagni's hernia*:
  - Soft tissue density in cardiophrenic angle
- Neoplastic
- *Soft tissue density mass*:
  - With discrete LN ± enhancement
  - ± calcification
  - LN elsewhere.

Lymphoma

- With calcifications fat, tooth, and cyst
- Teratodermoid tumor
- *Inflammatory*:
  - Lymph nodes with rim enhancement
  - Collection or abscess.

Adults
Widening of mediastinum on X-ray with lobulated soft tissue density mass on CT.

Lymphoma

Multiple discrete or matted LN ± enhancement, calcification, and LN elsewhere.

Thymoma

- Soft tissue calcification cysts
- Associated with myasthenia gravis
- Teratodermoid
- Cyst calcification
- Tooth, fat, young adult.

Thyroid

- Mixed attenuation contiguous with thyroid pole
- Widening with fat density on CT
- Epicardial fat pad.

Lipoma

- Widening with cystic density
- Pleuropericardial cyst
  - Abscess
- Vascular
  - Aortic aneurysm
  - Hemangioma
  - Mass.

MIDDLE MEDIASTINAL MASS
Children

- *Lymph nodes*:
  - Neoplastic
  - Inflammatory.
- *Foregut duplication cysts*:
  - Bronchogenic cyst
  - Esophageal duplication cyst
  - Neurenteric cyst.
- Cystic hygroma
- *Vascular*:
  - Vena cava enlargement.

Adult

- *Lymph nodes*:
  - Neoplastic
  - Inflammatory
  - Inhalation disease.
- *Primary tumors*:
  - Carcinoma of trachea
  - Bronchogenic carcinoma
  - Esophageal tumor
  - Leiomyoma and carcinoma
  - Mesothelioma.

- *Vascular lesions*:
  - Aortic aneurysm
  - Distended arteries or veins.
- Bronchogenic cyst.

LYMPH NODES

- 90% of masses in the middle mediastinum are malignant.
- Paratracheal, tracheobronchial, subcarinal, and bronchopulmonary groups. Middle mediastinal lymph node groups.
- Often asymptomatic, may produce cough, dyspnea, and weight loss.
- It appears as widening of right paratracheal stripe, bulge in aortopulmonary window, lateral displacement of azygo-esophageal line, lobulated widening of mediastinum and unilateral or bilateral lobulated hilar soft tissue mass.

Neoplastic

Hodgkin's disease, non-Hodgkin's disease, and the lymphatic leukemias produce middle mediastinal lymphadenopathy, which is often unilateral.

Hodgkin's Disease

- On CT, nodal involvement ranges from enlarged discrete lymph nodes to large conglomerate masses.
- Thymic involvement is seen in 70% of the cases.
- Involvement of superior mediastinal lymph node was seen in 98% of patients with intrathoracic disease.

Non-Hodgkin's Disease

- Noncontiguous spread, more advanced disease, other sites involvement more common.
- Involvement of superior mediastinum in less than 75% cases.
- Parenchymal involvement of lungs also occurs and calcification occasionally develops in Hodgkin's disease after radiation.

- Fungal infections like histoplasmosis, coccidioidomycosis, and blastomycosis produce hilar or paratracheal mediastinal adenopathy with or without pulmonary involvement.
- Other infective and inflammatory causes include infectious mononucleosis, measles, whooping cough, mycoplasma, adenovirus, and lung abscess.

Inhalation Disease

- Silicosis—eggshell calcification
- Coal worker's pneumoconiosis
- Berylliosis.

Foregut Duplication Cyst

Bronchogenic cyst: It is a thin-walled foregut cyst lined by ciliated columnar epithelial cells of respiratory origin that contains viscid mucoid material.

- Usually seen as an incidental mass in a young adult.
- Rarely the cyst can become infected in children and rupture into the bronchial tree and hemorrhage into the cyst can also occur.
- Majority occurs around carina in subcarinal region but can occur in right paratracheal or posterior mediastinum.
- Appear as well-defined round or oval soft-tissue mass that can alter in shape on respiration.
- Diagnosis is confirmed by CT or MRI. CT shows a thin-walled cyst containing fluid of either low attenuation (0–20 HU) or mucinous material containing cysts (20–50 HU).

Esophageal Duplication Cyst

- Less common than bronchogenic cysts, usually larger and usually situated to the right of the midline extending into the posterior mediastinum.
- May be incidental finding or produce symptoms related to esophageal or respiratory compression. It may contain ectopic gastric mucosa causing ulceration, hemorrhage or perforation.

Neurenteric Cyst
- Located in middle or posterior mediastinum.
- Contains neural tissue and maintains a connection with spinal canal.
- Commonly right-sided and associated with vertebral body anomalies like hemivertebrae, butterfly vertebrae, and scoliosis which are usually superior to it.
- CT, MRI—for defining extent, relationship to other structure and defining intrinsic contents that may be watery or viscous.

Cystic Hygroma
- 5% cases extend into the mediastinum from the neck.
- Mostly present at birth.
- Cystic with septation and some solid components on all imaging modalities.

Thoracic Aortic Aneurysm
- Usually seen as an incidental mediastinal abnormality on a chest radiograph in elderly patients.
- It appears as either widening of the mediastinum or as a well-defined round or oval soft tissue mass in any part of the mediastinum often with curvilinear calcification in its wall.
- Displacement of rim of calcification—aortic dissection.
- Pressure erosion of sternum or vertebral bodies.
- Diagnosis confirmed by CT or MRI which shows—aorta more than 4 cm and containing contrast-enhanced blood in its lumen with surrounding mural thrombus of lower attenuation and calcification in its wall.

Other Arterial Abnormalities
- Dilatation of the main pulmonary artery due to pulmonary artery hypertension, pulmonary valve stenosis with post-stenotic dilatation or a pulmonary artery aneurysm also produces an apparent left hilar mass.
- A tortuous innominate artery produces widening of the superior mediastinum on the right and an aneurysm of the innominate or subclavian arteries produce widening of the mediastinum on the left, often simulating a left hilar mass.

Venous Abnormality
- Dilated SVC produces slight widening of the mediastinum on the right usually caused by congestive, cardiac failure, tricuspid valve disease, etc.
- A persistent left-sided SVC produces slight widening of the mediastinum on the left side.
- A dilated azygos vein—oval soft tissue mass in the right tracheobronchial angle.

Metastasis
- Most mediastinal lymph node metastases arise from a primary thoracic neoplasm, most commonly bronchogenic carcinoma.
- Generally, the lymph nodes are on the same side.
- In patients with central squamous cell carcinoma or small cell carcinoma, the hilar/mediastinal mass may be the only abnormality on plain X-ray or CT.
- In patients with extrathoracic neoplasms, intrapulmonary metastases are 10 times more common than nodal metastases.
- *Most common tumors associated with nodal metastasis are*:
  – Genitourinary (renal and testicular)
  – Head and neck
  – Breast
  – Melanoma.
- Isolated lymph node involvement seen in 60% cases.
- Hilar and right paratracheal are most commonly involved.

Inflammatory
Tuberculosis

Primary tuberculosis produces an area of consolidation in one lobe with unilateral

enlargement of the bronchopulmonary, paratracheal, and subcarinal lymph node.
- Pleural effusion also occurs and complete calcification of the lymph node may develop as healing occurs.

Sarcoidosis (Fig. 1.9)
- Enlargement of the bronchopulmonary and paratracheal lymph node, which usually are bilateral.
- Enlarged lymph node in locations such as subcarinal, anterior, and posterior mediastinum may be seen particularly if CT is performed.

DIFFERENTIAL DIAGNOSIS OF POSTERIOR MEDIASTINAL MASSES

Mediastinum (Fig. 1.10)
- Anterior—in front of the anterior pericardium and trachea.
- Middle—within the pericardium including the trachea.
- Posterior—lies behind the posterior pericardium and trachea.

Differential Diagnoses
- *Region 5*:
  – Neurogenic tumors
  – Pharyngoesophageal pouch

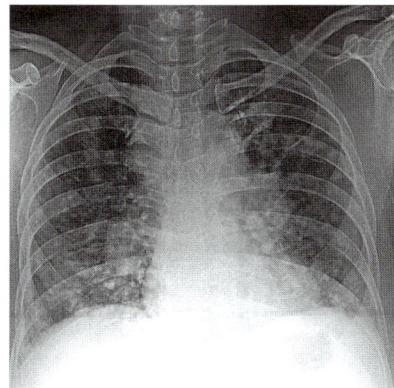

Fig. 1.9: Posteroanterior (PA) radiograph of chest shows superior mediastinal and bilateral adenopathy along with reticulonodular shadowing in bilateral lungs in a case of sarcoidosis.

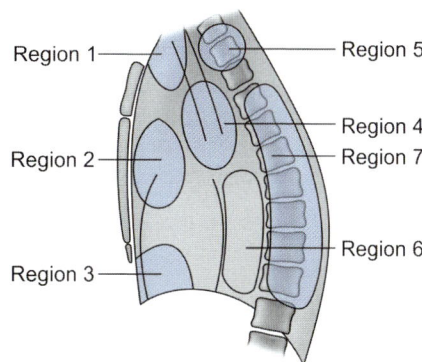

Fig. 1.10: Shows different regions in mediastinum. **Note:** There are different regions of mediastinum as discussed in text.

- *Region 6*:
  – Hiatus hernia
  – Neurenteric cyst
  – Aneurysm of descending aorta
  – Sequestrated lung segment
  – Esophageal dilatation
  – Dilatation of azygos vein.
- *Region 7*:
  – Neurogenic tumors
  – Bochdalek's hernia
  – Paravertebral mass
  – Extramedullary hematopoiesis.

Neurenteric Cyst
- Partial or complete persistence of the neurenteric canal or its incomplete resorption.
  – Gastrointestinal reduplication
  – Enteric cysts
  – Neurenteric cysts
  – Anterior meningocele
  – Cysts of the cord.
- *Associated spinal anomalies*:
  – Block vertebra
  – Hemivertebra
  – Butterfly vertebra
  – Spina bifida.
- Usually present in infants.
- Respiratory distress.
- Feeding difficulties.

- Cysts—appear as oval or rounded soft tissue mass in posterior mediastinum.
- *Anterior meningocele*: Diagnosed by CT—myelography and prone scan.
- *Esophageal duplication cyst*—barium swallow—ectopic gastric mucosa—Tc 99m positive.

Pertechnetate Scan
- Neurenteric cyst can be diagnosed by USG/CT/MRI—usually right-sided.

Dilated Azygos Vein
- Oval soft-tissue mass in right tracheobronchial angle.
- Caused by—increased central venous pressure.
  - Superior or inferior vena cava obstruction
  - Portal hypertension
  - Congenital azygos continuation of inferior vena cava (IVC)
  - Differential diagnosis—enlarged azygos lymph node
  - Azygos vein—decrease in size—in erect position
  - On deep inspiration
  - During maneuver.

Esophageal Lesions
- *Pharyngoesophageal pouch or Zenker's diverticulum*:
  - Round mass containing air-fluid level in the superior part of posterior mediastinum usually in the midline displaying the trachea anteriorly.
- Leiomyoma/leiomyosarcoma—soft tissue mass.
- Lower esophageal diverticulum—rounded mass with air-fluid level behind the heart.
- *Dilated esophagus*—widening of the posterior mediastinum on the right side from thoracic inlet to diaphragm with lateral displacement of azygoesophageal line. Dilated esophagus displaces the trachea anteriorly.
- Air-fluid level with non-homogeneous mottled appearance of food mixed with air diagnosis confirmed by barium swallow or CT.

Paravertebral Lesions
- Traumatic wedge compression fracture of vertebral body with paraspinal hematoma—history of trauma.
- Pyogenic/tubercular paravertebral abscess—narrowing of disk space with involvement of vertebral endplates.
- Smooth fusiform bilateral or unilateral soft tissue mass.
- Metastasis—bone destruction with pathological fracture.
- Extramedullary hematopoiesis—lobulated mass in chronic hemolytic anemia.
- Lymphoma.

Bochdalek's Hernia
- Developmental defect in posterolateral part of left hemi-diaphragm.
- Contents of the hernial sac include retroperitoneal fat, kidney, spleen, and splenic flexure.
  Large or small intestine, stomach, and colon may also herniate.
- Mediastinal shift/ipsilateral hypoplastic lung.
- Thirteen pairs of ribs may be associated.

Neurogenic Tumors
- Peripheral nerves
  ↓

I. Nerve sheath tumors:
- Neurofibroma
- Schwannoma or neurilemmoma
- Neurofibrosarcoma
- Malignant schwannoma

II. Ganglion cell tumors:
- Ganglioneuroma benign (>10 years)
- Ganglioneuroblastoma (5–10 years)
- Neuroblastoma (<5 years) (most malignant).

III. Paraganglionic nerve tissue tumors
↓ (rarest)
- Chemodectomas.
- Pheochromocytomas:
  - 30% malignant
  - Childhood or young adult patient
  - Asymptomatic, back pain, and spinal cord compression
  - Can be multiple in the setting of neurofibromatosis—association with lateral thoracic meningocele.
- Radiological features—well-defined oval soft tissue mass in paravertebral gutter.
- Nerve sheath tumors—circular and calcification—rare.
- Ganglion cell tumors—elongated, central spicules or nodules of calcification, enlargement of intervertebral foramen, and scoliosis.

Hiatus Hernia

- Usually an incidental finding in an elderly patient
- Often asymptomatic
- Clinical features—dyspnea, retrosternal chest pain, epigastric discomfort, and iron deficiency anemia
- CXR—round soft tissue mass with air or air-fluid level, behind heart, usually to the left of midline
  - Larger hernias may contain small intestine, colon, and liver.
  - Diagnosis—confirmed by lateral CXR, barium or CT (Fig. 1.11).

CHEST WALL ABNORMALITIES (TABLE 1.7)

Pectus Excavatum
- Most common congenital anomaly of sternum.
- Decreased prevertebral space—left hand deviation of heart with axial rotation.
  - Increased parasternal soft tissue in right inferomedial hemithorax
  - Lateral CXR and CT quantify the severity.

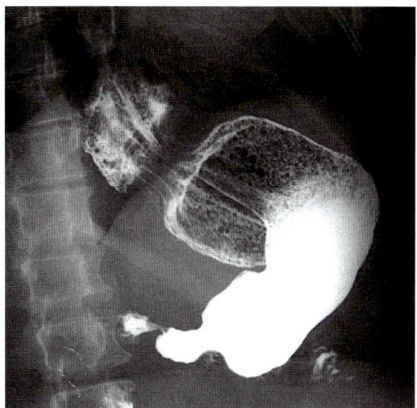

Fig. 1.11: Barium study radiograph shows hiatus hernia.

Table 1.7: Chest wall abnormalities.

Congenital and developmental anomalies	Tumors
	Soft tissue tumors

• Pectus excavatum
• Pectus carinatum
• Poland syndrome
• Cervical rib
• Cleidocranial dysplasia
	• Lipomas
	• Neurogenic tumors
	• Hemangiomas
	• Desmoid tumors
	  – Lymphomas
	• Sarcomas
	  – Osseous tumors

Inflammatory and infectious	
• Pyogenic • Tuberculosis (TB) • Actinomycosis • Aspergillosis	• Osteochondroma • Enchondroma • Osteoblastoma • Chondrosarcoma • Myeloma • Plasmacytoma
Non-neoplastic osseous	
	• Fibrous dysplasia • Paget's disease • Giant cell tumor • Aneurysmal bone cyst

Pectus Carinatum
- Protrusion of sternum anteriorly.
- May be seen in isolation or with cyanotic congenital heart disease.

Cervical Rib
Supernumerary rib that articulates with cervical type of transverse process.

Cleidocranial Dysostosis

Incomplete ossification of ribs with defective development of pubic bones, vertebral column, and long bones.

Poland Syndrome

- Partial/total absence of greater pectoral muscle and ipsilateral syndactyly.
- Atrophy of ipsilateral fifth ribs, absence of smaller pectoral muscle, aplasia of ipsilateral breast/nipple, simian crease of affected extremity.

Inflammatory and Infectious Disease

- Primary infection rare and seen in diabetes mellitus, immunosuppression, trauma, and intravenous drug abusers
- Secondary infection due to disease processes in lung or to pleurae, empyema more common
- May produce parenchymal infection, pleural effusion, chest wall masses, rib destruction, and even cutaneous fistula, air-fluid levels may be seen in soft tissues. Patients usually have febrile cause.

Tumors of Chest Wall

- Primarily soft tissue tumors are rare.
- In adults, most common benign soft tissue neoplasm is lipoma and most common malignant neoplasms are fibrous sarcoma and malignant fibrous histiocytomas (MFH).
- In children, primitive neuroectodermal tumor (PNET) (Askin) tumor, rhabdomyosarcoma and extraosseous Ewing's sarcoma are most common malignant soft tissue tumors.
- Secondary tumors are more common in thoracic skeleton.
- Majority of osseous lesions are in ribs, large numbers are metastatic.
- Osteochondroma is most common benign tumor of cartilage bone. Most common malignant tumor is chondrosarcoma.
- Majority of lesions arising from sternum are malignant and represent chondrosarcoma most often.
- Lesions of thoracic vertebrae are invariably metastatic.
- Most common tumors to produce pattern of chest wall mass with bone destruction are metastases and small round cell tumors (multiple myeloma), Ewing's tumor and neuroblastoma. The differential diagnosis in adults is metastases versus myeloma, whereas in a child, pattern is more suggestive of Ewing's tumor or metastatic neuroblastoma.

Radiological Differentiation of Chest Wall Tumors

Radiological differentiation of chest wall tumors has been shown in Table 1.8.

SUPERIOR RIB NOTCHING

Classification (Sargent et al.)

1. *Normal.*
2. *Disturbance of osteoblastic activity with decreased or deficient bone formation*
   - Paralytic poliomyelitis
   - Collagen diseases
     – Scleroderma
     – Rheumatoid arthritis
     – Systemic lupus erythematosus (SLE)
   - Exostosis
   - Neurofibroma
   - Surgery
   - Osteogenesis imperfecta
   - Coarctation of aorta
   - Marfan's syndrome
   - Radiation damage
   - Quadriplegia.
3. *Disturbance of osteoclastic activity with increased bone resorption*
   - Hyperparathyroidism
   - Hypovitaminosis D.
4. *Idiopathic.*

Table 1.8: Radiological differentiation of chest wall tumors (benign and malignant).

Benign	
Imaging findings	Tumor type

• Fat attenuation/intensity
• Calcification
  – Skeletal
  – Amorphous
  – Cartilaginous apical cap
  – Extraskeleton, punctate
• Cortical thinning—fluid-fluid levels
• Cortical expansion, sclerotic band
 	
• Rib erosion, well-defined contours, extraskeletal location
• Location at costochondral junction
• Location in paravertebral
• Location in shoulder region
	• Lipoma
	
	• Fibrous dysplasia
	• Osteochondroma
	• Cavernous hemangioma
	• ABC or GCT
	• Ossifying fibromyxoid tumor or chondromyxoid fibroma
	• Schwannoma or nonossifying fibroma
	• Osteochondroma
	• Ganglioneuroma or regional paraganglioma
	• Spindle cell lipoma

Malignant	

• Fat component
• Calcification
  – Skeletal
  – Rings and arcs
  – Flocculent or stippled
  – Centrally dense
• Extraskeletal
  – Heterogeneous
 	
  – Speckled
• Diffuse osteolytic changes
• Ill-defined mass
  – Eccentric growth, in children and young adults
  – Fluid-fluid levels and calcifications in adolescents and adults
  – Chronic lymphedema
  – Infiltrative growth
• Nonspecific findings
	• Liposarcoma
	
	• Chondrosarcoma
	
	• Osteosarcoma
	
	• Ganglioneuroma or neuroblastoma
	• Proximal type epithelioid sarcoma
	• Myeloma
	
	• Ewing's sarcoma
	
	• Synovial sarcoma
	
	• Angiosarcoma
	• Malignant lymphoma
	• Liposarcoma leiomyosarcoma (LMS), rhabdomyosarcoma (RMS), malignant fibrous histiocytoma (MFH), etc.

Salient Features

Poliomyelitis

- Limb deformities and muscle atrophy seen particularly involving the pectoral muscles and shoulder girdle.
- Rib notching seen in chronic cases usually involving 3rd–9th ribs.
- Unilateral hypertransradiant hemithorax.
- Scoliosis.

Rheumatoid Arthritis

- More common in females.
- Symmetrical arthritis especially involving the metacarpophalangeal (MCP) and proximal interphalangeal (PIP) joints of hands and feet and wrist.
- Absence of lateral end of clavicle or pencil pointing may be seen.
- Caplan's syndrome—multiple nodules in lung.
- Subcutaneous nodules.

Systemic Sclerosis

- Raynaud's phenomenon.
- Subcutaneous calcification—especially in the fingertips.
- Esophageal abnormalities—dilatation, atonicity, poor or absent peristalsis.

- Symmetric erosions on superior surface, predominantly along the posterior aspect of 3rd–6th ribs.
- Terminal phalanx resorption.
- Skin thickening.

Systemic Lupus Erythematosus
- Mostly females, butterfly rash.
- *Polyarthritis*: Bilateral and symmetrical involving the small joints of the hand, knee, and wrist.
- MCP and PIP joint involvement—no erosions.
- Recurrent pleural effusion often with pleurisy resulting in elevation of a hemidiaphragm and plate atelectasis at base.

Osteochondroma
- 10–20 years of age.
- Well-defined protrusion with the patent cortex and trabeculae continuous with that of parent bone. Cartilage cap.
- Most common distal femur and proximal tibia.
- Lesions arising from ribs and scapulae cause rib notching.
- Diaphyseal achalasia—multiple lesions.

Neurofibromatosis
- One or more primary relatives with neurofibromas
- Café au lait spots
- Optic gliomas
- Typical bone lesions—sphenoid dysplasia (absent greater wing or lesser wing, absent posterolateral wall of orbit)
- Tibial pseudarthrosis
- Rib notching, twisted ribbon ribs, and splaying of ribs
- Cerebral and cerebellar calcification, heavy calcification of choroid plexus.

Marfan's Syndrome
- Tall stature, long slim limbs
- Arachnodactyly
- Joint laxity—dislocation of sternoclavicular joint and hip joint
- Scoliosis and kyphosis
- Pectus excavatum and carinatum
- Aortic sinus dilatation and aortic regurgitation.

Osteogenesis Imperfecta
- Osteoporotic, fragile bones often with deformities secondary to fractures and mechanical stress
- Often in infant or child with blue sclerae
- Flattened or biconcave vertebrae
- Wormian bones
- Rapid fracture healing with exuberant callus
- Wavy, thin, and ribbon-like ribs with notching.

Hyperparathyroidism
- Subperiosteal bone erosion—particularly affecting the radial side of middle phalanx of middle finger, medial proximal tibia, and lateral end of clavicle
- Diffuse cortical damage—pepper-pot skull
- Brown tumors—mandible, ribs, and pelvis
- Ribs
  - Characteristically show random notching
  - Coarse sclerosis of trabecular pattern of clavicles and ribs.

INFERIOR RIB NOTCHING
Unilateral
- Blalock-Taussig operation
- Subclavian artery occlusion
- Aortic coarctation left subclavian artery or anomalous right subclavian artery.

Bilateral
- Aorta coarctation, occlusion, and aortitis
  - Subclavian
    - Takayasu's disease, atheroma
  - Pulmonary oligemia
    - Fallot's tetralogy
    - Pulmonary atresia
    - Stenosis

- Venous
  - SVC, IVC obstruction
- Shunts
  - Intercostal-pulmonary fistula
  - AV fistula
- Others
  - Hyperparathyroidism (HPT)
  - Neurogenic
  - Idiopathic.

Pleural effusion (Fig. 1.12 and Table 1.9).

ELEVATION OF DIAPHRAGM

Small Hilum (Table 1.10)

Unilateral (U/L)

- *Causes above the diaphragm*:
  - Phrenic nerve palsy
  - Pulmonary collapse
  - Pulmonary infarction
  - Pleural disease (Table 1.11)
  - Hemiplegia:
    - Diaphragmatic cause
  - Eventration:
    - Causes below the diaphragm
    - Gaseous distension of stomach/splenic flexure
    - Subphrenic inflammation of diaphragm
    - Scoliosis
    - Decubitus.

Bilateral (B/L)

- Poor inspiratory effort
- Obesity
  Above the diaphragm
  - B/L basal pulmonary collapse
  - Small lungs
  Below the diaphragm
  - Ascites
  - Pregnancy
  - Pneumoperitoneum
  - Hepatosplenomegaly
  - Intra-abdominal tumor
  - B/L subphrenic abscess.

Table 1.9: Types of effusion.

	U/L, B/L	Biochemical derangement	Consolidation
Transudate			
Cardiac failure	B/L	+	–
Hepatic failure	B/L	+	–
Nephrotic syndrome	B/L	+	–
Meigs' syndrome	U/L	–	–
Exudate			
Infection	U/L, B/L	–	+
Malignancy	U/L, B/L	–	+
Pulmonary infarction	U/L,	–	+
Collagen vascular disease	–	–	
Subphrenic abscess	U/L	–	+
Pancreatitis	U/L	–	+
Hemorrhagic			
CA bronchus	U/L, B/L	–	+/–
Trauma	U/L	–	–
Pulmonary infarction	–	–	+
Bleeding disorders	–	–	–
Chylous			
Obstructive thoracic duct	–	–	–

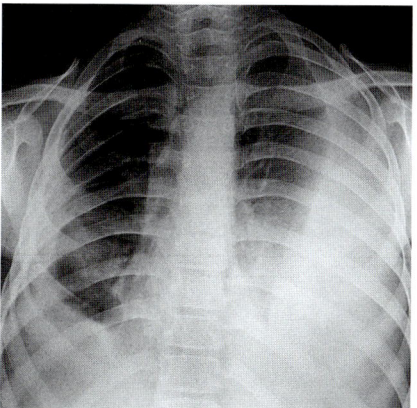

Fig. 1.12: Posteroanterior (PA) radiograph of chest shows bilateral pleural effusion causing compression atelectasis of underlying pulmonary parenchyma (L >R).

Table 1.10: Cases of small hilum

Apparent rotation, scoliosis	Volume loss	Soft tissue	Consolidation
Unilateral	+	–	–
Normal or left side lobar collapse, lobectomy	–	+	–
Hypoplastic pulmonary artery	–	–	+
McLeod's syndrome	–	–	–
Unilateral pulmonary embolus			
Bilateral			
Cyanotic congenital heart disease	–	–	–
Central pulmonary embolus	–	–	+

Table 1.11: Pleural lesions.

Pleural calcification	Local pleural mass
Old empyema	Loculated pleural effusion
Old hemothorax	Metastasis
Asbestosis inhalation	Malignant mesothelioma
Silicosis	Pleural fibroma
Talc exposure	

Unilaterally Elevated Diaphragm

- *Phrenic nerve palsy*: Smooth hemidiaphragm, no movement on respiration. Paradoxical movements on sniffing.
- *Pleural disease*: Especially old pleural disease, e.g. hemothorax, empyema, tuberculosis, and thoracotomy.
- *Splinting of the diaphragm*: Associated with rib fracture or pleurisy due to any cause.
- *Hemiplegia*: Associated with an upper motor neuron lesion.
- *Eventration*: More common on the left side.
  - Heart is shifted to the contralateral side
  - Paradoxical movements on sniffing.
- *Gaseous distension of stomach or splenic flexure*: Only the left hemidiaphragm.
- *Subphrenic inflammatory disease*: Subdiaphragmatic abscess or infection, inflammation.
- *Scoliosis*: Raised hemidiaphragm on the side of the concavity.
- *Decubitus*: Raised hemidiaphragm is on the dependent side.

Bilaterally Elevated Diaphragm

- *Bilateral basal pulmonary collapse*—which may be secondary to infarction or subphrenic abscess.
- Small lung due to fibrotic lung disease.
- Hepatosplenomegaly in patients of lymphoma, anemia, and many infectious pathologies.
- Large intra-abdominal tumors either located in the midline or in any of the superior abdominal quadrants. Ascites in ovarian tumor can also cause this.

Pneumothorax

- Spontaneous
- Iatrogenic
- Traumatic
- Secondary to mediastinal emphysema
- *Secondary to lung disease*:
  - Emphysema
  - Honeycomb lung (Fig. 1.13)

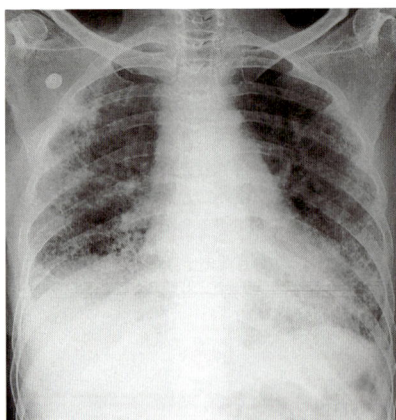

Fig. 1.13: Anteroposterior (AP) radiograph of chest shows honeycombing in both lungs with reduced volume of right lung.

- Pneumonia
- Bronchopleural fistula
- Pneumoperitoneum.

Pneumomediastinum

- Lung tear
- Perforation of esophagus, trachea, bronchus, perforation of hollow viscera.

PNEUMOMEDIASTINUM

It may be associated with pneumothorax and subcutaneous emphysema.

- *Lung tear*: A sudden rise in the intra-alveolar pressure, often with airway narrowing, causes air to dissect through the interstitium to the hilum and then to the mediastinum.
    - *Spontaneous*: Following severe bout of cough or a severe strenuous exercise
    - *Asthma*: Usually not before 2 years of age
    - *Diabetic ketoacidosis*: Secondary to severe and protracted vomiting
    - Childbirth—due to repeated Valsalva maneuvers
    - Artificial respiration
    - Chest trauma
    - Foreign body aspiration.
- *Perforation of esophagus, trachea or bronchus*:
    - Spontaneous
    - Boerhaave's syndrome
    - Following severe and protracted vomiting
    - Trauma
    - Foreign body aspiration or inhalation

    Ruptured esophagus also produces left-sided pneumothorax, hydropneumothorax.
- Perforation of a hollow abdominal viscus with extension of gas via the retroperitoneum.

Right-sided Diaphragmatic Humps

At Any Site

- Collapse/consolidation of the adjacent lung
- Localized eventration
- Loculated effusion

- Subphrenic abscess
- Hepatic abscess
- Hydatid cyst
- Hepatic metastasis.

Medially

- Pericardial fat pad
- Aortic aneurysm
- Pleuropericardial cyst
- Sequestrated segment.

Anteriorly

- Morgagni's hernia.

Posteriorly

- Bochdalek hernia.

LUNG TUMORS

Carcinoma: Approximately 50% of lung cancers arise centrally, i.e. in or proximal to segmental bronchi.

- Obstruction of lumen leads to collapse and often infection.
- Peripheral tumors appear as soft tissue nodules or irregular masses and invade the adjacent tissues. Signs of collapse and consolidation may occur.
- Peripheral tumors may arise in the scar. These mass lesions may present as hilar enlargement, airway obstruction, peripheral mass lesion, mediastinal involvement, pleural and bone involvement.

Alveolar cell carcinoma: Arises more peripherally, probably from the type II pneumocytes. It arises within the alveoli and produces areas of consolidation.

Metastases

- *Hematogenous*: Breast, skeleton, and urogenital
- *Lymphatic*: Less common, breast
- *Endobronchial spread*: Alveolar cell carcinoma

Metastasis is usually bilateral, affecting both lungs equally, with basal predominance. They are often peripheral and may be subpleural.

Cavitary Metastases
- Squamous cell carcinoma
- Sarcoma.

Calcifying Metastases
- Osteogenic sarcoma
- Chondrosarcoma
- Mucinous adenocarcinoma.

Endobronchial Metastases
- Carcinoma kidney and breast
- Large bowel.

Lymphangitis Carcinoma

Most common sites—lung, breast, stomach, pancreas, cervix, and prostate.

It is usually bilateral, but lung and breast cancers may cause unilateral lymphangitis.

Hodgkin's/Non-Hodgkin's Lymphoma

Present as nodal enlargement, which is usually bilateral, asymmetric and involves anterior mediastinal glands. These may calcify following therapy. Pulmonary infiltration may appear as areas of consolidation or areas of miliary nodules. Pleural effusion may be present in 30% of cases.

Leukemia

Mediastinal lymph node enlargement and pleural effusion are the most common radiologic abnormalities.

Sarcoma

- Kaposi's sarcoma may appear as segmental or lobar consolidation.
- Other primary pulmonary sarcomas include fibrosarcoma, leiomyosarcoma—which appear as solitary pulmonary masses, radiographically indistinguishable from a carcinoma of the lung.

Adenoma

Carcinoid accounts for approximately 90% of bronchial adenomas and adenoid cystic tumors for about 10%. These appear as well-circumscribed round or ovoid solitary nodules. On CT, calcification may be seen within the tumor.

Hamartoma

They are seen in childhood as a solitary pulmonary nodule. Thirty percent of these show calcification, often with a characteristic "popcorn" appearance.

Lung Abscess

Radiographically, an abscess may or may not be surrounded by consolidation. Appearance of an air-fluid level indicates that a communication with the airway has developed. It shows thick irregular wall, which shows postcontrast enhancement.

Bronchiectasis

It is the irreversible dilatation of one or more bronchi and is usually the result of severe, recurrent and chronic infection. It is frequently basal but in tuberculosis and cystic fibrosis, it usually involves the upper zone. Dilated bronchi produce tramline shadows or ring shadows, and dilated, fluid-filled bronchi may cause "gloved finger" shadows.

Asthma

During an attack, the CXR may show signs of hyperinflation, with the depression of the diaphragm and expansion of the retrosternal air space. The peripheral pulmonary vessels appear normal, but if the central pulmonary arteries are enlarged, the irreversible pulmonary arterial hypertension is probably present.

Chronic Bronchitis

Fifty percent of these patients may have normal CXR. In patients with a plain film abnormality, the signs are due to emphysema, superimposed infection or possibly bronchiectasis. "Dirty chest" appearance is seen.

Emphysema (Fig. 1.14)

With emphysema, air trapping is present, the lung volumes increase, the diaphragm becomes flattened, and the retrosternal air space increases. The number and size of the peripheral vessels decrease. Central pulmonary arteries may enlarge suggestive of cor pulmonale.

Bronchiolitis

It results due to infection (often in childhood) or due to inhalation of toxic fumes, drug therapy and rheumatoid disease. Radiologically, the appearances are most frequently of hyperinflation of lungs and perihilar prominence and indistinctness.

HILAR ENLARGEMENT (TABLES 1.12 AND 1.13)

Unilateral Hilar Enlargement (Fig. 1.15)

Carcinoma bronchus: The hilar enlargement may be due to the tumor itself or due to the involved lymph nodes.
- *Lymphoma*:
  - Unilateral is very unusual
  - Anterior mediastinal nodes are also involved.

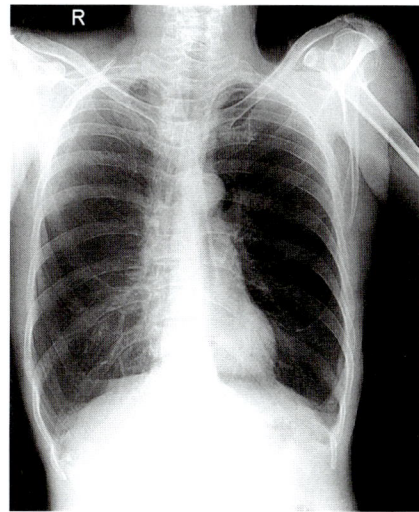

Fig. 1.14: Posteroanterior (PA) radiograph of chest shows bilateral pulmonary emphysema.

- *Infective*: Due to the nodal enlargement.
- *Poststenotic dilatation of the pulmonary artery*: Usually on the left side.
- *Pulmonary embolus*: Peripheral oligemia is characteristic.
- *Aneurysm*: In chronic pulmonary arterial hypertension. Calcification may also be present.
- *Mediastinal mass*: Middle mediastinum masses may superimpose.
- Perihilar pneumonia, ill-defined borders with presence of air bronchogram.

Bilateral Hilar Enlargement

- *Sarcoidosis*: Symmetrical, lobulated. Associated bronchotracheal, tracheobronchial and paratracheal lymphadenopathy
- *Lymphoma*: Asymmetrical, but multiple sites
- *Infective*:
  - Viral, mainly in children
  - TB—Bilaterally is rare
  - Histoplasmosis pulmonary nodules (multiple) accompany
- *Pulmonary arterial hypertension*:
  - Bilaterally is rare
  - Peripheral oligemia is characteristic
- *Silicosis*:
  - Symmetrical
  - Pinpoint multiple pulmonary nodules are present.

APICAL SHADOWS

Differential diagnosis of apical shadows has been shown in Table 1.14.

CALCIFICATION ON CHEST RADIOGRAPH

Intrapulmonary (Figs. 1.16 and 1.17)

- Granuloma, infection
- Chronic abscess
- Tumor:
  - Metastases
  - Hamartoma
  - AVM

Table 1.12: Unilateral hilar enlargement.

	Egg shell calcification	Air broncho-gram	LN	Angio
Lymph Node				
Carcinoma	–	–	+	–
Lymphoma	–	+	+	–
Infective				
TB				
Histoplasmosis	–	–	+	–
Coccidioidomycosis	–	–		
Sarcoidosis	+	–	–	–
Pulmonary Artery				
Poststenotic dilatation	–	–	–	+
Pulmonary embolus	–	–	–	+
Aneurysm	+	–	–	+
Mediastinal mass—superimposed on a hilum	–	–	–	–
Perihilar pneumonia		+	+/–	–

Table 1.13: Bilateral hilar enlargement.

	Symmetrical	Occupational	Lobulated
Idiopathic	+	–	+
Sarcoidosis			
Neoplastic			
Lymphoma	–		+
Lymphangitis carcinomatosis		–	–
Infective	±		+
Viruses	–	–	–
Primary tuberculosis (TB)	–	–	–
Histoplasmosis	–	–	–
Coccidioidomycosis			
Vascular	–	–	–
Pulmonary arterial hypertension			
Immunological	–	+	–
Extrinsic allergic alveolitis			
Inhalation	–	+	–
Silicosis			
Berylliosis			

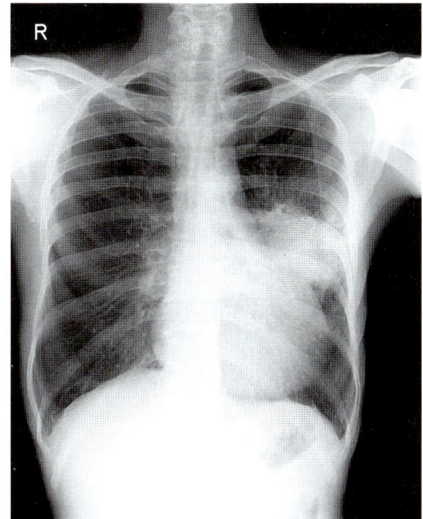

Fig. 1.15: Posteroanterior (PA) radiograph of chest shows left hilar mass.

- Hematoma
- Infarct
- Broncholith
- Alveolar microlithiasis
- Idiopathic.

Lymph Nodes

Tuberculosis, histoplasmosis, sarcoidosis, and silicosis.

Pleural

- Tuberculosis, asbestosis, and talcosis
- Hemothorax and empyema.

Mediastinal

- Cardiac
- Vascular
- Tumors.

Pulmonary Artery

- Hypertension
- Aneurysm
- Thrombus.

Chest Wall

- Costal cartilage
- Breast
- Bone tumor and callus
- Soft tissues.

AIR-FLUID LEVELS ON CHEST X-RAY

- *Intrapulmonary*:
  - Hydropneumothorax:
    - Trauma
    - Bronchopleural fistula
  - Esophageal:
    - Pharyngeal pouch, diverticulae
    - Obstruction—tumor, achalasia esophagectomy
  - Mediastinal:
    - Infections
    - Perforation—esophageal
  - Pneumopericardium: Diagnostic, trauma
  - Chest wall: Infection
  - Diaphragm: Hernia, eventration, and rupture.

Table 1.14: Differential diagnosis of apical shadows.

	U/L, B/L	Ellis curve	Pleural outline seen	Rib destruction	Symmetry
Pleural caps	U/L	–	–	–	+/–
Pleural fluid	U/L or B/L	+	–	–	±
Bullae	U/L	–	+	–	–
Pancoast's tumor	U/L	–	–	+	–
Infections—tuberculosis (TB)	U/L or B/L	–	–	–	
Pneumothorax	U/L	–	+	–	–
Soft tissue	B/L	–	–	+	+

Differential Diagnosis in Radiology

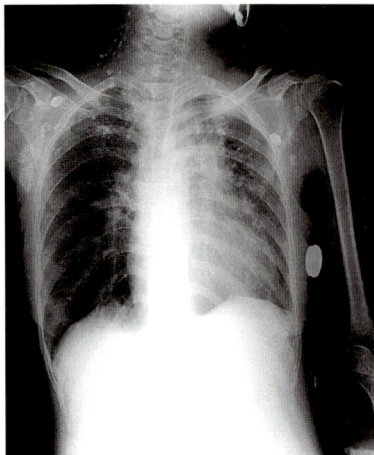

Fig. 1.16: Posteroanterior (PA) radiograph of chest shows multifocal pulmonary parenchymal, bilateral axillary and right cervical nodal calcifications associated with fibrotic changes in a case of healed Koch's chest.

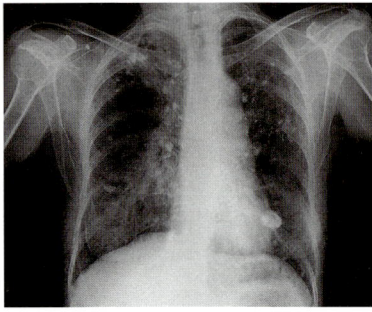

Fig. 1.17: Posteroanterior (PA) radiograph of chest shows multifocal pulmonary parenchymal and hilar calcifications associated with fibrotic changes in a case of healed Koch's chest.

Crescent Sign

- Fungal ball
- Blood clot in tubercular cavity
- Bronchial adenoma, carcinoma
- Hamartoma
- Hydatid cyst
- Pulmonary infarct.

CAVITATING PULMONARY LESIONS

Infection

- *Staphylococcus*
- *Klebsiella*
- Tuberculosis
- Histoplasmosis
- Amebic
- Hydatid
- Fungal.

Malignant

- Primary
- Secondary
- Lymphoma.

Abscess

- Blood borne
- Aspiration
- Pulmonary infarct
- Pulmonary hematoma
- Pneumoconiosis.

Collagen Diseases

- Rheumatoid nodules
- Wegener's granulomatosis.

Developmental

- Sequestrated segment
- Bronchogenic cyst
- Congenital cystic adenomatoid malformation
- Sarcoidosis
- Bullae, blebs
- Pneumatocele
- Traumatic lung cyst.

MASS WITHIN CAVITY (TABLE 1.15)

- Mycetoma—aspergilloma
- Tissue fragment from carcinoma
- Necrotic lung within abscess
- Disintegrating hydatid cyst
- Intracavitary blood clot.

CAVITATING PULMONARY LESIONS

Causes

- *Malignant*:
  – Primary
  – Secondary
  – Lymphoma

Chest

Table 1.15: Differential diagnosis of mass within cavity.

	1	2	3	4	5
Thick, irregular walled cavity	+	+	+	−	+
Adjacent lung parenchymal reaction	+	±	+	±	±
Clinical history	of infection	of weight loss	Infection	Infection	±
Mobile	+	±	±	+	+
Contrast enhancement in CT of mass	+	+	−	±	−
Calcification	−	±	−	−	± if chronic

- *Infections*:
  - Tuberculosis
  - *Staphylococcus*
  - *Klebsiella*
  - Amebic
  - Hydatid
  - Fungal
- *Abscess*:
  - Aspiration
  - Blood borne
- Pulmonary infarct
- Hematoma
- *Pneumoconiosis*:
  - Pulmonary massive fibrosis
  - Rheumatoid nodular
  - Collagen diseases
  - Wegener's granulomatosis
- *Developmental*:
  - Sequestration
  - Bronchogenic cyst
  - Congenital cystic adenomatoid malformation
- Sarcoidosis
- Bullae, blebs
- Traumatic lung cyst
- Pneumatocele.

Carcinoma

Primary

Very frequently cavity nodules turn out to be malignant.

Mechanism

Obstruction of an artery
(Infection of a nodule)
- In 2–10%, especially peripheral upper lobe involvement
- Most cavities are thick-walled, irregular inner surface
- Thickness more than 15 mm—85–90% malignant
- Cavitation—centric or eccentric
- Multiple cavitations
- More common in squamous cell carcinoma and then may be thin-walled.

Metastasis—Cavitation

- More common in upper lobe, may involve few nodules
- Thin or thick-walled
- Seen especially in squamous cell carcinoma—head and neck (uncommon in adenocarcinoma—especially colon)
- Sarcoma—osteosarcoma.

Hodgkin's Disease

- Thick or thin-walled
- Typically in an area of infiltration
- Hilar or mediastinal LN.

Tuberculosis

- Thick-walled and smooth, sometimes fluid level
- Mainly affects upper lobes and apical segment of lower lobe
- Usually surrounded by consolidation and fibrosis
- Typically there is large cavity surrounded by smaller satellite cavities
- Cavity walls are lined by tuberculous granulation tissue
- Cavities traversed by fibrotic remnants of bronchi and vessels
- Rasmussen aneurysm.

Staphylococcus aureus
- Mostly children, multiple
- Thick-walled cavities with a ragged inner lining
- No lobar predilection
- Associated with effusion and empyema.

Hydatid Cysts
- Complicated hydatid cyst
- Rupture into a bronchus-air crescent sign/ air cap
- Water lily sign.

Aspergillosis
- Any pulmonary cavity—TB, histoplasmosis, sarcoidosis
- Forms a ball which changes position, ball is seen to be mobile
- Almost always pleural thickening related to mycetoma
- Vascular granular tissue-bleeding may occur.

Abscess (Aspiration)
- Multiple or single
- Usually thick-walled
- Following aspiration
- Posterior segment or apical segment—U/L
- In sitting-right lower lobe.

Pulmonary Infarct

(Infection—may be)

Primarily:
1. Septic embolus

Secondary to:
2. Initially sterile, infarct, and infection

Tertiary to:
3. As aseptic cavitating infarct infected
   - Aseptic cavitation is usually solitary and arises in a large area of consolidation after about 2 weeks.
   - Cavity has scalloped inner margins and cross cavity band shadows/effusion.

Cystic Bronchiectasis (Fig. 1.18)
- Thin-walled lower lobes

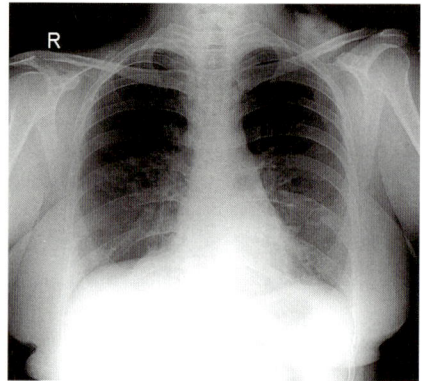

Fig. 1.18: Posteroanterior (PA) radiograph of chest shows bilateral perihilar cystic bronchiectasis.

- Air-fluid levels, peribronchial thickening and retained secretions
- Crowded vessels and retained secretions.

Sequestered Lung
- Thin- or thick-walled
- 66% in left lower lobe, 33% in right lower lobe
- Air-fluid level, surrounding pneumonia.

Wegener's Granulomatosis
- Bilateral and widely spread
- Nodules, cavitation in some nodules (1/3)
- Cavities are thick-walled, shaggy/irregular lining
- Become thinner with time
- After therapy may disappear.

Rheumatoid Nodules
- Thick-walled with a smooth inner lining and well-defined
- Lower lobes and peripherally
- Become thinner with time.

Progressive Massive Fibrosis
- Predominantly in mid and upper zone
- Begin peripherally and move centrally
- Nodule formation which cavitates into thick- and irregular-walled cavities in a background nodularity of pneumoconiosis.

Sarcoidosis

- In early disease, necrosis of coalescent granuloma and check valve mechanism beyond partial obstruction
- Thin-walled cavities
- B/L hilar lymph nodes.

Infected Emphysematous Bullae

- Thin-walled and air-fluid level
- Usually seen in emphysema, particularly paraseptal and scar associated
- Apical asymptomatic and those associated with scarring [throughout the lungs—chronic obstructive pulmonary disease (COPD)]
- Associated changes of inflammation in surrounding lung.

TRAUMA

Hematoma—Peripheral

- Air-fluid level—communication with bronchus.

Traumatic Lung Cyst

- Single or multiple
- Peripheral and thin-walled
- Uni- or multilocular
- Within hours of injury.

Bronchogenic Cyst

- Medial one-third of lower lobes
- If ruptures into a bronchus, thin-walled, air-fluid level, and surrounding pneumonia.

Cystic Adenomatoid Malformation

- Causes neonatal respiratory distress
- Cavities of various shapes and sizes scattered in an area of opaque lung with well-defined margins.

LUCENT LUNG LESIONS

Multiple Lucent Lung Lesions

Cavities

- *Infection*:
  - Bacterial pneumonia

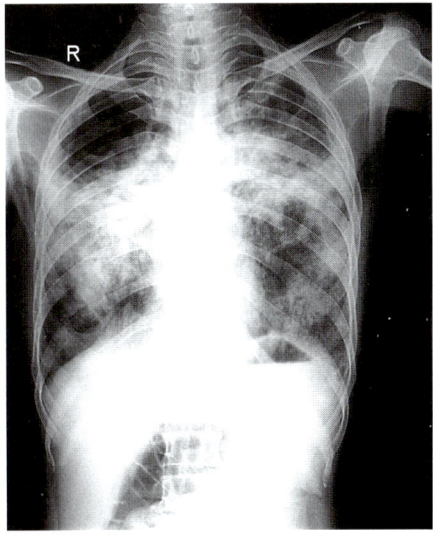

Fig. 1.19: Posteroanterior (PA) radiograph of chest shows right upper lobe cavitation in a patient of Koch's chest.

  - Granulomatous infection (Fig. 1.19)
  - Parasites.

Neoplasm

Vascular

- Wegener granulomatosis
- Rheumatoid arthritis
- *Thromboembolic or septic infarct*:
  - Cystic fibrosis
  - Tuberculosis
  - ABPA
  - Recurrent bacterial pneumonia.

Cysts

- Cystic bronchiectasis
- Pneumatocele
- *Congenital lesions—multiple bronchogenic cysts*:
  - Intralobar sequestration
  - CCAM type I
  - Diaphragmatic hernia.
- Centrilobular emphysema
- Honeycomb lung disease.

Differential Features are Same as Localized Lucent Defects (Table 1.16)

Cyst	Cavity
Thin-walled	Thick-walled > 1 cm
Clear, smooth	Irregular, ragged wall
Well-defined wall	Adjacent lung parenchyma
	May show reactive changes
±	
±	Air-fluid level ±

SOLITARY PULMONARY NODULE

- *Malignant*:
  - Primary
  - Secondary
  - Lymphoma
  - Plasmacytoma
  - Alveolar cell carcinoma
- *Benign*:
  - Hamartoma
  - Adenoma
  - Connective tissue tumor
- *Granuloma*:
  - Tuberculosis
  - Histoplasmosis
  - Sarcoidosis
- *Infection*:
  - Round pneumonia
  - Abscess
  - Hydatid
  - Amebic
  - Fungal
- *Pulmonary infarct*:
  - Pulmonary hematoma
- *Collagen disease*
  - Rheumatoid arthritis
  - Wegener's granulomatosis
- *Congenital*:
  - Bronchogenic cyst
  - Sequestration segment
  - Congenital bronchial atresia
  - AVM
  - Impacted mucus
- *Amyloidosis*:
  - Intraparenchymal lymph node

Table 1.16: Localized lucent defect.

Infection	Location	Air-fluid level	Cong/acq.	Uni/multicystic	Specific points
Bacterial	Any zone	+	Acquired	Multicystic with areas of breakdown	
Granulomatous	Apical	+	-do-	+ve	Fibrosis and cavitating
Fungal	Less likely to be apical	Fungal ball	-do-	Cystic	
Sarcoidosis	Upper zone	-	-do-	-	B/L hilar and R paratracheal LNs
Cystic bronchiectasis	Lower lobes	Air-fluid level	Cong./acquired	+	
Pneumatocele	In area of infection	±	Acquired	+	Staph. infection Sequelae
	Previous pneumonia/post-traumatic hematoma				
Intralobar sequestration	Lower lobes	±	Cong.	+	Vascular drainage is altered
Honeycombing lung congenital cystic adenomatoid malformation	Any zone	-	Acq./ Cong. end state disease	+	
		±		Multicystic	Cartilage development is defective

- *Pleural*:
  - Fibroma
  - Tumor
  - Loculated fluid
- *Nonpulmonary*:
  - Skin and chest wall lesions
  - Artifacts.

SOLITARY PULMONARY NODULE (TABLE 1.17)

Definition (Fig. 1.20)

Single, round intraparenchymal opacity, at least moderately well-marginated and not greater than 3 cm in maximum diameter.

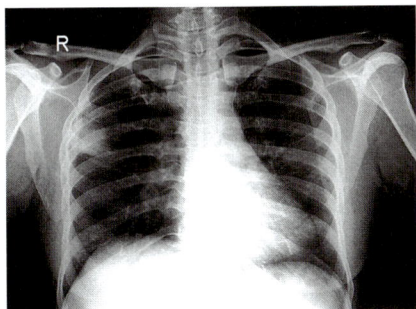

Fig. 1.20: Posteroanterior (PA) radiograph of chest shows solitary pulmonary nodule in right upper lobe peripherally.

Neoplasm

- Benign—hamartoma, inflammatory pseudo-tumor (Table 1.17)
- Malignant—bronchogenic carcinoma, carcinoid tumor, and metastasis (Figs. 1.21 and 1.22).

Infection

- Granuloma—tuberculoma
- Fungal—histoplasmoma
- Abscess
- Round pneumonia
- Parasites—*Echinococcus*.

Inflammatory

- *Connective tissue—Wegener's granulomatosis*:
  - Rheumatoid nodule
  - Sarcoidosis (rare).

Vascular

- Arteriovenous malformation
- Hematoma
- Pulmonary infarct
- Pulmonary artery aneurysm.

Airway

- Congenital lesion—bronchogenic cyst
- Mucocele

Table 1.17: Clinical and radiographic criteria for differentiating benign and malignant solitary pulmonary nodule (SPN).

Clinical	Benign	Malignant
Age	<40 years except hamartomas	>45 years
Sex	Female	Male
History	• High incidence of granuloma in area • Exposure to tuberculosis	Primary lesion elsewhere
Radiographic		
Size	Small (<2 cm)	Large (>2 cm)
Location	No predilection except for tuberculosis	Predominantly on upper lobes except for lung metastases
Definition and contour	Well-defined and smooth	Ill-defined, lobulated umbilicated
Calcification	More common	Less common
Doubling time	<30 to >450 days	30–450 days
Presence of fat	(+) symptoms of hamartoma	

Differential Diagnosis in Radiology

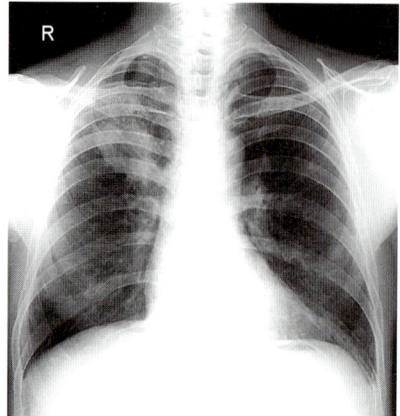

Fig. 1.21: Posteroanterior (PA) radiograph of chest shows bronchogenic carcinoma in right upper lobe with pulmonary metastases in left lower lobe.

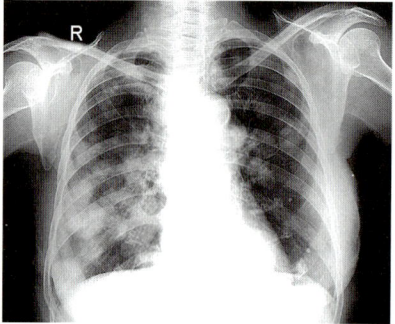

Fig. 1.22: Posteroanterior (PA) radiograph of chest shows multifocal pulmonary metastases from breast carcinoma.

- Infected bulla
- Pseudonodules
- ECG pads
- Cutaneous lesions
- Mole
- Nipple shadow
- Hemangiomas
- Neurofibromas
- Lipomas.

Characteristics of Solitary Pulmonary Nodule

- *Size*:
  - No size criteria that clearly distinguishes benign from malignant solitary pulmonary nodule (SPN)
  - 80% of benign SPN less than 2 cm in diameter
  - 15% of malignant SPN less than 1 cm in diameter
  - 42% of malignant SPN less than 2 cm in diameter.
- *Growth*:
  - Benign lesions—<30 days or <450 days (doubling time) SPN with doubling time between 30 days and 450 days require further evaluation
  - Doubling time for spherical lesions is defined as 25% increase in diameter.
- *Calcification*:
  - Approximately one-third of noncalcified SPNs have calcification on CT
  - Complete/central/laminated: Granulomas
  - Popcorn: Hamartoma
  - Amorphous/eccentric calcifications: Malignancy.
- *Fat*:
  - Fat within a smooth/lobulated SPN is suspected benignity of hamartoma—50% show presence of fat.
- *Cavitation*:
  - Cavities with greatest wall thickness less than 5 mm are benign
  - More than 15 mm are malignant.
- *Air bronchogram/bubbly lucencies*:
  - Presence of air bronchogram within SPN is suggestive of adenocarcinoma, particularly bronchoalveolar cell carcinoma
  - *Other causes*: Lymphoma, organizing pneumonia, pulmonary infarcts, and mass-like sarcoidosis.
- *Margins*:
  - Smooth, well-defined margins, symptoms of benign nodule although 21% of malignant nodules smooth margin
  - Lobulated/ill-defined/spiculated symptoms of malignant nodule, 25% of benign nodules may have undefined margins

- Presence of a small satellite nodule surrounding the periphery of a smooth SPN is symptom of granulomatosis infection.

Computed Tomography Nodule Enhancement

- Enhancement less than 15 HU symptom of benign nodule
- *False +ve*: Central necrosis, mucin-producing malignant neoplasm
- Enhancement more than 15 HU—nonspecific.

Pulmonary Hamartomas

- These consist of masses of cartilage with clefts lined by bronchial epithelium which may contain large calcification (popcorn) of fat; age group: 45–50 years.
- *Triad*: Pulmonary chondromas.
- *Carney's triad*: Gastric epithelioid leiomyosarcomas.
- Functioning extra-adrenal paragangliomas.
- 90% peripheral and 10% within a major bronchus.
- Spherical lobulated SPN with popcorn calcification, size less than 4 cm, fat density positive.

Inflammatory Pseudotumor (Plasma Cell Granuloma)

- Caused histology by mixture of fibroblasts, histiocytes, lymphocytes, and plasma cells.
- Age range is wide and includes children.
- SPN (2–5 cm) or as an area of consolidation, calcification is occasionally present. Endobronchial tumor can cause obstructive pneumonitis.

Bronchial Carcinoid

Bronchial carcinoids can invade locally, may metastasize to hilar and mediastinal lymph nodes as well as to brain, liver, and bone.
- *Age*: Age range is wide; peak—5 decades.
- *Clinical features*: Wheeze, Cushing's syndrome [ectopic adrenocorticotropic hormone (ACTH) secretion], carcinoid syndrome.
- Hilar/parahilar mass.
- 80–90%, central (endobronchial).
- 10–20%, peripheral with features of bronchial obstruction, pneumonia, calcification ±.
- Spherical/lobular SPN (2–4 cm) smooth well-defined margin calcification ±.

Bronchial Carcinoma (Fig. 1.23)

- Squamous cell carcinoma (30–50%)
- Adenocarcinoma (30–50%)
- Undefined small cell carcinoma (20–30%)
- Large cell carcinoma (10–15%)
- *Peak incidence*: 50–60 years
- *Radiological features*: Size more than 2 cm
  - Undefined margins
  - Umbilicated/notched margin
  - Corona radiata/speculations (+)
  - Pleural tail sign (+)
  - Doubling time between 30 days and 450 days
  - Lesion crosses fissure
  - *Cavitation*: (>15 mm thick wall)
  - Calcification rare if present—eccentric
- Associated findings—hilar/mediastinal lymph nodes, bone mets, pleural effusion, visceral mets (+)

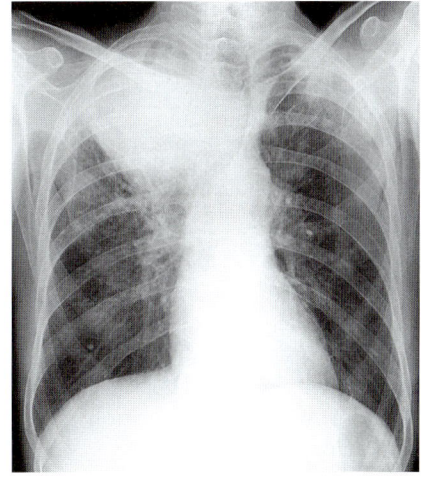

Fig. 1.23: Posteroanterior (PA) radiograph of chest shows bronchogenic carcinoma in right upper lobe.

- *Bronchoalveolar carcinoma*: Air bronchogram/bobby lucencies
  - Grows slowly
  - Cavitation is unusual.

Metastasis

Pulmonary metastasis is usually from breast, GI tract, kidney, testes, head, and neck tumors or from a bone and soft tissue sarcomas.
- *Site*: Usually in the outer portions of lung.
- Radiological features (R/f)—solitary/multiple.
- Spherical well-defined, occasionally irregular edge.
- Calcification—unusual except metastases from osteosarcoma, chondrosarcoma.
- *Rate of growth*: Variable—explosive in choriocarcinoma and osteosarcoma.
- Cavitation—unusual (squamous cell carcinoma +).

Tuberculoma

- Occurs in the setting of primary or postprimary tuberculosis and is considered to represent localized parenchymal diseases that alternatively activate and heal.
  - Nodule is 10–15 mm in diameter
  - Situated most commonly in the right upper zone
  - Single or multiple (confined to a single segment)
  - Margins well-defined
  - Satellite lesions (+)
  - Calcification frequent
  - Cavitation ±.

Hydatid Cyst

Caused by tapeworm (*Echinococcus granulosus* or *E. alveolaris*)
- Humans are accidental host
- Infection occurs by ingestion of ova by fomites/contaminated water.

Radiological features unruptured cyst: Homogeneous spherical/oval, well-defined lesion. Size 1–10 cm occurs particularly in middle zone/lower zone.

Ruptured cyst: Usually associated with secondary infection
- Meniscus sign—pericyst—ruptures ectocyst and endocyst intact appearance is that of an intracavitary body.
- *Disruption of inner layers*:
  - Air-fluid level
  - Floating membranes (water lily, camalote sign)
  - Double wall appearance
  - Dry cyst with crumpled membranes lying at its bottom (rising sun, serpent sign)
  - Cyst with all its contents expectorated (empty cyst sign).

Histoplasmoma

Caused by *Histoplasma capsulatum*, which is a fungus found in moist soil and in bird or bat excreta.

Histoplasma represents a small necrotic focus of infection surrounded by a massive fibrous capsule consisting of concentric lamination, some or all of which may calcify.
- Sharply-defined nodular shadow
- Less than 3 cm in diameter
- Most common site is in the lower lobe
- Satellite lesions (+)
- Calcification (+) central/eccentric
- Target lesion is pathognomonic—homogeneous density with central punctate deposit of calcium
- Associated findings—calcified hilar/mediastinal lymph nodes.

Pneumonia

Round pneumonias are usually pneumococcal which are usually seen in children, air bronchogram.

Lung Abscess

Cavitation secondary to necrosis is seen in:

Bacterial Pneumonias—S. aureus
- Gram-negative bacteria—*Klebsiella pneumoniae, Proteus, Pseudomonas*

- Anaerobes
- Amebic and fungal infections.

Cavitary Lesion with Adjacent Consolidation

- Size—2–12 cm
- Wall thickness less than 15 mm
- Inner aspect of cavity is smooth.

Wegener's Granulomatosis

- Necrotizing granulomatous vasculitis
- Lungs involved in 95% cases and late renal involvement is seen in 85% cases
- Men more than women
- Single/multiple nodules
- Size = 1 cm to several centimeter
- Well-defined margins
- Wax and wane
- Frequently cavitate
- Associated findings—granulomas in upper respiratory tract and glomerulonephritis.

Rheumatoid Nodules

Pleuropulmonary is seen in 5–54% cases of rheumatoid arthritis.
- Pulmonary, necrobiotic nodules are uncommon features of rheumatoid arthritis
- Associated with subcutaneous nodules
- Single/multiple
- Variable in size
- Wax and wane in size
- Cavitation (+)/(–) more common in lower lobe and in periphery
- Similar nodule may be seen in patients of rheumatoid arthritis who have been exposed to silica. It is known as Caplan's syndrome.

Pulmonary A-V Fistula

- Congenital—50% have hereditary hemorrhagic telangiectasia (Osler-Weber-Rendu disease)
- Acquired—liver diseases (cirrhosis), schistosomiasis, and metastatic thyroid cancer
- Round/lobulated nodule
- Prominent adjacent vascular shadow
- Most common site—lower lobe
- Variation in size with Valsalva (size)
- CT and pulmonary angiography show the feeding artery and vein and vascular nature of nodule.

Pulmonary Artery Aneurysm

Most pulmonary artery aneurysms are acquired as a result of septic embolization or an extension from a pulmonary parenchymal calcification.
- Peripheral aneurysms may mimic SPN pulsations of mass seen on fluoroscopy.
- Confirmation done by CT or pulmonary angiography.

Pulmonary Hematoma

History of (H/o) trauma (+); usually appears following resolution of contusion:
- Peripheral in location
- Smooth and well-defined
- Slow resolution over several weeks
- A pocket of air or fluid level (+).

Pulmonary Infarct

- Becomes visible 12–24 hours after embolic episode
- Lesions are more frequent in the lower lobe
- Hump-shaped opacity with its base applied to the pleural surface because of partial collapse, hemorrhagic congestion
- Cavitation is rare
- Matched defect is seen on ventricular perfusion scan
- Associated pleural effusion (+).

Bronchogenic Cyst

- Peak incidence is in 2nd and 3rd decades
- Two-thirds are intrapulmonary and occur in the medial one-third of the lower pulmonary region
- Round to oval
- Smooth-walled and well-defined
- CT shows thin-walled water density cyst.

PULMONARY EDEMA ON THE OPPOSITE SIDE TO A PRE-EXISTING ABNORMALITY (TABLE 1.18)

- Congenital absence or hypoplasia of a pulmonary artery
- McLeod's syndrome
- Thromboembolism
- Unilateral emphysema
- Lobectomy
- Pleural disease.

Localized Air Space Disease

- Pneumonia
- Infarction
- Contusion
- Edema
- Radiation
- Alveolar cell carcinoma.
- Differential features are discussed in alveolar shadowing.

Unilateral Pulmonary Edema

- Pulmonary edema on the same side as a pre-existing abnormality
- Prolonged lateral decubitus
- Unilateral aspiration
- Pulmonary contusion
- Rapid thoracocentesis of air or fluid
- Bronchial obstruction
- Clinical history is most important in the differential diagnosis of all the above entities.
  Bronchial obstruction:
- Respiratory distress ±
- *Examination of (E/o) occlusion*: It is seen in the form of luminal obstruction, atelectasis, and fissural displacement.

Alveolar Shadowing

Acute

Pulmonary edema
Cardiac
- *Noncardiac*:
  – Hypoproteinemia
  – Fluid overload
  – Drowning
  – Aspiration
  – Inhalation
  – Acute respiratory distress syndrome (ARDS), uremia
  – Infection
- At birth
- Aspiration
- Hyaline membrane disease (Fig. 1.24)
- Alveolar
- Blood pulmonary hemorrhage
- In hematoma
- Goodpasture's syndrome
- Pulmonary infarction.

Chronic

- Tumors
- Alveolar cell carcinoma
- Lymphoma
- Alveolar proteinosis
  – Microlithiasis
- Radiation pneumonitis
- Sarcoidosis
- Eosinophilic lung.

Characteristics

- 4–10 mm diameter
- Ill-defined margins
- Coalescence
- Nonsegmental.

Air Bronchogram

Common

- Consolidation pneumonic
- Pulmonary edema
- Hyaline membrane disease.

Rare

- Lymphoma
- Sarcoidosis
- Alveolar proteinosis
- Alveolar cell carcinoma
- Adult respiratory distress syndrome.

Chest

Table 1.18: Causes of pulmonary edema.

	Congenital absence or hypoplasia of a pulmonary artery	McLeod's syndrome	Thromboembolism	Unilateral emphysema	Lobectomy	Pleural disease
Lack of soft tissue outline	+	+	–	–	–	–
Prominent hilum	–	–	+	–	–	–
Subpleural consolidation	–	–	+	–	–	–
Elevated diaphragm	–	–	+	–	–	+
Pleural reaction	–	–	+	–	–	+
Cavitation	–	–	+	–	–	–
Mediastinal shift	–	–	–	+	+	–
Linear outline of pleura	–	–	–	+	–	+

	Location	Duration	Effusion	LNs	Air bronchogram			
Infection	Any	Rapid resolution	±	±		Reticulo-nodular pattern	Peripheral, center	
Hyaline membrane disease	Whole lung	-do-	±	–	+	–	Any	Usually presents with unusual features
Aspiration	Right UL in erect right LL in supine	-do-	–	–	±	During resolution	Any	White out lung
Hemorrhage/contusion	Any	–	–	–	–	–	–	Clinical h/o
Alveolar cell carcinoma	Any	Nonresolving pneumonia	++	–	+	–	–	Clinical h/o
Lymphoma	-do-	+	++	–	–	Any	Any	
Embolism/infarct	Any	1–2 days post-trauma resolves in 1–4 weeks	–	–	–	–	Any	
Sarcoidosis	UL		–	+	–	–	Peripheral	
Loffler's syndrome	UZ	Rapid	–	–	–	–	Central	
Metastasis	Any	No	+/–	+/–	–	–	Peripheral	
Consolidation	Follow the exposure history	Slow	+/–	–	+ in acute in chronic	–	P/C	Usually from chronic CA

Differential Diagnosis in Radiology

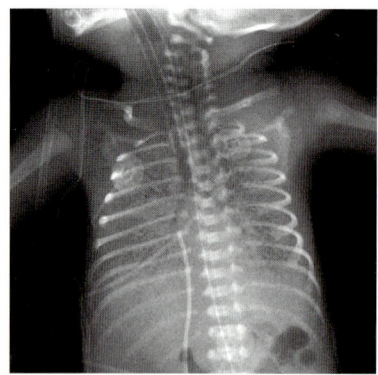

Fig. 1.24: Anteroposterior radiograph of chest in neonate shows hyaline membrane disease.

Mesothelioma

- Asymmetrical, irregular
- Thickening
- Calcification ±
- U/L.

Pneumonectomy

- Rib resection ±
- Thoracoplasty asymmetrical bony contour
- H/o present.

Pulmonary Agenesis

- Congenital anomaly
- Respiratory distress +
- Status of diaphragm.

Location and Zones of Different Lung Lesions (Table 1.19)

- Normally – Scaphoid abdomen
- Absent bowel loops with air ±
- Opaque thorax A few lucencies +.

Consolidation

- Air bronchogram
- Confined to one segment
- Air alveologram.

Collapse

- Vessels not seen
- Crowding of fissure and ribs
- Hilar and diaphragmatic displacement.

Fibrosis

Examination of (E/o) volume loss +.

Cardiomegaly

Cardiac contour conforming of uni/multi-chamber enlargement.

MILIARY SHADOWING

Differential Diagnosis of Miliary Shadowing

Disseminated pulmonary opacities
- Acinar
- Interstitial

Table 1.19: Location and zones of different lung lesions.

	1	2	3	4	5	6	7	8
Location	Any zone	Perihilar	Any zone	Any zone	UL	Any	Any	Any
Pleural effusion	±	+	±	±	–	–	±	+
Hilar enlargement	±	–	–	+	+	–	±	–
Silhouette with cardiac	±	+	+	±	–	–	±	–
Diaphragm	±	–	+	+/–	–	–	±	+
LNs	±	–	–	+	+	–	±	–
Crazy pavement pattern	–	–	–	–	–	+	–	–
White out lung	–	–	+	–	–	–	–	+
Vascular markings visualized	–	+	–	–	+	–	–	–
Resolution	+	+	+	–	+	+	–	+

Acinar—poorly-defined, round, parenchymal opacities
- 4–8 mm in diameter
- Represent an anatomical acinus filled with fluid.

Interstitial (Fig. 1.25)

Pulmonary interstitium is a network of connective tissue fibers that supports the lung. It includes alveolar walls, interlobular septa and peribronchovascular interstitium.

Interstitial nodules may take various patterns:
- Linear and septal lines
- Miliary shadows
- Reticulonodular shadows
- Honeycomb shadows
- Peribronchial cuffing and ground-glass pattern

Alveolar	Interstitial
Fluffy, ill-defined	Sharply-defined
4–8 mm	2–4 mm
Coalescent	Discrete
Segmental/lobar	Widespread
Air bronchogram	Usually 1 week
Time from onset of nodules is less	Usually more than one week
Higher density	Lower density

Miliary Shadowing

It is the presence of small, discrete, rounded pulmonary nodules of almost similar size measuring 2–4 mm in the interstitium.

Causes

- *Infectious diseases:*
    - Tuberculosis
    - Fungal infections—histoplasmosis, coccidioidomycosis, blastomycosis
    - Chickenpox.
- *Inhalational diseases:*
    - Silicosis
    - Barytosis
    - Stannosis
    - Coal miner's pneumoconiosis
    - Berylliosis
- *Granulomatous diseases:*
    - Sarcoidosis
    - Histiocytosis-X
- Metastases
- Secondary hyperparathyroidism
- Oil embolism
- Alveolar microlithiasis
- Hemosiderosis
- Bronchiolitis obliterans.

Miliary Tuberculosis (Fig. 1.26)

- Due to hematogenous spread of infection
- May be seen in both primary and post-primary disease

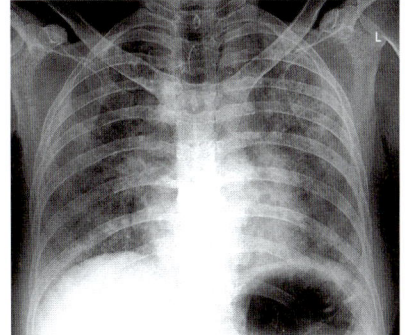

Fig. 1.25: Posteroanterior radiograph of chest shows bilateral interstitial pulmonary disease.

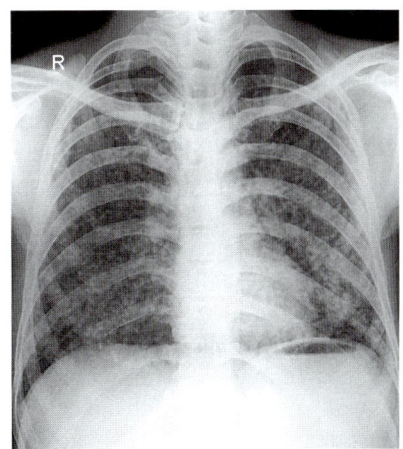

Fig. 1.26: Posteroanterior radiograph of chest shows miliary tuberculosis.

- Small discrete nodules 1–2 mm in diameter, evenly distributed throughout both lungs
- These are of soft tissue density and are well-defined
- Other tubercular manifestations as consolidation, pleural effusion, and lymphadenopathy may be present.

Histoplasmosis
- Due to infection with *Histoplasma capsulatum*
- Infection is usually subclinical and heals spontaneously leaving small calcified nodules or calcified mediastinal nodes
- Infection in immunocompromised patient may produce multiple nodules scattered throughout the lung, resulting in miliary shadowing
- Hilar nodes enlargement is common
- Consolidation, fibrosis and cavitation may occur.

Silicosis
- Multiple nodular shadows 2–5 mm in diameter
- Affects mainly mid and upper zones, relatively sparing the bases
- Hilar adenopathy which may calcify, fibrosis, cavitation may occur.

Coal Miner's Pneumoconiosis
- Small, faint nodules 1–5 mm in diameter appear in mid-zone spreading to whole lung
- Progressive massive fibrosis—mid and upper zones—in complicated cases
- Emphysematous bullae may appear.

Sarcoidosis
- Multisystem granulomatous disorder affecting young adults
- 75–90% patients show small, rounded or irregular nodules 2–4 mm in diameter, bilaterally symmetrical with upper and mid-zone preponderance
- Bilateral symmetrical lymphadenopathy, hilar and paratracheal
- Air trapping, pleural thickening and effusion may be positive.

Histiocytosis X
- Granulomatous disorder affecting young or middle-aged adults
- Pulmonary involvement is bilaterally symmetrical
- Chest X-ray shows diffuse nodular pattern in upper and mid-zones, 1–5 mm in size. Progress of disease leads to ring shadows, honeycombing and linear shadows.

Miliary Metastasis
- Rare cause of miliary shadowing
- Primary tumors most likely to provide miliary nodulation are thyroid, renal carcinoma, bone sarcomas and choriocarcinomas.

Hemosiderosis
In patients with heart disease which elevates left atrial pressure, e.g. in mitral stenosis, there is permanent miliary stippling due to focal nature of bleeding.

Alveolar Microlithiasis
- Multiple fine sand-like calculi in the alveoli
- Produce widespread dense opacities on chest X-ray
- Clinically there is relative lack of symptoms.

MILIARY SHADOWING (0.5–2 mm)
Soft Tissue Densities
- Miliary tuberculosis
- Fungal disease
- Pneumoconiosis
- Sarcoidosis
- Extrinsic allergic alveolitis
- Fibrosing alveolitis.

Greater than Soft Tissue Density
- Hemosiderosis
- Silicosis
- Siderosis

- Stannosis
- Barylosis.

Pneumoconiosis

These are diseases caused by inhalation of inorganic dusts. The diagnosis depends on a history of exposure to the dust and an abnormal chest radiograph and respiratory function tests.

Silicosis

- Gold-mining, sand-blasting, foundry, ceramic and pottery workers
- Multiple, nodular shadows 2–5 mm in diameter mid and upper zones
- Linear lines and septal lines may also be seen.

Coal Workers

- Pneumoconiosis
- Small, faint, indistinct nodules 1–5 mm in diameter appear in the mid-zones
- Coalescence of these nodules is common
- Develop bilaterally
- Fibrotic masses may calcify.

Asbestosis (Fig. 1.27)

Asbestosis mining and processing. In construction and demolition workers, ship-building.
- Lower zones nodules
- Pleural plaque, calcification, diffuse thickening and effusion— mid-zone, bilaterally

- Pulmonary fibrosis is marked
- Initially reticulonodular pattern results— which with progression becomes coarser and there is loss of clarity of the diaphragm and heart.

Berylliosis

In the acute stage, produces noncardiogenic pulmonary edema, while in the chronic stage, produces widespread noncavitating granulomas.

MULTIPLE OPACITIES [TABLES 1.20 (2–5 mm) AND 1.21 (Pinpoint)]

- Postlymphogram
- Silicosis
- Stannosis
- Baryltosis
- Alveolar microlithiasis.

Septal Lines

- Pulmonary edema
- Mitral valve disease
- Pneumoconiosis
- Lymphangitis carcinomatosa
- Sarcoidosis
- Infection
- Lymphoma.

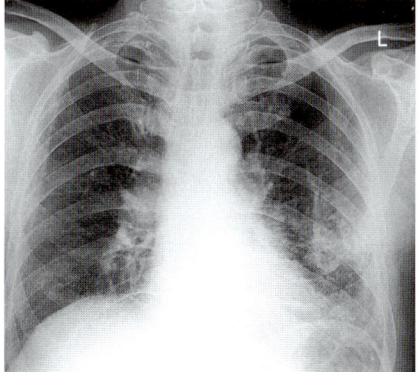

Fig. 1.27: Posteroanterior radiograph of chest shows calcified pleural plaque in left hemithorax.

Table 1.20: Multiple opacities (2–5 mm).

Remaining discrete	LN	Location	Size
Carcinomatosis	+/–	Any	Variable
Lymphoma	+	Any	Same
Sarcoidosis	+	Mid-zone	Variable
Tending to confluence and varying rapidly			
Multifocal pneumonia	+/–	Any	Variable
Pulmonary edema	–	Perihilar	Variable
Extrinsic allergic	–	Basal	Same
Alveolitis			
Fat emboli	–	Peripheral	Same

Table 1.21: Spectrum multiple pinpoint opacities.

	1	2	3	4	5
At the termination of the thoracic duct	+	–	–	–	–
In gold miners	–	+	–	–	–
Inhalation of tin oxide	–	–	+	–	–
Distribution	Near thoracic duct	–	–	Bases and apices spared	–
Kerley lines	–	–	+	–	–
Inhalation of barytes	–	–	–	+	–
Miliary	+	+	+	–	+
Negative shadows	–	–	–	–	+

COMPLETE OPAQUE HEMITHORAX

Causes (Figs. 1.28 and 1.29)

Technical	Rotation, scoliosis
Pleural	Hydrothorax, lung effusion thickening, mesothelioma
Surgical	Pneumonectomy, thoracoplasty
Congenital	Pulmonary agenesis
Mediastinal	Gross cardiomegaly, tumors
Pulmonary	Collapse, consolidation, fibrosis

Diaphragmatic Hernia

Scoliosis
- Lucency on   Vertebral
- Concave side   Anomaly
- Rotated side   Clavicular asymmetry

Effusion
- Blunted cardiophrenic angle
- Fluid along the lateral chest wall

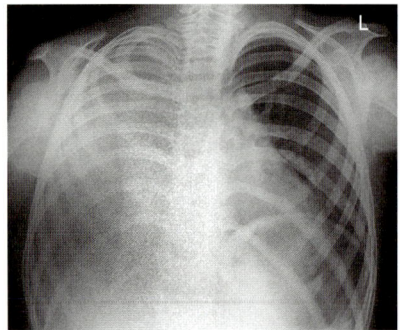

Fig. 1.28: Posteroanterior radiograph of chest shows opaque right hemithorax with fairly preserved hemithoracic volume.

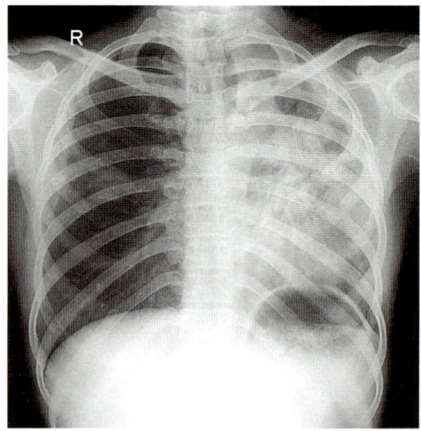

Fig. 1.29: Posteroanterior radiograph of chest shows opacities in left hemithorax with loss of volume with subsegmental pneumonitis in right middle zone in a case of Koch's chest.

- Silhouette with cardiac and diaphragm
- Changes with change of posture
- Thickening
  – Does not follow
  – Ellis curve.

OPAQUE HEMITHORAX (TABLE 1.22)

Causes

- Technical   Rotation, scoliosis
- Pleural   Pleural effusion
  – Pleural thickening
  – Mesothelioma
- Surgical   Pneumonectomy
  – Thoracoplasty

- Congenital
- Mediastinal
- Pulmonary

Pulmonary agenesis
Gross cardiomegaly, tumors
Collapse, consolidation, fibrosis

- Diaphragmatic hernia

Rotation
- In well-centered film, medial ends of clavicle are equidistant from spinous process of T4/5 level
- Lung nearest to the film, less translucent.

Pleural Effusion
- A massive effusion may cause complete radiopacity of a hemithorax
- Mediastinal shift to contralateral side
- Inversion of diaphragm
- If effusion without mediastinal shift, collapse of underlying lung.

Exclude Carcinoma Bronchus
- Ultrasound reveals fluid in pleural cavity. In AP-CXR—with patient supine a small effusion gravitates posteriorly—generalized increased density with apical cap
- Erect or decubitus film confirms the diagnosis
- Pulmonary agenesis/aplasia/hypoplasia.

Agenesis
- Complete absence of the lobe as well as its bronchus
- Absent vascular supply.

Aplasia
- No lung tissue
- Rudimentary bronchus.

Hypoplasia
- Bronchi and alveoli are present, but the lobe is underdeveloped
- More common on right side
- Mediastinal shifts present. Absence of a lobe is more common than absence of whole lung
- Loss of silhouette on the right side of the heart and ascending aorta due to deposition of extrapleural alveolar tissue
- If whole lung absent—completely opaque hemithorax with mediastinal shift and diaphragmatic shift
- Unlike acquired pneumonectomy, gross loss of lung volume, external diameter is not considerably less than normal side in congenital absence
- Bronchography—diagnostic
- Scintigraphy—absent ventilation and perfusion on the affected site
- Angiography —absent/hypoplastic pulmonary artery.

Table 1.22: Signs to help in interpreting a white out (opaque) hemithorax.

White out (opaque)		
CXR findings		Most likely cause
A	• Mediastinum displaced to the opposite side • Trachea central or deviated to the opposite side	Large pleural effusion with minimal secondary compression collapse of the underlying lung
B*	• Mediastinum central • No tracheal deviation	Large effusion with major collapse of the underlying lung
C	• Mediastinum displaced to the ipsilateral side • Trachea deviated to the same side	Collapse of the entire lung. Minimal or no pleural fluid
D	Features as for C above, and: • Ribs missing/distorted	Pneumonectomy. The clinical history is conclusive

*Exceptionally… these findings may be due to an extensive pneumonia affecting all the lobes of a lung, or to extensive tumor infiltration of the entire lung.

Diaphragmatic Hernia

- L > R more common in the left side
- If large hernia in early neonatal period may lead to opaque hemithorax
- Bochdalek hernia—posterolaterally due to persistent pleuroperitoneal canal
- It may contain fat, omentum, spleen, kidney and bowel—associated with pulmonary hypoplasia and contralateral mediastinal shift
- In older age group—hemithorax not opaque due to gas in bowel loops.

Consolidation

- Parenchymal opacification caused by replacement of air in the distal air spaces by fluid (transudate, exudate or blood) or tissue (e.g. bronchoalveolar cell carcinoma, lymphoma) is defined as consolidation
- Usually no volume loss
- Expansile consolidation pneumococcal and *Klebsiella pneumoniae*
  - Neoplasms
  - Air bronchogram.
- In older age group—hemithorax not opaque due to gas in bowel loops.

Pleural Thickening

If extensive—may lead to opaque hemithorax
- Previous thoracotomy
- Empyema
- Hemithorax
- Viewed en profile–appears as a band of soft tissue density
- En face—ill-defined veil-like shadowing
- USG—not so sensitive pleural thickening, not reliably detected unless 1 cm in thickness
- CT—very sensitive
- May calcify, involve visceral pleura
- If entire lung is surrounded by fibrotic pleura—fibrothorax
- *Fibrothorax is defined by criteria*
- If uninterrupted pleural density that extends over at least a fourth of the chest wall
- On CT—8 cm craniocaudal
  - 5 cm laterally
  - 3 mm thick
- No mediastinal shift
- Reduced ventilation due to decrease in volume
- If on X-ray—decreased vascularity, significant ventilatory restriction is present
- Surgical decortication is required.

Mesothelioma

More common primary pleural malignancy:
- Prolonged exposure to asbestos dust—crocidolite (MC)
- Nodular pleural thickening ± hemorrhagic pleural effusion around all or part of lung
- With central mediastinum
- Volume loss due to ventilatory restriction
- Bronchial stenosis by tumor compression at hilum
- Malignant pleural thickening is nodule and extends into fissures or over the mediastinal surface, may surround whole lung
- MRI better than CT in assessing involvement of mediastinum and chest wall. Signal intensity slightly more than muscles on both T1 and T2 WI.

Postpneumonectomy

- 2–3 months after surgery
- H/o of pneumonectomy
- ± Rib resection
- ± Opaque bronchial sutures.

HYPERTRANSRADIANT LUNG FIELD

Bilateral

- *Faulty radiologic technique*
  - Overpenetrated films
- *Decreased soft tissues*
  - Thin body habitus
  - Bilateral mastectomy
- *Cardiac causes of decreased pulmonary blood flow*
  - Right to left shunts (Tetralogy of Fallot, Ebstein's malformation, tricuspid atresia)
  - Eisenmenger physiology

- *Pulmonary causes of decreased pulmonary blood flow*
  - Pulmonary embolism
  - Air trapping
  - Emphysema
  - Bulla
  - Bleb
  - Interstitial emphysema.

Unilateral

- *Faulty radiologic technique*
  - Rotation of patient
    - Incorrect centering
    - Unequal compression of the chest wall soft tissue
- *Chest wall defects*
  - Mastectomy
  - Poland syndrome (congenital absent or underdeveloped pectoralis major)
- *Air trapping*
  - Extrinsic compression of main bronchus: compensatory emphysema of opposite side
  - Endobronchial obstruction: foreign body
  - Bronchiolitis obliterans
  - McLeod syndrome
  - Asymmetric emphysema
  - Pneumothorax
- *Vascular causes*
  - Pulmonary arterial hypoplasia
  - Pulmonary embolism
  - Congenital lobar emphysema (Fig. 1.30)
  - Compensatory over-aeration.
- *Skeletal abnormality:*
  - Scoliosis.

Tetralogy of Fallot

Congenital disease presenting as left to right shunt with four components VSD, infundibular narrowing of the right ventricular outflow tract, right ventricular hypertrophy, overriding aorta.

Plain Skiagram Chest

- Boot-shaped heart
- Hypoplasia of pulmonary artery
- Pulmonary oligemia leading to translucent lungs
- Right-sided aortic arch.

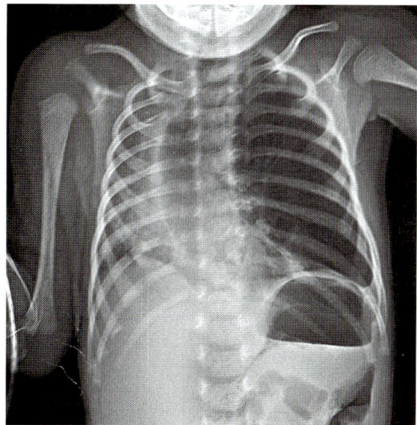

Fig. 1.30: Anteroposterior radiograph of chest shows congenital emphysema of left lung with herniation to right side midline.

ECHO

- Discontinuity between anterior aortic wall and IV septum due to overriding aorta
- Small left atrium
- RV hypertrophy with small outflow tract
- Doppler USG can quantify severity of VSD and pulmonary stenosis.

Ebstein's Anomaly

- Congenital disease with left to right shunt with atrialization of right ventricle due to downward displacement of the dysplastic incompetent tricuspid valve leading to a small right ventricle. There is associated ASD or PDA
- Patient presents early reversal of the shunt from right to left, leading to cyanosis.

Plain Skiagram Chest

- Massive globular "funnel-like" cardiomegaly with small pedicle due to hypoplastic aorta and pulmonary trunk (the only CHD with this feature)
- Extreme RA enlargement
- Dilated IVC and azygous vein
- Severe pulmonary oligemia leading to translucent lung fields
- Calcification of tricuspid valve may occur.

ECHO

- Large sail-like tricuspid valve
- RA enlargement
- Doppler USG can quantify tricuspid regurgitation.

Tricuspid Atresia

Congenital disease with atresia of the tricuspid valve and pronounced cyanosis at birth and is associated with ASD and a small VSD. Pulmonary stenosis may or may not be present. It may present with or without transposition of great vessels.

Plain Skiagram Chest

- Left ventricular contour of the heart with rounding due to both enlargement and hypertrophy of left ventricle
- RA enlargement
- Concave pulmonary bay
- Pulmonary oligemia leading to translucent lung fields.

Eisenmenger Physiology

Occurs when there is reversal of left to right shunt as a consequence of pulmonary arterial hypertension

Plain Skiagram Chest

- Pronounced dilatation of central pulmonary arteries
- Pruning of peripheral pulmonary arteries leading to increased translucency
- Enlargement of RV
- Return of LA and LV to normal size
- Normal pulmonary venous pressure.

Pulmonary Embolism

- The embolism is usually a result of DVT in the lower limbs
- There is a classic triad seen in 33% of cases of hemoptysis, pleural rub and thrombophlebitis
- Hypertranslucency is seen bilaterally in cases presenting with acute massive embolic episode, which blocks the main pulmonary artery before the development of infarction. The development of infarction leads to segmental, lobar or wedge-shaped areas of consolidation. Pleural effusion is usually present
- Unilateral hypertranslucency may occur in cases where the embolus blocks one of the major pulmonary arteries.

Air Trapping

- There is trapping of air in the lungs due to valve mechanism acting at the level of the trachea or major bronchi
- In children, this is usually due to a foreign body. In adults, an endotracheal or endo-bronchial growth of extrinsic pressure is the usual cause
- On plain skiagram chest, there is hyper-translucency with evidence of increased volume like splaying of ribs, long tubular heart, barrel-shaped chest due to increased AP diameter of the chest and depressed domes of diaphragm. These findings may be unilateral or bilateral depending on the etiology. However, in unilateral increase in volume, these findings are unilateral except for the contralateral shift of mediastinum and largely normal cardiac contour
- *Bulla, Blebs and Pneumatoceles*: When very large, it may compress the surrounding normal lung and may lead to either unilateral or bilateral hypertranslucency
- *Bronchiolitis obliterans*: Also known as constrictive bronchiolitis or obliterative bronchiolitis is a result of inflammation of bronchioles leading to obstruction of bronchial lumen
- Chest X-ray may be normal
- Hyperinflated lungs leading to increased lucency may be seen in up to 60% of cases
- There is decrease in pulmonary blood flow
- On HRCT, there is mosaic perfusion and lobular air trapping may be seen, bronchial wall thickening and bronchiectasis may also be seen.

McLeod syndrome: Also known as Swyer-James syndrome, it is a result of acute viral bronchiolitis in infancy, leading to constrictive bronchiolitis
- There is increased translucency of the affected lung
- Small hemithorax with decreased or normal volume of the lung
- Air trapping during expiration
- Small ipsilateral hilum
- Reduced pulmonary vasculature with pruning of vessels.

Emphysema: This term is broadly used to define pulmonary diseases characterized by permanently enlarged air spaces distal to terminal bronchioles accompanied by destruction of alveolar walls and local elastic fiber network.

Plain Skiagram Chest

- Hyperinflated translucent lungs
- Low or flat hemidiaphragms
- Increased retrosternal air space
- Barrel chest
- Pulmonary vascular pruning
- Right heart enlargement
- Bullae.

Compensatory emphysema or over-aeration is a distinct clinical entity where there are unilateral findings of emphysema seen due to diseased nonfunctional contralateral lung.

Pneumothorax

Can be unilateral or bilateral and is a result of collection of air in the pleural cavity

Plain Skiagram Chest

- There is increased translucency with loss of bronchovascular markings
- There is contralateral shift of mediastinum in the unilateral types
- In tension pneumothorax, there may be inversion of diaphragm
- Congenital lobar emphysema

- Result of congenital insult leading to constriction of bronchi supplying one lobe leading to air trapping and increase in volume
- The enlarged lobe compresses the remaining normal lobes
- Contralateral mediastinal shift.

Pulmonary Arterial Hypoplasia

- Small or absent main pulmonary artery
- Concave pulmonary bay
- Pulmonary oligemia.

HYPERTRANSLUCENT LUNG FIELD

Causes of Bilateral Hypertranslucency

Faulty Radiologic Technique
Overpenetrated film.

Decreased Soft Tissues
- Thin body habitus
- Bilateral mastectomy.

Cardiac Causes
- Right to left shunt
- Eisenmengerization of left to right shunt.

Pulmonary Causes
- Decreased vascular bed
  - Pulmonary embolus.
- Increase in air space
  - Air trapping—asthma, acute bronchitis, emphysema
  - Bullae, blebs
  - Interstitial emphysema.

Localized Lucent Lung Defect
- Cavity
  - Infection
  - Neoplasm
  - Vascular occlusion
  - Inhalational—silicosis with coal worker's pneumoconiosis.

- Cyst
  - Cystic bronchiectasis
  - Pneumatocele
  - Centrilobular/bullous emphysema
  - Honeycomb lung
  - Diaphragmatic hernia
  - CCAM Type I, CLE, bronchogenic cyst.

Hyperlucent lung (Unilateral):

Normal	Increased density contralateral lung
	Over-penetrated film
Technical	Over-penetrated film
	Rotation, scoliosis
Soft tissue	Mastectomy
	Congenital absence of pectoralis major
	Poliomyelitis (Poland's syndrome)
Emphysema	Compensatory: Lobar collapse, lobectomy
	Obstructive: Foreign body, tumor
	McLeod's syndrome
	CLE
	Bullous
Vascular	Absent/hypoplastic pulmonary artery, obstructed pulmonary artery
	< Tumor embolus
Pneumothorax	McLeod's syndrome

HONEYCOMB LUNG (TABLE 1.23)

Common	Rare
Histiocytosis-X	Tuberous sclerosis
Scleroderma	Amyloidosis
Rheumatoid disease	Neurofibromatosis
Fibrosing alveolitis	Lymphangioleiomyomatosis
Pneumoconiosis	—
Sarcoidosis	—
Similar appearance	—
Bronchiectasis	Connection with bronchus +
Cystic fibrosis	Pancreatic anomalies + Achlorhydria

Multiple Pinpoint Opacities

Postlymphogram	: Iodized oil emboli. Contrast medium is seen at the site of termination of the thoracic duct
Silicosis	: Located in upper and mid-zones, seen in gold miners
Stannosis	: Evenly distributed throughout the lung with Kerley A and B lines
Baryltosis	: Inhalation of barytes Very dense, discrete opacities May be slightly larger in size Bases and apices are spared
Alveolar microlithiasis	: Familial, black pleura, enlarged heart size is positive.

Lobar Pneumonia (Fig. 1.31)

Consolidation involving the air spaces of an anatomically recognizable lobe. The entire lobe may not be involved and there may be a degree of associated collapse.

- *Streptococcus pneumoniae*: The most common cause, unilobar in distribution. No cavitation. Little or no collapse. Pleural effusion is uncommon.
- *Staphylococcus*: Especially in children. Sixty percent develop pneumatocele. No lobar predilection, effusion, empyema and pneumothorax and bronchopleural fistulae are common.

Table 1.23: Honeycomb lung.

Location	Upper zones	Extrinsic allergic alveolitis
	Upper and mid-zones bases	Histiocytosis
		Rheumatoid
		Scleroderma
		Cystic bronchiectasis
		Cryptogenic fibrosing alveolitis
	Mid and bases	Sarcoidosis

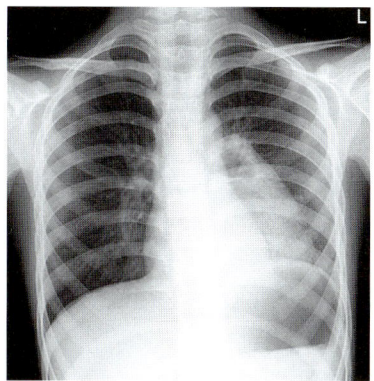

Fig. 1.31: Posteroanterior radiograph of chest shows left lower lobe consolidation collapse.

- *Klebsiella pneumoniae*: Multilobar involvement, cavitation and lobar enlargement is common.
- *Tuberculosis*: Associated collapse is common. Right lung is more frequently involved. Anterior segment of the upper lobe and the medial segment of the middle lobe are the most common sites.
- *Streptococcus pyogenes*: Lower lobe predominates, often associated with pleural effusion.

Consolidation with Bulging Fissures

Homogeneous or inhomogeneous air-space opacification with bulging of the bounding fissures:
- *Infection with abundant exudates: Klebsiella, Streptococcus pneumoniae*, tubercular bacilli.
- *Abscess*: When air-area of consolidation breaks down.
  Common organisms include *Staphylococcus aureus*, *Klebsiella* and other gram –ve organism.
- Cancer of the bronchus.

Lung Disease Associated with Honeycombing

Collagen Disorders

Rheumatoid lung : Basal predominance Infiltrates and effusion are common

Scleroderma basal
Preceded by fine, linear basal streaks.
Extrinsic allergic alveolitis upper zones
Sarcoidosis sparing of extreme apices
- Hilar lymph adenopathy
- Egg shell calcification.
  Pneumoconiosis : Mainly due to asbestosis
  Cystic bronchiectasis lower and middle zones
  Bronchial wall thickening
  Localized areas of consolidation
Histiocytosis—mid and upper zones.
Disseminated nodules followed by honeycomb pattern
Tuberous sclerosis : Rare
Neurofibromatosis : Rib notching + Ribbon ribs + Scoliosis

HONEYCOMB PATTERN

- A generalized reticular pattern or miliary mottling which when summated produces the appearance of air containing 'cysts' 0.5–2 cm in diameter.
- Obscured pulmonary vasculature.
- Late appearance of radiological signs after the onset of symptoms.
- Complications
  – Pneumothorax is frequent
  – Cor pulmonale later in the course of the disease.

Causes

- Collagen diseases—rheumatoid arthritis, scleroderma
- Extrinsic allergic alveolitis
- Sarcoidosis
- Pneumoconiosis
- Cystic bronchiectasis
- Cystic fibrosis
- Drugs—nitrofurantoin, busulfan, methotrexate, adriamycin, vincristine, cyclophosphamide, bleomycin and melphalan
- Langerhans cells histiocytosis

- Lymphangioleiomyomatosis
- Tuberous sclerosis
- Idiopathic interstitial fibrosis (cryptogenic fibrosing alveolitis)
- Neurofibromatosis.

Rheumatoid Arthritis
- Most pronounced at the bases
- Its severity does not parallel to that of joint involvement
- In the earlier stages, it is characterized by radiologic appearance of patchy area of air space consolidation (multifocal ill-defined densities)
- In the intermediate stage, there is fine reticular pattern or reticulonodular pattern
- As the progress decreases, there is appearance of cystic spaces of honeycomb lung
- All the above features may be preceded by basal infiltrates ± small effusion.

Scleroderma
- Predominantly basal
- Less regular 'honeycomb' pattern which is preceded by fine, linear, basal streaks, cor pulmonale is unusual
- Other clinical signs which include skin changes, soft tissue calcification, disturbances of esophageal motility and dilatation of the esophagus
- Radiologically, an upper GIT series may demonstrate both esophageal dilatation and decreased motility as well as small bowel dilatation.

ASBESTOSIS
- It produces a basilar distribution that may progress from a fine reticular interstitial pattern to a coarse interstitial pattern with honeycombing
- The basilar reticular or honeycomb pattern is also frequently associated with pleural thickening, pleural calcification.

Silicosis
- It has predominant upper lobe distribution
- It may be associated with hilar or mediastinal lymphadenopathy with pleural thickening. The fine reticular pattern is seen which progresses to honeycomb lung.

Extrinsic Allergic Alveolitis
Predominantly seen in the upper lobes of the lung.

Sarcoidosis
Sparing of extreme apices:
- Honeycombing of the lung is usually preceded by some classic findings including hilar adenopathy and an interstitial nodular or fine reticular interstitial pattern
- As the interstitial disease, progresses, there is regression of hilar adenopathy.

Langerhans Cell Histiocytosis
- 'Honeycomb' pattern preceded by disseminated nodules
- May be predominantly in the mid and upper zones
- Cor pulmonale is uncommon.

Usual Interstitial Pneumonitis/ Cryptogenic Fibrosing
Alveolitis
- More marked in the lower lobes of the lungs initially and progresses to involve the whole of the lungs
- In HRCT, there is honeycombing and fibrosis. It shows a uniform and patchy distribution.

Tuberous Sclerosis
- Symptoms, when they appear, usually first appear in adult life
- Pneumothorax, pulmonary insufficiency and cor pulmonale may complicate the syndrome
- The clinical and radiological manifestation of the disease in the brain, kidneys and skin readily establishes the diagnosis.

Neurofibromatosis

Honeycomb lung ± rib notching ribbon ribs and/or scoliosis is seen in 10% cases but not before adulthood.

PLEURAL DISEASES OR LESIONS (FLOWCHART 1.2)

Serous membrane which covers the surface of lung and lines the inner surface of chest wall.

Common conditions are:
- Pleural effusion
- Pleural thickening
- Pneumothorax
- Pleural masses
- Pleural calcification.

Pleural Effusion

May be transudate, exudate, pus, blood or chyle.

Transudate

Contains less than 3 g/dL of protein, usually bilateral
- *Increase hydrostatic pressure:* Main cause is congestive cardiac failure (CCF)—1st on right side and then bilateral, constrictive pericarditis.
- *Decrease colloid osmotic pressure*
  - Decrease protein product—cirrhosis with ascites
  - Protein loss/hypervolemia
  - Nephrotic syndrome
  - Overhydration
  - Peritoneal dialysis
- Meig-Salmon syndrome
  - Ovarian fibroma, thecoma, GCT, Brenner's tumor, etc.
  - Ascites
  - Pleural effusion resolves with tumor removal.

Exudate

Increased permeability of abnormal pleural capillaries with release of high-protein fluid into pleural space. More than 3 g/dL of protein.
- Infection
  - *Empyema:* Pleural effusion with presence of pus. +/– positive culture. Microorganisms are anerobic bacteria Gross pus (WBC >15000/cm^3)
  - *Parapneumonic effusion:* Less with pneumonia, abscess, bronchiectasis.
  - *TB:* Increase protein content >75 g/dL
  - *Fungi and parasite:* Amebiasis, secondary to liver abscess.
- *Malignant disease:* Lung carcinoma (Ca), lymphoma, breast, ovarian Ca and malignant mesothelioma. Positive cytological result.
- *Vascular:* Pulmonary embolism (15–30%)
- *Abdominal disease*
  - *Pancreatitis:* Left side pleural effusion (68%), right side (10%).
  - *Boerhaave's syndrome:* Left side
  - *Subphrenic abscess:* Pleural effusion—79%, elevation and restriction of diaphragmatic movement

Endometriosis plate-like atelectatic or pneumonia.
  - *Connective tissue disorder.*

RA—UL (R>L) recurrent alternating sides relatively unchanged in size for months.

Systemic Lupus Erythematosus (SLE)

Bilateral (B/L) in 50% (L>R), increased cardiac size.

Wegener's Granuloma

Hemothorax
- Bleeding into the pleural space may be trauma
- Hemophilia or excessive anticoagulation—rare
- Pulmonary infarction—blood stained
- Lung carcinoma—blood stained.

Chylothorax

- Chyle is milky fluid high in neutral fat and fatty acid.
- Secondary to damage or obstruction of the thoracic lymphatic vessels.

Causes: Most common cause—trauma—surgery. Carcinoma of lung, lymphoma, filariasis.

Radiological Features

Plain film: Frontal view less sensitive < Lateral view < Lateral, decubitus view.

Differential Diagnosis in Radiology

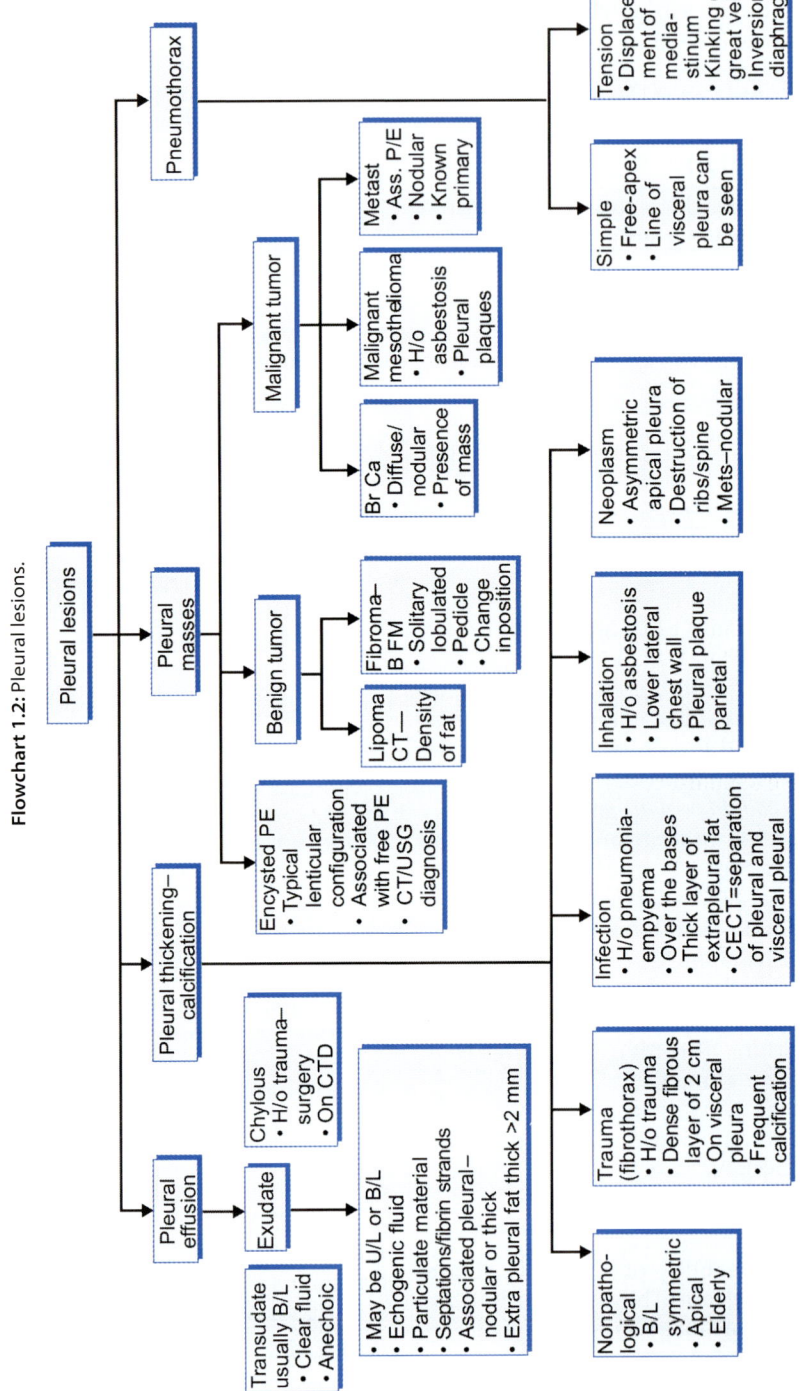

Flowchart 1.2: Pleural lesions.

- Moderate effusion with mediastinum is shifted towards the side of collapse—likely due to carcinoma of bronchus.
- Empyema may be suspected by the appearance of a fluid level.
- Septations.

Ultrasonography (USG)

Very sensitive, can detect few mL of fluid.

Transudate—clear fluid separating the visceral and parietal pleura.

Moving lung suspended within the pleural space.

Exudate—Echogenic fluid, containing floating particulate material, septations or fibrin strands may be associated with pleural nodule or thickening more than 3 mm.

CT—simple pleural effusion—sickle-shaped disease in the most dependent part of thorax posteriorly
- As regard to tissue density—CT is rarely helpful
- Exudate— >water density septation
- Parietal pleural thickening on CECT
- Extrapleural fat thickening of more than 2 mm
- Chylous—decreased density than H_2O.

Acute hemorrhage—increased density of fluid with presence of fluid-fluid level.

Pleural Thickening

- Nonpathological
  - Bilateral symmetrical apical pleural thickening
  - Elderly patient
  - Probably ischemia is the cause
- *Trauma*: If the entire lung is surrounded by the fibrotic
  - Fibrothorax is secondary to organized effusion, hemothorax or pyothorax
- Dense fibrous layer of 2 cm thickness almost always on visceral pleura
- Frequent calcification on inner aspect of pleura.

Infection
- Chronic empyema—history of pneumonia with presence of parenchymal scars. Usually seen over the bases.
- Frequently a thickened layer of extrapleural fat can be seen separating the parietal and visceral layer.
- Calcification may be seen.

Tuberculosis (TB)
- Lung apex
- Can be associated with apical cavity
- Calcification may be seen.

Inhalation Disorder

Asbestos exposure involves the lower lateral chest wall, basilar interstitial disease.

Pleural plaque: Involves the parietal pleura with sparing of visceral pleura.

Neoplasm

Asymmetric apical pleural thickening may represent Pancoast tumor destruction of adjacent ribs and spine penetrated film will be helpful.
- Metastasis—often nodular.

Pleural Calcification

Has the same causes as pleural thickening.

Unilateral (U/L) pleural calcification—result of previous empyema, hemothorax or pleurisy and also occur in visceral pleura associated with pleural thickening.
- Calcification may be in a continuous sheet or in discrete plaque.

Bilateral (B/L) calcification seen in asbestos exposure, more delicate, frequently visible over the diaphragm and adjacent to axilla located in parietal pleura.

Pleural Masses

- Incomplete border and tapered superior and inferior borders
- Usually make obtuse angle with chest wall
- Displacement of adjacent lung parenchyma with compressive atelectasis and blowing of bronchi and pulmonary vessels around the mass
- Vanishing tumor and encysted pleural effusion fluid may become loculated in interlobar fissure seen in heart failure lateral film typical lenticular configuration. Encysted pleural effusion—often associated with free pleural effusion

- Water density
- Neoplasm.

Benign
- *Lipoma*—CT detects the origin of mass of fat density.
- Benign lipoma confirms fat density with few fibrin strands.
- Thymolipoma, angiolipoma, teratoma, characterized by islands of soft tissue density, interspersed with fat.
- Fibroma/benign fibrous mesothelioma—most common benign tumor may be associated with hypoglycemia and HPOA solitary lobulated noncalcification mass. If pedicle is seen—diagnostic, shape changes with the change in patient's position.

Malignant Pleural Thickening
Bronchogenic carcinoma: Most common cause. When a bronchogenic carcinoma involves the pleura diffusely with resultant pleural effusion, the tumor is considered unresectable.

Malignant Mesothelioma
- Rare tumor
- 70% of cases—history of asbestos exposure
- Nodular pleural thickening around all or part of lung with pleural effusion
- Pleural—plaque
- Metastatic disease—breast and gostrointestinal tract (GIT)
- Most common manifestation is malignant pleural effusion
- Pleural thickening is nodular and frequent. Encase the entire lung including mediastinum.
- Pleural lymphoma
- Pleural effusion
CT—localized broad-based lymphomatous pleural plaque.

Pneumothorax
- *Spontaneous*—most common type.
- Male: female ratio: 8:1, young male with tall thin stature.
- Due to rupture of a congenital pleural bleb, such blebs are usually in the lung apex and may be bilateral.
- *Iatrogenic*—for example, postoperative, after chest aspiration during artificial ventilation, after lung biopsy.
- *Traumatic*—result of a penetrating chest wound, closed chest trauma, associated finding like rib fracture.

Hemothorax
Surgical/mediastinal emphysema
Secondary to lung disease:
- Emphysema
- Chronic bronchitis
- Common factor in an elderly patient
- Rupture of a tension cyst in *Staphylococcus pneumoniae*
- Rupture of a subpleural TB focus
- Rupture of a cavitating subpleural metastases
- Pneumoperitoneum—air passes through a pleuroperitoneal foramen
- Generalized
- Localized—if pleural adhesions are present.

Open
If air can move freely in and out of pleural space during respiration.

Closed
If no movement.
Valvular: If air enters the pleural space on inspiration but does not leave on expiration, it is valvular—as intrapleural pressure increase, it leads to development of tension pneumothorax.

Radiological features: Small pneumothorax in an erect patient collects at the apex.
Expiratory film—useful in closed pneumothorax. Lateral decubitus film with affected side uppermost.

Tension pneumothorax: Massive displacement of mediastinum.
- Kinking of great veins
- Acute cardiac and respiratory embarrassment

Chest

- Ipsilateral lung may be squashed against the mediastinum and herniate across the midline
- Depression of ipsilateral diaphragm.

Loculated pneumothorax—pleural adhesion may result in loculated pneumothorax.

Diffenrtial diagnosis—subpleural bullae, thin-walled pulmonary cavity/cyst.

Few linear strands can be seen in these but not in pneumothorax.

Hydropneumothorax containing a horizontal fluid level (Fig. 1.32).

PLEURAL FLUID

Radiological Appearances of Pleural Fluid

- Most dependent recess of the pleura is the posterior costophrenic angle (100–200 mL of fluid is required to fill this). Small effusions are hence seen earlier on a lateral film and now on ultrasound
- Decubitus view with a horizontal beam is being the most sensitive view
- The effusion casts a homogeneous opacity spread upwards. Typically, this opacity has a fairly well-defined, concave upper edge, which is higher laterally than medially and obscures the diaphragmatic shadow
- A massive effusion may cause complete radiopacity of a hemithorax
- In the presence of a large effusion, lack of displacement of the mediastinum suggests that the underlying lung is completely collapsed
- Lamellar effusions are shallow collections between the lung surface and the visceral pleura
- Large effusions may accumulate between the diaphragm and the undersurface of a lung—this is called subpulmonary pleural effusion. The apex is more lateral than normal. This collection moves fully with changes of posture
- Empyema usually has a lenticular shape, irregular thick walls and may compress the underlying lung
- Loculated effusions tend to have comparatively little depth, best considerable width, rather like a biconvex lens.

Pneumothorax (Fig. 1.33)

It collects in a free pleural space in an erect patient at the apex. On the frontal film, sharp white line of the visceral pleura will be visible, separated from the chest wall by the radiolucent pleural space, which is devoid of lung markings.

An expiratory film will make a closed pneumothorax easier to see since on a full

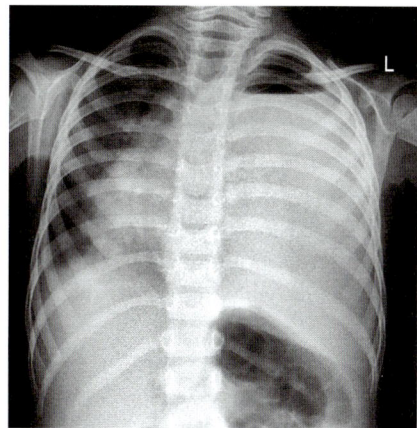

Fig. 1.32: Posteroanterior radiograph of chest shows hydropneumothorax on left side with mediastinal shift to right side.

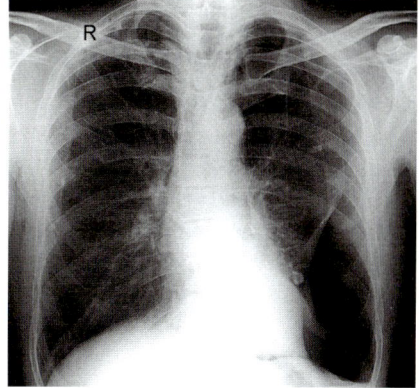

Fig. 1.33: Posteroanterior radiograph of chest shows loculated pneumothorax in left lower hemithorax causing compression atelectasis of left lower lobe.

expiration, the lung volume is at its smallest, while the volume of pleural air is unchanged.

In tension pneumothorax, the ipsilateral lung may be squashed against the mediastinum, or herniate across the midline, and the ipsilateral hemidiaphragm may be depressed.

Nodular extension into the fissures, pleural effusion, and volume loss of the ipsilateral lung, all suggest malignancy.

Metastatic: The most frequent primary tumors being of the bronchus and breast.

PLEURAL TUMORS

Benign: Mesothelioma: Well-defined, lobulated mass adjacent to chest wall, mediastinum, diaphragm.

Lipoma: Well-defined, lobulated mass may change shape with respiration on CT, presence of fat is diagnostic.

Malignant: Mesothelioma—due to prolonged exposure to asbestosis.
Nodular pleural thickening with pleural effusion. Rib involvement may occur, but is rare.

PLEURAL CALCIFICATION (FLOWCHART 1.3)

The common conditions are:
- Old empyema
- Old hemothorax
- Asbestos inhalation
- Silicosis.

Old Empyema and Old Hemothorax
- Calcification is irregular, resembles a plaque or sheet and is contained within thickened pleura
- En face, it is hazy and veil-like but in profile, it is dense and linear, paralleling the chest wall
- Usually unilateral
- Most common site: Lower posterior half of chest
- In tuberculous empyema—both visceral and parietal pleura may be calcified, which are sometimes separated by a soft tissue opacity which may contain fluid.

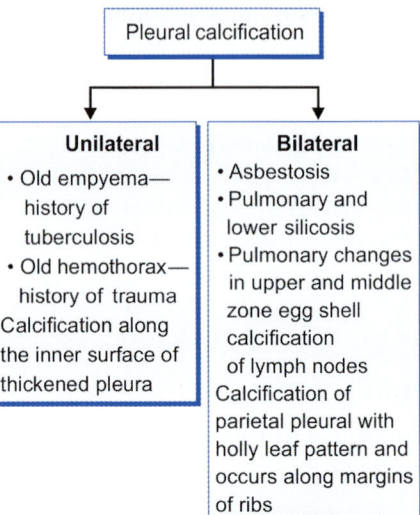

Flowchart 1.3: Pleural calcification.

Asbestos Inhalation
- A feature of asbestosis is pleural plaque which is a well-defined soft tissue sheet originating in the parietal pleura (latent period is 10 years).
- Latent period for calcification to develop is 20 years.
- Lesions are usually bilateral, lying in the middle zone, lower zone and diaphragm.

When calcified, 'holly leaf pattern' with sharp and often angulated outlines and often follow the margins of the ribs.
- Usually less than 1 cm thick.

Diffuse pleural thickening: Unlike pleural plaques, the margins are well-defined and tapered; may reach several centimeters in thickness.
Pleural effusion—uncommon.

Malignant Mesothelioma
Latent period: 40 years
Pulmonary changes (peripheral lower zone):
- Fibrosis
- Bronchial carcinoma
- Pseudotumor (fibrotic atelectasis).

Extrathoracic Manifestation
Peritoneal mesothelioma, malignancy of upper GIT.

Silicosis

- Inhalation of silica (SiO_2)
- Pleural calcification is similar to asbestosis.

Other Features

- Multiple small nodules in upper zone and middle zone
- Hilar lymph nodes with egg shell calcification
- Progressive massive fibrosis
- Caplan's syndrome also occurs in patients with rheumatoid arthritis and silicosis.

HIGH RESOLUTION CT-PATTERN OF PARENCHYMAL DISEASE

Peripheral, Base

- Cryptogenic fibrosing alveolitis
  - Early   : Ground glass appearance
                 Subpleural reticular shadows
  - Later   : Reticulations extend centrally
  - Chronic   : Small cyst formation, commencing at subpleural site.
- Asbestosis
  - Early   : Changes are seen at the lung base.
                 Posteriorly.
                 Thickened curvilinear, subpleural lines are seen.
                 Thickened subpleural septal lines, coarse parenchymal lines extending centrally.
  - Chronic   : Honeycombing
                 Rounded atelectasis with comet tail sign

Central Upper Fluid Zones

- *Sarcoidosis*: Thickened bronchovascular markings with perivascular beading present centrally.
- Patchy alveolar opacification.
- Subpleural and peribronchovascular nodules.

Peripheral and Central

- *Lymphangitis*: Bronchovascular markings and septal line thickening.
- No alveolar opacification is seen.

Widespread

- *Lymphangioma*: Characteristic widespread distribution.
- *Leiomyomatosis*: More common in women.
- Uniform-sized well-defined cysts with normal parenchyma surrounding them.
- *Tuberous sclerosis*
  - Variable-sized cyst
  - No feminine predilection.

CARDIOPHRENIC ANGLE MASS (FLOWCHART 1.4)

Solid

- Fat density
  - Epicardial fat pad
    - Obese, Cushing's syndrome
    - Uncapsulated, homogeneous extrapleural fat.
  - Lipoma
    - Uncommon, well-defined, encapsulated thin fibrous septae.
- Liposarcoma
  - Ill-defined
  - Inhomogeneous.
- Morgagni hernia
  - Soft tissue
- Lymph nodes
  - Lymphoma
  - Carcinoma—breast, lung, colon

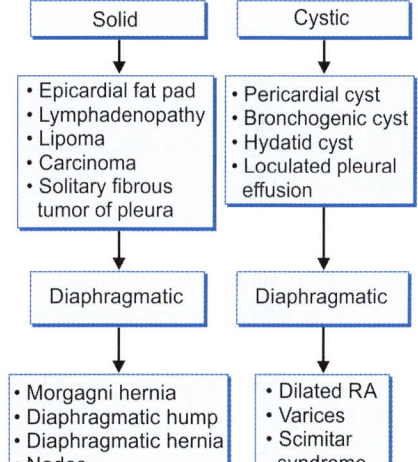

Flowchart 1.4: Cardiophrenic angle masses.

- Traumatic—diaphragmatic hernia
  - History of trauma
  - Mostly left sided
  - Single entry and exit
  - Barium or other studies—useful in diagnosis
- Diaphragmatic hump
  - Herniation of liver through the gap
  - Liver scan or USG
- Fibrous tumors of pleura
  - Pleura-based, well-defined, homogeneously enhancing, stalked
- Primary or secondary malignancy
  - Well-defined smoothly marginated lung-based.

Cystic or Vascular

Pericardial cyst
- Well-defined, round to oval, fluid density, non-enhancing, right CP angle

Hydatid cyst
- Unilocular, associated with hepatic cyst or may be bilateral
- Meniscus sign, water lily sign
- Loculated pleural effusion
- USG—makes the diagnosis
- Varices
- Delayed phase scanning is needed
- Portal hypertension, more on right
- Scimitar syndrome
- Abnormal vessel draining into IVC or hepatic vein
- Lobar agenesis or aplasia
- Accessory diaphragm, pulmonary sequestration.

Pericardial cyst
- *Etiology*—embryogenesis, parietal recess, diverticulum, sequelae
- 30–40 years, asymptomatic

Plain film chest—well-defined, round to oval mass
- Cardiophrenic angle mass usually right
- Changes shape with respiration and body position.

Ultrasound
Well-defined, anechoic to hypoechoic, no septae.

Computed Tomography (CT)
- 3–8 cm in size
- May extend into fissures
- No enhancement, no perceptible wall.

Hydatid Cyst

- *Three layers:* Adventitia, friable ectocyst, inner germinal layer
- *Lung cyst:* Unilocular, 20% bilateral, 10% associated with hepatic cyst
- Well-defined, round-oval, homogeneous masses up to 10 cm in diameter
- Calcification is rare
- Meniscus sign, water lily sign.

Morgagni Hernia

- Defect between septum transversum and right and left costal margins of diaphragm
- Usually asymptomatic, more common in obese people
- Right-sided, small lesions may only have omental fat, and then it may be difficult to distinguish from epicardial fat pad
- Large lesion—colon, liver, stomach or small intestine may herniate
- Barium study—tenting of colon or loop above the diaphragm.

CT—omental fat, omental vessels and abdominal viscera are seen in the mass.

Diaphragmatic Hump and Hernia

- Trauma—hernia mostly seen on left side (posterior and central)
- Colon or less commonly stomach are the contents
- Barium—entry and exit through the defect are closely apposed
- Obstruction is frequent probably because of angular margins of the defect but are detected late because of subtle changes in plain film

- On right side—liver may herniate in severe trauma
- A liver scan is helpful.

Congenital Hernia
- More common on right side
- It has a hernial sac.

Scimitar Syndrome
- Presence of partial anomalous pulmonary venous return below the diaphragm, mostly right side
- Lobar agenesis or aplasia, other systemic artery from aorta in lower thorax or upper abdomen
- Pulmonary artery may be small or entirely absent, accessory diaphragm, hepatic herniation, pulmonary sequestration.

Fibrous Tumors of Pleura
- Solitary, sharply-defined, sometimes lobulated soft tissue pleural-based mass without evidence of chest wall invasion, homogeneous enhancement
- Pedicle or stalk—pathognomonic and indicator of benign lesion, mobility
- May grow very large than obtuse or acute angle may be formed with pleura.

Primary or Secondary Carcinoma
- Well-defined, smoothly marginated
- Lung-based
- Multiple.

Epicardial Fat Pad
- Excessive deposition of fat in mediastinum
- Obese patient
- Cushing syndrome or excessive corticosteroid intake
- Uncapsulated and extrapleural fat.

Lipoma
- Uncommon
- Well-defined, encapsulated, generally homogeneous
- May contain thin fibrous septae
- Inhomogeneous, poorly-defined.

Lymph Nodes
Anterior diaphragmatic group of LN—2 nodes, <5 mm is normal.

Causes of enlargement are:
- Unilateral or bilateral
  – Lymphoma
  – Lung, breast or colon cancer—metastasis.

Chapter 2

Breast: Mammographic Differential Diagnosis

DENSITY OF LESION ON MAMMOGRAM

The density of lesion on mammogram is given in Figure 2.1.

MARGINS OF LESION

The margins of lesion are described in Figure 2.2.

CIRCUMSCRIBED RADIOLUCENT LESION (FLOWCHART 2.1)

Lipoma

- Usually solitary, presents usually in older women
- Usually have a thin capsule
- Frequently large at diagnosis
- Difficult to palpate due to soft consistency.

Oil Cyst

- Single or multiple
- Usually small 2–3 cm
- *History of (H/o) trauma:*
  - Surgical
  - Seat belt injury
- ± Mural calcification

Galactocele

- During lactation—milk containing cyst caused by obstruction of a duct by inspissated milk in a woman who has abruptly stopped breastfeeding 2–3 cm in diameter.

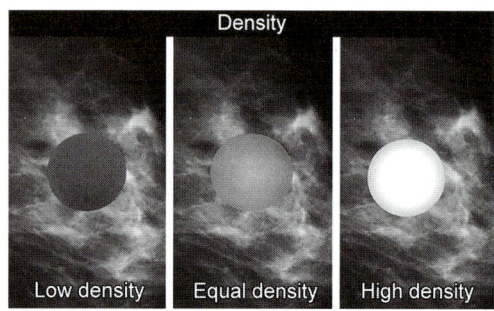

Fig. 2.1: Density of lesion on mammogram.

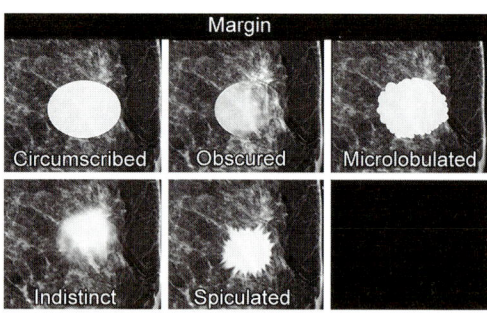

Fig. 2.2: Margins of lesion.

- Lucent or mixed density mass.
- Characteristic fat-fluid level when imaged with horizontal beam.

MIXED DENSITY LESIONS (FLOWCHART 2.2)

- *Fibroadenolipoma (hamartoma)*: Mammographic appearance is determined by the relative amount of fat and glandular tissue.
- Uncommon benign tumor composed of normal or dysplastic mammary tissue,

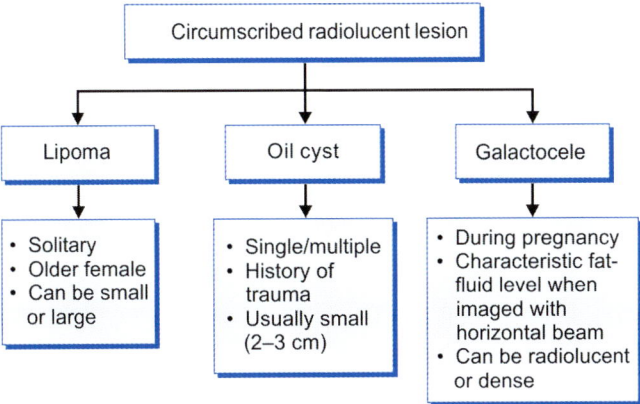

Flowchart 2.1: Circumscribed radiolucent lesion.

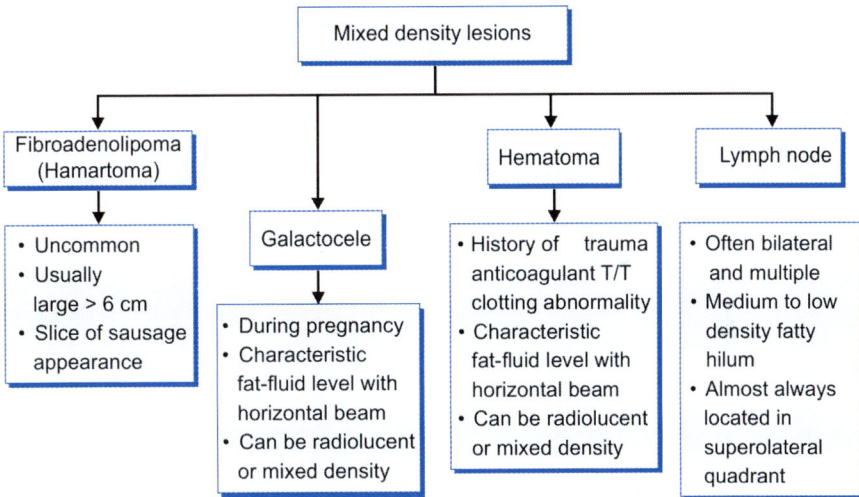

Flowchart 2.2: Mixed density lesions

including adipose and fibrous tissues and ducts and lobules in varying amount.
- Often large at diagnosis, often 6 cm in diameter at the time of diagnosis.
- Lack of normal architecture with lack of orientation of glandular tissue toward the nipple results in an appearance resembling a "slice of sausage".
- There may be a thin soft tissue density capsule visible.

Galactocele

Discussed earlier.

Hematoma

- *History of trauma:* Blunt or surgical
- History of anticoagulant intake
- History of clotting abnormalities
- Medium to high density mass, often having irregular margins
- Overlying skin edema present in acute stage
- Gradual decrease in size or disappearance of the lesion on follow-up.

Lymph Node

- Medium to low-density lesion with a fatty notch or center

- Often bilateral (B/L) and multiple
- Almost always located in the superolateral quadrant
- Pathological nodes have ± loss of central fatty hilum, ± enlargement.

Causes

- *Rheumatoid arthritis:* After gold treatment ± fine dense gold deposits
- *Sarcoidosis:* ± Punctate calcification
- *Infection:* Tuberculosis—(coarse calcification ±)
- *Malignancy:*
  – Leukemia
  – Lymphoma
  – Metastasis from carcinoma breast carcinoma ovary (± irregular microcalcification).

RADIOPAQUE (SOFT TISSUE DENSITY LESION)

Simple Cyst (Fig. 2.3)

- Most common cause of a circumscribed mass arising in a female 40 years or more in age
- Sharply circumscribed low soft tissue density mass ± radiolucent halo (halo sign)
- Often multiple and B/L (Bilateral)
- Most commonly 1–3 cm in diameter
- *Calcification:* Uncommon rarely peripheral thin eggshell calcification may be present
- Cyst may develop quickly prior to menses and diminish in size just as rapidly
- *Ultrasonography:* Oval or round echo-free lesion with smooth well-defined walls.

Strict sonographic criteria for simple cysts are:
- Well-circumscribed margins
- A bright posterior wall
- Round or oval contour
- Absence of internal echoes
- Through transmission.

Fibroadenoma (Figs. 2.4 to 2.6)

- Common benign estrogen sensitive tumor composed of fibrotic and glandular tissues in varying proportion that usually appears in adolescent and young women before the age of 30 years.
- Usually solitary, round, ovoid, or smoothly lobulated mass of medium density.
- Calcification, which is coarse, popcorn like, or primarily peripherally distributed is characteristic.
- *Ultrasonography:* Typical appearance is of a well circumscribed, round, or oval mass showing posterior acoustic enhancement and with a homogeneous internal echo pattern—usually of low reflectivity compared to the surrounding breast tissue.

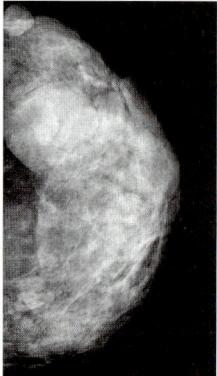

Fig. 2.3: Craniocaudal mammogram shows multiple well-defined, simple breast cysts.

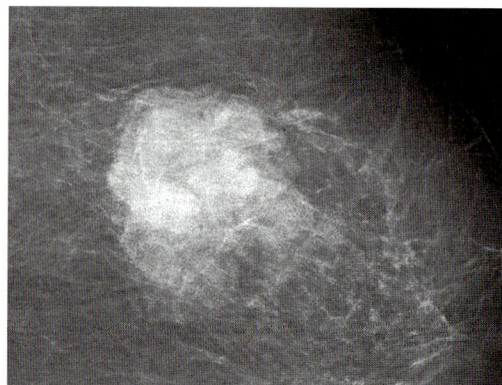

Fig. 2.4: Magnified mammogram shows lobulated fibroadenoma.

Breast: Mammographic Differential Diagnosis

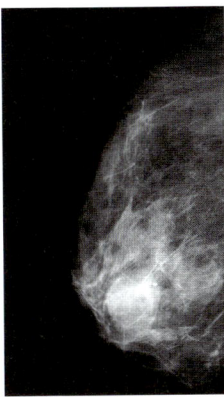

Fig. 2.5: Craniocaudal mammogram shows well-defined fibroadenoma with focal calcification.

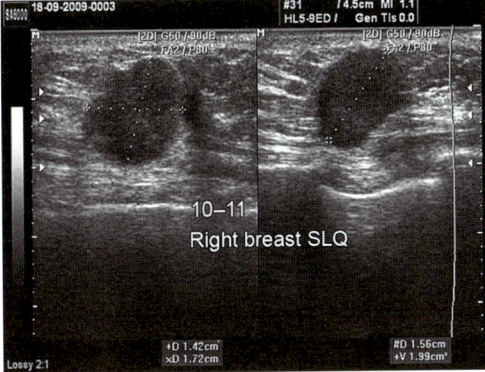

Fig. 2.6: High-resolution sonogram of breast shows well-defined fibroadenoma with posterior acoustic enhancement.

Papilloma

- Usually occurs in the retroareolar region.
- May cause a serous or serosanguineous nipple discharge.
- Usually the lesion is several millimeters in size. The mammogram may show a slight bulging of a retroareolar duct or may appear normal.
- Crescent, rosette, or eggshell calcification may occur.

Phylloides Tumor (Cystosarcoma Phylloides)

- Fibroepithelial tumor which is usually large when diagnosed.
- 30–50 years old female; grows rapidly.
- On mammography solitary large, round, oval or polylobulated, and sharply outlined lesion, ± radiolucent halo.
- May develop plaque-like calcification (rarely).
- Can recur, if not completely excised.

Metastasis

Lymphoma and other hematologic malignancies, melanoma, and lung cancer are the three most common blood-borne hematologic sources, followed by ovarian cancer, soft tissue sarcomas, and other gastrointestinal and genitourinary cancer.

- Seen on mammograms as discrete nodules, usually solitary (85%) and less often multiple (15%).
- Unilateral in 75% and B/L (Bilateral) in 25% cases.
- Diffuse involvement is much less frequent.
- Majority are found in upper-outer quadrant.
- Cannot be differentiated from other benign nodules, such as cysts or fibroadenomas. However, the presence of one or more nodules in patient with known primary should alert one to the possibility of blood-borne metastasis.
- A spiculated mass indicates the presence of a second primary breast cancer and not metastasis.
- With the exception of psammomatous calcification in metastatic ovarian carcinoma, metastases to the breast do not calcify.

Lymphoma

- Primary lymphoma of the breast is rare (B-cell is m/c than T-cell lymphoma).
- Secondary involvement of the breast with lymphoma is more frequent.
- The most common form of involvement is a circumscribed mass that is well defined or shows minimal irregularity (solitary, uncalcified relatively circumscribed mass with indistinct margins).
- Moderate to marked spiculation may or may not be present.

- In the absence of known or suspected lymphoma, the mammographic findings are nonspecific.
- Bilateral axillary lymphadenopathy suggests the possibility of lymphoma.

CIRCUMSCRIBED MALIGNANT LESIONS (CIRCUMSCRIBED CARCINOMA)

- Circumscribed carcinoma is a descriptive term referring to any ductal carcinoma that appears as a circumscribed mass on mammogram.
- Circumscribed malignant lesions are most commonly medullary, mucinous, papillary, or intracystic carcinoma, and rarely invasive ductal carcinoma (Fig. 2.7).
- Medullary carcinomas may grow rapidly and mostly occur in women less than 50 years old.
- Mucinous and papillary carcinomas have a favorable prognosis and mostly occur in women over 50 years.
- Medullary carcinoma exhibit varying degrees of lobulations. Invasive papillary carcinoma frequently appears as a cluster of smooth or irregular nodules, nodules in several quadrants, or as a solitary nodule.
- The outline of malignant circumscribed lesion is usually less sharply defined than benign circumscribed masses, and malignant lesions are typically of high soft tissue density (see Flowchart 2.1).

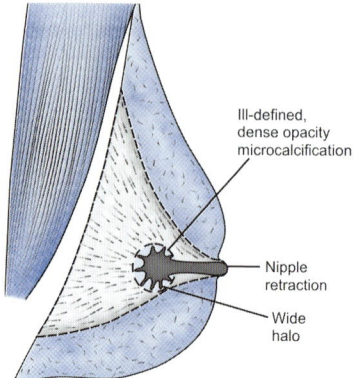

Fig. 2.7: Typical carcinoma.

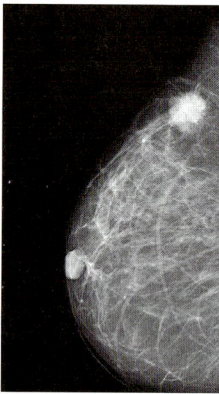

Fig. 2.8: Mediolateral mammogram shows spiculated breast carcinoma.

Spiculated Breast Masses (Figs. 2.8 and 2.9)

Invasive Carcinoma

- Approximately 95% of spiculated masses are due to invasive breast cancer.
- On mammography, there is evidence of a distinct irregular, central tumor mass from which dense spicules radiate in all directions.
- Spicules that reach the skin or muscles cause retraction and localized skin thickening.
- This sunburst appearance is most commonly seen in scirrhous infiltrating ductal carcinoma.

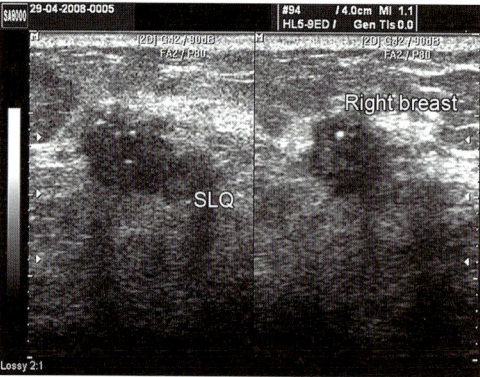

Fig. 2.9: High-resolution sonogram of breast shows spiculated breast carcinoma with posterior acoustic shadowing and internal microcalcifications.

- A web-like pattern of spicules may be seen with invasive lobular carcinoma.
- Most spiculated carcinomas of 1 cm diameter or more can be demonstrated by ultrasound. The typical ultrasound features are of an echo-poor mass, with poorly-defined margins, and posterior acoustic shadowing.

Postsurgical Scar

- Surgical scar can be diagnosed from the appropriate clinical history and physical examination, showing the position of incision site corresponds to the position of the stellate lesion, if necessary, by carrying out mammogram with skin marker on the incisional skin scar.
- Postsurgical scarring usually will regress with time, whereas spiculated carcinoma usually will grow.
- Postsurgical scarring will characteristically lack a central density and will appear different on the craniocaudal and oblique lateral views. It will have a planar configuration corresponding to the incisional plane rather than a three-dimensional one.
- A central lucency due to fat necrosis, when present, is a reliable sign that a lesion is due to previous surgery.

Fat Necrosis

- Fat necrosis may assume any one of several mammographic appearances, stellate mass, circumscribed mass, amorphous density, or architectural distortion.
- When present, central lucency in the mass or lipid cysts seen as a round lucent areas surrounded by a thin fibrotic capsule suggests the correct diagnosis.
- Fat necrosis may occur secondary to blunt trauma, surgical procedures, or on an idiopathic basis, especially in older women who have pendulous, fatty breasts.

Radial Scar (Complex Sclerosing Lesion)

- It is characterized histologically by a fibroelastic center surrounded by ducts and lobules arranged in a radiating fashion.
- On mammograms, the lesion is fairly small, 10–15 cm in diameter. Some appear solid in the center, but in most, there is a radiolucent center or no solid central core.
- Although seen on both mammographic views, the lesion tends to occur in one plane both on mammogram and histologic sections. It typically varies in appearance from one projection to another.
- All patients have normal physical findings. Skin thickening and retraction over the lesion are infrequent.
- Even when the mammographic findings are suggesting a radial scar, they are not diagnostic. Thus, biopsy is required.

Breast Abscess

- Usually caused by *Staphylococcus* and *Streptococcus*.
- May also appear as a spiculated or poorly defined mass.
- The clinical diagnosis is usually clear, as there is pain, swelling, and erythema.
- Usually retroareolar and occurs in young primiparous women during lactation.

Sclerosing Adenosis

- It may also appear as a small stellate tumor, which may be difficult to distinguish from radial scar or cancer on mammography.
- *Extra-abdominal dermoid (fibromatosis)* is a rare benign condition that can appear as a spiculated or poorly-defined mass as on mammography.
- *Granular cell myoblastoma:* It is a rare benign tumor that produces a palpable lump with ill-defined stellate margins on mammography, suggestive of malignancy.

Pseudomass (Summation Shadows)

- Overlapping glandular tissue may simulate a mass on one projection, but no similar mass is seen on an orthogonal view.
- Therefore, an area of asymmetric tissue must be identified on two views before it can be considered abnormal.

The Edematous Breast (Fig. 2.10)

The mammographic features are:
- Skin thickening, initially affecting mainly the lower part of the breast.
- Diffuse increased density.
- Coarse trabecular pattern.
- Enlargement of the breast.

Differential Diagnosis

- *Carcinoma of the breast:* An edematous breast may be caused either by an advanced primary tumor, lymphatic spread from a primary tumor, or inflammatory carcinoma.
    - Extension of tumor into lymphatic vessels can produce focal skin thickening and increased density of the subcutaneous tissue. In inflammatory carcinoma, intense edema causes rapid enlargement and tenderness of the affected breast with diffuse skin thickening.
- *Axillary lymphatic obstruction:* Axillary lymphatic obstruction can occur secondary to metastasis from ipsilateral breast or contralateral breast or from nonbreast. Primary advanced gynecologic malignancies (ovarian, uterine), rarely may block primary lymphatic drainage in the lesser pelvis, causing lymph flow through thoracoepigastric collaterals and overloading the axillary and supraclavicular lymphatic drainage.
- *Postoperative axillary lymph node removal or dissection:* It may also lead to edematous breast. Edema of the breast may persist mammographically even when it is not obvious clinically.
    - If axillary lymph node dissection has been performed for metastatic disease and skin thickening occurs, it may be impossible to determine whether this appearance represents metastatic involvement of the breast or impaired lymphatic drainage from surgery.
- *Radiation therapy:* The features of edema develop progressively following radiotherapy treatment, reaches maximum at about 6 months, and has resolved approximately 18 months following treatment.
    - If skin thickening and breast edema recur after the initial edema has resolved or decreased, recurrent carcinoma should be considered.
- *Mastitis or breast abscess:* Focal or diffuse skin thickening may be related to lactation, skin, or nipple infection with extension into the breast or hematogenous spread of infection.
- *Fluid overload state:* Edematous breast may develop in patients with cardiac failure, renal failure, cirrhosis, and hypoalbuminemia. It is usually bilateral. The thickening occurs mostly in the dependent aspect of the breast. In a bedridden patient lying on one side, the skin thickening may be unilateral and involve only the dependent breast.

BREAST CALCIFICATION TYPES (FIGS. 2.11 AND 2.12)

Characteristically Benign Calcification

- *Eggshell calcification:* It represents hollow spherical structure with a thin calcific rim.
- Can occur in:
    - Idiopathic fat necrosis: Small, several centimeters across the breast.
    - Common in large fatty breast.
- *Post-traumatic or postsurgical:* Larger.
- Rarely in the wall of the "garden variety", type of breast cysts which occur in fibrocystic disease.

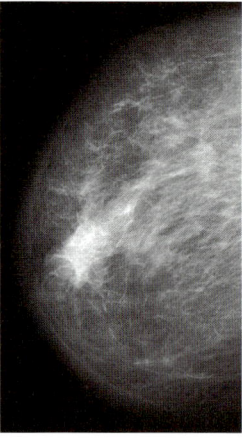

Fig. 2.10: Mediolateral mammogram shows breast edema and skin edema in erysipelas.

Breast: Mammographic Differential Diagnosis

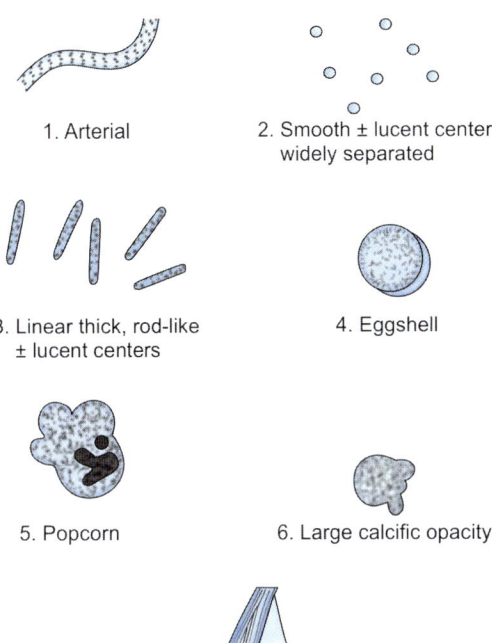

Fig. 2.11: Schematic diagram showing types of calcification.

- *Tram tracks calcification:* Railroad track calcification.
- The typical appearance of vascular calcification is that of two parallel calcific lines, along the vessel walls.
- These calcifications may be seen to be continuous with noncalcified soft tissue shadows of the vessels.
- *Large rod-like calcification:* These follow the course of the ducts branching out in a series of orderly areas which radiate from the retroareolar area.

- These occur in the duct lumen as solid cores, and are due to benign secretory involvement.
- These are distinguishable from malignant linear calcification by being longer, wider, and more variable in width, and being more frequently B/L (Bilateral).
- *Popcorn calcification:* It is characteristic of fibroadenoma.
- *Dystrophic calcification:* Dystrophic calcification resulting from surgery and/or radiation therapy often has a bizarre or plaque-like shape and is frequently large.
- *Milk of calcium:* It represents calcium that layers out in the dependent portion of tiny microcysts.
- Best seen on horizontal beam lateral view—which demonstrates a calcium-fluid level or meniscus (the tea-cup sign) while a craniocaudal view will show a round smudge shadow often, but not always B/L (Bilateral).
- *Skin calcifications:* There may be punctate or tiny hollow spheres of 1–2 mm diameter each.
  – These occur in sebaceous glands
  – Most common locations are in the periareolar, axillary, and medial breast areas.
- Sometimes may present as localized cluster of punctate calcification, rather than diffuse calcification.
  In these cases, findings that raise the possibility that clustered calcification may be in the skin and do not require biopsy, in comparison to clustered parenchymal calcification that do require biopsy, include a peripheral location (frequently in the subcutaneous tissue), or a location in the periareolar region, axillary area, or medial breast. The presence of one or more tiny hollow spherical calcifications within the cluster also suggests skin calcifications.
- True nature can be confirmed by tangential view, which projects the cluster in the skin.
- *Pseudocalcification:* These include aluminum chloride deodorant seen in the axilla or talcum powder seen in the inframammary area or in the medial side of breasts.

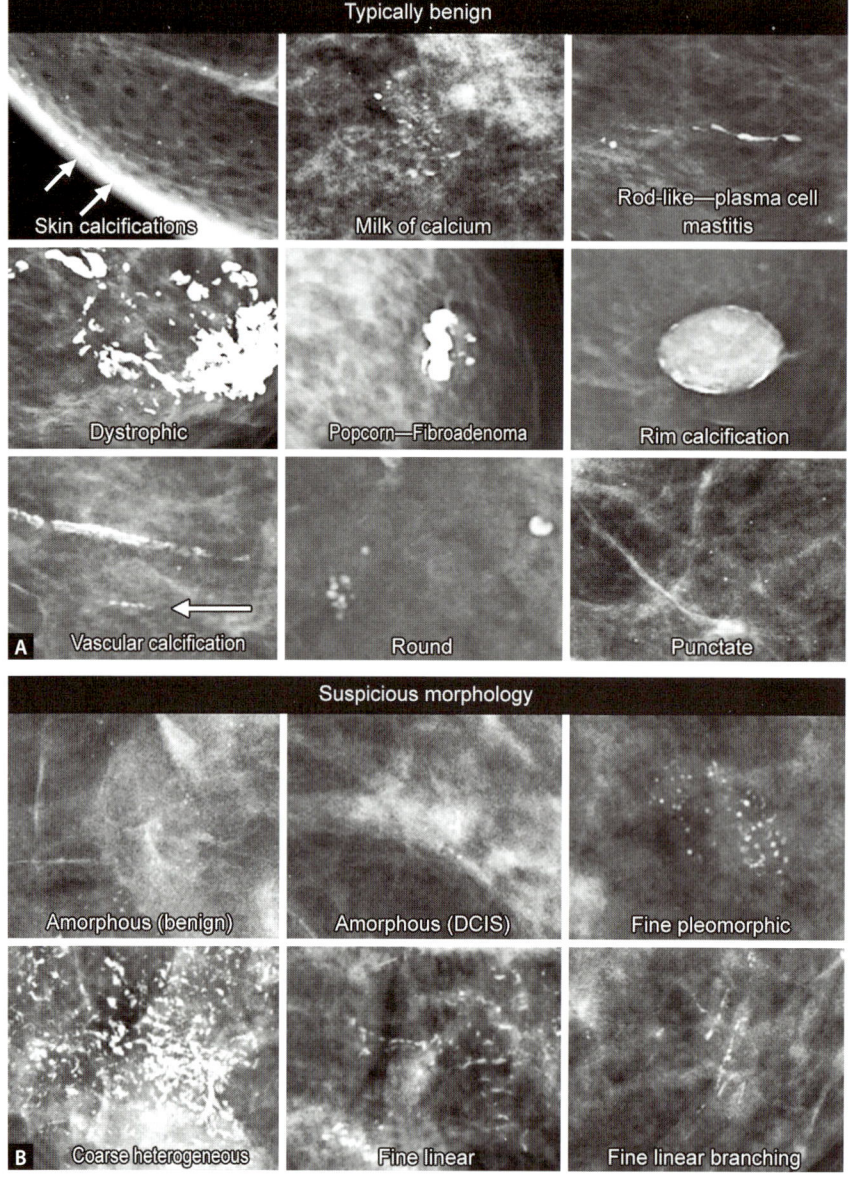

Figs. 2.12A and B: Images showing different types of calcification.

- Confirmation can be obtained when necessary, by repeating the appropriate view, after the area has been cleaned.
- *Calcification suspicious for malignancy:*
  - Characteristics required for suspicion of malignancy:
    - Linear (casting shape)
    - Linear distribution
    - Segmental distribution
    - Markedly clustered distribution.
  - *Characteristics not specific for malignancy but increasing degree of suspicion:*
    - Variation in shape (pleomorphism)
    - Variation in size

- Irregular margins of individual particles
- Irregular boundaries of areas of calcification.

Malignant (Fig. 2.13)
- Linear (casting type)
- Linear distribution
- Segmental distribution
- Markedly clustered distribution
- Pleomorphism in size and shape
- Irregular margins of individual particles
- Irregular boundary with areas of calcification.

Calcification
- Microcalcification is defined as individual calcific opacities measuring less than 0.5 mm in diameter.
- *Macrocalcification:* Opacities more than 0.5 mm in diameter.
- Microcalcification is not specific to carcinoma.
- Microcalcification is seen in 30-40% of carcinomas on mammography.
- Macrocalcification may be found in carcinoma.

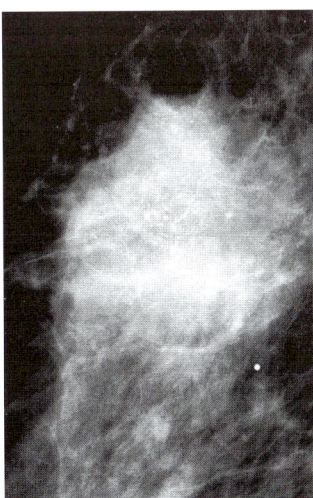

Fig. 2.13: Magnified mammogram shows multiple microcalcifications in breast carcinoma.

Definitely Benign
- *Arterial*—tortuous, tramline.
- Smooth, widely separated, and some with radiolucent center.
- Linear thick, rod like, widespread, and some with radiolucent center.
- *Eggshell curvilinear:* Margin of cyst, fat necrosis.
- "Popcorn" in fibroadenoma.
- Large individual calcific opacity more than 2 mm, e.g. involutional fibroadenoma.
- *Floating calcification*—seen as calcific/fluid level seen on lateral oblique projection in "milk of calcium" cysts.

Probably Benign
- *Widespread*—one/both breasts.
- Macrocalcification of one size.
- Symmetrical distribution.
- Widely separated opacities.
- Superficial distribution.
- Normal parenchyma.

Possibly Malignant—Biopsy is Indicated (Fig. 2.13)
- *Microcalcification*—particularly segmental, cluster distribution (>five particles in 1.0 cm³ space; of these 30% will be malignant).
- *Mixture of sizes and shapes*—linear, branching, and punctate.
- Associated suspicious soft tissue opacity.
- Microcalcification eccentrically located in soft tissue mass.
- Deterioration on serial mammography.

Benign Conditions that Mimic Malignancy
- Microcalcification
- *Sclerosing adenosis:* One/both breasts, widely separated opacities.
- Suspicious soft tissue opacity.
- *Fibroadenoma*—when one margin is ill defined.
- *Fat necrosis*—ill defined, sometimes with radiolucent center.
- Postbiopsy scar.

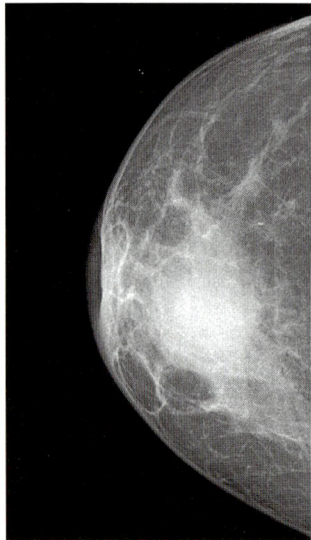

Fig. 2.14: Craniocaudal mammogram shows skin edema and retraction of nipple in carcinoma breast.

- Radial scar.
- Plasma cell mastitis.
- Hematoma.
- Summation of normal tissues.
- Irregular skin lesion, e.g. wart.

CARCINOMA

Primary Features

- *Opacity*—ill defined, spiculated outline, and comet tail. Usually dense.
- *Microcalcification*—mixture of sizes, and shapes; linear, branching, and punctate cluster arrangement. Eccentric to and/or outside soft-tissue opacity.

Secondary Features (Fig. 2.14)

- *Distortion*—adjacent tissues, obliteration subcutaneous, and retromammary spaces.
- Skin, nipple retraction.
- Edema—all or part of breast.
- Halo—wide around primary opacity.
- Duct dilatation.
- Venous engorgement.

Note: Approximately 10% of palpable carcinomas in premenopausal women are not diagnosable on mammography.

Chapter 3

Cardiovascular System

DIFFERENTIAL DIAGNOSIS OF CARDIOVASCULAR DISORDERS

Pericardial Effusion (Flowchart 3.1)

- Pericardial fluid more than 50 mL.
- Change in size and shape of the cardiac contour on chest X-ray (CXR) occurs only when the fluid is more than 250 mL.
- It is difficult to differentiate between pericardial effusion and chamber enlargement.
- An important clue favoring effusion is rapid enlargement of cardiac silhouette without significant changes in the lung.

Causes

- Malignancy
  - Secondaries normally from breast, lung
  - May cause tamponade
  - Usually hemorrhagic.
- Inflammatory: Bacterial, viral, tuberculous infection. Exudative in nature.
- Heart diseases
  - Cardiac failure—transudative in nature
  - Myocardial infarction—known as Dressler's syndrome.
- Endocrine diseases
  - Myxedema causes substantial pleural effusion, often asymptomatic.
- Collagen diseases: All collagen diseases may cause pericardial effusion. Systemic lupus erythematosus (SLE) causes large pericardial effusion.
- Uremia
  - 18% in acute uremia
  - 51% in chronic uremia
  - May lead to tamponade.
- Hemopericardium
  - Traumatic
  - Rupture of heart in course of myocardial infection (MI). Dissecting aneurysm leading into pericardium (Flowchart 3.1).

INVISIBLE MAIN PULMONARY ARTERY

Underdeveloped Main Pulmonary Artery (Table 3.1)

- Tetralogy of Fallot
  - Obstruction of right ventricular outflow tract due to pulmonary stenosis.
  - Associated ventricular septal defect (VSD) and right ventricular hypertrophy.
  - Overriding of aorta.
- Pulmonary stenosis
  - Due to reduced flow.
  - Associated right ventricular hypertrophy.
  - Decreased pulmonary vascularity.
- Tricuspid stenosis
  - Due to reduced blood flow into the right ventricle and pulmonary artery.
  - Enlarged right atrium.
  - Hepatic congestion–anasarca.

Misplaced Pulmonary Artery

- Complete transposition of great vessels.
  - Pulmonary trunk is absent in 99%—pulmonary artery is located posteriorly in midline.
  - "Egg on its side" appearance of heart with narrow superior mediastinum.
- Persistent truncus arteriosus—single artery giving rise to pulmonary and systemic aortic stenosis (AS).
  - Cardiomegaly with enlarged left atrium.

Differential Diagnosis in Radiology

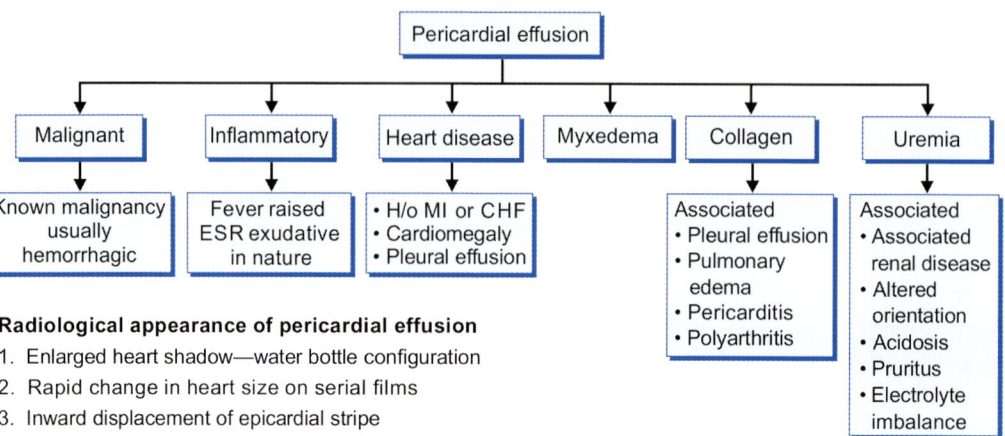

Flowchart 3.1: Pericardial effusion.

Radiological appearance of pericardial effusion
1. Enlarged heart shadow—water bottle configuration
2. Rapid change in heart size on serial films
3. Inward displacement of epicardial stripe
4. Loss of retrosternal clear space in lateral view
5. Differential density sign—increase in lucency at heart margin

Table 3.1: Causes of differential features of underdeveloped pulmonary artery.

Causes of underdeveloped pulmonary artery	Clinical features	Main pulmonary artery	Heat shadow	Pulmonary flow	Associated features
Tetralogy of Fallot	Cyanosis, fainting spells on exertion	Underdeveloped	RVH concave pulmonary bay, upward prominence of cardiac apex, cor-En-sabot appearance	Decreased	Pulmonary stenosis, VSD, Right aortic arch
Pulmonary stenosis	Mostly asymptomatic cyanosis, heart failure	Underdeveloped	Right ventricular hypertrophy	Decreased	Cor pulmonale
Tricuspid atresia	Progressive cyanosis from birth	Underdeveloped	Right atrial enlargement, enlarged LV small pulmonary bay	Decreased	ASD, small VSD
Complete transposition of great arteries	Cyanosis, symptomatic 2 wks. After birth	Located in midline posteriorly	Right heart enlargement, "egg on side" appearance	Increased	PDA and patent foramen ovale, VSD in 50%
Truncus arteriosus	Cyanosis, CHF systolic murmur	Arising from single trunk Along with system arteries		Markedly increased	Right aortic arch in 35%, forked ribs

- Large aortic shadow.
- Markedly increase pulmonary blood flow.

PULMONARY ARTERIAL HYPERTENSION (FIG. 3.1)

Sustained Pulmonary Artery Pressure more than 30 mm Hg (Flowchart 3.2)

- Primary
  - Idiopathic, 3rd decade M<F dyspnea, syncope.
- Secondary
  - Parenchymal pulmonary disease
    * Cor pulmonale, chronic obstructive pulmonary disease (COPD), chronic bronchitis, asthma, emphysema, and interstitial fibrosis.
    * Alveolar hypoxia and hypercapnia— pulmonary vasoconstriction— pulmonary arterial hypertension.
  - Congenital heart disease
    * Large left to right shunt (Eisenmenger's syndrome) ASD, ventricular

Cardiovascular System

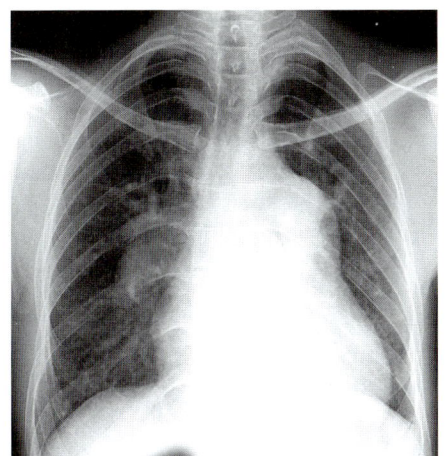

Fig. 3.1: Posteroanterior radiograph of chest shows cardiomegaly with enlarged pulmonary trunk and right inferior pulmonary artery in pulmonary arterial hypertension.

septal defect (VSD), patent ductus arteriosus (PDA) lead to increased pulmonary blood flow, leading to increased pulmonary resistance—pulmonary arterial (PA) hypertension.
  ♦ Tetralogy of Fallot.

- Pulmonary thromboembolism: Thrombus impacted in pulmonary arteries—rise in pulmonary arterial pressure—pulmonary arterial hypertension.
  ♦ Modest increase in heart size.
  ♦ Pulmonary oligemia.
  ♦ Right ventricular enlargement.
- Arteritides, e.g. Polyarteritis nodosa: Narrowing of pulmonary arteries causes increase in pressure—PHT.

Radiographic Appearance of Pulmonary Arterial Hypertension

- Large triangular heart
- Large main and central pulmonary artery
- Pruning of pulmonary arteries
- Calcification of central pulmonary vessels.

ENLARGED LEFT VENTRICLE (ELV)

Volume Overload

- Ventricular septal defect (VSD) (Fig. 3.2)
  - Most common congenital heart disease. Bouts of respiratory infection, feeding problems, failure to thrive.

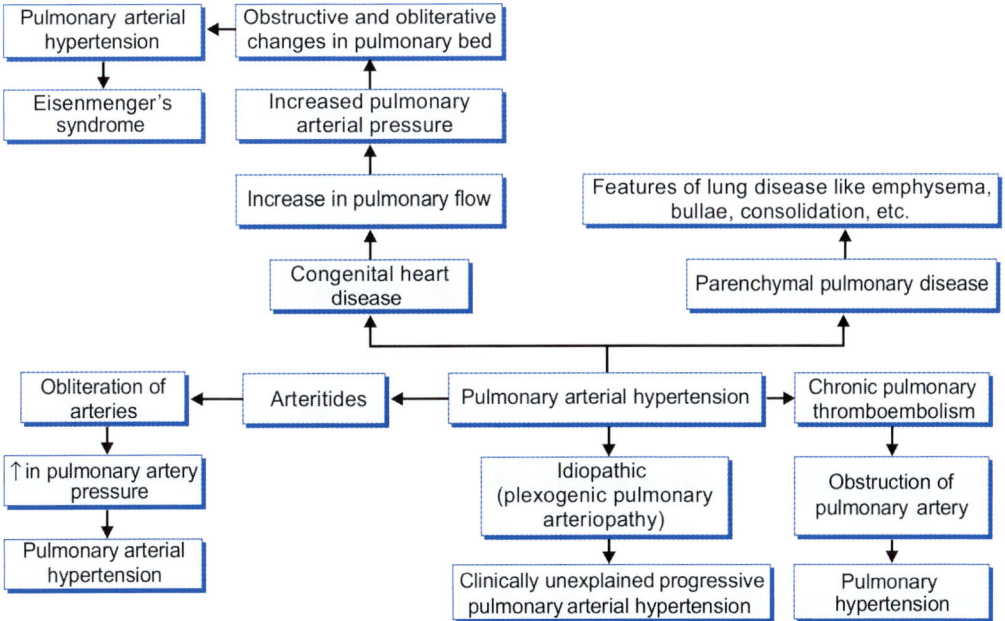

Flowchart 3.2: Pulmonary arterial hypertension.

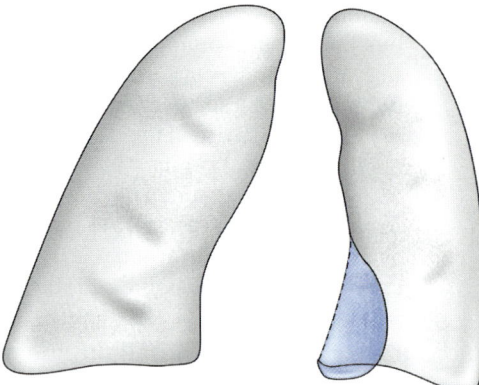

(PA view: Chest shows prominent LT heart border (inferior part). Rounding of LT heart border (apex of heart).

Fig. 3.2: Apex displaced inferiorly – ventricular septal defect.

- Increased pulmonary vascular resistance causes left ventricle (LV) enlargement.
• Patent ductus arteriosus (PDA)
  - Mostly asymptomatic. Congestive heart failure usually by 3 months of age. Continuous murmur. Enlarged RV, LV and LA, enlarged pulmonary artery segment and enlarged aorta.
• Mitral incompetence
  - Backward flow of blood from LV into LA during systole with consequent increase in LV volume.
  - LA + LV enlargement, mitral annular calcification.
• Aortic incompetence
  - Water hammer pulse with systolic ejection and high pitched diastolic murmur.
  - LV enlargement with dilatation of aorta.

Pressure Overload

• Aortic stenosis
  - Angina, syncope, heart failure with systolic murmur.
  - Calcification of aortic valve.
  - Enlarged LV with post-stenotic dilatation of ascending aorta in 90% cases.
• Coarctation of aorta
  - Shelf-like narrowing of aorta usually beyond the origin of left subclavian artery.
  - Small irregular contour of upper descending aorta on X-ray.
  - Rib notching.
• Systemic hypertension
  - Due to increased resistance to blood flow.
  - May lead to congestive heart failure (Fig. 3.3).
  - Dyspnea on exertion, headache.

High Output States

• Anemia.
• AV fistula.
• Hyperthyroidism.

Myocardial Causes

• Cardiomyopathy
  - Cardiomegaly with poor contractility of ventricular wall.
  - Global heart enlargement.
• Ischemic heart disease.
  - Coronary artery calcification.
  - Left ventricular aneurysm may be present.

ENLARGED LEFT ATRIUM

Volume Overload (Table 3.2)

• Mitral regurgitation
  - VSD Refer to cause of enlargement of left.
  - PDA Ventricle for salient features.
  - ASD with shunt reversal.

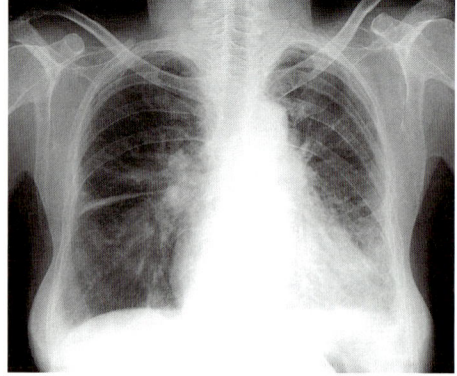

Fig. 3.3: Posteroanterior radiograph of chest shows cardiomegaly with signs of pulmonary edema, bilateral minimal pleural effusion and right fissural fluid in congestive cardiac failure.

Cardiovascular System

Pressure Overload (Table 3.3)

- Mitral stenosis (Figs. 3.4 and 3.5)
  - History of rheumatic fever.
  - Shortness of breath on exertion.
  - Left atrial enlargement with universal enlargement of left atrial appendage.
  - Changes in pulmonary circulation with pulmonary venous hypertension.
- Left atrial myxoma
  - Dyspnea, chest pain, fever, myalgia, weight loss, raised ESR.
  - Enlargement of LA, no enlargement of atrial appendage.

Table 3.2: Volume overload.

	Clinical features	Chamber enlargement	Pulmonary artery	Pulmonary veins	Pulmonary vasculature	Associated features
Mitral incompetence	Fatigue, exertional dyspnea orthopnea	LA + LV	Normal	Mild pulmonary venous HT	Normal	Frequent mitral annular calcification
Aortic incompetence	Collapsing pulse, early diastolic murmur	LV enlargement dilated aorta	Normal	Pulmonary venous HT	Normal	Dilatation + calcification of ascending aorta
VSD	Dyspnea, syncope, chest pain, hemoptysis	LA + LV + RV	Enlarged	Pulmonary venous HT in shunt reversal	Pulmonary plethora	Small aorta
PDA	CHF by 3 months of age	LV + LA + RV	Enlarged	—	Increased	Enlarged ascending aorta and arch
Aortic stenosis	Angina syncope, systolic murmur	LV hypertrophy	Normal	Pulmonary venous congestion		Post-stenotic dilatation of aorta
Coarctation of aorta	Lower extremely cyanosis, headache, cold extremities	LV hypertrophy, dilated left subclavian artery and dilated ascending aorta	Normal	Normal	—	Enlarged pulsatile collateral in intercostal spaces
Cardiomyopathy	Congestive cardiac failure	LV enlargement or globular heart	Normal	Prominent	—	Rib notching

Table 3.3: Pressure overload.

	Clinical features	Chamber enlargement	Pulmonary artery	Pulmonary veins	Aorta	Associated features
Mitral stenosis	Dyspnea, cough orthopnea	Esp. left atrial appendage RV enlargement LV enlargement	Prominent	Prominent with pulmonary venous HT	Small	Ossific nodules in lung, Kerley's lines
Mitral regurgitation	Fatigue, exertional dyspnea	LA + LV	Normal	Prominent but mild venous HT, then MS	Enlargement	Kerley's lines, less frequent
VSD	Dyspnea, syncope, chest pain, hemoptysis	LA, LV, RV	Enlarged pulmonary plethora	Pulmonary venous HT occurs in Eisenmenger's syndrome	Small	
PDA	CHF by 3 months of age	LA, RV + LV	Enlarged		Enlarged	Obscured aortopulmonary window
Myxoma	Dyspnea, weight loss, fever, increased ESR	LA, No enlargement of left atrial appendage		Pulmonary venous HT	Small	

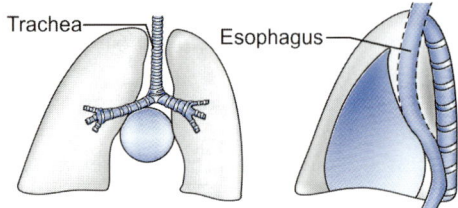

PA view: 1. Obliteration of concavity on LT heart border. 2. Double RT cardiac border. 3. Elevated LT carinal angle more than 70° and splaying of carina. 4. Prominent LT atrial appendage and straigtening of LT heart border

RAO view: Barium swallow shows LT atrial enlargement shadow or impression

Fig. 3.4: Mitral valvular disease.

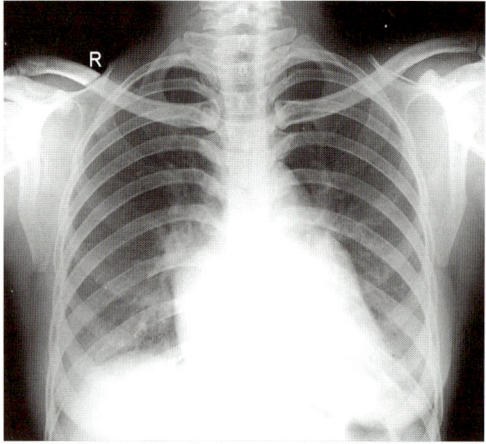

Fig. 3.5: Posteroanterior radiograph of chest shows cardiomegaly with enlarged left atrium and its appendage in rheumatic heart disease.

Secondary to Left Ventricular Failure

Radiographic features of enlarged left atrium are mentioned as follows:
- Straightening of left heart border or discrete bulge below the pulmonary conus.
- Double heart shadow progressing to form the right heart border.
- Displacement of barium-filled esophagus backwards (in lateral view).
- Splaying of carina and elevated left main bronchus.

DILATATION OF PULMONARY TRUNK

- Idiopathic
  - Unexplained dilatation of main pulmonary artery.
- Pulmonary regurgitation
  - High-pitched diastolic blowing murmur.
  - Enlarged RV.
- Poststenotic dilatation in pulmonary valve stenosis
  - Mostly asymptomatic.
  - Enlarged pulmonary trunk and left pulmonary artery.
  - Hypertrophy of RV with elevation of cardiac apex.
- Congenital L-R shunts
  - Due to volume overload in RV and pulmonary artery.
  - RV enlargement.
- Pulmonary artery hypertension
  - Large and often triangular heart.
  - Main and central pulmonary arteries are large.
  - Pruning of pulmonary arteries, i.e. tapering to periphery.
- Pulmonary artery aneurysm
  - Can be traumatic or mycotic.
  - Focally dilated main pulmonary artery with convex pulmonary bay.

ENLARGEMENT AORTA

- Volume overload
  - Aortic regurgitation
    - Water hammer pulse, diastolic murmur.
    - LV enlargement.
  - Patent ductus arteriosus (PDA)
    - Continuous murmur.
    - Enlargement RV, LV and LA. Enlargement of pulmonary artery segment, and pulmonary plethora.
- Poststenotic dilatation in aortic stenosis
  - Angina, syncope.
  - Calcification of aortic valve.

- Left ventricular enlargement.
- Enlarged ascending aorta.
- Pressure overload
  - Coarctation of aorta
    - Shelf-like narrowing of aorta beyond the origin of left subclavian artery.
    - Small irregular contour of upper descending aorta on X-ray with rib notching.
  - Systemic hypertension
    - May lead to left ventricular failure.
    - Dyspnea on exertion.
- Aneurysm of aorta (Fig. 3.6)
  - Congenital.
  - Mycotic.
  - Syphilitic—there is widening of mediastinum.
  - Atherosclerotic or round or oval soft tissue mass.
  - Traumatic in mediastinum with or without dissecting aneurysm with peripheral rim of calcification.

SMALL AORTA

- Aortic stenosis
  - Angina, syncope, heart failure with systolic murmur.
  - Calcification of aortic valve.
  - Left ventricular hypertrophy.
- Mitral stenosis
  - History of rheumatic fever (Fig. 3.5).
  - Shortness of breath on exertion.
  - Left atrial enlargement with universal enlargement of left atrial appendage.
  - Pulmonary venous hypertension with pulmonary ossific nodules.
- Left to right shunts
  - Most of the blood flows into right-sided chambers and into the pulmonary circulation causing pulmonary plethora.
  - Left ventricle recovers less blood and aorta is small.
- Hypertrophic obstructive cardiomyopathy
  - Asymmetrical hypertrophy of the left ventricle with difficulty in filling of LV.
  - Shortness of breath, angina, arrhythmias, jerky pulse.
  - Left ventricle has a chunky outline.
- Long segment coarctation of aorta (infantile or tubular hypoplasia)
  - Hypoplasia of long segment of aortic arch after origin of innominate artery.
  - Co-existent cardiac anomalies are common.
  - Congestive heart failure (CHF) in neonatal period (in 50%).

ENLARGED RIGHT ATRIUM (TABLE 3.4)

- Volume overload
  - Tricuspid regurgitation
    - There is systemic venous congestion and reduction of cardiac output.
    - Right-sided heart failure, hepatomegaly, ascites, and anasarca.
    - RV and RA enlargement (Fig. 3.7).
  - Atrial septal defect
    - Most common congenital heart defect in subjects more than 20 years of age.
    - Usually presents more than 40 years.
    - Mildly symptomatic, dyspnea, fatigue, palpitations.
    - Chest X-ray hilar dance (increased pulsations of central pulmonary arteries).

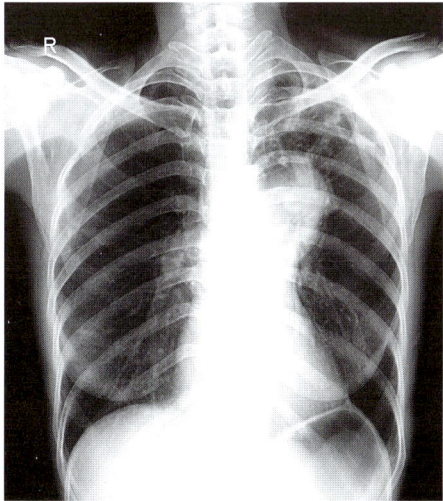

Fig. 3.6: Posteroanterior radiograph of chest shows aneurysm of arch of aorta. Incidental note is made of the fibrotic changes in left upper lobe.

Table 3.4: Enlarged right atrium.

	Clinical features	Chamber enlargement	Pulmonary vasculature	Pulmonary arteries	Pulmonary veins	Associated features
Tricuspid regurgitation	Systemic venous congestion, hepatomegaly, ascites	RV and RA	Normal or diminished	Normal or small	Normal	Right heart failure, pleural effusion edema, systolic pulsations of liver
ASD	Respiratory infections, feeling difficulties, arrhythmias	RA + RV	Hilar dance due to → pulsations of pulmonary arteries	Prominent		Loss of visualization of SVC
Total anomalous pulmonary venous return	Cyanosis, right ventricular heave	RA + RV figure of 8 appearance, dilated SVC	Increased pulmonary flow		Absent connection of pulmonary veins to LA	Neck veins undistended
Tricuspid stenosis	Fatigue refractory edema, ascites, hepatomegaly	RA and SVC enlargement	Oligemia	Small with flat concave pulmonary segment	Normal	
Right atrial myxoma	Systemic venous congestion	Enlarged RA, SVC, IVC and azygous vein	Decreased	Normal		Pulmonary emboli may arise
Secondary to LVF	Dyspnea, orthopnea, PND fatigue edema, ascites	LV, LA → RV and RA → Congestive heart failure	Redistribution of flow to upper lobes	Elevated pulmonary arterial pressure with PHT	Dilatation of pulmonary veins	Pleural and interlobar effusion

- RA and RV enlargement and pulmonary plethora.
  - Total/Partial anomalous pulmonary venous return.
    * Pulmonary veins drain blood into right atrium.
    * Increased pulmonary blood flow.
    * ASD restores oxygenated blood to left side.
    * Volume overload to RV: Cyanosis, right ventricular heave (i.e. increased contact of RV with sternum).
    * Figure of '8' or Snowman configuration of cardiac silhouette.
- Pressure overload
  - Tricuspid stenosis/Atresia.
    * Pulmonary oligemia, small pulmonary bay.
    * Right atrial enlargement, bulging the heart shadow to the right.
  - Myxoma of right atrium.
    * Causes occlusion of tricuspid valve and RA enlargement.
    * Systemic symptoms of fever, increased ESR, weight loss.
- Secondary to right ventricular failure (Fig. 3.8)
  - Congestive hepatomegaly, anasarca and systemic venous distension.

Cardiovascular System

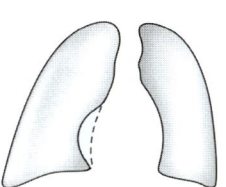
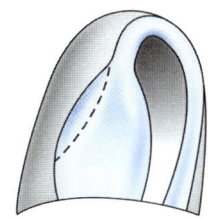

PA view: Prominent right heart border

Lateral view: Anterosuperior part of cardiac outline is promient

Fig. 3.7: Enlarged right atrium.

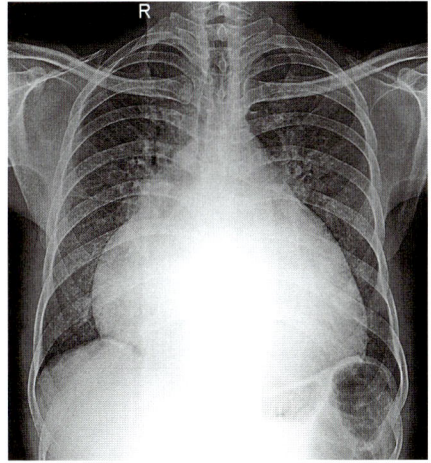

Fig. 3.8: Posteroanterior radiograph of chest shows biventricular enlargement in case of rheumatic heart disease with mitral stenosis and mitral regurgitation.

ENLARGED RIGHT VENTRICLE (TABLE 3.5)

Volume Overload

- Atrial septal defect
  - Increased amount of blood entering the right atrium and hence right ventricle.
  - Increased pulmonary flow with prominent pulmonary arteries.
  - Right atrial and right ventricle enlargement.
- Total/Partial anomalous pulmonary venous return
  - Pulmonary vein drains blood to the right atrium.
  - Volume overload of right ventricle with pulmonary over circulation/plethora.
- Tricuspid regurgitation
  - Increased amount of blood entering RV during diastole.
  - Right heart failure with systemic venous congestion.
- Pulmonary regurgitation
  - High-pitched diastolic murmur.
  - Enlarged RV (Fig. 3.9).
- Ventricular septal defect
  - Flow of blood from LV to RV—increased output of RV— increased size.
  - Enlarged RV, pulmonary artery.
  - Pulmonary plethora.

Pressure Overload

- Pulmonary stenosis.
  - Increased contractility of RV—RVH.
  - Pulmonary oligemia, small pulmonary bay.
- Pulmonary hypertension.
  - Increased resistance to right ventricular outflow—RVH.
  - Pruning of pulmonary arteries with enlarged proximal part.
- Tetralogy of Fallot.
  - Due to associated pulmonary stenosis.
- Ventricular septal defect.

Secondary to Left Heart Disease/Mitral Stenosis (Fig. 3.10)

- Increased left atrial pressure—pulmonary venous hypertension—pulmonary arterial hypertension—RVH.

RIGHT AORTIC ARCH

- Mirror image type—brachiocephalic branches being the mirror image of normal.
  - Tetralogy of Fallot (refer to the previous section for features)
  - Truncus arteriosus
  - Transposition of great vessels
  - Tricuspid atresia
  - Large VSD—refer to previous section for salient features.

Transposition of Great Vessels

- Right aortic arch in 3%
- Pulmonary artery originating from LV and aorta from RV

Differential Diagnosis in Radiology

Table 3.5: Enlarged right ventricle.

	Clinical features	Chamber enlargement	Pulmonary vasculature	Pulmonary arteries	Pulmonary veins	Associated features
ASD	Respiratory infections, feeding difficulty	RA + RV	Overcirculation	Prominent		Loss of visualization of SVC due to clockwise rotation of heart due to RVH
Total anomalous pulmonary venous return	Cyanosis, right ventricular heave	RA + RV "figure of 8" appearance of heart	Increased flow		Absent connection of pulmonary veins to LA	Neck veins undistended
Tricuspid regurgitation	Systemic venous congestion	RV + RA	Normal or diminished	Normal or small Enlarged	Normal	Right heart failure, pleural effusions
Pulmonary regurgitation VSD	High pitched diastolic murmur dyspnea, syncope, chest pain	RV + RA LA, LV, RV	Increased pulmonary plethora	Enlarged	Pulmonary venous hypertension in reversal of shunt	Small aorta
Pulmonary stenosis	Angina, syncope	RV, RA	Oligemia	Small with concave pulmonary bay		
Pulmonary hypertension, tetralogy of Fallot	Syncope, angina, shortness of breath	RV enlargement with large triangular heart	Clear lung fields	Enlarged central pulmonary artery with peripheral pruning		
Left heart disease	Dyspnea, orthopnea fatigue edema, ascites	LA, LV, RV, RA and congestive heart failure	Redistribution of flow to upper lobes	Elevated pulmonary arterial pressure with PHT	Dilatation of pulmonary veins	Pleural and interlobar effusion

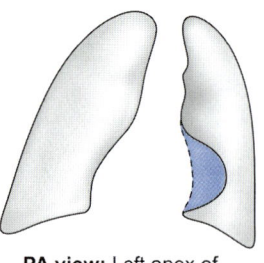 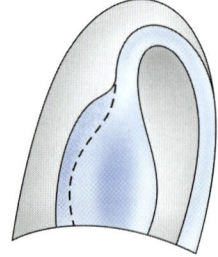

PA view: Left apex of heart is prominent and elevated

Lateral view: Whole anterior part of cardiac shadow is prominent

Fig. 3.9: Enlarged right ventricle.

- Egg on its side appearance of heart with narrow superior mediastinum
- Right heart enlargement.

Right Aortic Arch with Anomalous Left Subclavian Artery

- Bulbous configuration of origin of LSA—retro-esophageal aortic diverticulum (from descending aorta)
- Small rounded density left lateral to trachea
- Right aortic impression on tracheal air shadow.

Cardiovascular System

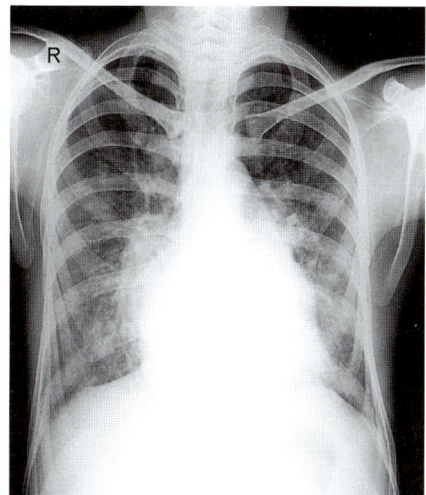

Fig. 3.10: Posteroanterior radiograph of chest shows cardiomegaly with signs of pulmonary venous hypertension in case of rheumatic heart disease.

Causes

- Tetralogy of Fallot
- ASD ± VSD Refer to previous sections for
- Coarctation salient features.

PULMONARY VENOUS HYPERTENSION

- Increased pulmonary venous pressure.
- Pulmonary capillary wedge pressure more than 15 mm Hg.

Causes

Left Ventricular in Flow Tract Obstruction

- Proximal to mitral valve—normal left atrium
  - Total anomalous pulmonary venous return (below the diaphragm).
    * Pulmonary venous return into portal vein/IVC/ductus venosus/left gastric vein with constriction of descending pulmonary vein by diaphragm, enroute through esophageal hiatus—pulmonary venous hypertension.
    * Pulmonary edema + pulmonary venous congestion.
  - Constrictive pericarditis
    * Fibrous thickening of pericardium interfering with filling of ventricular chambers.
    * Dyspnea, peripheral edema, neck vein distension.
    * Dilatation of SVC, azygos vein, and pulmonary venous hypertension.
  - Fibrosing mediastinitis
    * Widening of upper mediastinum
    * Compression of SVC + pulmonary veins.
  - Primary pulmonary veno-occlusive disease
    * Fibrous narrowing of intrapulmonary veins
    * Pulmonary edema, pleural effusion
- At mitral valve level—enlarged left atrium (Fig. 3.10)
  - Mitral stenosis
    * Redistribution of pulmonary blood flow to upper lobes due to back pressure.
    * Interstitial pulmonary edema and alveolar edema.
  - Left atrial myxoma.
  Obstructs the mitral valve with pulmonary back pressure similar to MS.
- Ball valve thrombus.

Left Ventricular Failure

- Increased preload, increased after load, high output failure.
- Transmission of back pressure to left atrium—pulmonary veins—pulmonary venous hypertension.

ENLARGED SUPERIOR VENA CAVA

Increased Volume of Blood Flow

- Tricuspid regurgitation
  - Systemic venous congestion and reduction of cardiac output.
  - Right-sided heart failure.
  - RV and RA enlargement.
  - Congestive hepatomegaly and anasarca.

- Supracardiac total anomalous pulmonary venous return
  - Pulmonary veins drain into superior vena cava.
  - Superior vena cava is dilated.

Obstructive Causes (Superior Vena Cava Syndrome)

- Bronchogenic carcinoma.
  - Lymphoma.
  - Mediastinitis.
  - Constrictive pericarditis.
  - Retrosternal goiter.
  - Ascending aortic aneurysm.
    - Head and neck edema.
    - Cutaneous enlarged venous collaterals.
    - Superior mediastinal widening.
    - Encasement/compression/occlusion of SVC.

CARDIAC CALCIFICATIONS

Pericardial Calcifications

- Idiopathic pericarditis
  - Calcification occurs at front and sides, not at back as fluid does not collect here.
  - There may be pleuropericardial adhesions roughening the outline of heart.
- Rheumatoid arthritis
  - Pericarditis occurs in 20–50% cases.
  - Features of bones involvement—osteoporosis, erosions.
  - Pleural effusion, interstitial fibrosis.
- Tuberculosis
  - Most important infectious cause.
  - Causes constrictive pericarditis.
- Viral infection
- Chronic renal failure
  - Associated pleural effusion, ascites, pericardial effusions.
- Radiotherapy to mediastinum
  - May lead to pericarditis, pericardial fibrosis and calcification.

Myocardial Calcifications

- Infections—viral or bacterial.
  - This can be suspected when CHF occurs in relation to viral pyrexia and bacterial sepsis.
- Myocardial aneurysm—may show wall calcification.
- Rheumatic fever—causes myocarditis.
  - May produce pericardial effusion, pleural effusion.

Intracardiac

- Valvular—(See in valvular calcifications).
- Cardiac tumors—atrial myxoma, rhabdomyoma and fibroma.

CARDIAC VALVE CALCIFICATIONS (FIGS. 3.11A AND B)

- *Aortic valve:* Indicates significant aortic stenosis.
  - Congenitally bicuspid valve = 70% to 85%
  - Atherosclerotic degeneration
  - Rheumatic AS
  - Syphilis.
- Mitral valve
  - Rheumatic heart disease
  - Mitral valve prolapse.
- Pulmonary valve
  - Tetralogy of Fallot
  - Pulmonary stenosis
  - Atrial septal defect.

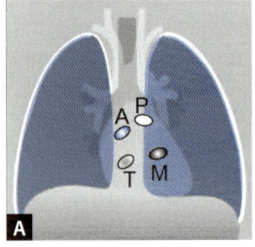 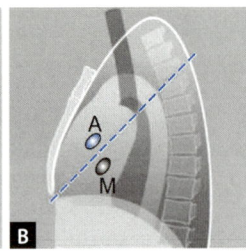

Figs. 3.11A and B: (A) The position of the valves on the frontal CXR. P = Pulmonary; A = Aortic; M = Mitral; T = Tricuspid. (B) The position of the aortic (A) and mitral (M) valves on the lateral CXR. The dotted line extends from the carina to the anterior costophrenic angle. A useful rule of thumb: calcification situated mainly above this line will lie in the aortic valve calcification situated mainly below this line will lie in the mitral valve.

- Tricuspid valve
  - Rheumatic heart disease
  - Atrial septal defect
  - Infective endocarditis.

SITUS

Term describing position of atria, tracheobronchial tree, pulmonary arteries, thoracic and abdominal viscera.

Situs Solitus—Normal Situs

- Abdominal
  - Liver and IVC are right-sided.
- Cardiac
  - Morphologic right atrium is right-sided.
  - Morphologic left atrium is left-sided.

Situs Inversus (Fig. 3.12)

Mirror image of normal.
- Abdominal
  - Mirror image position of abdominal organs.
- Cardiac
  - Morphologic right atrium is left-sided.
  - Morphologic left atrium is right-sided.

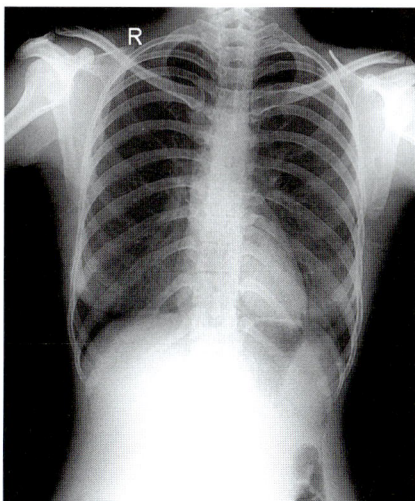

Fig. 3.12: Posteroanterior radiograph of chest shows situs inversus with dextrocardia and gastric shadow under right dome of diaphragm.

Situs Intermedius/Ambiguous

- Abdominal
  - Liver may be midline.
  - Bowel malrotations.
- Cardiac
  - Indeterminate atrial morphology.
  - Bilateral right atria/Bilateral left atria.

CYANOTIC HEART DISEASE

Cyanotic Heart Disease

- Increased pulmonary flow
  - Complete transposition of great arteries.
  - Truncus arteriosus.
  - Total anomalous pulmonary venous connection.
  - Common atrium.
  - Double outlet right ventricle.
  - Single ventricle without pulmonic stenosis.
- Normal or decreased pulmonary blood flow
  - Tricuspid atresia.
  - Tetralogy of Fallot.
  - Pulmonary arteriovenous fistula.
  - Pulmonary atresia with intact interventricular septum.
  - Pulmonary stenosis with right to left atrial shunt.
  - Double outlet right ventricle with pulmonic stenosis.

Acyanotic Heart Disease (With Left to Right Shunt)

- Atrial level
  - Atrial septal defect.
  - ASD with mitral stenosis (Lutembacher's syndrome).
  - Partial anomalous pulmonary venous return.
- Ventricular level
  - Ventricular septal defect.
  - VSD with aortic regurgitation.
  - VSD with LV to RA shunt.
- Aortic root to right heart shunt
  - Ruptured sinus of Valsalva aneurysm.
  - Coronary AV fistula.
  - Anomalous origin of left coronary artery from pulmonary trunk.

- Aortopulmonary shunt
  - Patent ductus arteriosus.
  - Aortopulmonary window.
- Multiple level shunts
  - ASD with VSD.
  - VSD with PDA.
  - Common atrioventricular canal.

Acyanotic without Shunt

- Left heart malformations
  - Congenital left atrial inflow obstruction
    - Pulmonary vein stenosis.
    - Mitral stenosis.
    - Cor triatriatum.
  - Mitral regurgitation
    - Congenitally corrected transposition of arteries.
    - Atrioventricular septal defect.
    - Primary dilated endocardial fibroelastosis.
    - Aortic stenosis/Regurgitation.
    - Coarctation of aorta.
- Right heart malformations
  - Acyanotic Ebstein's anomaly.
  - Pulmonic stenosis.
  - Congenital pulmonary regurgitations.
  - Idiopathic dilatation of pulmonary trunk.

Chapter 4

Soft Tissue Lesions

DIFFERENTIAL DIAGNOSIS OF SOFT TISSUE LESIONS

Increased Heel Pad Thickness or Heel Pad Sign (Flowchart 4.1)

- Normal < 21 mm
- Males > 23 mm
- Females > 21.5 mm.

Acromegaly

- Osseous enlargement, flared ends of long bones.
- Spade-like hands, widening of terminal tufts, prognathism, enlargement of paranasal sinuses, sellar enlargement.
- Posterior scalloping of vertebrae.

Myxedema

- Clinical features—fatigue, lethargy, constipation, cold intolerance, stiffening of muscles.
- Dull, expressionless facies, periorbital puffiness.
  - Calvarial thickening, wedging of dorsolumbar vertebrae, coxa vara.

Peripheral Edema

- Edema due to any reason will increase the heel pad thickness (Fig. 4.1).

Obesity

- Especially in children—heel pad is thick, because of fat deposition.

Epanutin Eptoin Therapy

- Erythematous eruptions, gingival hyperplasia may occur.

Infection/Injury

- Due to pus collection or hematoma formation, heel pad thickness may be increased.
- Increased heel pad thickness.

Mnemonic: MADCOP

- **M:** myxedema
- **A:** acromegaly
- **D:** phenytoin therapy
- **C:** callus
- **O:** obesity
- **P:** peripheral edema.

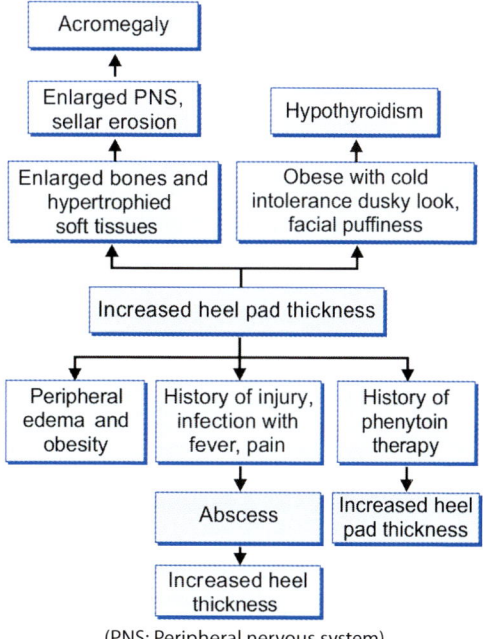

Flowchart 4.1: Increased heel pad thickness.

(PNS: Peripheral nervous system)

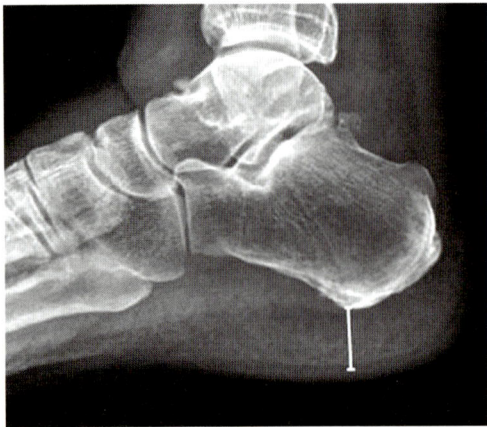

Fig. 4.1: Heel pad thickness is measured as shortest perpendicular distance from the lowest point of the calcaneal tuberosity to the plantar surface.

SOFT TISSUE OSSIFICATION

Leading to Formation of Trabecular Bone

- Myositis ossificans
- Burns
- Paraplegia
- Liposarcoma
- Parosteal osteosarcoma
- Congenital myositis ossificans progressiva
- Tumoral calcinosis
- Surgical scar.

Myositis Ossificans

- Benign solitary self-limiting ossifying soft tissue mass typically occurring in skeletal muscle
- Adolescents, young athletic adults
- Located in large muscles of extremities in 80%
- Well-defined partially ossified soft tissue mass after 6–8 weeks
- Radiolucent zone separating lesion from bone
- Periphery more denser than center.

Liposarcoma

- Second most common soft tissue sarcoma in adults
- Age: 5th-6th decade
- Usually painless, mass located in trunk, lower extremity–upper extremity, head and neck
- Amorphous calcification.

Parosteal Osteosarcoma

- Large lobulated cauliflower-like homogeneous ossific mass extending away from cortex
- Large soft tissue component with osseous and cartilaginous elements
- Periphery is less dense than center
- Located commonly at posterior aspect of distal femur, either end of tibia, proximal humerus and fibula.

Burns

- Ossification in relation to joints, commonly hips, elbows and shoulders
- May occur at sites distal to injury
- The cause is unknown.

Paraplegia

- Occurs in adults with spinal lesions and children with spinal dysraphism
- Particularly in relation to pelvis
- Woolly appearance.

Congenital Myositis Ossificans Progressiva

- Autosomal dominant or primary mutation
- Ossification in perimuscular fascia, not in muscles
- Sheets of bone in neck, thorax, and limb
- Abnormally short metacarpal of thumb and metatarsal of big toe.

Tumoral Calcinosis

- Masses of bones in soft tissue near joints
- May cause discomfort and limitation of movement.

Surgical Scar

- True bone may form away from any preexisting bone structure or periosteum.

LINEAR CALCIFICATION OF SOFT TISSUES

Arterial

- Diabetes
  - Occurs commonly in calf-region
  - Associated diabetic nephropathy or cystopathy.
- Hyperparathyroidism
  - Calcification in arterial tunica media
  - Cornea, vessels, and periarticular region
  - Chondrocalcinosis
  - Associated bone erosions, brown tumors.
- Werner's syndrome
- Atheroma (Fig. 4.2)
  - Plaque-like calcification, linear calcification of walls.
  - Commonly femoral and popliteal arteries.

Venous

- Thrombosed veins
  - Phleboliths are present.
- Varicose veins.

Nerves

- Leprosy
  - Areas of calcification, reticulated pattern.
  - Joint space preserved.
  - Absorption of nasal spine, alveolar ridge.
  - Neurotrophic joints.
- Neurofibromatosis
  - Soft tissue masses.
  - Optic nerve gliomas.
  - Ribbon ribs, sphenoid dysplasia, and pseudoarthrosis.

Ligamentous (Fig. 4.3)

- Tendinitis
  - Pellegrini-Stieda lesion—calcification of medial collateral ligament of knee.
- Ankylosing spondylitis (Fig. 4.4)
  - Posterior longitudinal/anterior longitudinal ligament calcification.
- Fluorosis (Figs 4.5 and 4.6)
  - Sacrotuberous and sacrospinous ligamentous calcification, increased bone density
  - Interosseous membrane calcification.
- Alkaptonuria
  - Calcification in paravertebral soft tissues and tendon insertion
  - Disk calcification
  - Massive osteophytosis.

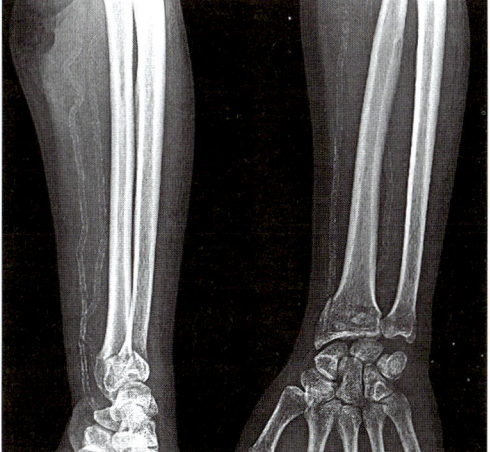

Fig. 4.2: Anteroposterior and lateral radiographs of forearm show arterial calcification.

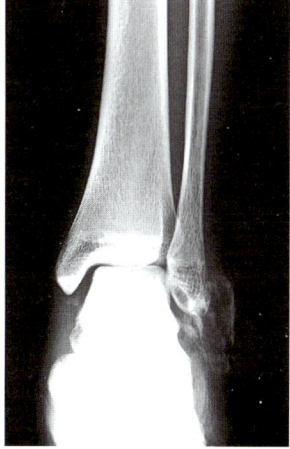

Fig. 4.3: Anteroposterior radiograph of ankle shows soft tissue ligamentous calcification adjacent to lateral malleolus.

PARASITIC CALCIFICATION (TABLE 4.1)

Cysticercus Cellulosae (Figs. 4.7 and 4.8)
- Calcified cysts produce oval shadow 10–15 mm long and 2–3 mm broad with a translucent center
- Number of cysts usually in hundreds
- Arranged in direction of muscle fibers
- May be associated with cysts in brain.

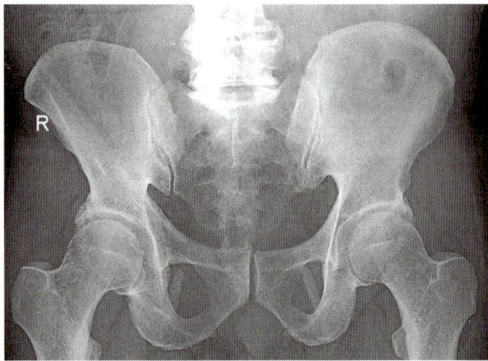

Fig. 4.6: Anteroposterior radiograph of pelvis shows calcification in bilateral sacrotuberous ligament and osteosclerosis of lower lumbar spine in fluorosis.

Loiasis (Calabar Swelling)
- Caused by microfilaria
- Found in subcutaneous tissues and undergoes calcification after death
- Commonly in hands, in web spaces
- Coiled thread-like opacities with amorphous calcification.

Guinea Worm
- Calcifies after its death.
- Elongated or coiled strip of calcium density.
- May be crushed by muscle action into a round irregular mass.

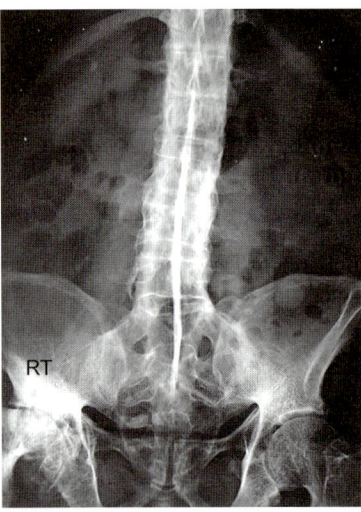

Fig. 4.4: Lateral radiograph of dorsolumbar (DL) spine in ankylosing spondylitis shows anterior longitudinal ligament calcification.

Armillifer Armillatus
- Curved in one plane (comma-shaped)
- Chest and abdomen.

AREAS OF DECREASED DENSITY

Fat
- Lipomas
- Normal sites
  - In front of lower end of humerus, below patella (Fig. 4.9), in front of Achilles tendon.
- Lipohemarthrosis
  - Following fractures
  - Particularly around knees and shoulders.

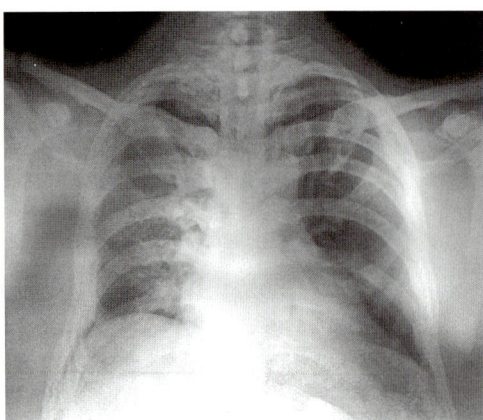

Fig. 4.5: Posteroanterior radiograph of chest shows diffuse osteosclerosis in fluorosis.

Soft Tissue Lesions

Table 4.1: Periarticular soft tissue calcification.

Features	Gout	Sarcoidosis	Secondary HPT	Hyper-vitaminosis D	Synovial osteochondro-matosis	Synovioma
Age	> 40 years	20–40 years	–	–	20–50 years	20–50 years
Type of calcification	Large nodular calcification in gouty tophi	–	Periarticular, arterial walls, chondrocalci-nosis, viscera	Metastatic calcinosis in periarticular areas—putty-like premature falx calcification	Multiple calcified bodies	Large sphenoid well-defined soft tissue mass with amorphous calcification
Site	Hands and feet, 1st MTP most common ear > bones, tendons and bursae	Small bones of hands and feet	Around hip, knee, shoulder, wrist	Periarticular + arterial walls + nephrocalcinosis	Large joints knee > elbow > hip > shoulder > ankle	Knee most common, hip ankle, elbow, wrist, hands, feet
Bone changes	Punched out lytic bone lesions, mouse bite erosions with overhanging margins joint space is preserved	Reticulated lace-like trabecular pattern in middle and distal phalanges with cystic lesions acro-osteolysis	Osteosclerosis, especially axial skeleton, pelvis, ribs, clavicles, Rugger-Jersey spine	Cortical + trabecular dense calvaria widening of provisional zone of calcification	Pressure erosion of bone or secondary degenerative changes widening of joint space and accumulation of loose bodies	Periosteal reaction, bone remodeling due to pressure invasion of cortex and juxta-articular osteopenia
For	Dermatomyositis Scleroderma Tumoral Calcinosis	Refer to generalized calcinosis.				

(HPT: Hyperparathyroidism; MTP: Metatarsophalangeal)

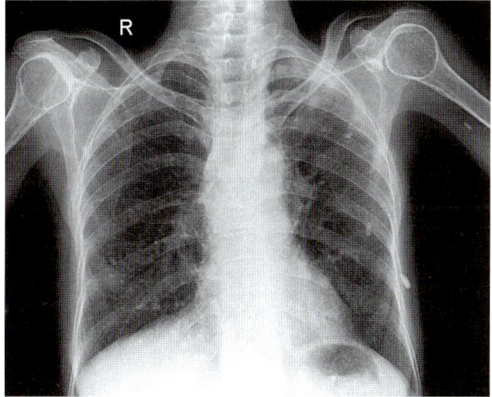

Fig. 4.7: Posteroanterior radiograph of chest shows multiple oval calcifications in soft tissues in cysticercosis.

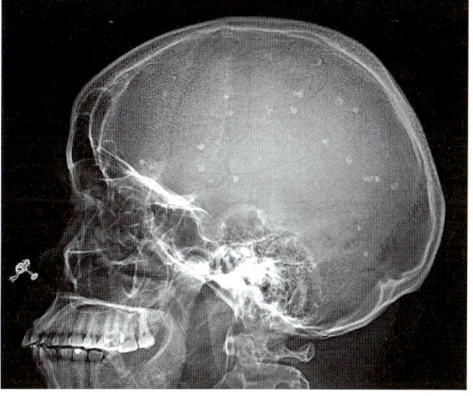

Fig. 4.8: Lateral radiograph of skull shows multiple calcified lesions in neurocysticercosis.

Differential Diagnosis in Radiology

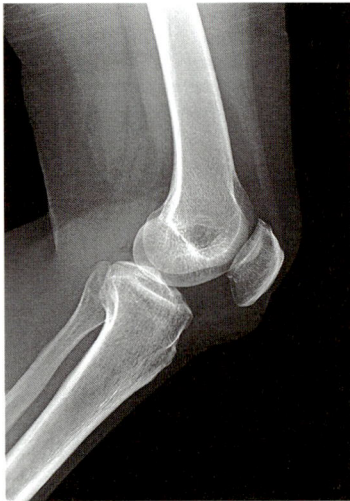

Fig. 4.9: Lateral radiograph of knee joint shows infrapatellar lipoma.

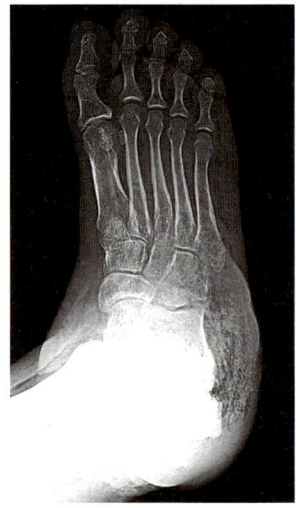

Fig. 4.10: Anteroposterior radiograph of foot shows aeroceles in soft tissues in gas gangrene.

Gas

- Hernias
  - Containing intestine
  - Seen below inguinal ligament or in scrotum.
- Air entering from outside
  - Air bubbles near compound fractures.
  - Fractures of peripheral nervous system (PNS)—air in facial soft tissues.
  - Soft tissues of chest from lungs—after rib fractures, laceration of lung, thoracocentesis or after surgery.
  - From mediastinum.
- Lower abdominal wall or thigh—following rupture of pelvic abscess or after perforation of a hollow viscus.
- Gas formed in tissues (Figs. 4.10 and 4.11)
  - Infection in diabetes, by *Clostridium welchii*.
  - Anerobic myositis.

PERIARTICULAR SOFT TISSUE CALCIFICATION

Inflammatory

- Scleroderma
- Dermatomyositis
- Gout.

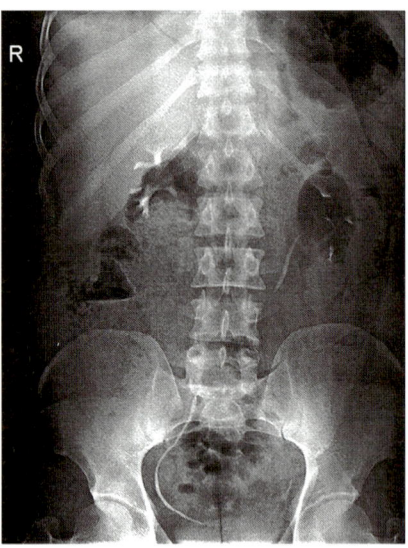

Fig. 4.11: Anteroposterior radiograph of abdomen shows aeroceles with air fluid level in right lumbar region in right paracolic abscess.

Degenerative

- Calcium pyrophosphate dihydrate deposition disease.

Renal Failure

- Secondary hyperparathyroidism.

Table 4.2: Sheet-like calcification.

Features	Congenital myositis ossificans progressiva	Dermatomyositis
Type	Autosomal dominant	Inflammatory myopathy
Calcification	In perimuscular fascia and not in muscles	Necrosis, fibrosis and calcification in muscles
Parts commonly affected	Sheets of bone in neck, thorax and limbs	Extremities, elbows, knees, hands abdominal wall and chest wall
Age	Early childhood	5–15 years and 50–60 years
Bone changes	Short metacarpal of thumb and metatarsal of big toe + abnormality of vertebrae	Pointing and resorption of terminal tufts

Hypercalcemia

- Sarcoidosis
- Hypervitaminosis D
- Milk alkali syndrome.

Neoplastic

- Synovial osteochondromatosis
- Synovioma.

Idiopathic

- Tumoral calcinosis.

GENERALIZED CALCINOSIS

- Collagen vascular disorders
  - Scleroderma
  - Dermatomyositis
- Idiopathic tumoral calcinosis
- Idiopathic calcinosis universalis.

Scleroderma

- Calcinosis of skin
- Raynaud's phenomenon
- Esophageal dysmotility
- Sclerodactyly
- Telangiectasia.

Dermatomyositis

Inflammatory myopathy with linear and confluent calcifications in soft tissues.
- Pointing and resorption of terminal tufts
- Respiratory muscle weakness
- Dysphagia.

Idiopathic Tumoral Calcinosis

- Progressive large nodular juxta-articular calcified soft tissue masses
- Normal serum calcium and phosphorus and no metabolic/renal or collagen disease
- Diaphyseal periosteal reaction with patchy areas of calcification in medullary cavity
- Calcinosis cutis.

Idiopathic Calcinosis Universalis

- Children and young adults
- Plaque-like calcium deposits in skin and subcutaneous tissues
- Sometimes in tendons and muscles
- No true bone formation.

SHEET-LIKE CALCIFICATION IN SOFT TISSUE (TABLE 4.2)

- Congenital myositis ossificans progressiva.
- Dermatomyositis.

Chapter 5

Abdomen and Gastrointestinal Tract and Hepatobiliary System

DILATED ESOPHAGUS

Normal versus Abnormal Appearance of Esophagus

Normal
- Wall thickness 3 mm when adequately distended
- 5 mm when incompletely distended

Abnormal
- Greater or eccentric thickness
- AP diameter esophagus – more than 16 mm
  Lateral diameter esophagus – more than 24 mm

Abnormal
- Air-filled level–obstructive or motility disorders
  Fluid-filled lumen
  Lumen caliber more than 10 mm

Strictures

Smooth
Inflammatory
Peptic, Barrett's
Scleroderma
Corrosive

Neoplastic
Carcinoma
Mediastinal tumors
–Cancer bronchus
Leiomyoma

Others
Achalasia
Iatrogenic

Irregular
Neoplastic
Carcinoma
Leiomyosarcoma
Carcinosarcoma
Lymphoma

Inflammatory
Reflux (rarely)
Crohn's disease

Iatrogenic
Radiotherapy
Fundoplication

Prolonged use of nasogastric tube

Skin disorders
- Epidermolysis bullosa
- Pemphigus

Peptic Stricture

- Situated most frequently in the distal esophagus near the G-E junction.
- Associated with reflux and hiatus hernia.
- Most peptic strictures are circumferential. Occasionally may be asymmetrical with radiating folds or a pseudo-diverticular appearance.
- If luminal diameter less than 13 mm—associated with dysphagia.
- 14–19 mm – 50% cases—dysphagia.

Barrett's Esophagus

- The normal squamous epithelium is replaced by columnar epithelium. This usually begins in distal esophagus and progresses proximally.
- Esophagogram (nonspecific)—reflux, hiatus hernia, stricture, thickened folds, shallow ulcers and erosions.
- More specific finding—(double contrast) fine reticular mucosal pattern distal to a stricture (seen in < 1/3rd cases)
- In Barrett's esophagus—strictures usually develop at the junction of squamous and columnar epithelium.

Scleroderma

- Esophageal involvement seen in 75–85% cases.

- Caused by atrophy of smooth muscle and its replacement by connective tissue.
- Radiological features: Dilatation, atonicity, poor or absent peristalsis of gastroesophageal reflux through a widely open G-E junction—stricture.

Other Associated Features

- Raynaud's phenomenon
- Skin thickening
- Terminal phalanx resorption with soft tissue atrophy
- Erosions of distal interphalangeal, first carpometacarpal, metacarpophalangeal and metatarsophalangeal joints
- Respiratory system: Aspiration pneumonitis, interstitial lung diseases and fibrosis in left lower zone
- Small bowel-dilated, atonic with thickened folds and pseudosacculations.

Corrosives

- Ingestion of sodium hydroxide/acid ingestion
- Site of involvement—aortic arch, left main bronchus and above diaphragmatic hiatus
- Acute phase—edema, spasm, ulceration, loss of mucosal pattern at hold-up points
- After several weeks—smooth stricture develops—symmetrical and longitudinal.

Achalasia (Figs. 5.1 and 5.2)

Esophageal motor disturbance caused by failure of lower esophageal sphincter to relax.
- Loss of primary and secondary peristalsis
- Intermittent emptying.

Causes

- Idiopathic (absence of smooth muscle ganglionic cells).
- Secondary to Chagas disease.
  - Malignancy—with invasion of myenteric plexus, chest X-ray—dilated esophagus with air-fluid level. Barium examination—dilated sigmoid-shaped esophagus.

- "Bird Beak" appearance of distal esophagus.
- Loss of primary and secondary peristalsis in distal two-thirds of esophagus.
- Feature of esophagitis.
- Intermittent spurting of barium into the stomach, stricture classically occurs below diaphragm.

Leiomyomas

- Most common benign esophageal neoplasm, these are usually intramural in origin
- *Barium examination*: Sharply-defined smooth/lobulated defect with superior and inferior margins that form right angles with the luminal wall.

CT—shows the intra-luminal and extrinsic component.

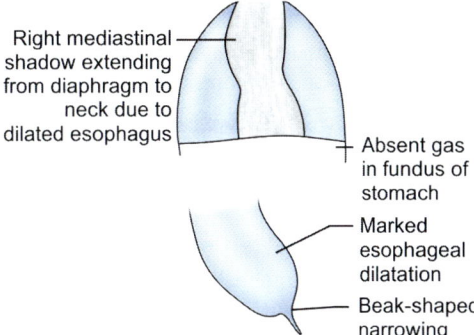

Fig. 5.1: Achalasia cardia—on barium study.

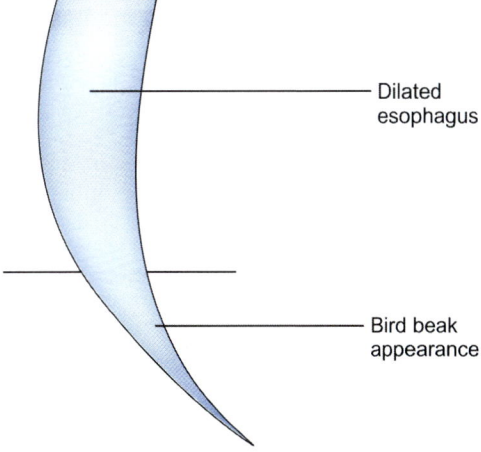

Fig. 5.2: Achalasia cardia.

Carcinoma Esophagus

Incidence, commonly seen in—Plummer-Vinson syndrome, Barrett's, cardiac disease, asbestosis and dye-ingestion.
- (10–20%) Adenocarcinoma—distal 1/3rd.
- (80–90%) Squamous (sq) cell carcinoma (ca)—middle 1/3rd.

Types
- Polypoidal, infiltrative, ulcerative and superior spreading
- Radiological features: Irregular filling defects.

Annular/Eccentric
- Extra-luminal soft tissue mass
- Proximal and distal shouldering
- Proximal dilatation
- Mucosal destruction/ulcerations
- Satellite lesions in esophagus.

Chest X-ray
- Mediastinum widening
- Tracheal deviation, anterior bowing of posterior tracheal wall
- Widened retrotracheal stripe (> 3 mm)
- Air-fluid level in esophagus.

Computed Tomography (CT)
For the extent of involvement: Tracheobronchial, aortic, pericardial invasion, mediastinal lymphadenopathy.

Esophageal Lymphoma (Rare)

Both non-Hodgkin's and less commonly Hodgkin's lymphoma may involve esophagus.

Invasion
- Mediastinal lymph nodes with esophageal invasion.
  - Extrinsic compression with irregular, serrated margins.
- Contiguous spread of lymphoma from gastric fundus (cannot be differentiated from carcinoma).
- Synchronous development of lymphoma in the wall of esophagus.
  - Submucosal nodules, enlarged folds, polypoidal masses, strictures.

Secondary Esophageal Neoplasms

Most common neoplasms that spread directly to esophagus are gastric and bronchial carcinoma.

Others
Hypopharyngeal, thyroid and primary mediastinal.
- Esophageal invasion from neoplasmatically-laden adjacent lymph node is more common than direct metastasis to the esophagus. (Most common primary sites are—lungs in males and breast in females).

Radiological Features
Extrinsic impression with regular/irregular margins and displacement of esophagus.

Radiation Esophagitis
Occurs when dose exceed 20 Gy (2000 rad) leading to ulceration, stricture and rarely perforation.

ESOPHAGEAL CARCINOMA

Predisposing Factors
- Achalasia 2–8% cases of long-standing achalasia undergo malignant degeneration because of chronic stasis induced esophagitis.
- Lye-like strictures (2–16%).
- Head and neck tumors (2–8%).
- Celiac disease.
- Plummer-Vinson syndrome (4–16%).
- Radiation (> 20 to 50 gray; Latent period—20 years).
- Tylosis autosomal dominant condition characterized by hyperkeratosis of palms and soles (95% cases > 65 years).
- Smoking and alcohol.
- Barrett's esophagitis (15%) predisposing factors for Adenocarcinoma.
- Scleroderma.

Pathology

Gross

- *Infiltrating*: Most common, irregular narrowing and constriction of lumen.
- *Polypoidal*: Lobulated/Fungating mass protrudes into the lumen.
- *Superficial Spreading*: Spreads superficially without invading deeper layers.
- *Ulcerative*: Flat masses in which the bulk of the tumor is replaced by ulceration.

Histology

Squamous cell carcinoma—80–90%
Adenocarcinoma—10–20%.

Japanese Society of Esophageal Disease

- Early esophageal carcinoma: Mucosa and submucosa involved
- Superficial esophageal carcinoma: Mucosal and submucosal involvement with lymph node metastasis
- Small esophageal carcinoma: Growth less than 3.5 cm regardless of depth of invasion of lymph node metastasis.

Distribution

- Squamous cell carcinoma has a relatively even distribution in the upper, middle and distal third of esophagus
- 75% of adenocarcinoma arise in the distal one-third at or adjacent to the gastroesophageal junction.

Routes of Spread

- *Direct extension*: Esophagus lacks mucosa, therefore, carcinoma spreads readily into adjacent structures—thyroid, larynx, trachea, bronchus, lungs, aorta, pericardium and diaphragm.
- *Lymphatic extension:* "Jump" metastasis can occur in the neck, mediastinal lymph nodes in the absence of segmental lymph node involvement because of rich interconnecting lymphatics in esophagus.
    - Sub-diaphragmatic lymph nodes—pericardial, lesser curvature and celiac lymph node.
    - Lymphatic metastasis can also occur within the esophagus which presents as submucosal nodules.
- *Hematogenous metastasis*: Lung, liver, adrenal, kidney, pancreas, peritoneum and bones.

Clinical Aspects

Dysphagia, odynophagia, anorexia, weight loss, persistent substernal chest pain, hoarseness of voice and chronic cough (aspiration and tracheoesophageal fistula), hematemesis.

Radiographic Findings

Early esophageal carcinoma: Double contrast esophagography is the best radiological technique and has increased sensitivity but less specificity.

Early esophageal cancer is seen as small protrusions less than 3.5 cm which may appear as:

- Plaque-like with central ulceration
- Sessile polyp with smooth/lobulated contour
- Focal irregularity/nodularity
- Superficial spreading carcinoma extends longitudinally in the wall without invading beyond the mucosa/submucosa and is seen radiographically as tiny coalescent nodules or plaques causing nodularity/granularity.

Advanced Carcinoma

- Chest X-ray shows mediastinal widening
- Hilar/retrohilar/retrocardiac mass
- Tracheal deviation, anterior bowing of posterior tracheal wall
- Widened retrotracheal stripe
- Air-fluid level in esophagus
- Barium studies
    - Irregular narrowing, nodular or ulcerated mucosa, proximal and distal shouldering, proximal dilatation (Fig. 5.3).
- Lobulated/fungated mass (intraluminal) usually more than 3.5 cm with areas of ulceration
- Well-defined meniscoid ulcer with a radiolucent rim of tumor surrounding the ulcer

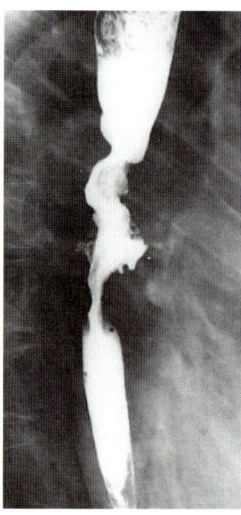

Fig. 5.3: Barium esophagogram in anteroposterior projection shows esophageal narrowing with proximal shouldering in a patient of esophageal carcinoma.

- Thickened, tortuous or serpiginous long filling defects because of submucosal spread which are known as varicoid carcinoma
  – Smooth extrinsic impression with gently sloping obtuse borders because of mediastinal lymphadenopathy.
  – Satellite lesions in esophagus and stomach because of lymphatic metastasis.
- Detection of complications on barium study
  – Esophago-airway fistula—lateral film.
  – Necrotic tumor containing cavity in lung/mediastinum communicating with the esophagus.

Computed Tomography (CT)

Best imaging modality for staging patients (Mediastinal invasion, mediastinal adenopathy and distant metastasis).
- Criteria for tracheobronchial invasion
  – Displacement of trachea/bronchus from the spine.
  – Indentation on the posterior wall of trachea/bronchus.
  – Bowing of posterior wall of trachea/bronchus.
  (Absence of fat plane between the trachea and/or bronchus and esophagus cannot be used to predict invasion).

- Criteria for aortic invasion
  – Area of contact more than 90% or 1/4th of aortic circumference.
  – Obliteration of the triangular fat space between aorta, spine and esophagus suggests of invasion.
- Criteria of pericardial invasion
  – Presence of mass effect with concave deformity of the heart associated with loss of normal fat plane in this region.
- Mediastinal adenopathy
  Limitations—CT cannot demonstrate lymph node metastasis that has not caused significant lymphadenopathy.
- Enlarged periesophageal lymph node cannot be detected because they are inseparable from the primary cancer.
- CT cannot differentiate benign from malignant lymph-adenopathy.

Sub-diaphragmatic Lymphadenopathy

Frequently the lymph nodes at or above the celiac axis are involved (>8 mm—Enlarged).

MRI

Superior to CT in detecting mediastinal invasion.

Endoscopic Ultrasound

- *Advantage*: Evaluates the depth of tumor invasion. Periesophageal lymph node can also be identified.
- *Disadvantage*: Esophageal ultrasound probe is unable to pass through a malignant stricture.

Differential Diagnosis of Esophageal Carcinoma

Early Esophageal Carcinoma

- *Squamous papilloma*: Small, sessile lobulated polyp.
- *Candida esophagitis*: Multiple plaque-like defects with intervening normal mucosa.
- *Pseudomembranes/inflammatory exudates*: Multiple plaque-like defects are present.

Abdomen and Gastrointestinal Tract and Hepatobiliary System

Advanced Carcinoma
- Benign stricture
  - Smooth, no mucosal destruction
  - No shouldering.
- *Esophageal varices:* On full column film the varicoid appearance disappears, and valsalva increases the varicoid appearance.
- *Leiomyoma*: Submucosal mass lesion with smooth margins which forms right angle.

THICKENED MUCOSAL FOLDS ESOPHAGUS AND STOMACH

Q. What are mucosal folds?
Ans. Folds are convolutions of mucosa, made so in order to the functional assimilative capacity of gut keeping the structural needs to minimum. The total surface area thus increases greatly but the length of intestine is kept to a minimum. It consists of epithelium, lamina propria, muscularis mucosa.

Q. Why is their demonstration so important?
Ans. Because this is the basic functional layer of gastrointestinal tract (GIT) and most diseases either originate or involve this layer early on.

Q. How are they radiologically demonstrated?
a. Mucosal relief
b. Full barium
c. Double contrast

Ans. a and c are techniques of choice to demonstrate early involvement and diseases of mucosa, submucosa and even distal layers may be shown, through their effects on mucosa and submucosa.

Thickened Esophageal Folds

Causes
- Varices
- Esophagitis
- Varicoid carcinoma
- Lymphoma.

Varices: Due to:
- Portal hypertension: Known as Uphill varices.
- SVC obstruction: Known as Downhill varices.
- Idiopathic: Due to congenital wall weakness.
  - Uphill
  - Downhill   Superior vena cava, thyroid;
  Above   Bronchial; Mediastinal
                      ↓
  Azygos   SVC → Heart
                      ↓
  Below/At   Azygos + Hemiazygos
  Azygos   Periesophageal plexus
  - CF Uphill → Bleeding anemia
    Downhill → SVD Syndrome; Bleed rare.
  - Imaging: Plain X-ray → Dilated azygous; ± Show
    as posterior mediastinal mass.
  - Barium
    - Prone (RAO).
    - ± Buscopan.
    - Wait/Watch.
    - Mucosal relief.
    - Irregular serpiginous filling defects.
    - Faintly merge (differential diagnosis cancer).
  - CT → Nodular enhancing streaks in wall.
  - Angiography → Celiac, SMA, portal, splenic
  - Change with respiration, deglutition, Valsalva, position.
  - TES/Doppler → Abnormal dilated vascular channels seen.

Esophagitis

Infectious → Candida; HSV; HIV; CMV; TB; Actinomycetes.
Non-infectious → Drugs; Caustic; RTT; NG Tube; Crohn's; Skin Diseases; Alcohol; GVHD.
- Fold thickening is nodular and scalloped.
- Associated specific findings seen:
  CMV → Giant ulcers.
  Candida → Plaques.
  HIV, HSV → Multiple aphthoid ulcers.
  TB → Strictures.
  Actinomyces → Sinus.
  Doxycycline and tetracyclines → Temporary superficial ulcers.
  Caustic → Long segment stricture.

Varicoid Carcinoma
- Its basically a morphological variant seen radiologically as fold thickening.

- Its etiology, histopathology and management protocol are nearly the same.
- Usually involves the lower esophagus.

Lymphoma
- MC secondarily involved from mediastinal nodes.
- Radiologically
  – Smooth extrinsic impression
  Intrinsic
  – Smooth tapered stricture with achalasia.
  Large mass
  Varicoid (Rare).

THICKENED GASTRIC FOLDS

- Normal variant.
- Gastritis—alcoholic (Flowchart 5.1)
  – Hypertrophic
  – Antral
  – Corrosive
  – *H. pylori* and other infections
  – Post-radiation
  – Post-freezing.
- Peptic ulcer disease.
- Zollinger-Ellison syndrome (ZES).
- Ménétrier's disease.
- Lymphoma.
- Pseudolymphoma.
- Carcinoma.
- Varices and antral vascular ectasia.

- *Infiltrative process:*
  – Eosinophilic gastritis
  – Crohn's disease
  – Sarcoidosis
  – Tuberculosis
  – Syphilis
  – Amyloidosis.
- *Adjacent pancreatic disease*
  – Acute pancreatitis
  – Extension of carcinoma pancreas.
- *Alcoholic gastritis:*
  – Due to prolonged use of large volume; corrected by cessation.
  – MCC of acute exogenous gastritis.
  – Sometimes folds become so bizarre as to mimics malignancy.
  – Due to mucosal and submucosal edema.
  – May progress to atrophic gastritis.
- *Hypertrophic gastritis:*
  – Idiopathic local/diffuse hypertrophy of mucosa and glands without their destruction.
  – Neuromuscular disorder, increased acid output, chronic inflammation.
  – Increased secretions, poor coating.
  – Thick (4–5 mm; N—1–2 mm), polygonal and angular areae gastricae seen.
  – Associated peptic ulcer commonly present.

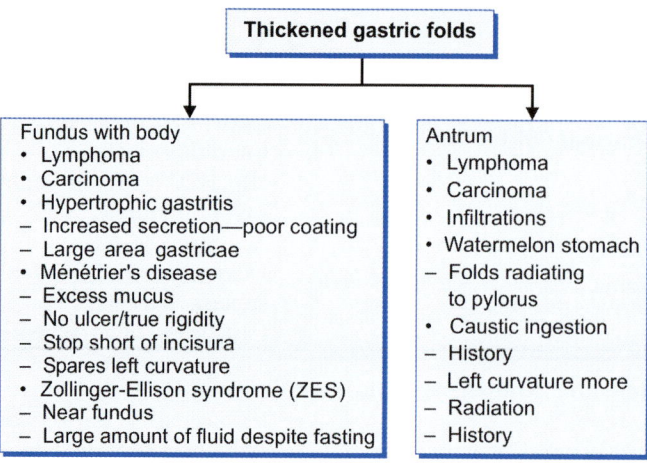

Flowchart 5.1: Thickened gastric folds.

- *Antral gastritis:*
  - Misnomer.
  - H. pylori, alcohol, tobacco, coffee.
  - ± a part of the spectrum of ulcer disease.
  - ± associated with antral spasm, with ± persistent/transient (Seen as loss of prepyloric shoulders).
  - Antral granulations seen.
- *Corrosive gastritis:*
  - Thick folds with ulcer, atony, rigidity.
  - Usually severe disease seen.
  - Fixed and gaping pylorus seen due to damaged muscles.
  - ± gas in the wall.
  - Antrum, body and LC most affected.
  - Acids more dangerous for stomach, alkaline for esophagus.
- *Helicobacter pylori* (and other infections):
  - Antrum and body affected more.
  - If fundus also involved d/d Ménétrier's disease.
  - On CT circumferential or focal thickening are seen points that need differentiation from malignancy.
  - CMV gastritis in AIDS leads to diffuse fold thickening and decreased distensibility.
  - Other infective processes causing similar changes are toxoplasmosis and cryptococcosis.
- *ZES and ulcer disease:*
  - Body and antrum (never fundus).
  - Increased acid output.
  - In ZES fundic mucosa is seen in antrum.
  - In ulcer disease only perilesional thickening is seen.
  - In ZES large amount of gastric fluid is seen despite adequate fasting.
- *Menetrier's disease*: (known as giant-hypertrophic gastritis)
  - Whole stomach especially fundus and body; diffuse or focal; ESP greater curve.
  - Abrupt transition between normal and abnormal folds.
  - Massive hypertrophy and hyperplasia of folds (i.e. glands) leading to brain-like appearance.
  - Decrease in acid.
  - Polypoidal appearance when seen end on.
  - Mottle/reticular appearance due to excess mucus.
  - Overall wall is thick and hypoperistalsis seen.
  - May be associated with or lead to adenocarcinoma.
  - 'Pediatric hypertrophic gastropathy' that presents as hypoalbuminemia in absence of any cause, thick mucosa and following viral infection is a distinct but related entity.
- *Lymphoma and pseudolymphoma:*
  - Pseudolymphoma is a benign proliferation of lymphoid tissue.
  - Gastric lymphomas are usually nodular in type, however other varieties may be ulcerative, polypoidal, infiltrative (that leads to fold thickening) and mixed types.
  - May lead to an associated ulcer, loss of wall pliability, lymphadenopathy (increased retrogastric space), splenomegaly, predominant involvement of distal stomach.
- *Carcinoma (Tables 5.1 and 5.2):*
  - As usually misunderstood, it is not the linitis plastica malignancies (diffuse infiltrative adenocarcinoma) that leads to fold thickening.
  - Malignancy leading to fold thickening is colloid carcinoma or mucinous adenocarcinoma which also have specks of calcification (Table 5.3).
  - Fold thickening with normal volume and pliability is seen.
  - Peristalsis is normal.

Table 5.1: Differentiating features between squamous cell carcinoma and adenocarcinoma.

Squamous cell carcinoma	Adenocarcinoma
Equal distribution in the distal esophagus	Most common, situated in upper, mid and lower esophagus
Rarely extends sub-diaphragmatically to involve stomach	Frequently extends and invades cardia/fundus
Most common type—Infiltrating	Most common type—Polypoidal and mixed polypoidal—infiltrative

Table 5.2: Differentiation features of lymphoma vs carcinoma.

		Lymphoma	Carcinoma
1.	Age	— Bimodal	— Mid-old
2.	CF	— Mass	— Mass + Bleed
3.	No.	— Multicentric +	— Rare
4.	Epicenter	— S/M	— Mucosa
5.	Distensibility	— N A/E HD	— (↓↓↓)
6.	Caliber	— N or ↓	— (↓↓↓)
7.	Loss of area Gastricae	— +	— –
8.	Enhancement	— ↑	— (↑↑↑)
9.	Perigastric fat	— N	— Involved
10.	Wall thickness	— ↑↑↑↑ (>3 cm)	— ↑↑
11.	HSM	— +	— ±/–
12.	Lymph node	— + (Above and below kidney)	— ±
13.	Extension to duo-denumesophagus	— ++	— ±
14.	Hemorrhage and necrosis	— ±	— +++
15.	Contour	— Regular	— Irregular
16.	Adjacent organ involvement	— +	— +++

Table 5.3: CT-differentiation of gastric adenocarcinoma from gastric lymphoma.

CT	Lymphoma	Adenocarcinoma
Wall thickness	4.0 cm	1.8 cm
Mean	1.1–7.7 cm	1.1–3.2 cm
Range	Regular 42%	Regular 27%
Contour	Irregular 58%	Irregular 73%
Extent	Diffuse 80%	Focal 87%
Direct spread to adjacent organs	42%	73%
Lymph node above/below renal hilum	42%	0%

- *Varices:*
    - In PHT are associated with esophageal varices but if isolated gastric varices are seen, then splenic vein thrombosis should be suspected.
    - Multiple, curvilinear, crescentic, smooth, lobulated filling defects with splenic impression.
    - Seen mainly in fundus extending to LC.
    - Charge in appearance.
    - Varices in antrum and body are due to obstruction of splenic vein proximal to patent coronary veins.
    - Watermelon stomach is a distinctive form of gastric antral vascular ectasia radiating to pylorus.
- *Infiltrative processes:* Conditions like eosinophilic gastroenteritis (eosinophilia with eosinophilic infiltration and exudation), Crohn's disease, amyloidosis, sarcoidosis, TB, syphilis cause diffuse rugal thickening.
- *Adjacent—pancreatic disease:*
    - Due to enzymatic mural irritation/spasm and due to perigastric inflammation.
    - Posterior wall and left coronary more.
    - Is an indicator of severe pancreatic inflammation.
    - Malignant infiltration causes distorted fold thickening.

Thickened Duodenal Folds

- *Inflammatory disease:*
    - Peptic ulcer disease
    - Brunner's gland hyperplasia
    - Zollinger-Ellison's syndrome (ZES)
    - Duodenitis
    - Pancreatitis
    - Cholecystitis:
        - Uremia
        - Tuberculosis (Fig. 5.4)
        - Crohn's disease (CD)
        - Parasitoses (Giardia, strongyloides)
        - AIDS
        - Non-tropical sprue.
- *Neoplastic:*
    - Metastasis to peripancreatic nodes
    - Lymphoma
    - AIDS-related malignancies.
- *Diffuse infiltrative disorders:*
    - Amyloidosis
    - Whipple's disease
    - Mastocytosis

- Eosinophilic enteritis
- Intestinal lymphangiectasia.
- *Vascular disorders:*
  - Varices
  - Mesenteric arterial collaterals
  - Intramural hemorrhage
  - Chronic duodenal congestion.
- *Cystic fibrosis (Mucoviscidosis):*
  - Peptic ulcer disease:
    * Most common cause.
    * May lead to Brunner's gland hyperplasia seen as nodular thickening of folds known as Cobblestone appearance.
    * These do not disappear on compression as compared to simple mucosal thickening.
  - Zollinger-Ellison syndrome (ZES):
    * Nonbeta is left cell tumor of pancreas.
    * Increased gastrin hyperstimulation of parietal cells and hypertrophy of rugae, hyperacidity and hypervolemic gastric secretions.

Ulcer Disease

Most common in bulb and stomach but also may occur in 2nd and 4th port of duodenum and jejunum.

Also giant ulcers due to excess acids that overwhelm the pancreaticobiliary secretions.

Also associated dilution and dilatation.

Disease may continue even after removal of primary and secondary or ectopic masses in stomach, duodenum, splenic hilum.

- *Duodenitis:*
  - Basically an endoscopic diagnosis.
  - Thick (>5 mm) duodenal folds are very sensitive but poorly- specific indicator (Fig. 5.5).
  - Hyperacidity leads to nodularity, deformity and spiculation.
  - Increased peristalsis is noted.
  - However, differentiation between different causes is not possible.
- *Pancreatitis/cholecystitis:*
  - Very important causes in everyday practice.

- Hyperirritable; poor filling; narrow lumen; widened sweep
- Thickening in periampullary and proximal second parts.
- *Uremia and chronic dialysis:*
  - First and second parts of duodenum show thick and irregular folds; rigid.
  - Due to associated pancreatitis; due to associated ulcer.

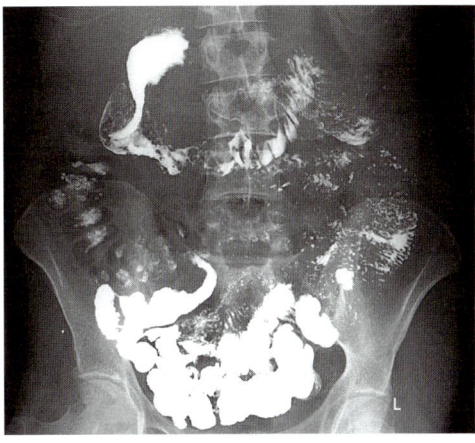

Fig. 5.4: Barium meal followthrough in anteroposterior projection shows duodenal narrowing in a patient of duodenal tuberculosis.

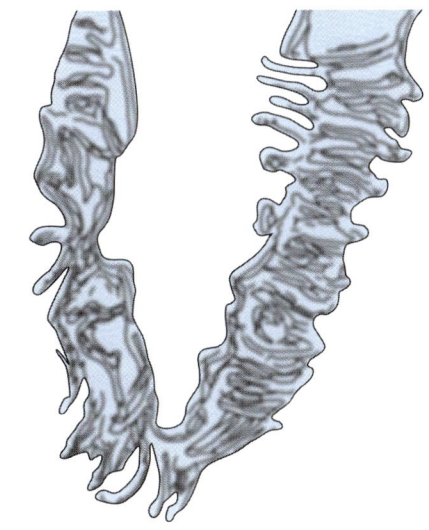

Fig. 5.5: Nodular and serpiginous thickening of duodenal mucosal fold involving 2nd port of duodenum.

- *Crohn's disease/tuberculosis:*
  - Associated ulcers and stenosis.
  - In tuberculosis associated antral/pyloric disease seen.
- *Other infection:*
  - Giardiasis—increased fluid, increased peristalsis and jejunal involvement.
  - Strongyloidosis—CD-like.
  - HIV-related cryptococcosis, MAIC, CMV-dilatation.
  - Non-tropical sprue—bizarre thickening with erosions in D1 and D2.
- *Neoplastic:*
  - Lymphoma—coarse, nodular, irregular.
  - Metastasis to lymph nodes—extrinsic impression mimicking thickened folds.
  - Kaposi sarcoma—submucosal infiltration.
- *Varices:*
  - Extrahepatic portal vein obstruction, intrahepatic portal vein obstruction, splenic vein obstruction.
  - Other associated varices.
    - Vertical compression on duodenum bulb 1 cm distal to pylorus by dilated posterosuperior pancreaticoduodenal vein.
    - Small variceal dilatation leading to Cobblestone appearance.
    - Large serpiginous varices.
    - An isolated varix on medial descending duodenal wall.
- *Mesenteric arterial collaterals:*
  - Atherosclerotic occlusive disease leading to blocked celiac trunk, SMA or both are the causes.
  - Basically from pancreaticoduodenal arcade and gastroduodenal artery, which are close to medial duodenal wall
    - Serpiginous filling defects.
    - C-loop widening.
    - Nodular defects may be seen.
    - Sharp impression on superior aspect of D1 due to aberrant right hepatic artery may be seen.
- *Intramural bleed/congestion:*
  - Stacked coin appearance
  - Bleeding disorder, trauma, anticoagulants
  - Congestion is due to cirrhosis and CHF.
- *Cystic fibrosis:*
  - Thick, coarse mucosa.
  - Nodules may be seen.
  - Smudging of coating.
  - Altered duodenal contour.
  - D1, D2 rarely jejunum.
  - Basically decreased HCO_3, increased H^+ leading to irritation.

THICKENED SMALL BOWEL
Folds (Flowchart 5.2 and Fig. 5.6)

- Thickened small bowel folds with dilatation—ZES; vascular insufficiency; infections; amyloidosis; abetalipoproteinemia; lymphoma; hypoalbuminemia; disease of intestinal wall and mesentery (secondaries, TB, CD).
- Thickened small bowel folds with gastric involvement—lymphoma; CD; eosinophilic enteritis; ZES; Ménétrier's disease; amyloid; Whipple's disease; varices.
- Thickened small bowel folds which are regular with no other feature.

Fold thickened: Jejunum more than 2.5 mm
Ileum more than 2.0 mm

Hemorrhage in Bowel Wall

Anticoagulants, ischemic bowel disease with infarction; vasculitis as thromboangiitis obliterans, Henoch-Schönlein purpura, collagen vascular disease hemophilia, idiopathic thrombocytopenic purpura; trauma; secondary clotting disorders as secondaries, myeloma, lymphoma, leukemia, hypofibrinogenemia.

Intestinal Edema

Hypoproteinemia—cirrhosis, protein losing enteropathy, nephrotic syndrome.

Lymphatic Block

Tumor, fibrosis, lymphangitis angioneurotic edema.
- *Intestinal lymphangiectasia:* Primary or secondary.
  - Abetalipoproteinemia.
  - Amyloidosis.

Abdomen and Gastrointestinal Tract and Hepatobiliary System

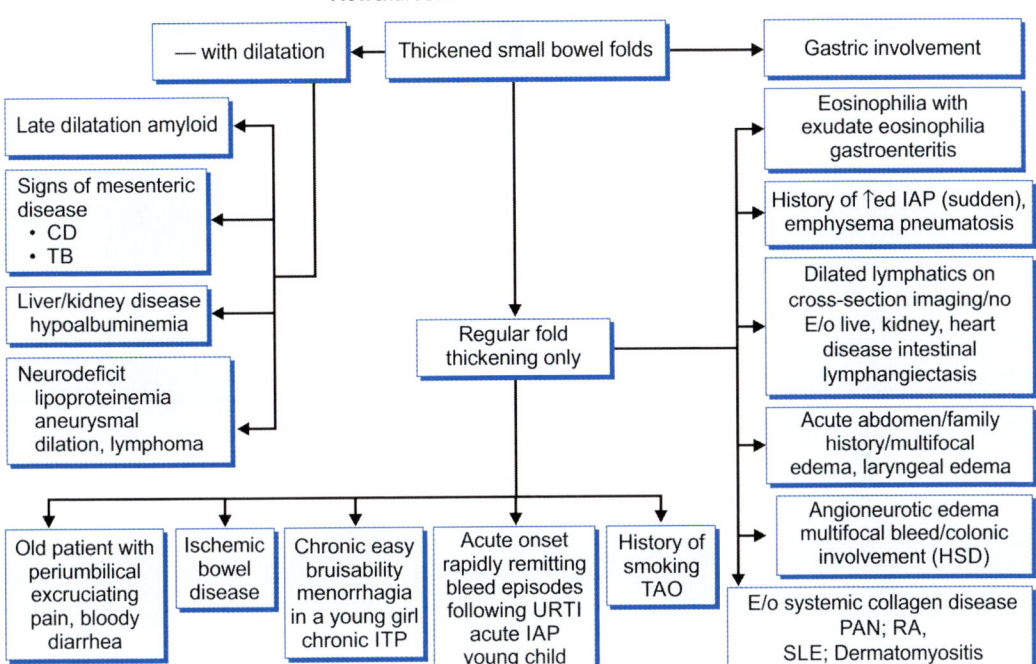

Flowchart 5.2: Thickened small bowel folds.

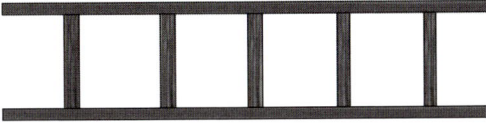

Fig. 5.6: Small bowel folds.

- Vasculitis.
- Pneumatosis intestinalis.
- Xanthomatosis.
- Eosinophilic gastroenteritis.
- *Vascular insufficiency:*
  - Acute catastrophic
    * Length
    * Collaterals
    * Severity
    * Chronic

Arterial/veno-occlusive disease.
Systemic hypovolemia.
Thickening of folds—hemorrhage + edema.
Dilatation—adynamic ileus.
- Disease of wall with mesentery
  - *Thickening*: Due to infiltration + Edema (Venous/lymphatic block)

(Metastatic, granulomatous, inflammatory)
- *Dilatation*: Mesenteric involvement leading to areas of obstruction.

Crohn's disease (CD), a disease that may involve any part of GIT from mouth to anus, has certain specific associated features like ulcer, stricture, fistula, sinus (also tuberculosis).

Crohn's disease, however, shows a poorly distensible stomach having irregular tubular narrowing and poor peristalsis, especially antral. If both sides of pyloric canal are involved, a characteristic Pseudo-Billroth I deformity results.
- *Infectious enteritis:*
  Nonspecific fold thickening and dilatation is seen in *Salmonella, strongyloidiasis, Candida, cytomegalovirus (CMV), Cryptococcus, Mycobacterium avium-intracellulare complex (MAIC).*
- *Hypoalbuminemia:*
  - Liver and kidney disease
  - Infiltration free of cells
  - Dilatation + thickening

- Gastric fundal rugae +–
- Albumin threshold more than 2.7 g%
- *Abetalipoproteinemia*
- *Amyloidosis and Whipple's disease:*
  - Show dilatation (late) with symmetric fold thickening and thickened gastric rugae
  - In amyloidosis, deposition is in between muscle fibers and in perivascular areas.
- *Lymphoma*: Submucosal infiltration.
  - Infiltrative
    - *Dilatation:*
      - Due to distal narrowing
      - Due to neural involvement known as aneurysmal dilatation
      - Fold thickening
      - Slow passage
      - Most common.
  - Exo- and endoenteric—large mass with ulcer, displaced loops and fistula.
  - Multinodular.
  - Polypoidal.
  - Mesenteric.
- *Ménétrier's disease:*
  - PLE with giant gastric folds.
  - Regular intestinal folds.
  - Altered surface metabolism.
- *Eosinophilic gastroenteritis:*
  - Immune/allergy.
  - Jejunum + distal stomach.
  - Initially regular but late, irregular due to spreading of edema.
  - Eosinophilia + Eosinophilic infiltration + Eosinophilic exudation.
  - Mural thickening may be associated with obstruction.
  - Good response to steroids (Only definite differential diagnosis to Crohn's disease).
  - *Folds are*:
    - Distorted
    - Irregular
    - Angulated
    - Saw-toothed
    - Rigid
    - Separated.
- *Xanthomatosis:*
  - Multicentric proliferation of lipid laden cells in bowel wall.
  - Regular fold thickening.
  - Narrowing of stomach and colon.
- *Pneumatosis:*
  - A mimicker and not true wall thickening.
- *Intestinal lymphangiectasia:*
  Primary
  Secondary
  Obstruction
  - Giant foam cells in walls.
  - Diffuse regular fold thickening + loss of protein-rich exudate in GIT + absent liver, kidney, heart disease.
  Lymphangiectasias
  - Thickening due to edema + lymphatic obstruction.
- *Angioneurotic edema:*
  - AD; multifocal mucosal edema attacks.
  - Focal changes, temporary during crisis, family history.
  - Regular fold thickening + mesenteric edema separated loops.
- *Vasculitis:*
  - Leads to infarcts, bleed, perforation, strictures associated with fold thickening.
  - Henoch-Schonlein purpura (HSP)—circumferential colonic wall thickening with luminal narrowing.
- *Hemophilia:*
  - Short-long segment fold thickening of bleed.
  - Colon may be involved.
- *Idiopathic thrombocytopenic purpura:*
  - *Acute*: Healthy young child, 1–2 weeks after sore throat
  - *Chronic*: Young adult female, insidious onset menorrhagia
    - Petechiae at GUT, GIT, skin, etc.

THICKENED GASTRIC FOLDS

Gastric folds are said to be thickened when they measure >1 cm in thickness.
- Thickened folds in fundus and body.
  - Hypertrophic gastritis
  - *Zollinger-Ellison syndrome:*
    - Gastrin producing tumor
    - Postbulbar ulcer in 1 and 2 part of duodenum is suggestive
    - Ulcers distal to 2nd part of duodenum are virtually diagnostic

- Excessive acid secretion causes mucosal edema and fold thickening.
- 50% multiple and 50% malignant.
- Ménétrier's disease
- Marked glandular hypertrophy
- Hypochlorhydria and hypoproteinemia are associated
- Course of disease is chronic and unremitting in adults but resolution occurs in children
– Varices—associated with esophageal varices.
– *Lymphocytic gastritis:*
  - Large
  - Varioli form erosions.
- Thickened folds predominantly in antrum. (The thickened rugal fold of more than 5 mm in antral area and of more than 1.5 cm along greater curvature. There are also prominent area gastricae of 4–5 mm which are polygonal or regular throughout stomach).
  – *Inflammatory/Infiltrative:*
  - Crohn's disease
    - Aphthous ulceration, fold thickening, deep ulcers, skin lesion and scarring are observed.
  - Amyloidosis, sarcoidosis, cystic fibrosis
    - Associated lung changes suggest the diagnosis in sarcoidosis.
  - *Tuberculosis*: Caseous lymphadenopathy is characteristic.
  - Eosinophilic gastritis
    - 50% have peripheral eosinophilia and 50% have allergic history.
  - Caustic ingestion.
  - Drugs like 5-fluorouracil.
  - Radiotherapy.
  - Watermelon stomach.
    - Vascular ectasia involving submucosal vessels.
  - Acute pancreatitis.
  - Pseudolymphoma
    - This is a benign reactive nodular hyperplasia.
    - 70% have ulcer near the center of affected area.

- Thickening involving any part of stomach
  – *Carcinoma:*
    - Thickened folds are irregular with signs of mucosal destruction
    - Loss of pliability of gastric wall
  – *Lymphoma:*
    - Usually NHL
    - Multifocal, usually large masses with coarse mucosal folds which may extend along GE junction or pylorus with preservation of wall pliability.

THICKENED DUODENAL FOLDS

- *Inflammatory:*
  – Duodenitis
  – Pancreatitis
  – *Crohn's disease:*
    - Precedes aphthous ulcer
    - Duodenal cap and D2 predominantly affected
      - Infections
    - HIV, CMV, MAI, *Cryptosporidium.*
- *Neoplastic:*
  – Zollinger-Ellison's syndrome
    - Associated ulcers are seen.
  – Lymphoma
  – Metastases—rare
    From melanoma, breast, ovary, etc.
- *Infiltrative disorders:*
  – Amyloidosis
  – Whipple's disease
  – Mastocytosis
    – Eosinophilic enteritis
    – Peripheral eosinophilia
    – History of allergy
    – Intestinal lymphangiectasia.
- *Vascular:*
  – Varices
    - Invariably associated with esophageal varices
  – Intramural hemorrhage
    - Trauma, bleeding diathesis
    - "Stacked-coin" appearance
  – Ischemia—seen in vasculitis, collagen disease.

- *Edema:*
    - Hypoproteinemia—Nephrotic syndrome, cirrhosis, etc.
    - Lymphatic obstruction
    - Venus obstruction
        - Budd-Chiari syndrome
        - Constrictive pericarditis
            - Angioneurotic edema.
- *Infestations:*
    - Giardiasis
        - Associated with hypermotility
        - Spasm producing narrowing
        - Associated with nodular lymphoid hyperplasia or hypogammaglobulinemia
    - Hookworm
        - *Ancylostoma duodenale*
    - Strongyloidosis stercoralis
    - Tapeworm
        - *Tenia saginata/Tenia solium.*

MASSIVELY DILATED STOMACH

Gas or food-filled stomach can be identified, with the wall of greater curvature convex caudally with pyloric antrum pointing cranially. Mottled translucencies can be seen due to air trapped within food residues.

Causes

- *Paralytic ileus:*
    - Common in elderly
    - Associated with fluid and electrolyte disturbance
    - High mortality rate:
        - Postoperative
        - Trauma
        - Peritonitis
        - Pancreatitis
        - Cholecystitis
        - Diabetic coma
        - Hepatic coma
        - Uremic coma
        - Hypokalemia
        - Drugs like anticholinergics.
- *Mechanical gastric outlet obstruction:*
    - Fibrosis/scarring secondary to ulceration
    - Malignancy in antrum
    - Gastric volvulus:
        - Organo-axial type is usually associated with hiatus hernia
        - Elevation of left hemidiaphragm
        - No gas beyond stomach
        - Collapsed small bowel loops
    - Proximal small bowel obstruction
    - Bezoars
    - Infantile/adult hypertrophic pyloric stenoses.

    US is diagnostic.
- *Miscellaneous:*
    - Air swallowing
    - Intubation.

TARGET LESIONS IN STOMACH ON BARIUM STUDY (FIG. 5.7)

Appearance is due to umbilication or ulceration at the apex of nodule.

- *Benign lesions:*
    - Leiomyoma—apical/central ulceration
    - Ectopic pancreatic rests
        - Primitive ductal system fills with barium producing a central niche at the apex of the tumor.
    - Neurofibroma
        - May be multiple and multifocal
        - Other stigmata of neurofibromatosis.
    - Acute erosive gastritis
        - Ulcer surrounded by halo of edema.
- *Malignant lesions:*
    - Leiomyosarcoma
        - Central ulceration but usually tumors are large
    - Lymphoma (Fig. 5.8)
    - Metastases from melanoma, carcinoid, breast, bronchus and pancreas.

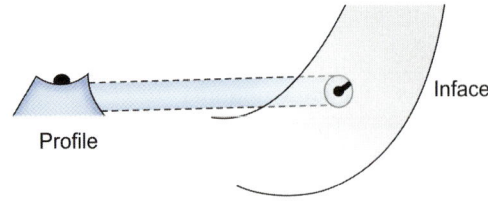

Fig. 5.7: "Bull's eye" (Target) lesions in the stomach.

GAS IN GASTRIC WALL

Interstitial Gastric Emphysema

- Appear as linear or curvilinear lucent shadows along the gastric wall.

Causes

- Raised intragastric pressure
- Post-endoscopy
- Peptic ulceration
- Necrotizing enterocolitis.

Emphysematous Gastritis

- Due to gas-forming organisms in wall
- Common in elderly, diabetes mellitus, alcohol abuse and following corrosive ingestion.

Cystic Pneumatosis

- Seen in elderly
- Associated with chronic obstructive pulmonary disease (COPD).

COBBLESTONE DUODENAL CAP ON BARIUM STUDY (FIG. 5.9)

- *Small size cap:*
  - Erosive duodenitis
    - Central fleck of barium with halo of edema.
    - Duodenal cap is irritable
  - Benign nodular lymphoid hyperplasia
    - 1–3 mm nodules involving entire duodenal loop.
  - Heterotopic gastric mucosa
    - 1–6 mm nodules extending from pylorus towards apex of cap.
  - Food residue/effervescent granules
    - Move to most non-dependent part.
- *Big polypoidal cap:*
  - Large ulcer with surrounding edema
  - Hypertrophied Brunner's gland
    - Uniform size
    - Extends from pylorus to ampulla of Vater
    - Associated with end-stage renal failure in 25%.

- *Crohn's disease*
  - Aphthoid ulcers are seen.
- *Varices:*
  - Base of cap is usually affected
  - Decrease in erect position
  - Invariably associated with esophageal varices.
- Lymphoma.
- Carcinoma.

DILATED DUODENUM/OBSTRUCTION OF DUODENUM

- *Congenital causes:*
  - Annular pancreas
  - Peritoneal bands—Ladd band
    - Most common cause in neonates
    - Associated with malrotation and midgut volvulus
      - Aberrant vessel
      - Atresia, webs and stenosis.

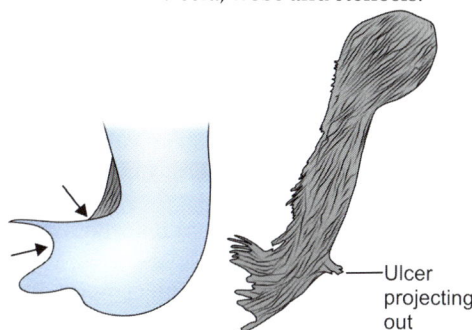

Gastric adenocarcinoma polypoid type—shows abrupt narrowing of the pyloric canal due to mural infiltration of adenocarcinoma polypoidal intraluminal component

Fig. 5.8: Gastric lymphoma UGI-marked thickening of gastric ruge giving "Cobblestone" appearance and shrunken stomach (arrows).

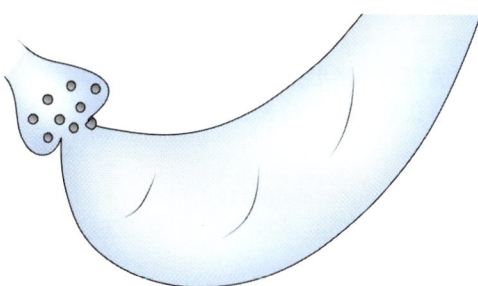

Fig. 5.9: "Cobblestone" duodenal cap.

- *Inflammatory narrowing:*
    - Chronic duodenal ulcer scar
    - Acute pancreatitis: Phlegmon, abscess, pseudocyst
    - Acute cholecystitis: Perforated gallstone
- *Intramural hematoma:*
    - Blunt trauma (Accident, child abuse)
    - Anticoagulant therapy
    - Blood dyscrasias.
- *Tumoral narrowing:*
    - Primary duodenal tumors
    - Tumor invasion from pancreas, right kidney, lymph node enlargement.
- *Extrinsic compression:*
    - Aortic aneurysm
    - Pseudoaneurysm.
- *Miscellaneous:*
    - Superior mesenteric artery syndrome from extensive burns, rapid weight loss, prolonged bed-rest
        - Hold-up of barium in third part of duodenum
        - Delay of 4–6 hours in gastroduodenal transit
        - Proximal dilatation and vigorous peristalsis with sharp cut-off sign
        - Barium passes easily in making the patient prone
        - Postprandial pain relieved by lying on left side
        - Decreased aorto-mesenteric angle of 6–25° as opposed to normal of 45° as on US and decreased aorto-mesenteric distance of 2–8 mm as opposed and normal 8–10 mm by CT
        - 20% associated with duodenal ulcer
        - Very-very rare in obese people
            - Bezoar
            - Scleroderma
            - Paralytic ileus.

DILATED SMALL BOWEL/JEJUNAL AND ILEAL OBSTRUCTION

Criteria

Jejunal diameter should not exceed 4 cm.
Ileal diameter should not exceed 3 cm on small bowel enema.
The criteria limits are 0.5 cm less on barium meal follow-through studies.

- *Congenital:*
    - Ileal atresia/stenosis
    - Enteric duplication cyst—most common ileum
        - Location—antimesenteric border
    - Midgut volvulus
    - Mesenteric cyst—most common ileum
        - Location—mesenteric side
    - Meckel's diverticulum.
- *Extrinsic bowel lesions:*
    - Fibrous adhesions from previous surgery/peritonitis
        - Most common cause in adults
    - Hernias (inguinal, femoral, umbilical)
    - Volvulus
    - Masses—neoplasms, abscess.
- *Luminal occlusion (Figs. 5.10A and B):*
    - Swallowed foreign body, bezoar, gallstone, etc.
    - Meconium ileus
    - Intussusception
    - Tumor, e.g. lipoma.
- *Intrinsic bowel wall lesion:*
    - Strictures from neoplasm, Crohn's disease, tuberculosis enteritis, parasitic disease, radiotherapy, amyloidosis
    - Intramural hemorrhage—blunt trauma, Henoch-Schönlein purpura
    - Vascular insufficiency—arterial/venous occlusion
    - Celiac disease, tropical sprue, dermatitis herpetiformis
    - Scleroderma
    - Lymphoma.
- *Miscellaneous:*
    - Postvagotomy and postgastrectomy
    - Rapid emptying of stomach produces small bowel dilatation
    - Extensive small bowel resection
    - Zollinger-Ellison's syndrome.

STRICTURES SMALL BOWEL

- *Neoplasms:*
    - Lymphoma
        - Usually secondary to lymph node involvement
        - Primary is usually NHL
        - Associated with thick folds.

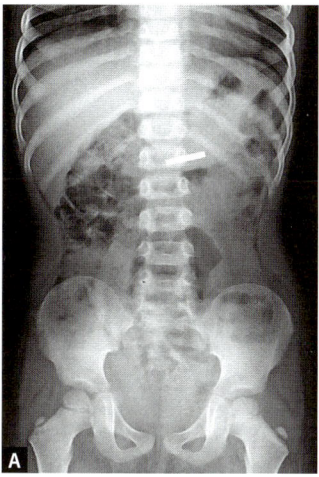 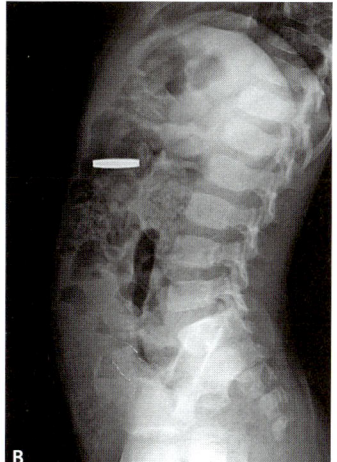

Figs. 5.10A and B: Anteroposterior and lateral radiograph of abdomen showing coin as a foreign body in upper jejunal loop.

- Carcinoid
  - Most common site distal ileum
  - Produces intense fibroblastic response.
- Carcinoma
  - Most common site is duodenum
  - Produces short segment stricture with mucosal destruction and ulceration.
- Sarcoma
  - Lympho- or leiomyosarcoma
  - Thick folds with eccentric lumen.
- Metastases
- Flattened mucosal folds.
- *Crohn's Disease:*
  - Aphthous ulcers
  - Skin lesions.
- *Tuberculous/Parasitic infestation:*
  - Long segment smooth strictures
  - Multifocal.
- *Ischemic:*
  - Ulcers rare
  - Evolution more rapid ± strictures.
- *Radiation enteritis:*
  - Produce endarteritis and fibrosis
  - Doses more than 4500 rads.
- Enteric-coated potassium chloride tablets
- Surgical anastomosis
- Amyloidosis.

SMALL INTESTINAL STRICTURE

Differential Diagnosis (Flowchart 5.3)

- Tuberculosis
- Crohn's disease
- Metastatic carcinoma
- End-stage radiation enteritis
- Endometriosis
- Eosinophilic gastroenteritis
- Post-traumatic
- Drug induced
- Primary malignancy.

Tuberculosis (Figs. 5.11A and B)

- Usually presents in a patient with a past or current history of pulmonary tuberculosis, either from swallowing of sputum or due to hematogenous spread.
- Sometimes primary, as from ingestion of infected cow's milk.
- Patient presents with loss of appetite, low-grade fever or sometimes subacute intestinal obstruction. Mantoux test may be positive and erythrocyte sedimentation rate (ESR) is usually raised.
- Ulcerative form is most frequent, with ulcers presenting in an axis perpendicular to the long-axis of intestines.
- Hypertrophic form present with gross thickening of bowel wall.

Flowchart 5.3: Small intestinal stricture.

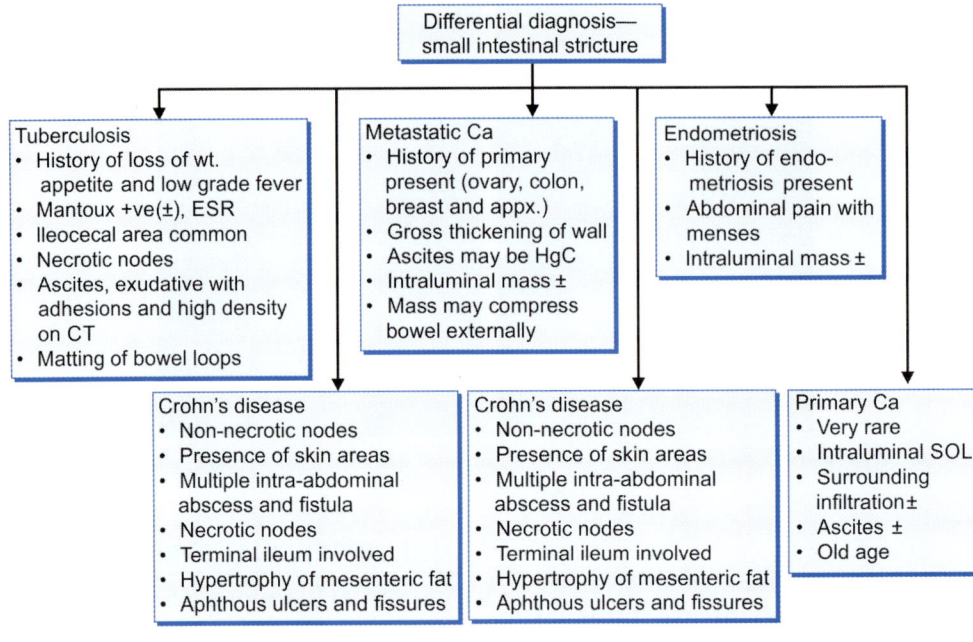

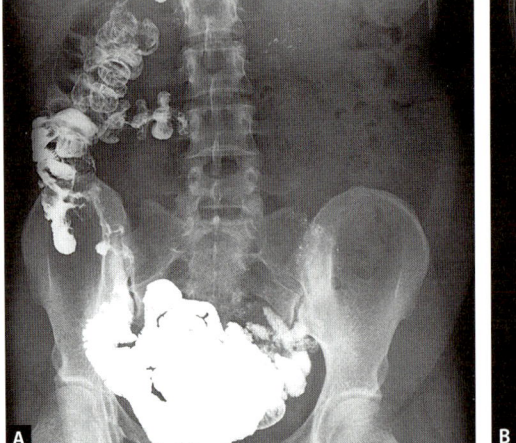
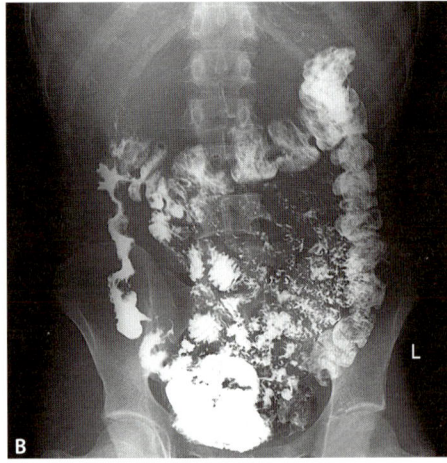

Figs. 5.11A and B: Barium meal followthrough studies with anteroposterior projection showing ileocecal and cecal with ascending colon involvement by tubercular process in two different patients.

- Most common in the region of terminal ileum and cecum, but may involve any part of the gastrointestinal (GI) tract. In the ileocecal area it usually presents with stricture and shortening of cecal pole. Multiple strictures may be seen in the small intestines or the whole of GI tract.
- Intestinal loops may be matted as seen on fluoroscopy, ultrasonography (USG) or CT.
- Mesenteric, peripancreatic or retroperitoneal adenopathy is seen with lymph nodes having caseous necrotic centers and peripheral enhancement on contrast-enhanced computed tomography (CECT).

- Ascites is usually present and is exudative with internal echoes and thick shaggy septations/adhesions seen on USG. On CT, the ascitic fluid is of high attenuation value (20–45 HU).
- Omentum may be rolled up or may have irregular masses of soft tissue density. Similar masses may also be seen in mesentery.

Crohn's Disease

- A kind of regional enteritis is a disease of unknown etiology
- Presents with discontinuous (skip areas) and asymmetric involvement of entire GI tract but most commonly involves the small intestines
- There is transmural inflammation, ulceration and formation of non-caseating granulomas and enlargement of abdominal lymph nodes
- Patients present with colicky abdominal pains, diarrhea, low-grade fever, weight loss and malabsorption
- There is cobblestone mucosae due to presence of abnormal edematous, ulcerated and fissured mucosa separated by normal uninvolved mucosa
- Perianal abscess and fistula formation is very common
- Terminal ileum alone or in combination with jejunum and ileum is most commonly involved
- There is intense fibrosis of involved loops with formation of 'string sign' due to stricture formation leading to marked narrowing of bowel loops
- There is ulceration (aphthous ulcers) and fissuring of mucosa leading to appearances of thorns (rose thorns or raspberry thorns) on barium studies
- Thickening of bowel loops leads to the "pseudo-kidney sign" seen on USG
- "Creeping fat" appearances on CT are due to massive proliferation of intestinal fat leading to separation of bowel loops
- Multiple intra-abdominal abscesses may also be seen
- Multiple fistulous tracts (enterocolic, perianal, colovesical, colovaginal, enterocutaneous), etc. may also be seen either on barium studies or on CT
- Extraintestinal manifestations, such as fatty infiltration of liver, sclerosing cholangitis, urolithiasis, digital clubbing, seronegative arthropathy, erythema and nodosum may also be the presenting features.

Metastatic Carcinoma

- There is usually a history of primary carcinoma elsewhere
- Intraperitoneal spread occurs from primary mucinous cancers of ovary, appendix, colon and breast.

Eosinophilic Enteritis

- Patients present with relapsing attacks of gastroenteritis, there is peripheral blood eosinophilia in 50% of cases and positive history of atopy can be elicited
- There is formation of eosinophilic granulomas and fibrosis
- Fibrosis leads to stricture formation
- There is separation of bowel loops and sometimes ascites may also be seen.

Post-traumatic

- The interval between trauma and onset of symptoms is usually 1–18 weeks
- The stenotic segment may vary in length and outline
- History may be suggestive and diagnosis is one of exclusion.

Drug Induced

- Usually due to non-enteric coated tablets of KCl and rarely NSAIDs
- The drugs induce small bowel ischemia leading to ulceration, then fibrosis and subsequently stricture formation
- The strictures are very short segments and diaphragm-like and may be multiple.

Primary Malignancy

- Very rare
- May produce appearances like colonic carcinoma

- There is evidence of mucosal destruction with overhanging edges
- Hematogenous dissemination is seen in malignant melanoma, breast carcinoma, lung carcinoma and Kaposi sarcoma
- Direct extension may be seen in carcinoma of ovary, uterus, prostate, pancreas, colon and kidney
- There may be a single mass protruding into the lumen of the bowel or encircling the bowel like an annular carcinoma leading to stricture formation
- Stricture may also form due to direct compression either by the primary carcinoma itself or by involved nodes
- On CT, there is presence of soft tissue nodules or masses, sheets of tissue causing thickening of bowel wall, fixation and angulation of bowel loops and ascites.

Radiation Enteritis

- There is a history of radiotherapy done for a primary intra-abdominal or pelvic carcinoma usually seen in women with carcinoma of ovary, cervix, and endometrium or in patients with carcinoma of bladder or colon
- There is a latent period of usually 1–2 years before a full-blown picture emerges
- There is irregular nodular thickening of folds with straight or transverse ulcers
- Bowel wall is thickened with luminal narrowing and stricture formation
- Strictures may be multiple and can be partial or complete
- There may be shortening of small bowel
- Bowel loops may be matted together due to intense desmoplastic reaction induced by radiation.

Endometriosis

- Rare but usually involves the rectum and colon, rarely small intestines are involved
- There may be a history of endometriosis or colicky abdominal pain during menstruation
- May present as an intraluminal mass or stricture of bowel wall due to intense desmoplastic reaction invoked by periodic loss of blood by the endometriotic deposits (Flowchart 5.3).

THICKENED FOLDS IN SMALL BOWEL (FLOWCHART 5.2)

Normal fold thickness — 1.5–2 mm
Abnormal fold thickness — Jejunum more than 2.5 mm
Ileum more than 2.0 mm
Caliber —
  Proximal jejunum   more than 3.5 cm (4.5 cm, if small bowel enema)
  Mid-small bowel   more than 3.0 cm (4.0 cm, if small bowel enema)
  Ileum   more than 2.5 cm (3.0 cm, if small bowel enema)

Divided into two categories:
1. With dilated small bowel—common causes
   – Vascular insufficiency
   – Lesions of bowel and mesentery
   – Z-E syndrome
   – Amyloidosis
   – Lymphoma
   – Abetalipoproteinemia
   – Extensive small bowel resection.
2. With non-dilated small bowel.

Localized (< 50% of Small Bowel)

Smooth and Regular
- *Vascular:*
  Intramural hematoma
   – Trauma
   – Bleeding diathesis
  Ischemia
   – Acute—embolus, Henoch-Schönlein purpura
   – Chronic—vasculitis, RT, atheroma, fibromuscular dysplasia
- *Edema:*
   – Adjacent inflammation or mass
- *Infiltrative disease:*
   – Early amyloidosis
   – Early eosinophilic enteritis.

Irregular and Distorted
- *Inflammatory:*
  - Crohn's disease
  - Z-E syndrome
- *Infective:*
  - Tuberculosis
- *Neoplastic:*
  - Lymphoma
  - Carcinoid
  - Melanoma or other metastases.

Generalized (> 50% Small Bowel Involved)

Smooth and Regular
- *Vascular:*
  - Bleeding diathesis
  - Vasculitis, RT, etc.
- *Edema:*
  - Hypoproteinemia
  - Venous congestion
  - Lymphatic obstruction
  - Angioneurotic edema
- *Infiltrative:*
  - Late amyloidosis
  - Eosinophilic enteritis
- Abetalipoproteinemia.

Irregular and Distorted
- Inflammatory
  - Crohn's disease
- *Infiltrative:*
  - Late amyloidosis
  - Eosinophilic enteritis
  - Whipple's disease
  - Mastocytosis
- *Infestation:*
  - Giardiasis
  - Strongyloidosis
- *Neoplastic:*
  - Lymphoma
- Primary lymphangiectasia.

THICKENED SMALL BOWEL FOLDS WITH GASTRIC ABNORMALITY

- Lymphoma/metastases
- Z-E syndrome
- Ménétrier's disease
- Amyloidosis
- Eosinophilic gastroenteritis
- Whipple's disease
- Crohn's disease.

NODULAR APPEARANCE OF SMALL BOWEL

- *Sand-like nodules (1 mm):*
  - Seen in following infiltrative disorders as:
    - Waldenström's macroglobulinemia
    - Associated with normal fold
  - Mastocytosis—associated with thick folds
  - Whipple's disease—associated with thick folds.
- *Small nodules (> 2 mm):*
  - Thickened folds
    - Inflammatory – Crohn's disease
      - Cobblestone mucosa
      - With skip areas
    - Neoplastic – lymphoma.

Normal Folds
- *Inflammatory:*
  - Nodular lymphoid hyperplasia
  - Associated with hypogammaglobulinemia
  - Associated malabsorption and giardiasis
- *Polyposis (Fig. 5.12):*
  - Peutz-Jeghers syndrome
  - Autosomal dominant
  - Multiple hamartomas
  - May be associated with intussusception.
Gardner's and Canada-Cronkhite syndromes may occasionally involve small bowel.
- Lymphoma.
- Metastases—on antimesenteric border, especially melanoma, breast, GIT and ovary.
- Infections as typhoid, yersinia, histoplasmosis.

MALABSORPTION

Defined as deficient absorption of any essential food materials within the small bowel.
- *Primary:*
  - The digestive abnormality is the only abnormality

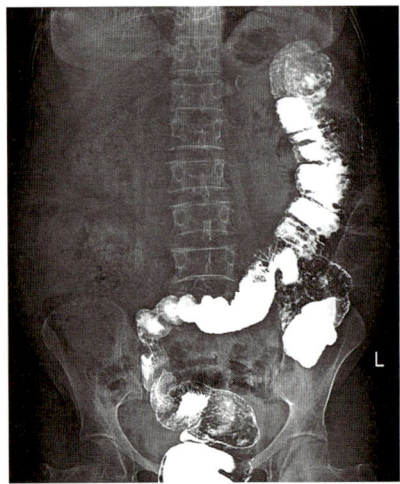

Fig. 5.12: Barium enema in anteroposterior projection showing multiple polypoidal filling defects in the left side of colon.

- Celiac or tropical sprue
- Disaccharidase deficiency.
- *Secondary:*
  - The abnormality occurs during the course of some disease
  - Enteric
  - Gastric—fistula, gastrectomy, pyloroplasty
  - Pancreatic—cystic fibrosis, pancreatitis, carcinoma
  - Hepatobiliary
  - Intra- or extrahepatic biliary obstruction
  - Acute and chronic liver disease.

Malabsorption

Clinical Features

- Diarrhea
- Steatorrhea
- Flatulence, abdominal distension
- Weight loss
- Other—paresthesia, bone pain, tetany, glossitis, cheliosis, anemia, lassitude.

Blood tests: Anemia, LFT, serum iron, folic acid, albumin, vitamins K, D and B_{12}.

Fecal fat: 72-hour quantitative fecal fat analysis estimation of 14c in breath after ingestion of radioactive triglyceride.

D-14[c]-xylose breath test: Test of choice for detecting bacterial overgrowth.
- Gram-negative bacteria metabolize D-xylose to 14 CO_2 hydrogen test for lactase deficiency
- A rise of more than 20 ppm in exhaled hydrogen above basal level after ingestion of lactose at 1 g/kg body weight.

Barium (Fig. 5.13)

- Dilution of barium, because of hypersecretion of fluid by bowel
- Flocculation
- Segmentation of the column of barium
- Moulage sign is the appearance of barium in a featureless tube due to effacement of mucosal folds.

Malabsorption describes impaired absorption of normal dietary constituents, namely protein, carbohydrates, fats, minerals and proteins.

Causes

- Mucosal:
  - Celiac disease
  - Inflammation—tropical sprue
    - Crohn's disease
    - Radiotherapy

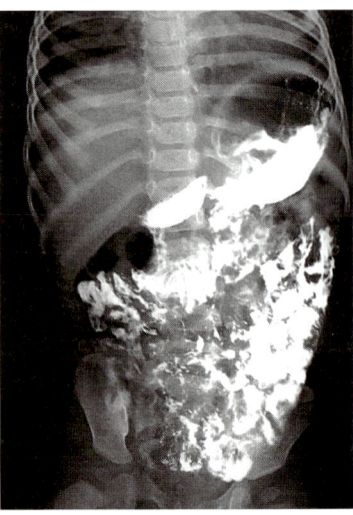

Fig. 5.13: Barium follow-through study in anteroposterior projection showing signs of malabsorption.

- Infiltrative disorder:
  - Whipple's disease
  - Mastocytosis
  - Amyloidosis
  - Eosinophilic enteritis
- Lymphangiectasias
- *Parasites:*
  - Giardiasis
  - Strongyloidosis
- Ischemia
- *Inadequate digestion:*
  - Postgastrectomy
  - Deficiency or inactivation of pancreatic lipase
  - Gastrinoma
  - Disaccharidase deficiency (lactose intolerance)
- *Reduced intestinal bile salt concentration:*
  - Liver disease
  - Blind loop syndrome
  - Pseudo-obstruction
  - Ileal resection
  - Ileal inflammatory disease (Crohn's, tuberculosis)
  - Drugs—by sequestration of bile salts
- Inadequate absorptive surface
- Intestinal resection or bypass (Short-bowel syndrome)
- *Major resection:*
  - Severe ischemia/infarction
  - Volvulus
  - Trauma
- Repeated resections
  - Crohn's disease
  - Peutz-Jeghers syndrome
- With or without colon: 150 cm
- With colon: 50–70 cm
- Normal ileum can assume the function of jejunum by adaptation
- Lost ileum is metabolically irreplaceable
- Resection of more than 100 cm of terminal ileum—interrupts extrahepatic circulation of bile salt.

Barium

- Shows indication of the length of residual small bowel
- Features of adaptation—increased lumen diameter, thickened folds, more numerous crinkled folds.

Cystic fibrosis: Exocrine pancreatic secretions are low in bicarbonate and viscid.
Acid with pH—maldigestion
- *Duodenum*—thickened or flattened folds, nodular filling defects, and lumen dilatation with sacculations along its lateral border
- In small bowel, particularly terminal ileum—normal fold pattern is replaced by an irregular network of curving lines.

Celiac Disease

- Antibodies to gliadin fraction of gluten HLA-DR3
- Gold standard in diagnosis—characteristic changes shown by mucosal biopsy
- Favorable clinical response to gluten-free diet
- Reversal to near normalcy on follow-up mucosal biopsies.

Radiological Features

Lumen dilatation more than 3 cm in follow through:
- Increased separation or even absence of jejunal folds
- Reversal of normal fold character between the ileum and the jejunum
- Increase in number and thickness of folds
- Mosaic mucosal pattern—network of barium containing grooves separating areas 1-3 mm in size
- In duodenum—fewer and irregular folds
- On gluten-free diet—number of folds in jejunum returns to normal
- Less improvement in number of ileal folds
- If bowel caliber increases while on gluten-free diet, suspect a complication, i.e. lymphoma, carcinoma or intersusception/intussusception (rare and non-obstructive).

Tropical Sprue

- Postinfective malabsorption with subtotal villous atrophy
- In tropical countries

- Extends throughout the small bowel
- Megaloblastic anemia, vitamin B_{12} and folate deficiency
- Dramatic response to broad-spectrum antibiotics and folate.

Barium: Lumen dilatation, thickened folds and flocculation.

Zollinger-Ellison's Syndrome

- Gastric acid hypersecretion—maldigestion of fat
- Severe peptic ulcer disease—steatorrhea
- Gastrinoma—damage of jejunal mucosa
- Radiological features (R/F)—dilated duodenum with coarse nodular folds with erosions
- Thickened folds increased fluid, particularly in the proximal jejunum
- 75–80% of gastrinomas pancreas
- 15% duodenum
- Endoscopic USG more than 50% of adjacent pancreatic gastrinomas
- CT/MR/somatostatin receptor scintigraphy.

Eosinophilic Gastroenteritis

- History of allergic disorders
- *Diagnostic criteria:*
  - Symptoms related to gastrointestinal tract (GIT)
  - Eosinophilic infiltration of mucosa on biopsy or a characteristic barium appearance with peripheral eosinophilia
  - Exclusion of parasitic or certain extra-intestinal disease like polynodosa arteritis
- Remissions and recurrences—typical
- *Predominantly mucosal:*
  - Nausea, vomiting, diarrhea
  - Fold thickening—antral
  - Straight thickened folds in small bowel
  - Patchy distribution
  - Predominant involvement of muscularis — thickening of muscularis with lumen narrowing—antral
  - Small bowel—segmental narrowing, not associated with fold thickening
  - Serosal—rare, ascites, pleural effusion.

Whipple's Disease

Tropheryma whippelii

- GIT (small bowel), heart valves, CNS, joint capsule involvement
- Lamina propria filled with macrophages containing PAS positive residue
- Enteroclysis—best radiological test for diagnosis of Whipple's disease
- Diffuse or patchy micronodules, predominantly in the jejunum and at the duodeno-jejunal junction.

Computed tomography—abdominal lymphadenopathy with fatty material.

Pseudo-obstruction

Signs/symptoms of obstruction without a mechanical cause:

- *Primary familial de novo:*
  - Visceral neuropathy
  - Myopathy
- Dilated aperistaltic bowel loops
- Antegrade barium study to exclude mechanical obstruction should be avoided
- To be evaluated by CT
- *Secondary collagen vascular disease:*
  - Scleroderma
  - Dermatomyositis/Polymyositis
  - SLE
- Amyloidosis
- Endocrine disorder: (a) Hypothyroidism, (b) Diabetes.
- Neurological disease—Chagas disease
- Paraneoplastic visceral neuropathy—small cell lung carcinoma
- Jejunal diverticulosis
- Drugs—narcotics, tricyclic antidepressants.

Systemic Sclerosis

- Most common cause of chronic intestinal pseudo-obstruction
- Esophagus—most common involved side, small bowel—60%
- 35% patients present with malabsorption
- Radiological feature—aperistalsis in distal two-third of esophagus with patulous lower esophageal sphincter and reflux esophagitis

- Involvement of 2nd and 3rd parts of duodenum and jejunum
- Hidebound appearance
- Sacculations.

Amyloidosis
- Deposition of insoluble glycoprotein
- GIT involvement—more common in primary amyloidosis
- Small bowel—non-specific dilatation, fold thickening, impaired motility, suspected of pseudo-obstruction
- Localized deposition—filling defects either macro- or micronodular.

Bacterial Overgrowth Syndromes
Normal 10^4 organisms/mL, aerobic—in jejunal aspirate—more than 10^6/mL abnormal.

Protective Mechanisms
- Gastric acid
- Peristalsis
- Mucus and rapid turnover of enterocytes
- Humoral and cellular immunity.

Causes
Stasis
- Strictures
- Diverticulosis
- Blind loop
- Bypassed bowel
- Pseudo-obstruction.

Increased Bacterial Entry
- Impaired gastric acid output—achlorhydria, hypochlorhydria
- Gastrectomy
- Atrophic gastritis
- Omeprazole.

Immunodeficiency
- Advanced age
- Hypogammaglobulinemia
- Malignancies
- AIDS.

Effects
- Deconjugation of bile salts
- Reduced absorption of amino acids and carbohydrates
- Bind and utilize B_{12}.

Jejunal Diverticulosis
Most common site of small bowel diverticulae.
- Along mesenteric border
- Erect X-ray abdomen—numerous air-fluid levels in the upper abdomen
- Supine film rounded air-filled space without valvulae conniventes
- Barium meal followthrough/enteroclysis/CT
- Active bleeding—Tc 99m sulfur colloid scanning.

Parasitic Infestations
- *Giardiasis*: Villous atrophy, disruption of microvilli, bile salt decomposition—cytotoxic T cell
- Acute self-limiting diarrhea/chronic diarrhea, malabsorption, weight loss
- *Diagnosis*: Stool examination/duodenal mucosal biopsy or duodenal aspirate
- Strongyloidosis: Increased or decreased motility, narrowing, ulceration, thickened folds, dilatation of lumen
- Pipestem appearance of jejunum—chronic cases
- Megaduodenum
- Intestinal tuberculosis and extensive small bowel involvement by Crohn's disease may also lead to malabsorption syndrome
- Radiation enteropathy—damage to mucosa malabsorption.

Lactose Intolerance
Primary
Acquired:
- Celiac and tropical sprue, regional enteritis, viral and bacterial infections of GIT, giardiasis, cystic fibrosis and VC

- Bloating, cramps, flatulence following milk ingestion
- Measurement of breath hydrogen after 50 g lactose ingestion.

Lymphangiectasia

- Congenital malformation
- Blockage of lymph drainage in the mesentery or retroperitoneum extensive abdominal or retroperitoneal carcinoma/lymphoma, carcinoid, cirrhosis, chronic pancreatitis, congestive heart failure
- Enteroclysis may reveal diffuse or patchy micronodules similar to Whipple's with thickened, edematous folds, with increased intraluminal fluid
- Younger patients are affected
- Mesenteric nodes are not enlarged except in patients with secondary cause, where primary pathology may be obvious.

Mastocytosis

- Mast cell infiltration
- Urticaria
- Mucosal and submucosal infiltration with histamine release pain, nausea, vomiting, and diarrhea
  - Thickened irregular folds, diffuse mucosal nodularity, large urticaria-like lesions.

PROTEIN LOSING ENTEROPATHY

- *Disease with mucosal ulceration:*
  - Carcinoma
  - Lymphoma
  - Villous adenoma
  - Inflammatory bowel disease
  - Peptic ulcer disease.
- *Non-ulcerative mucosal disease:*
  - Celiac disease
  - Tropical sprue
  - Whipple's disease
  - Allergic gastroenteropathy
  - Gastrocolic fistula
  - Villous adenoma of colon.
- *Associated with hypertrophic gastric rugae:*
  - Ménétrier's disease.

- *Lymphatic obstruction:*
  - Intestinal lymphangiectasia
  - Lymphoma
  - Retroperitoneal fibrosis.
- *Venous obstruction:*
  - Cirrhosis
  - Inferior vena cava thrombosis
  - Constrictive pericarditis.
- *Chronic arterial obstruction:*
  - Atherosclerosis.
- *Heart disease:*
  - Tricuspid insufficiency.

PATHOLOGIC LESIONS IN TERMINAL ILEUM

- Inflammatory lesions
  - *Crohn's disease*:
    - Asymmetric involvement with skip lesions
    - Predominates on the mesenteric border
    - Aphthoid ulcer—earliest sign
    - Fissure ulcer
    - Cobblestone pattern
    - Separation of bowel loops
    - Strictures and pseudosacculations.
  - *Ulcerative colitis:*
    - Involves ileum in 10% of total colitis cases known as backwash ileitis
    - Dilated ileum with granular mucosa
    - No ulcers.
  - *Radiation enteritis:*
    - Mural thickening with symmetrical stenosis
    - No ulceration or cobblestoning.
- Infective
  - *Tuberculosis:*
    - Cecum is predominantly involved
    - Contraction and retraction of cecum
    - Straightening of ileocecal angle
    - Ulcer is uncommon.
  - *Yersinia:*
    - Cobblestone mucosa with aphthous ulcers (resembles Crohn's disease)
    - No deep fissure ulcer
    - Spontaneous resolution in 10 weeks.

- Actinomycosis:
  - Very rare
  - Predominantly cecum is involved.
- Histoplasmosis
  - Very rare.
- Neoplastic:
  - Lymphoma:
    - Usually non-Hodgkin's lymphoma
    - Irregular, nodular, thickened mucosa
    - Irregular polypoidal mass
    - Long segment annular stricture
    - Multiple ulcers
    - May be difficult to differentiate from Crohn's disease radiologically.
  - Carcinoid:
    - Invariably malignant if > 2 cm
    - Annular fibrotic stricture
    - Intraluminal filling defect
    - Mesenteric mass (produces stretching, rigidity and fixation of loops)
    - Intense desmoplastic response produces stellate arrangement of loops.
  - Metastases
  - Ischemia:
    - Rare
    - Thickened
    - Folds, with 'cobblestoning' and 'thumb-printing'
    - Rapidly progressive, changes differentiate it from Crohn's disease.

COLONIC POLYPS

- *Polyp* is a mass projecting into the lumen of hollow viscus above the level of mucosa. Arises from mucosa but may be derived from submucosa/muscularis propria.
  - Neoplastic—adenomatous
  - Non-neoplastic—hamartomatous/inflammatory.
- *Pseudopolyp* refers to island of inflamed mucosa on a background of denuded mucosa.
  - Pseudopolyposis of ulcerative colitis
  - Cobblestoning of Crohn's disease.
- Postinflammatory/filiform polyps are finger-like projections of submucosa covered by mucosa on all sides following healing and regeneration.

- Adenomatous polyps:
  - *Single*: Tubular, tubulovillous, villous
    - These form a spectrum both in size and degree of dysplasia
    - Villous adenoma is the largest with severest dysplasia with highest premalignant potential
    - Size: < 5 mm—0% malignant
      5 mm—1 cm—1% malignant
      1 cm—2 cm—10% malignant
      more than 2 cm—50% malignant
    - Puckering of bowel wall occurs at the base of polyp
    - Villous adenomas are poorly coated because of mucous secretion; hence are associated with protein-losing enteropathy or hypokalemia.

Turcot's syndrome
- Autosomal recessive
- Increased risk of CNS malignancy.
  - *Multiple*: Familial adenomatosis coli, adenomatosis of GIT, Gardner's syndrome.
    - May form a part of spectrum of same disease
    - Adenomas more numerous in distal colon and rectum
    - *Colon carcinoma develops in:*
      - 30% by 10 years after diagnosis
      - 100% by 20 years after diagnosis.
    - *Carcinoma is multifocal in 50%*
    - *Extracolonic abnormalities include:*
      - Hamartomas and adenomas in stomach
      - Adenoma of duodenum
      - Periampullary carcinoma
      - Jejunal and ileal polyps
      - Mesenteric fibromatosis
      - Multiple osteomas in skull and mandible
      - Dental abnormalities—hypercementomas, odontomas, dentigerous cyst, etc.
      - Epidermoid cysts in leg, face, scalp, etc.
      - Pigmented lesion in fundi oculi
      - Rarely thyroid carcinoma.

- Non-adenomatous single polyps:
  - Carcinoid:
    - Most common in appendix
    - Leiomyoma
    - Lipoma
    - Hemangioma, lymphangioma
    - Fibroma, neurofibroma.
- Hamartomatous polyp:
  - Single juvenile polyp
    - Most common in rectum.
  - Multiple:
    - Juvenile polyposis—non-hereditary
    - Peutz-Jeghers syndrome—hereditary
    - Canada-Cronkhite syndrome—non-hereditary
    - Juvenile polyposis:
      - Seen in children <10 years of age.
      - Peutz-Jeghers syndrome
      - Autosomal dominant
      - 'Carpets' small bowel
      - Also affects colon and stomach in 30%
      - Pigmentation of mucosa and skin
      - Increased incidence of gastric, duodenal and ovarian carcinoma
      Canada-Cronkhite syndrome
      Predominantly affects stomach and colon
      Increased incidence of carcinoma of colon
      Skin pigmentation, nail atrophy and alopecia are associated features.
- Hyperplastic polyp:
  - Single/multiple—most common in rectum.
  - Nodular lymphoid hyperplasia.
    - Seen usually in children.
- Inflammatory/postinflammatory polyp
  - Single—benign lymphoid polyp
    - Fibroid granulation polyp.
  - Multiple:
    - Ulcerative colitis - Polyps at all stages
    - Crohn's disease - Less common than ulcerative colitis
    - Schistosomiasis - Predominantly, involves rectum
    - Amebiasis

COLONIC POLYPS

- Adenomatous
- Hyperplastic
- Hamartomatous
- Inflammatory
- Infective
- Others.

Adenomatous

Simple Tubular Adenoma, Tubulovillous Adenoma, Villous Adenoma

These three form a spectrum both in size and degree of dysplasia. Villous adenoma is the largest, shows most severe dysplasia and has the highest malignancy incidence.

Signs suggestive of malignancy are:
- Size:
  less than 5 mm - 0% malignant
  5 mm   - 1 cm–1% malignant
  1–2 cm   - 10% malignant
  More than 2 cm - 50% malignant
- Sessile—base is greater than height
- Puckering' of colonic wall at base of polyp
- Irregular surface.

Villous adenomas: These are typically fronded, sessile and are poorly coated by barium because of their mucus secretion. It may cause a protein losing enteropathy or hypokalemia.

Familial polyposis coli and Gardner's syndrome—AD: Both conditions may represent a spectrum of the same disease. Multiple adenomas of colon which are more numerous in distal colon and rectum. Colonic carcinomas develop in early adulthood (in 30% by ten years after diagnosis and in 100% by 20 years). Sixty percent of those who present with colonic symptoms already have colonic carcinomas. The carcinoma is multifocal in 50% of cases. Extracolonic abnormalities may occur:

- Hamartomas of stomach (40%).
- Gastric adenomas (more common in the Japanese).
- Adenomas of duodenum (25%).
- Periampullary carcinoma (12%).
- Jejunal and ileal polyps (in 60% of patients in Japanese literature).

- Mesenteric fibromatosis—a non-calcified soft tissue mass which may displace bowel loops and produce mucosal irregularity from local invasion. USG reveals a hypo- or hyperechoic mass and CT a homogeneous mass of muscle density.
- Multiple osteomas—most frequently in the outer table of the skull, the angle of mandible and frontal sinuses.
- Dental abnormalities—hypercementomas, odontomas, dentigerous cyst, supernumerary teeth and multiple caries.
- Multiple epidermoid cysts—usually on legs, face, scalp and arms.
- Pigmented lesions of the ocular fundus: in 90% of patients with Gardner's syndrome and other extracolonic manifestations.
- Thyroid carcinoma in 0.6%.

Hyperplastic

- Solitary/multiple—most frequently found in rectum.
- Nodular lymphoid *hyperplasia*—usually children. Filling defects are smaller than familial polyposis coli.

Hamartomatous

- *Juvenile polyposis*: ± Familial children under 10 years. Commonly solitary in rectum.
- *Peutz-Jeghers syndrome*: Autosomal dominant. 'Carpets' small bowel, but also affects colon and stomach in 30%. Increased incidence of carcinoma of stomach, duodenum and ovary.

Inflammatory

- *Ulcerative colitis*: Polyps can be seen at all stages of activity of the colitis (no malignant potential): *acute*: pseudo polyps (i.e. mucosal hyperplasia); *chronic*: sessile polyp (resembles villous adenoma); *quiescent*: tubular, filiform (wormlike) and can show branching pattern.

  Dysplasias in colitic colon is usually not radiologically visible. When visible, it appears as solitary nodule, several separate nodules (both nonspecific) or as a close grouping of multiple adjacent nodules with apposed, flattened edges (the latter appearances being associated with dysplasia in 50% of cases).
- *Crohn's disease:* Polyps less common than in ulcerative colitis.

Infective

- *Schistosomiasis*—predominantly involves rectum ± strictures.
- Amebiasis.

Others

- *Canada-Cronkhite syndrome*—not hereditary.

  Predominantly affects stomach and colon; but can occur anywhere in bowel. Increases incidences of carcinoma of colon.

  Other features are alopecia, nail atrophy and skin pigmentation.
- *Turcot's syndrome*: Autosomal recessive. Increased incidence of CNS malignancy.

COLONIC STRICTURES/NARROWING

Neoplastic

- *Carcinoma*:
  - Annular/scirrhous.
  - Associated with mucosal distinction.
  - Short segment less than 6 cm.
- *Lymphoma:*
  - Cecum and rectum more frequently involved.
  - Radiologically, polypoidal mass, diffusely infiltrative mass or annular lesion.
- *Metastatic:*
  - From prostate, cervix, uterus, kidney, stomach, pancreas, etc.

Chronic Stage of any Ulcerative Colitis

- Inflammatory—are symmetrical, smooth and tapering.
  - Ulcerative colitis.
  - Common in sigmoid colon.
  - Require more than 5 years.

- Malignant risk starts after 10 years and increases by 10% per decade.
- Crohn's disease—seen in 25% cases.
- 50% are multiple.
- Solitary rectal ulcer syndrome.
- *Infective:*
  - Tuberculosis.
  - Most common in ileocecal region.
  - Short 'hourglass' stricture.
  - Amebiasis.
  - Common in descending colon.
  - Occurs in 2–8% cases.
  - Multiple in 50%.
  - Improvement with metronidazole.
  - LGV.
  - Sexually transmitted disease caused by *Chlamydia*.
  - Long and tubular stricture.
  - Most common in rectosigmoid region.
  - Schistosomiasis.
  - Most common in rectosigmoid region.
  - Other.
  - H. zoster, CMV, strongyloidosis, etc.
- *Ischemic:*
  - Infarction heals rapidly by stricture formation.
  - Most common site is splenic flexure.
  - Have tapering ends.
- *Traumatic:*
  - Radiotherapy.
  - Latent period—several years.
  - Most common site—rectosigmoid.
  - Cathartic colon.
  - Pseudostricture—changes during exam.
  - Initially ascending colon is involved.
  - Caustic colitis.

Extrinsic Masses

- *Inflammation as in*:
  - Retractile mesenteritis
  - Diverticulitis
  - Pericolic abscess.
- *Deposits:*
  - Amyloidosis
  - Endometriosis
  - Pelvic lipomatosis.

Postsurgical
- Adhesive bands
- Surgical anastomosis.

Normal
- Cannon point.

PNEUMATOSIS INTESTINALIS

Also known by the name of:
- Pneumatosis cystoides intestinalis
- Bullous emphysema of intestine
- Intestinal gas cysts
- Peritoneal lymphopneumatosis.

Causes
- *Bowel necrosis/gangrene*:
  - Most common cause
  - There is damage and disruption of mucosa with entry of gas-forming bacteria.
    - Necrotizing enterocolitis—in neonate.
    - Ischemia and infarction as in mesenteric thrombosis.
    - Neutropenic colitis.
    - Sepsis.
    - Volvulus.
    - Caustic ingestion.
- *Mucosal disruption*:
  - Increased intraluminal gas pressure leads to overdistension and dissection of gas in bowel wall.
    - Intestinal obstruction as pyloric stenosis, annular pancreas, imperforate anus, Hirschsprung's disease, and meconium plug syndrome, etc.
    - Intestinal trauma as in endoscopy, rent, perforation, bowel surgery, barium enema, penetrating and blunt abdominal trauma, etc.
    - Infection and inflammation as peptic ulcer disease, tuberculosis, peritonitis, Crohn's disease, ulcerative colitis, Whipple's disease, etc.

- *Increased mucosal permeability:*
  - Defects in lymphoid tissue allows bacterial gas to enter bowel wall.
    - Immunotherapy
      - Graft versus host disease
      - Organ/bone marrow transplantation.
    - Miscellaneous
      - AIDS enterocolitides, steroid therapy, chemo- and radiation therapy, collagen vascular disease, diabetes mellitus.
- *Pulmonary disease:* Alveolar rupture with air dissection into interstitium and mediastinum, followed by retroperitoneal dissection and then along vascular bundles into bowel wall.
- Chronic obstructive pulmonary disease.
- Chest trauma.
- Positive pressure ventilation.

MEGACOLON IN ADULTS

Transverse colon diameter greater than 5.5 cm is known as megacolon.

Causes

- *Non-toxic (without mucosal abnormality):*
  - Distal obstruction as by carcinoma
  - Ileus—paralytic or secondary to hypokalemia
  - Pseudo-obstruction
    - No organic lesion evident
    - Few fluid levels and feces seen in rectum.
  - Purgative abuse.
- *Toxic:* Acute transmural fulminant colitis produces neuromuscular degeneration and loss of motor tone. Mortality is 20%.
  - Inflammatory
    - Ulcerative colitis
    - Crohn's disease
    - Pseudomembranous colitis
  - Ischemic colitis
  - Dysentery
    - Amebiasis
    - *Salmonella*.

Radiological Findings

- Colonic ileus with marked dilatation of transverse colon and few air-fluid levels
- Increasing caliber of colon on serial radiographs without redundancy
- Loss of normal colonic haustra and interhaustral folds
- Irregular mucosal surface with pneumatosis coli
- Barium enema is contraindicated due to risk of perforation.

THUMBPRINTING IN COLON (FIG. 5.14)

This is due to thickened mucosal folds because of submucosal edema/hemorrhage.

Causes

- *Colitides:*
  - Ischemic
    - Most common site is splenic flexure
    - Peroral pneumocolon may obliterate it.
  - Ulcerative colitis
  - Crohn's disease
  - Amebic colitis
  - Pseudomembranous colitis
  - Schistosomiasis.
- *Neoplastic:*
  - Lymphoma
  - Metastases
  Pseudo-thumbprinting is produced by mucosal indentation by mural air cysts. Careful examination will reveal intramural air.
- *Miscellaneous:*
  - Endometriosis
  - Amyloidosis
  - Diverticulitis/diverticulosis
  - Hereditary angioneurotic edema.

APHTHOUS ULCERS

These are fine erosions with a halo of edematous mucosa.

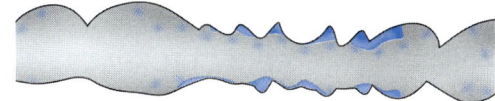

Fig. 5.14: Shows thumbprinting in colon.

Causes

- *In colon*:
  - Crohn's disease—earliest sign
  - Amebic colitis
  - *Yersinia* colitis:
    - Produces thick mucosal folds with ulceration
    - Lymphoid nodular hyperplasia
  - *Salmonella, Shigella* infection
  - Herpes virus infection
  - Behçet's disease:
    - Usually simulates Crohn's disease
    - Occasionally resembles idiopathic ulcerative proctocolitis.
  - Ischemic colitis
  - Lymphoma.
- *In small bowel:*
  - Crohn's disease
  - *Yersinia* enteritis
  - Polyarteritis nodosa.

ANTERIOR INDENTATION OF RECTOSIGMOID JUNCTION

- *Ascites:*
  - Most common cause
  - Especially in erect position.
- Abscess (pericolic).
- Hematoma.
- Endometriosis.
- Surgery
  - Sling repair for rectal prolapse.
- *Tumors:*
  - Peritoneal metastases—common site for gastric, colonic, pancreatic and ovarian metastatic deposits.
  - Primary pelvic tumor, especially adnexal/tubo-ovarian masses.
- *Hydatid cyst*
  - Metastatic from rupture of usually the hepatic cyst into peritoneal cavity with seedlings.

WIDENING/ENLARGEMENT OF PRESACRAL/RETRORECTAL SPACE

Normal width is less than 5 mm in 95%.
Width more than 1 cm is considered abnormal.

- *Normal variation:*
  - 40% cases and associated usually with obesity.
- *Rectal inflammation:*
  - Ulcerative colitis:
    - Seen in 50% cases
    - Width increases as disease progresses.
  - Crohn's colitis
  - Idiopathic proctosigmoiditis
  - Radiation therapy
- *Rectal infection:*
  - Proctitis (Tubercular, amebiasis, LGV, etc.)
  - Diverticulitis
- *Rectal tumor*

A. Benign	B. Malignant
1. Developmental—cyst dermoid, enteric cyst	1. Adenocarcinoma, cloacogenic carcinoma
2. Lipoma, neurofibroma	2. Lymphoma, sarcoma, lymph node metastases
3. Epidermal cyst	3. Prostatic, uterine, vesical, ovarian causes
4. Rectal duplication	

- *Body fluids/deposits:*
  - Hematoma
    - Surgery, sacral fracture
  - Pus
    - Perforated appendix, presacral abscess.
  - Serum
    - Edema, venous thrombosis.
  - Fat
    - Cushing syndrome, pelvic lipomatosis.
  - Amyloidosis.
- *Sacral tumors:*
  - Metastases, plasmacytoma, chordoma in adults.
  - Sacrococcygeal teratoma, anterior sacral meningocele in children.
- *Miscellaneous:*
  - Colitis cystic profunda.
  - Pelvic lipomatosis.

CYSTIC MESENTERIC MASSES

- *Benign cysts:*
  - Pancreatic pseudocyst:
    * Sequelae of pancreatitis
    * Cyst contents reveal P. amylase.
  - Non-pancreatic pseudocyst:
    * Sequelae of mesenteric/omental hematoma/abscess.
    * Thick-walled, usually septated with hemorrhagic/purulent contents.
  - Enteric duplication cyst.
  - Enteric cyst.
  - Mesothelial cyst.
- *Masses:*
  - Cystic lymphangioma (most common).
  - Pseudomyxoma peritonei.
  - Cystic mesothelioma.
  - Mesenteric cyst.
  - Mesenteric hematoma.
  - Benign cystic teratoma.
  - Cystic spindle cell tumor (leiomyoma/leiomyosarcoma).

NONVISUALIZATION OF GALLBLADDER ON ULTRASOUND

- Contracted gallbladder.
- Chronic cholecystitis.
- Gallbladder carcinoma.
- Perforation of gallbladder.
- Congenital absence of gallbladder.

Filling Defects in Gallbladder

- *Fixed:*
  - *Single and small:*
    * Calculus, wall adherent.
    * Adenomyomatosis:
      - Usually fundal
      - Stricture
      - Rokitansky-Aschoff sinuses
      - Visible after contraction
    * Polyp
    * Neurinoma
  - *Single and large:*
    * Calculus
    * Tumor—primary/secondary
  - *Multiple:*
    * Calculi:
      - 30% radiopaque
    * Cholesterolosis "strawberry" gallbladder:
      - Characteristic multiple mural filling defects.
- *Mobile:*
  - Tumefactive sludge, biliary balls
  - Blood clot
  - Calculus—usually non-shadowing.
- "Comet-tail" defect in gallbladder:
  - Rokitansky-Aschoff sinuses
  - Intramural stone
  - Cholesterolosis of gallbladder.

GAS IN BILIARY TREE

These appear as irregularly branching gas shadows not reaching liver edge. Bile duct is outlined; gallbladder may or may not be seen.

- *Within the bile duct:*
  - Incompetence of sphincter of Oddi. (after sphincterotomy/passage of stone/patulous as in elderly)
  - Postoperative (cholecystoenterostomy/choledocho-enterostomy)
  - *Spontaneous biliary fistula*:
    * Gallstone ileus—gallstone erodes the inflamed gallbladder wall to enter duodenum (60%) and colon (20%)
    * Duodenal ulcer perforates into bile duct
    * Malignancy
    * Trauma
- *Within the gallbladder:*
  - All of the above
  - Emphysematous gallbladder
    * Seen in diabetes due to infection by gas forming organism.
    * Air bile level seen on erect films.
    * Intraluminal and intramural gas.

GAS IN PORTAL VENOUS

- Branching gas shadows within 2 cm of liver capsule
- Gas may also be seen in portal and mesenteric venous and bowel wall
- Considered a life-threatening event and sign of bowel infarction and gangrene, unless proved otherwise.

- Children:
  - Necrotizing enterocolitis—10% cases.
  - Umbilical vein catheterization.
  - Erythroblastosis fetalis.
  - *Congenital GI obstruction*: Duodenal atresia, esophageal atresia, imperforate anus.
- Adults:
  - *Intestinal necrosis (in 74% of adults):*
    - Bowel infarction
    - Ulcerative colitis
    - Necrotizing enterocolitis due to mesenteric arterial thrombosis
    - Perforated ulcer (gastric/duodenal).
  - *Miscellaneous:*
    - Hemorrhagic pancreatitis
    - Sigmoid diverticulitis
    - Intraabdominal abscess
    - Pneumonia
    - Inadvertent gas injection during endoscopy
    - Dead fetus
    - Diabetes, diarrhea
    - During double contrast barium enema (DCBE), especially in severely ulcerated colon
    - Acute gastric dilatation (Fig. 5.15).

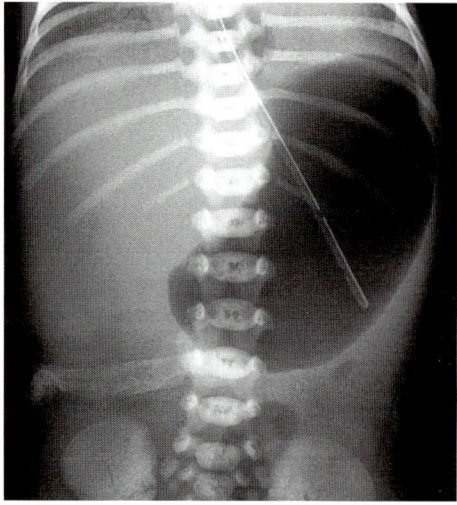

Fig. 5.15: Anteroposterior radiograph of abdomen showing dilatation of stomach.

DIFFUSE HEPATOMEGALY

- *Neoplastic:*
  - Diffuse metastases
  - Diffuse HCC
  - Lymphoma
  - Angiosarcoma
- *Metabolic/Storage:*
  - Fatty infiltration
  - Amyloidosis
  - Wilson's disease
  - Hemochromatosis
  - Glycogen storage disease
  - Lipid storage disease
  - Galactosemia
- *Congenita:*
  - Polycystic liver
- *Infective/inflammatory:*
  - Viral—infective and serum hepatitis, infectious mononucleosis
  - Bacterial—tuberculous, brucellosis
  - Fungal—histoplasmosis
  - Protozoal—malaria, ameba, kala-azar
  - Parasitic—hydatid
  - Spirochetal—syphilis
  - Other—sarcoidosis
- *Vascular:*
  Passive venous congestion as in:
  - CHF
  - Constrictive pericarditis
- *Degenerative*—cirrhosis
- *Myeloproliferative*—myelofibrosis Polycythemia rubra-vera.

HEPATIC CALCIFICATION

- *Multifocal and small:*
  - Healed granulomas (Tuberculosis, histoplasmosis, brucellosis)
  - Intrahepatic biliary calculi
- *Curvilinear:*
  - Hydatid seen in 20–30% cases
  - Congenital cyst
  - Abscess—especially amebic/old pyogenic
  - Porcelain gallbladder (Fig. 5.16)
- *Localized in mass:*
  - *Metastatic:*
    - Usually multifocal

Abdomen and Gastrointestinal Tract and Hepatobiliary System

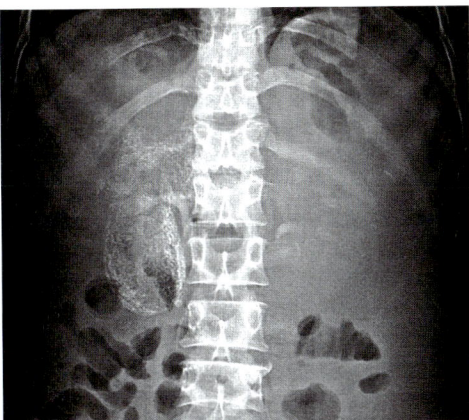

Fig. 5.16: Anteroposterior radiograph of abdomen shows porcelain gallbladder.

- Seen with mucinous carcinoma of colon, breast, stomach, ovarian carcinoma, melanoma, pleural mesothelioma, osteosarcoma and carcinoid.
- Amorphous/flaky/stippled/granular.
- May be seen following chemotherapy/RT.
  - *Hepatoma:*
    - Punctate, stippled or granular.
  - Hepatoblastoma
  - Cholangiocarcinoma.
- *Sunray speculation:*
  - Hemangioma/infantile hemangioendothelioma.
  - Metastatic as colloid carcinomas.
  - Rarely hepatoma.
- *Irregular:*
  - Hepatic artery aneurysm.
  - Portal vein thrombosis.
  - Capsule of regenerating nodules.
  - Chronic granulomatous disease of childhood.
- *Diffuse increased attenuation:*
  - *Iron accumulation:*
    - Primary/secondary hemosiderosis.
  - *Copper accumulation:*
    - Wilson's disease.
  - *Iodine accumulation:*
    - Amiodarone therapy as an anti-arrhythmic.
  - *Gold:*
    - Gold therapy for rheumatoid arthritis.
  - *Thallium:*
    - Ingestion of rodenticides.
  - Glycogen storage disease.
  - Thorotrast.

PRIMARY HEPATIC MASSES

- *Primary benign:*
  - *Epithelial:*
    - *Hepatocellular:*
      - Regenerative nodules
      - Adenomatous hyperplastic nodules
      - FNH
      - Hepatocellular adenoma
    - *Cholangiocellular:*
      - Bile duct adenoma
      - Biliary cyst adenoma
  - *Mesenchymal:*
    - *Tumor containing adipose:*
      - Lipoma
      - Myolipoma
      - Angiomyolipoma
    - *Tumor of muscle:*
      - Leiomyoma
    - *Tumor of vessels:*
      - Infantile hemangioendothelioma
      - Hemangioma
      - Peliosis hepatis
    - *Miscellaneous*—mesothelioma
  - *Mixed tissue tumor:*
    - Mesenchymal hamartoma
    - Benign teratoma
  - *Miscellaneous:*
    - Adrenal rest tumor
    - Pancreatic rest tumor
- *Malignant:*
  - *Epithelial:*
    - *Hepatocellular:*
      - Hepatoblastoma (in pediatric age)
      - HCC
    - *Cholangiocellular:*
      - Cholangiocarcinoma
      - Biliary cystadenocarcinoma
  - *Mesenchymal:*
    - *Tumor of vessel:*
      - Angiosarcoma

- Epithelioid hemangioendothelioma
- Kaposi sarcoma
  - *Miscellaneous:*
    - Embryonal sarcoma
    - Fibrosarcoma
  - *Tumor of muscle:*
    - Leiomyosarcoma
    - Rhabdomyosarcoma
- *Miscellaneous:*
  - Carcinosarcoma
  - Teratoma
  - Yolk sac tumor
  - Carcinoid
  - Squamous carcinoma
  - Lymphoma.

NEONATAL OBSTRUCTIVE JAUNDICE

- *Infections:*
  - *Bacterial:*
    - *E. coli*, syphilis
  - *Viral:*
    - TORCH, HBV, Coxsackie

  On USG—liver echogenicity and size normal or increased.
  TBIDA scan—may reveal delayed uptake by hepatocytes.
- *Metabolic:*
  - *Inherited:*
    - α-1 antitrypsin deficiency, cystic fibrosis, galactosemia, hereditary tyrosinemia
  - *Acquired*
    - Inspissated bile syndrome (secondary to erythroblastosis): Cholestasis due to total parenteral nutrition.
- *Biliary tract abnormalities:*
  - *Extrahepatic:*
    - Biliary obstruction/hypoplasia/atresia.

Biliary Atresia

- Correctable type with patent intrahepatic ducts
- Non-correctable type with occluded intrahepatic ducts
- Normal size, contractible gallbladder rules out the diagnosis
- Absence of small gallbladder favors the diagnosis
- Liver echogenicity on US may be normal or increased
- Normal uptake by hepatocytes but no excretion into bowel on TBIDA scan favors the diagnosis but is not diagnostic.

Choledochal Cyst

- May present in neonate or early childhood.

Todani's Type

- (Most common)—fusiform or focal dilatation of CBD
- Diverticulum of CBD
- Choledochocele—outpouching of CBD in wall of duodenum
- Dilated CBD with focal dilatation of intrahepatic ducts
- Focal dilatation of CBD
- Focal dilatation of intrahepatic ducts (Caroli's disease).

TBIDA scan: Photopenic areas with delayed uptake of tracer. Complications include calculi, pancreatitis, abscesses, cirrhosis, portal hypertension, malignancy.

- "Bile-plug" syndrome
- *Intrahepatic:*
  - *Ductular hypoplasia/atresia*
  - *Alagille syndrome:*
    - Autosomal dominant
    - Dysmorphic facies with ocular abnormalities
    - CVS anomalies, especially pulmonary stenosis
    - Hypoplasia of intrahepatic ducts
    - Butterfly vertebra
    - Radioulnar synostosis.

FETAL/NEONATAL HEPATIC CALCIFICATION

- Peritoneal—on hepatic surface
  - *Meconium peritonitis:*
    - Most common cause of abdominal calcifications

- Solid or cystic masses with calcified walls seen on USG.
  - *Ruptured hydrometrocolpos:*
    - Appearance similar to meconium peritonitis
    - Dilated fluid-filled uterus and vagina.
- *Parenchymal:*
  - *Congenital infections:*
    - TORCH complex
    - Scattered nodular calcification
    - Other stigmata of disease process.
  - *Hepatic tumors:*
    - Hemangioma, hamartoma, hepato_blastoma, teratoma, metastatic neuroblastoma.
- *Vascular:*
  - Portal vein thromboemboli
    - Seen as subcapsular branching calcification
  - *Ischemic infarcts:*
    - Calcification in branching pattern distributed throughout liver.

DIFFUSELY HYPOECHOIC LIVER

- *Acute hepatitis:*
  - Hepatomegaly with normal echo pattern.
- *Diffuse malignant infiltration:*
  - Hepatomegaly with coarse or altered echo pattern.

DIFFUSELY HYPERECHOIC LIVER (BRIGHT LIVER)

Fatty infiltration	Hepatomegaly +/–	Echopattern Normal
Cirrhosis (fibrosis + fatty)	– (Shrunken liver in late stage)	Coarse and nodular
Hepatitis (Chronic)	+/–	Coarse
Infiltration/ deposition	+	Coarse (Malignant, glycogen may be storage granuloma) and nodular Coarse
Steatohepatitis	+	

FOCAL AND HYPERECHOIC HEPATIC LESIONS

- Metastases from GIT, ovary, pancreas, GUT.
  - Usually multiple and larger than 2 cm
  - Hypoechoic halo around lesions.
- *Capillary hemangioma:*
  - Usually single and less than 2 cm
  - Central arteriole may be seen.
- *Adenoma:*
  - Especially in case of associated hemorrhage.
- Focal nodular hyperplasia.
- *Focal fatty infiltration:*
  - Especially around ligamentum teres and GB fossa.
- *Debris within lesions:*
  - Abscesses and hematoma.
- *Miscellaneous:*
  - Hepatoma, lipoma, hemochromatosis.

FOCAL, HYPOECHOIC AND HEPATIC LESIONS

- Hepatoma
- Metastases, especially cystic from ovary/stomach
- Lymphoma
- Cavernous hemangioma
- *Cysts:*
  - Hydatid
- *Abscesses:*
  - Including complicated/infected cysts
- Hematoma is acute stage.

PERIPORTAL HYPERECHOGENICITY

- Air in biliary tree
- Recurrent pyogenic cholangitis
- Cholecystitis
- Schistosomiasis
- Periportal fibrosis.

THICKENED GALLBLADDER WALL

- Diffuse (anterior wall more than 3 mm except physiologically contracted)
  - *Intrinsic:*
    - Acute cholecystitis
    - Chromic cholecystitis
    - Xanthogranulomatous cholecystitis
    - Hyperplastic cholecystosis
    - Sepsis
    - GB carcinoma
    - AIDS cholangiopathy
    - Sclerosing cholangitis
    - GB varices.
  - *Extrinsic*
    - Hepatitis
    - Hypoalbuminemia
    - Renal failure
    - CHF
    - Hepatic vein obstruction
    - Benign ascites
    - Cirrhosis
    - GVH disease
    - Lymphatic obstruction.
- Focal:
  - *Metabolic:*
    - Hyperplastic cholecystosis.
  - *Benign tumor:*
    - Adenoma
    - Neurinoma
    - Papilloma
    - Carcinoid
    - Fibroadenoma.
  - *Malignant:*
    - Adenocarcinoma
    - Leiomyosarcoma
    - Metastases.
  - *Inflammation/infection:*
    - Polyp
    - Parasitic granuloma as in ascaris, filariasis, etc.
    - Retention cyst
    - Xanthogranulomatous cholecystitis.
  - *Miscellaneous:*
    - Impacted gallstone
    - Heterotopic mucosa.

FOCAL HYPODENSE LESIONS ON NECT LIVER

Lesions	Enhancement on CECT
1. *Malignant*	
– Heterogeneous pattern of hemangiosarcoma, intrahepatic cholangio-carcinoma	Hepatoma, metastasis enhancement especially in early arterial phase
2. *Benign*	
a. Hemangioma	Usually peripheral nodular enhancement advancing peripherally; persistent enhancement on delayed scans
b. Adenomas—seen in young females	Early arterial phase enhancement which fades rapidly
c. Focal nodular hyperplasia – Seen in young females – Asymptomatic unless large	Early arterial phase enhancement which fades rapidly Central stellate scar may be seen
3. *Cyst*—benign, simple, hydatid, VHL, polycystic liver disease	No enhancement but margins clearly demarcated; imperceptible walls
4. *Abscesses*—pyogenic, amebic, fungal	Peripheral enhancement with heterogeneous perilesional enhancement due to edema in adjacent hepatic parenchyma
5. *Focal fatty infiltration* – No mass effect	No change but increased conspicuousness
6. *Vascular* – Infarction, hematoma, laceration – Hepatic artery aneurysm	 No change but increased conspicuousness Intense enhancement No change
7. *Biliary tree dilatation* – Biloma, Caroli's disease, choledochal cyst	

HYPERPERFUSION ABNORMALITIES OF LIVER

There are areas of early enhancement on arterial-dominant phase due to decreased portal blood flow/formation of intrahepatic arterioportal shunts/increased aberrant drainage through hepatic veins.
- *Lobar/segmental:*
  - Portal vein thrombosis
  - Obstruction by malignant neoplasm
  - Ligation of arterioportal shunt
  - Hypervascular GB disease
- *Sub-segmental:*
  - Obstruction of peripheral portal branches
  - Acute cholecystitis
  - FNAB
- *Generalized heterogeneous:*
  - Cirrhosis
- *Subcapsular:*
  - Idiopathic
- *Miscellaneous:*
  - Aberrant venous drainage as gastric or cystic veins.

HEPATIC TUMORS WITH VASCULAR "SCAR"

- FNH
- Hepatic adenoma
- Giant cavernous—hemangioma
- Fibrolamellar HCC
- Intrahepatic cholangiocarcinoma
- Hypervascular metastases.

DIFFUSELY HYPODENSE LIVER ON NECT

- Fatty infiltration (obesity, early cirrhosis, Cushing's disease, late pregnancy, CCl4 poisoning, etc.
  - No change on postcontrast scans
  - No mass effect on vascular channels.
- *Malignant infiltration:*
  - Heterogeneous enhancement on CECT.
- *Amyloidosis:*
  - No change on CECT.

- *Budd-Chiari syndrome:*
  - On CECT, non-visualized hepatic veins and/or IVC, multiple collaterals at porta
  - Hepatomegaly in acute cases
  - Shrunken liver with hypertrophied caudate lobe in chronic cases.

MRI in Important Hepatic Lesions

Lesions	T1W	T2W	Gadolinium
1. HCC	↓, Iso, ↑	↑	↑
2. Metastases except melanoma	↓	↑	± ↑
3. Melanoma metastasis	↑	↓	± ↑
4. Hemangioma	↓	↑	↑
5. Adenoma	↑	↓	–
6. FNH			
Central scar	↓	↑	↑
margin	Isointense	↑	± ↑
7. Regenerating nodules	↓, Isointense Hyperintense	↓	–
8. Hemochromatosis	↓	↓ ++	–

SPLENOMEGALY

- *Massively:*
  - CML
    - Kala-azar
  - Myelofibrosis
    - Gaucher's disease
  - Malaria
    - Lymphoma
- *Moderately:*
  - All the above
  - Storage disorders (Niemann-Pick disease, DM)
  - Hemolytic anemia (TTP, Spherocytosis)
  - Portal hypertension
  - Leukemias
- *Mildly:*
  - All of the above
  - Infection:
    - Viral—infectious mononucleosis
    - Bacterial—brucellosis, enteric fever

- Fungal—histoplasmosis
- Rickettsial—typhus
- Sarcoidosis
- Amyloidosis
- Rheumatoid arthritis
- SLE
- Splenic trauma.

SPLENIC CALCIFICATION

- *Diffusely disseminated:*
  - Phleboliths:
    - May have central lucencies
  - Granulomas:
    - Most common multiple, small nodular
    - Seen in tuberculosis, histoplasmosis and brucellosis.
- *Vascular:*
  - Splenic artery calcification—curvilinear
  - Splenic artery aneurysm.
- *Calcified cyst wall (Curvilinear):*
  - Congenital cyst
  - Post-traumatic cyst
  - Echinococcal cyst
  - Cystic dermoid
  - Epidermoid.
- *Miscellaneous:*
  - Sickle cell anemia—fine granular
  - *Pneumocystis carinii*
  - Healed abscess or infarct or hematoma.

HYPERECHOIC SPLENIC LESION

- *Granulomas:*
  - Miliary tuberculosis, histoplasmosis
- Phleboliths
- Myelofibrosis
- Gamma-Gandy nodules in portal hypertension.

FOCAL HYPOATTENUATING LESIONS IN SPLEEN

- Lymphoma/leukemia
- Metastases
- Abscesses

- *Cystic lesions:*
  - Congenital cyst/epidermoid
  - Pseudocyst (Post-traumatic)
  - Cystic degeneration of infarct/hematoma
  - Cavernous hemangioma/lymphangioma.

PANCREATIC CALCIFICATION

- *Chronic pancreatitis:*
  - Numerous tiny stippled calcifications usually intraductal.
    - Alcoholic
      - Calcification limited to head and tail.
    - Biliary
    - Idiopathic
    - Hereditary
      - Autosomal dominant.
      - Calcification is typically rounded and large.
      - Diagnosis considered in young, non-alcoholics.
    - Pancreatic pseudocyst
      - Curvilinear rim calcification is addiction.
- *Neoplastic:*
  - Microcystic adenoma—"sunburst" appearance
  - Macrocystic cystadenoma—amorphous and peripheral
  - Adenocarcinoma (rare)
  - Cavernous hemangioma—multiple phleboliths
  - Metastases from colon, ovarian carcinomas.
- *Hyperparathyroidism:*
  - Similar to chronic pancreatitis
  - Concomitant nephrocalcinosis or urolithiasis.
- *Cystic fibrosis*
  - Typically fine and granular
  - Occurs late in disease and suggests advanced pancreatic fibrosis.
- *Kwashiorkor*
  - Similar to chronic pancreatitis

Tropical pancreatitis appears before adulthood.
- *Intraparenchymal hemorrhage:*
  - Old hematoma/abscess/infarct.
- *Hemochromatosis.*

PANCREATIC MASSES

Focal pancreatitis
History of:
- Usually in pancreatic head
- Calcification/cystic areas
- May be difficult.

Serous cystadenoma (Microcystic)
- Benign.
- Females > males, 1.5:1, elderly female abdominal pain and/or mass.
- Hypervascular, multilocular cystic tumor with small cyst—with clear watery glycogen-rich fluid.
- Central scar with sunburst pattern of calcification.
- USG—homogeneous hyperechoic solid looking encapsulated mass.

Mucinous cystadenoma (Macrocystic)
- Malignant/premalignant
- Uni/multilocular
- Females > males, body and tail of pancreas.
- Large cystic areas may contain curvilinear calcification in cyst wall.
- Epigastric pain/abdominal mass.

May be difficult to differentiate from necrotic adenocarcinoma but carcinoma has thick, irregular wall with calcification.
- *Intraductal papillary mucinous tumor:*
  - Abdominal pain/recurrent pancreatitis
  - Males > females
  - Ductal dilatation.
- *Islet cell tumors:*
  - 80% functionally—small
  - 25% nonfunctioning—large.
- *Most common insulinoma:*
  - 90% benign, 10% malignant, 90% solitary
  - Whipple triad-1 decrease blood glucose, (hypoglycemia) relief by glucose.
  - CT- hypervascular-arterial phase
  - Post Gd. MR-Rim enhancement.
- Endoscopic—relatively hypoechoic with well-defined smooth margins.
  - 2nd MC Gastrinoma—ZES—(Acid hypersecretion diarrhea, peptic ulcer)
  - 60% multiple, 60% malignant
  - Hypervascular
  - Gastrinoma triangle-cystic and CD superior, 2nd and 3rd parts of duodenum, pancreatic head and neck.

Adenocarcinoma
More than 80% of all primary pancreatic neoplasms.
- Males > females
- Risk factors
  - Cigarette smoking
  - Alcohol and coffee—not associated with increased adenocarcinoma.

Clinical features
- Pain
- Weight loss
- Jaundice—cancer head of pancreas
- Unexplained venous thrombosis
- 60% head, 13% body, 5% tail, 22% diffuse.

Imaging
- CT most popular means of determining the local tumor extent and assessing candidates for potential curative surgery.
- Should be the initial diagnostic procedure.

Ultrasonography

Echo poor homogeneous highly attenuating masses, becoming heterogeneous as they enlarge, with irregular lobulated margins.
- Double duct sign, chain of lakes appearance of main pancreatic duct.

Doppler

Involvement of PV, SV, hepatic and gastroduodenal arteries.

NECT

Most adenocarcinoma have attenuation pattern similar to normal pancreas unless necrosis/cystic change present.
- Detected only as contour deformity
- Calcification usually absent.

Contrast Enhanced CT

Hypovascular, with tumor-pancreas contrast being maximum in pancreatic phase.

Other Features

- Focal contour change with or without discrete mass
- Focal lesion of soft tissue density in an otherwise fatty replaced gland
- Spherical enlargement of the head
- Convex rounded border of the uncinate process
- Abrupt termination of CBD
- Double duct sign.

Criteria for Unresectability

- Tumor diameter 5 cm or more
- Extra pancreatic invasion of adjacent tissues and organs, with the exception of the duodenum
- Distant metastasis > nodal hematogenous
- Occlusion, stenosis or encasement of vessels portal vein SMA, celiac trunk.

TNM staging

T Tx—primary tumor cannot be assessed
    T0—no e/o any primary tumor
    T1—tumor limited to pancreas
    T1a—less than 2.0 cm
    T1b—more than 2.0 cm
    T2—extension into duodenum, bile duct or peripancreatic tissue.
    T3—extension into stomach, spleen, colon or adjacent large vessels.
N Nx—could not be assessed
    N0— –ve
    N1— +ve
M Mx— could not be assessed
    M0— –ve
    M1— +ve

MRI—useful in tumor detection, staging, identification of level of obstruction and site of tumor.

Gradient echo and T1W spin echo—used to evaluate vascular invasion.

T1WI: To evaluate lymphadenopathy.
T2W: For hepatic metastases.
T1WI: Hypointense relative to normal pancreatic parenchyma.
T2WI: Variable signal intensity. Postgadolinium-hypovascular.
MRCP: Heavily T2WI-level and degree of duct obstruction.

Endoscopic Retrograde Cholangio-Pancreatography (ERCP):
- When CT/MR findings unclear.
- Ductal dilatation without identification of mass.
- To differentiate duodenal and ampullary tumors from periampullary tumors.

Endoscopic Ultrasound

- Currently under evaluation.

Advantages

- To visualize pancreas and surrounding structures with high resolution
- To guide FNAC
- Vascular and LN invasion.

Disadvantages

- Invasive
- Operator dependence
- Inability to detect distant metastases.

Solid and Papillary Epithelial Neoplasm

- Young female: 11–47 years
- 84% less than 35 years
- Large size tumor with solid and cystic areas with well-defined capsule in the body and/or tail of pancreas. Common intralesional hemorrhage and necrosis
- This unusual neoplasm is considered when characteristic CT findings are seen in young female patients.

Lymphoma

- Usually secondary to systemic disease
- Primary very rare
- Large homogeneous solid mass, infrequently with central cystic areas
- Lymphadenopathy
- Displacement and stretching of peripancreatic vessels.

Metastasis

- Most common from melanoma—hyperintense on T1
- Also from—Breast, lung, kidney, prostate, GIT
- Multiple with H/o primary (known primary)
- If solitary, may be indistinguishable from primary.

FOCAL PANCREATIC MASSES

Lesions	Features	Findings on CT
Neoplastic		
Adenocarcinoma	Most common in head and tail	Isodense of NECT followed by body calcification very rare. Presence of metastasis and invasion of vessel distinguish it from focal pancreatitis Hyper attenuating in early arterial phase
Islet cell tumor	– 80% are functioning, except functioning insulinomas, all are malignant 75% of nonfunctioning tumors are benign, calcification common, diagnosis is usually by clinical symptomatology and hormonal markers	– β-cell tumor–90% benign and < 2 cm – Usually isodense on NECT with marked contrast enhancement – Gastrinoma–60% malignant, marked contrast enhancement – Associated with MEN-I – Glucaganoma – > 4 cm
Cystadenoma carcinoma	Usually females > 60 years	Multiple small cysts in head (<2 cm)
Cystadenoma	Frequently calcified	
Cystadenocarcinoma	Calcification less common	Multiple large cysts (> 5 cm) in body and tail.
Lymphoma	Usually secondary	Large homogeneous solid mass with peri-pancreatic lymphadenopathy causing displacement and stretching of vascular structures
Solid and papillary	Rare *epithelial neoplasm*	—
Metastases	Usually form RCC, HCC, bronchogenic	Known primary at other site breast, ovarian cancer melanoma
Inflammatory		
Focal pancreatitis	Usually in head of pancreas Calcification may be seen	Absence of associated metastases and adjacent invasion
Pancreatic abscess	Secondary to infected phlegmon/pseudocyst	Ring enhancing mass occurring as complication of pancreatitis
Pseudocyst	Complication of acute pancreatitis.	Thick wall cystic mass, may be multiple with H/o acute pancreatitis

ADRENAL MASS

Width of normal limb is less than 1 cm
- Bilateral large adrenals:
  - Hodgkin's disease
  - Adrenal hyperplasia
  - Adrenal hemorrhage
  - Wilms' tumor
  - Infection as histoplasmosis/tuberculosis
  - Pheochromocytoma
  - Metastases
- Unilateral adrenal mass
  - CT attenuation
    < 0HU = benign mass
    0–15 HU = probably benign
    >15 HU = indeterminate
  - On 15 minutes delayed contrast enhanced scan.
    <25 HU = benign lesion
    >25 HU = malignant lesion
  - Size of mass
    <3 cm in diameter = likely benign (90%)
    >5 cm in diameter = likely malignant

Small solid mass	Large solid mass	Cystic masses
Cortical adenoma usually <10HU	– Cortical carcinoma – Pheochromocytoma	Pseudocyst (old hemorrhage infarction)
Metastases usually from lung, breast, RCC, etc.	– Neuroblastoma/ganglioneuroma – Myelolipoma	– Lymphangioma/hemangioma
Pheochromocytoma Granulomatous disease	– Metastase – Hemorrhage	– True cyst – Hydatid cyst
Myelolipoma (Typically fat density)	– Abscesses – Hemangioma	– Cystic degeneration of tumor/hemorrhage – Cortical adenoma with low density

ADRENAL CALCIFICATION

Child

- *Tumor:*
  - Neuroblastoma (90%)
  - Ill-defined, non-homogeneous, stippled calcification
  - Ganglioneuroma (20%)
  Inhomogeneous and stippled
  - Dermoid (Tooth/calcified focus).
- *Vascular:*
  - Hemorrhage (secondary to sepsis, birth trauma)
  Partial or complete ring-like calcification in cyst wall formed secondarily.
- *Miscellaneous*
  - Wolman's disease—AR lipidosis
  Punctate cortical calcifications.

Adults

- Tumors
  - Pheochromocytoma (rare) but when present, is usually in "eggshell pattern"
  - Carcinoma—irregular and punctate
  - Adenoma—punctate and small
  - Ganglioneuroma—flocculent calcification.
- Vascular
  - Hemorrhage (trauma)
  - Similar to that in a child.
- Infection
  - Tuberculosis, histoplasmosis, Waterhouse-Friderichsen syndrome
  - Irregular and punctate.
- Endocrinal
  - Addison disease
  - Commonly due to tuberculosis.

EXTRALUMINAL INTRA-ABDOMINAL GAS

- Pneumoperitoneum
  - Gas within the peritoneal cavity.
- Gas in bowel wall
  - Pneumatosis coli
  - Pneumatosis intestinalis—ischemia/infarction of bowel wall as in necrotizing enterocolitis.

- Gas in biliary tree
  - Irregular branching gas shadows which do not reach the liver edge. It is seen in conditions as patulous sphincter, following passage of gallstones and following postoperative procedures in biliary tree, enterobiliary fistulas, etc.
- Gas in urinary tract
  - Fistula between urinary tract and intestine (Congenital, postoperative, trauma, etc.) emphysematous pyelonephritis and cystitis, etc.
- Gas in portal vein
  - Branching gas shadows which extend to within 2 cm of the liver capsule.
  - Following bowel/mesenteric infarction, air embolus following DCBE.
- *Abscess*
  - Mottled gas pattern. Lack of normal mucosal/haustral pattern help differentiate it from gas in fecal matter.
- Necrotic tumor
  - Usually in large tumors especially following treatment.
- Retroperitoneal gas
  - Secondary to bowel perforation, postoperative procedures/diagnostic retroperitoneal air insufflation.

PNEUMOPERITONEUM

The collection of free air in the peritoneum because of a diverse group of diseases is known as pneumoperitoneum. An erect chest film is preferred to an erect abdominal film for this diagnosis. With careful radiographic techniques, as little as 1 mL of free gas in the peritoneum can be demonstrated. The views done usually to detect this little amount of gas are either an erect chest or left lateral decubitus abdominal film. A patient should be at least in position 10 minutes before the radiograph is taken so that the gas collects in the desired highest point in the abdomen. A pneumoperitoneum can be detected in 76% of cases using an erect chest film. However, if a left lateral decubitus suspected of having pneumoperitoneum are critically ill, an erect film may not be obtained. So it is important to identify the signs of pneumoperitoneum on a supine abdomen film.

Signs on a Supine Film

- Collection of gas in the right upper quadrant adjacent to liver lying mainly in the subhepatic space and the hepatorenal or Morrison's pouch (Doge's sign), and is visible as an oval, linear or triangular collection of gas
- Visualization of outer as well as inner wall of a bowel loop (Rigler's sign)
- Small triangular collection of gas in between three loops of bowel (stellate triangle sign)
- Reflection of peritoneum like the falciform ligament, the medial and lateral umbilical ligaments and the urachus can occasionally be identified when very large amount of free gas is present
- Very large amount of gas may accumulate beneath the diaphragm (cupola sign) or in the center of abdomen (football sign)
- Ligamentum teres sign is air outlining fissure of ligamentum teres hepatis seen as vertically-oriented sharply-defined slit-like area of hyperlucency between 10th and 12th ribs within 2.5–4.0 cm of vertebral border, 2–7 mm wide and 6–20 mm long
- Gas bubbles may be seen lateral to right edge of liver.

Etiology

- *Disruption of wall of a hollow viscus*:
  - Infectious bowel diseases like typhoid, tuberculosis. Typhoid being the commonest cause.
  - Perforated gastric/duodenal ulcer.
  - Blunt/penetrating trauma.
  - Iatrogenic: Laparoscopy, laparotomy, leaking surgical anastomosis, and endoscope induced perforations, enema tip injury, diagnostic pneumoperitoneum.
  - Perforated appendix.
  - Ingested foreign body perforation.
  - Diverticulitis (ruptured Meckel's diverticulum).
  - Necrotizing enterocolitis with perforation.

- Inflammatory bowel disease (Toxic megacolon).
- Intestinal obstruction secondarily leading to perforation (Figs. 5.17A and B).
- Ruptured pneumatosis cystoides intestinalis with 'balanced pneumoperitoneum' (free intraperitoneal air act as tamponade of pneumatosis cysts, thus maintaining a balance between intracystic air and pneumoperitoneum.
- Idiopathic gastric perforation, i.e. spontaneous perforation in premature infants (congenital gastric wall defects).

- *Through peritoneal surface:*
  - Transperitoneal manipulations like needle biopsy, catheter placements.
  - Mistaken thoracocentesis/chest tube placement.
  - Extension from chest as in dissection of pneumomediastinum, bronchopleural fistula.
  - Penetrating abdominal injury.
- *Through female genital tract:*
  - Iatrogenic as in culdocentesis, Rubin test for tubal patency and pelvic examinations
  - Spontaneous as during intercourse, douching, horse-back riding and knee-chest exercises.
- *Intraperitoneal pathologies*:
  - Peritonitis by gas-forming organisms
  - Ruptured abscess.

Pseudopneumoperitoneum

These are processes that mimic free gas in the peritoneum:
- *Pseudo wall sign*: This is seen when two gas distended bowel loops come in close apposition
- *Chilaiditi's syndrome*: It is a specific radiological abnormality seen in very thin asthenic individuals due to interposition of colon between the liver and diaphragm leading to a false impression of free gas. The colon can however be recognized on careful inspection of presence of the haustral pattern
- Sub-diaphragmatic intraperitoneal fat or interposition of omental fat between liver and diaphragm
- *Curvilinear collapse*: Sometimes a band of curvilinear collapse with a crescent of normal lung between it and diaphragm may simulate free gas
- Sub-pulmonary pneumothorax
- Uneven diaphragm
- Retroperitoneal air
- Sub-diaphragmatic abscess (Fig. 5.18).

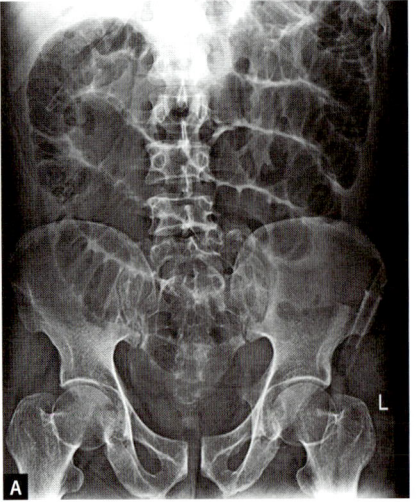 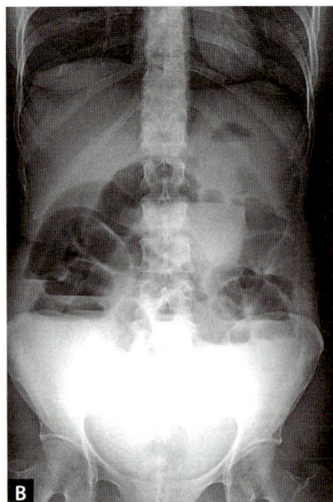

Figs. 5.17A and B: Anteroposterior radiograph of abdomen in supine and erect posture in a case of intestinal obstruction.

Abdomen and Gastrointestinal Tract and Hepatobiliary System

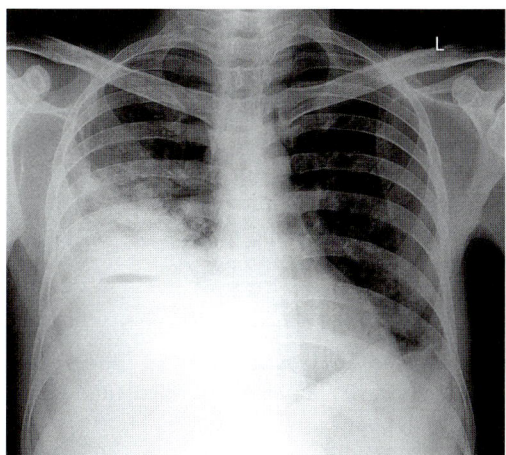

Fig. 5.18: Posteroanterior radiograph of chest shows right subphrenic abscess causing pneumonic consolidation with pleural effusion on right side associated with minimal pleural effusion on left side.

PNEUMOPERITONEUM (FLOWCHART 5.4)

- It indicates presence of gas within the peritoneal cavity
- As little as 1 mL of free gas may be detected on erect chest or left lateral decubitus abdominal films, but gas may take up to 10 minutes to rise
- On erect films, gas accumulates beneath the domes "cupola or moustache" sign
- On supine films, gas may be seen in subhepatic space (dolfin sign); outlining falciform ligament; outlining outer margin of bowel wall (Rigler's sign); and at times gas may collect in the center of the abdomen over a fluid collection (football sign) (Fig. 5.19).

Causes

- *Perforation:*
  - Peptic ulcer—75–80% shows pneumoperitoneum.
  - Inflammation toxic megacolon, diverticulitis.
  - Infarction (bowel or mesentery).
  - Obstruction (volvulus, neoplasms, etc.)
  - Pneumatosis coli/intestinalis.
- *Iatrogenic:* Postprocedure (following peritoneal dialysis, endoscopy, embolization) or postoperative. It may take 2–3 weeks for reabsorption of air; however, serial radiographs will show a definite decrease.
- *Associated chest conditions:*
  - Pneumonia.
  - Emphysema.
  - Carcinoma of lung.
  - Pneumomediastinum.
  - Intermittent positive pressure ventilation.
  - Pulmonary peritoneal fistula.

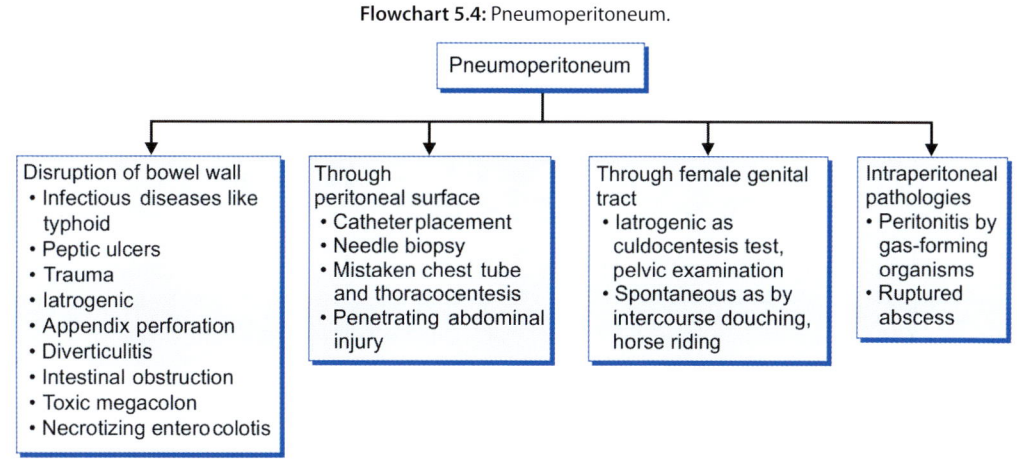

Flowchart 5.4: Pneumoperitoneum.

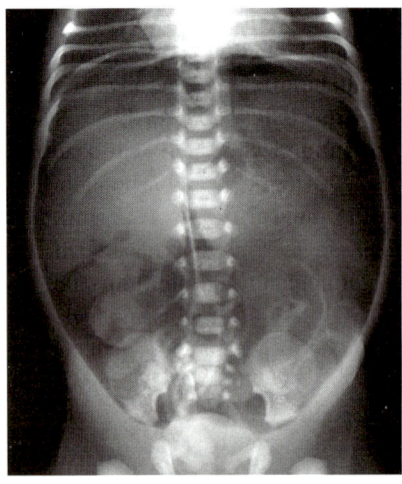

Fig. 5.19: Anteroposterior radiograph of abdomen in supine posture shows diffuse pneumoperitoneum.

- Introduction per vaginum as following vaginal douches.
- Idiopathic.

GASLESS ABDOMEN

Characterized by Ground-glass Haziness in Abdominal Radiograph with Normal Properitoneal Fat Lines or Bulging of Flank Lines in Some Cases

In Children

- *High obstruction:*
  - Isolated esophageal atresia.
  - Duodenal atresia.
  - Annular pancreas.
  - Hypertrophic pyloric stenosis.
  - Choledochal cyst.
  - Volvulus.
- Excessive vomiting.
- Excessive nasogastric aspiration.
- Fluid-filled bowel loops as closed loop obstruction, bowel wash out.
- Relative absence of bowel loops in abdomen as in congenital diaphragmatic hernia.

In Adults

- *High obstruction:*
  - Volvulus.
  - Benign and malignant strictures.
- Ascites.
- Pancreatitis and other acute abdominal conditions producing excessive vomiting.
- *Fluid-filled bowel:*
  - Mesenteric/bowel infarction.
  - Active colitis.
- Large abdominal mass pushing and collapsing the bowel loops laterally.
- Normal variant.

ASCITES

It is defined as accumulation of fluid in the peritoneal cavity. Smaller amount of fluid is first detected in pelvis.

Radiographic Signs

- Obliteration of fat lines at the superior border of bladder.
- Linear lucency of pelvic fat between the fluid density and bony pelvis.
- Symmetric densities on both sides of bladder due to fluid in peritoneal recesses (dog's ears) appearance.
- With larger amounts of fluid.
  - Elevation of both domes of diaphragm.
  - Homogenous shadow of soft tissue density called "ground-glass appearance".
  - Poor visualization of psoas and renal outline.
  - Obliteration of right lateral inferior margin of liver.
  - Displacement of ascending and descending colon medially with obliteration of haustral markings and of the flank stripes.
  - Visualization of lateral lucent band between the lateral abdominal wall and right lobe of liver.
    ♦ Hellmer's sign.
- On barium study—separation of small bowel loops is seen.
- Ultrasonography is very sensitive in detecting ascites, even the minute amounts, especially with a full bladder.

Technique

However, small amount of fluid collections in pelvis are more sensitively detected by

transvaginal/transrectal ultrasound than transabdominal approach. Hyperechoic reflections are seen with complicated ascites.
- On CT/MRI, ascites appear as extra-visceral collection and, in addition, may reveal the underlying cause in some instances.

Causes
- *Neonatal ascites:*
  – Urinary causes
    • Bladder/renal rupture.
    • Posterior urethral valves.
  – Chylous ascites
    • Perforation of GB/CBD.
    • Intestinal lymphangiectasia.
  – Hemoperitoneum
    • Ruptured adrenal/spleen/liver.
    • Ruptured congenital neuroblastoma.
    • Ruptured hepatic tumor or hemangioma.
  – Intestinal contents (Bowel perforation)
    • Meconium ileus.
    • Atresia.
    • Stress ulcer.
  – Transudate
    • Fetal hydrops.
    • Cardiac failure.
    • Idiopathic.
- *Adults*
  – Cirrhosis with portal hypertension.
  – Hypoalbuminemia.
  – Infectious peritonitis—particularly tubercular.
  – Perforation peritonitis (Fig. 5.20).
  – Tumoral ascites.
  – Malignancy
    • Mesothelioma, peritoneal metastases, carcinoma of GIT and ovary.
  – Benign
    • Fibroma of ovary (Meig's syndrome).

Increased Pressure in the Vascular System
- CHF
- Constrictive pericarditis.
- Thrombosis of IVC.

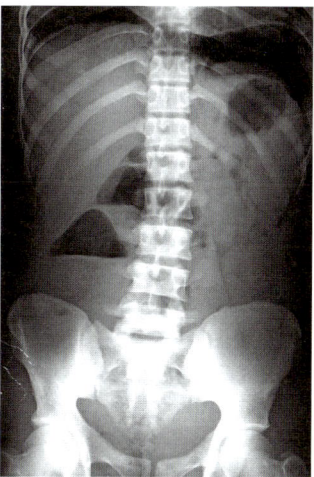

Fig. 5.20: Anteroposterior radiograph of abdomen in erect posture shows pneumoperitoneum under both domes of diaphragm associated with air-fluid levels in right abdomen.

Lymphatic Obstruction
- Obstruction of visceral lymphatic drainage or of the origin of lymphatic duct at the level of cistern of Pecquet.
- Lymphoma.
- Postradiotherapy.
- Trauma.
- Filariasis
  – Miscellaneous as myxedema, extrahepatic causes of portal hypertension.

ABDOMINAL MASS IN NEONATE

- *Renal (55%):*
  – *Hydronephrosis*: Dilated pelvicalyceal system. It may be associated with hydroureter and bladder hypertrophy. It may be due to PUJ obstruction, posterior urethral valves, ectopic ureterocele, prune-belly syndrome and UVJ obstruction.
  – *Multicystic dysplastic kidney.*
  – *Infantile polycystic kidney.*
  – *Mesoblastic nephroma.*
  – *Renal vein thrombosis.*
  – *Renal ectopia.*
  – *Paranephric collection (urinoma).*
  – *Wilms' tumor (rare).*

- *Genital (15%):*
  - Hydrometrocolpos—dilated fluid-filled vagina and/or uterus.
  - Adnexal cysts—follicular cysts (most common), corpus luteal cyst, theca lutein cyst, para-ovarian cyst, teratoma, cystadenomas.
  - Gastrointestinal (15%) commonly associated with obstruction.
    - Duplication cyst—most common bowel mass.
    - Mesenteric cyst.
    - Meconium pseudocyst.
    - Dilated bowel.
  - *Non-renal retroperitoneal (10%):*
    - Adrenal hemorrhage—commonly due to neonatal stress.
    - Neuroblastoma.
    - Teratoma.
  - *Hepato/Spleno/Biliary (5%):*
    - Hepatoblastoma.
    - Hepatic cyst.
    - Splenic cyst.
    - Splenic hematoma.
    - Choledochal cyst.
  - *Miscellaneous:*
    - Urachal cyst.
    - Meningocele in lower abdomen.
    - Sacrococcygeal teratoma.

ABDOMINAL MASS IN CHILD

- Renal 55%:
  - Wilms' tumor.
  - Hydronephrosis—due to PUJ obstruction, PU valves, reflux disease, associated with UTI.
  - Cyst—multicystic dysplastic kidney, polycystic disease, simple cysts, cystic nephroma, calyceal cyst, etc.
- *Non-renal retroperitoneal 23%:*
  - Neuroblastoma.
- *Gastrointestinal 18%:*
  - Appendicular abscess.
  - Hepatoblastoma commonly in right lobe, 40% are bilateral lobes and 40% calcify.
  - Hemangiomas—multiple, involving entire liver ± CHF and may be associated with cutaneous hemangiomas.
  - Choledochal cyst—10% present with a classical triad of mass, pain and jaundice. Dynamic radionuclide scintigraphy with 99Tc—TBIDA is diagnostic.
  - Omental cyst (greater omentum/lesser sac, multilocular).
  - Mesenteric cyst (between leaves of small bowel mesentery).
  - Duplication cyst.
  - Pancreatic pseudocyst.
  - Meckel diverticulum.
  - Mesenteric lymphoma.
- *Genital:*
  - Ovarian cyst.
  - Teratoma.
- *Miscellaneous:* Cystic lymphangioma.

DD of Wilms' Tumor and Neuroblastoma

		Wilms' Tumor	*Neuroblastoma*
•	Age	80% <3 years	15–30% <1 year; 75% <5 years
•	Site	Kidneys	Adrenal (40%), sympathetic chain in abdomen (25%), chest (15%), neck (5%), pelvis (5%)
•	Plain Film		
	– Calcification	10%	2/3 cases
	– Renal outline	Lost or enlarged	Maintained but displaced
	– Intervertebral foramina	Normal	May be enlarged
	Bone lesion	Uncommon	Common

- On USG/CT/MRI

– Major vessels	Displaced	Encased
hemorrhage/ necrosis	Common	Uncommon
– IVC/renal vein thrombosis	Common	Uncommon

- Radionuclide scanning: Not useful / MIBG scanning is useful for skeletal metastases
- Associated syndrome: Beckwith synd. (macroglossia, organomegaly, exomphalos hemihyper-trophy) Cryptorchidism, hypospadias, aniridia, hemi-hypertrophy may also be associated / Opsomyoclonus (cerebellar ataxia and jerky eye movement), hypertension and ± diarrhea due to VIP secretion

INTESTINAL OBSTRUCTION IN NEONATE

- *Duodenal—most common:*
  - Stenosis/Atresia—"double-bubble" sign; may be associated with annular pancreas, mongolism or with other abnormalities of GIT.
  - Annular pancreas—may not present until adulthood.
  - Peritoneal bands—congenital fibrous bands of Ladd connect cecum to posterior abdominal wall and commonly cross duodenum.
  - Aberrant vessel as preduodenal portal vein.
  - Congenital web.
  - Choledochal cyst.
- *Jejunal and ileal obstruction.*
  CT is best modality for evaluation (95% accurate with 94% sensitivity and 96% specificity).
  - Atresia/stenosis.
  - Midgut volvulus results from arrest in rotation and fixation of small bowel in fetal life.
  - Meconium ileus—mottled lucencies are seen due to gas entrapment in meconium. Peritoneal calcification secondary to perforation is seen in 30% cases.
  - Inguinal hernia.
  - Inspissated milk—dense amorphous intraluminal masses surrounded by rim of air with or without mottled lucencies within them. Resolves spontaneously.
  - Paralytic ileus usually due to drugs administered during labor.
  - Enteric duplication cyst—located on antimesenteric side, mostly in ileum.
  - Mesenteric cyst from meconium peritonitis located on mesenteric side.
- *Colonic:*
  - Hirschsprung's disease (Fig. 5.21).
  - Small left colon syndrome.
  - Meconium plug syndrome.
  - Atresia.
  - Anorectal malformation (Fig. 5.22).
    - *High type*—with or without sacral agenesis and gas in bladder (due to rectovesical fistula)
    - *Low type*—perineal/urethral fistula may be associated.

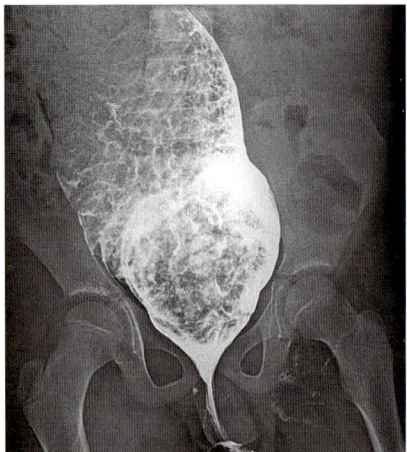

Fig. 5.21: Barium enema in anteroposterior projection shows anorectal narrowing with proximal megacolon in Hirschsprung's disease.

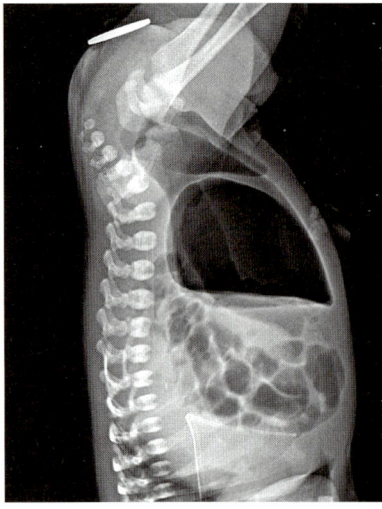

Fig. 5.22: Lateral invertogram shows high type of anorectal malformation with signs of intestinal obstruction.

ABNORMALITIES OF BOWEL ROTATION

- *Exomphalos:* It refers to total failure of bowel to return to the abdomen from the umbilical cord, which are contained within a sac. This is a midline lesion.
  - *Differential diagnosis:* Gastroschisis—paramidline abdominal wall defect through which the bowel protrudes.
- *Non-rotation:*
  - Asymptomatic.
  - Small bowel located on right side of abdomen.
  - Colon located on left side of abdomen.
  - Small and large bowel lies on either side of SMA with a common mesentery.
  - Superior mesenteric vein (SMV) is situated to the left of superior mesenteric artery (SMA).
- *Malrotation*—DJ flexure lies to the right of midline and caudal to its usual position.
  - The cecum is more cephalad than normal.
  - Invariably complicates left-sided diaphragmatic hernia.
  - SMV is anterior to SMA.
- *Reverse rotation:*
  - Colon is dorsal to SMA with jejunal and duodenum anterior to it.
- *Paraduodenal hernias (rare):*
  - Through fossa of Landzert on left side (3/4)
    - Lateral to 4th part of duodenum and behind descending and transverse mesocolon.
  - Through fossa of Waldeyer on right side (1/4)
    - Caudal to SMA and inferior to 3rd part of duodenum.
- *Extroversion of cloaca—rare:*
  - No rotation of bowel.
  - Ileum and colon open separately onto the extroverted area in the midline below the umbilical cord.

INTRA-ABDOMINAL CALCIFICATION IN NEONATE

- *Extraluminal:*
  - Peritoneal calcification following fetal bowel perforation and meconium peritonitis.
- *Intraluminal:*
  - Intestinal obstruction following imperforate anus, small bowel atresia or Hirschsprung's disease.
  - Multifocal gastrointestinal atretic sites.

HEMATEMESIS

It occurs due to upper GI bleed where the bleeding site is proximal to the ligament of Treitz. Mortality is approximately 10%. Barium exam should be avoided in acute cases.

Causes

- *Esophageal causes:*
  - Hiatus hernia (Figs. 5.23A and B)
  - Esophageal varices—mortality 50%
  - Esophageal neoplasms
  - Mallory-Weiss tears—very low mortality.
- *Gastric causes*—mortality less than 10% if less than 60 years and more than 35% if more than 60 years.
  - Acute hemorrhagic gastritis—secondary to steroids, NSAIDs or alcohol intake.
  - Gastric ulcers.
  - Malignancy especially leiomyosarcoma.
- *Duodenal causes:*
  - Blood dyscrasias.
  - Hereditary telangiectasia—autosomal dominant.
  - Connective tissue disorders as Ehlers-Danlos syndrome, pseudoxanthoma elasticum.
- Visceral artery aneurysm.
- Vascular malformation.

DYSPHAGIA IN ADULTS

Difficulty in swallowing can be due to:
- *Intrinsic causes:*
  - Benign strictures.
    - Peptic strictures due to reflux esophagitis.
    - Ingestion of corrosive acids and alkalis or foreign bodies.
    - Iatrogenic following prolonged nasogastric intubation or fibrosis secondary to radiotherapy.
    - Cutaneous diseases such as epidermolysis bullosa and pemphigus.
    - Syndromes as Plummer-Vinson syndrome, which produces anterior indentation in the form of web. It is common in females with iron deficiency anemia and in males with postgastrectomy status. Web can occur from C4 to D1 level. The condition is premalignant.
    - Tumors as leiomyomas.
  - Malignant strictures.
    - Carcinomas
    - Lymphomas.
  - Miscellaneous:
    - Infections as moniliasis, HSV or CMV infections. They all produce

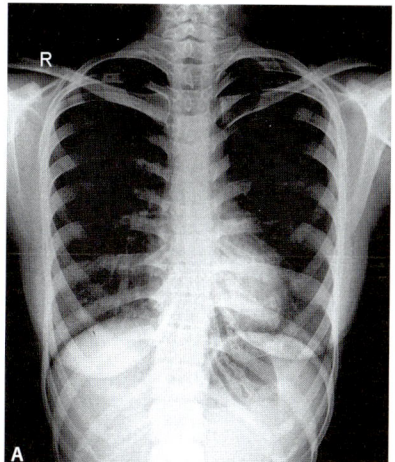 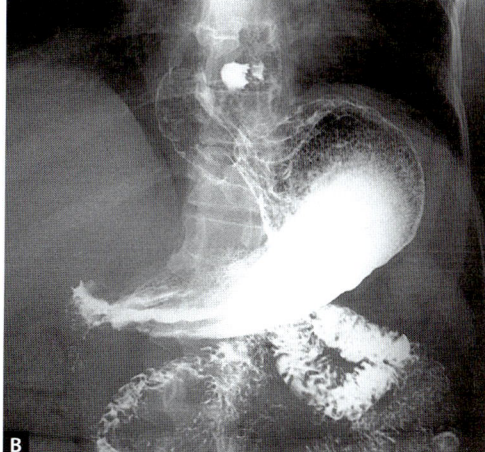

Figs. 5.23A and B: Plain posteroanterior radiograph of chest and oblique view of barium meal study shows hiatus hernia.

shaggy ulcerated appearance and odynophagia (painful deglutition)
- Schatzki's ring may produce dysphagia if internal diameter is less than 6 mm.
- *Extrinsic causes:*
  - Tumors:
    - Mediastinal lymphomas and other tumors, mediastinal lymphadenopathy.
  - Vascular:
    - Aortic aneurysm.
    - Aberrant right subclavian artery produces posterior indentation (dysphagia lusoria).
    - Aberrant left pulmonary artery produces anterior indentation.
    - Right-sided aortic arch produces right lateral and posterior indentation.
  - Pharyngeal pouch may indent the esophagus. It may produce air-fluid level with signs of aspiration pneumonitis on chest radiograph.
  - Goiter.
  - Enterogenous cyst lies adjacent to the esophagus. Evidence of associated hemivertebra and anterior meningocele may be there.
  - Prevertebral abscess/hematoma.
- *Neuromuscular disorders:*
  - Megaesophagus as in Chagas disease, achalasia cardia.
  - Systemic disease as scleroderma, myasthenia gravis.
  - Bulbar/pseudobulbar palsy.
- *Psychiatric disorder:*
  - Globus hystericus.

NEONATAL DYSPHAGIA

- *Congenital anomalies:*
  - Cleft palate.
  - Macroglossia associated with syndromes as Pierre Robin or Beckwith-Wiedemann syndrome.
  - Esophageal atresia.
  - Brain malformation as Chiari malformation.
  - Vascular anomalies.
    - Aberrant right subclavian artery compressing the esophagus from behind.
    - Aberrant left pulmonary artery indenting the esophagus anteriorly.
    - Right-sided aortic arch producing a posterior and right lateral indentation over esophagus.
  - Choanal atresia.
- *Miscellaneous:*
  - Delayed/subnormal mental development.
  - Prematurity.

PHARYNGEAL/ESOPHAGEAL DIVERTICULA

Diverticulum is a blind sac or pouch arising from pharynx or esophagus.
- *Upper third:*
  - Zenker's/Pharyngoesophageal/Hypopharyngeal diverticulum.
    - Present in middle-aged and elderly, especially more than 50 years of age.
    - Arises through the posterior wall of hypopharynx usually on the left side through Killian's triangle (weak area between the inferior constrictor and cricopharyngeus sphincter).
    - Causes oropharyngeal dysphagia, regurgitation, aspiration and hoarseness of voice.
    - May present as a mass in neck or superior mediastinal mass on chest X-ray with or without an air-fluid level.
    - It is a pulsion type of diverticulum.
  - *Lateral pharyngocele:*
    - Congenital—is remnant of 2nd branchial arch.
    - Acquired—Seen in trumpeters, glassblowers.
- *Middle third:*
  - Traction:
    - Usually at the level of carina.
    - Secondary to mediastinal inflammation or adenopathy as in tuberculosis and histoplasmosis.
  - Developmental as in tracheoesophageal fistulas.

- Lower third:
  - Epiphrenic:
    Causes include:
    - Long standing peptic esophagitis and strictures.
    - Iatrogenic—postendoscopy or surgical injury.
    - Motility disorders as diffuse esophageal spasms, achalasia, hypertensive lower esophageal sphincter.
    - Collagen disorders—Ehlers-Danlos syndrome.
    - Miscellaneous.

Esophageal

Intramural Pseudodiverticulosis

- Very rare.
- There is dilatation of submucosal glands producing numerous tiny out-pouching within the wall.
- Segmental/diffuse.
- Strictures/dysmotility of esophagus is usually associated.

ESOPHAGITIS/ESOPHAGEAL ULCERS

Signs of Esophagitis

- Fine mucosa with nodularity in double contrast studies.
- Thickening of longitudinal folds (wider than 3 mm).
- Thickening of transverse folds.
- Reduced or absent peristalsis.

Reflux Esophagitis

Part of Esophagus Involved

- Lower third esophagus.

Features

- Blurring of squamocolumnar junction
- Fine, punctate ulcer which ultimately becomes punched out immediately above the esophagogastric junction.

Comments/Additional Features

- Hiatus hernia is commonly associated.

Barrett's Esophagitis

Part of Esophagus Involved

- Lower third.

Features

- Ulceration at junction of columnar and squamous esophageal mucosa.
- Fine reticular pattern of mucosa resembling area gastricae due to islands of columnar mucosa.

Comments/Additional Features

- Increased risk of carcinomatous change.

Moniliasis

Part of Esophagus Involved

- Any part but mainly upper-third.

Features

- Early:
  - Mucosal plaques.
  - Folds become nodular.
- Late:
  - Deep marginal ulceration, perforation, fistula and stricture may occur.

Comments/Additional Features

- Common in immunocompromised.

Herpetic Esophagitis

Part of Esophagus Involved

- Mid esophagus.

Features

- Sessile filling defects.
- Punched out ulcers on a background of normal mucosa.
- Ultimately, diffuse ulceration.

Comments/Additional Features

- Common in immunocompromised.
- Oral herpetic lip-lesions suggest the diagnosis.

Cytomegalovirus Esophagitis

Part of Esophagus Involved

- Any part.

Features
- Discrete, superficial ulcer.
- Giant ulcers on a normal mucosal background.

Comments/Additional Features
- Seen invariably in AIDS patients.
- Endoscopic biopsy differentiates them from similar looking HIV ulcers.

Tuberculous Esophagitis

Part of Esophagus Involved
- Any part.

Features
- Deep ulcers and fistulas.
- Scarring and stricture formation.

Comments/Additional Features
- Caseating mediastinal nodes are associated.

Drug-induced Esophagitis

Part of Esophagus Involved
- Mid-esophagus.

Features
- Ulceration.

Comments/Additional Features
- Prolonged contact with certain drugs at sites of esophageal impression above the aortic arch or that produced by left main bronchus, above the impression caused by dilated left atrium and left ventricles (tetracycline, KCl, quinidine, aspirin, phenylbutazone).

Caustic Esophagitis

Part of Esophagus Involved
- Sites of anatomical holdup.

Features
- Ulceration with mucosal sloughing.
- Fibrosis, long-segment smooth strictures.
- Perforation into pleural/pericardial cavity.
- Ultimately, esophagus may be atonic, especially if myenteric plexus is destroyed.

Comments/Additional Features
- Dyes include sodium hydroxide and carbonate, iodine and bleaches.
- Increased risk of squamous cell carcinoma latent period = 20–40 years.

Radiation Esophagitis

Part of Esophagus Involved
- Part included in radiation field.

Features

Doses more than 2500 and less than 4500 rads produce transient changes as:
- Mucosal granularity.
- Minute ulcers.
- Narrowing of lumen from mucosal edema.

Doses more than 4500 rads produce transient changes as:
- Severe esophagitis due to obliterative endarteritis.
- Long smooth tapered strictures.

Comments/Additional Features
- Drugs like adriamycin and actinomycin-D potentiate esophagitis.

Nasogastric Tube Esophagitis

Part of Esophagus Involved
- Lower-third.

Features
- Features of peptic esophagitis.

Comments/Additional Features
- Nasogastric intubation for as short as 3 days can make LES incompetent.

Miscellaneous

Causes include Crohn's disease—intramural diverticulosis.

ESOPHAGEAL STRICTURES

	Inflammatory	Neoplastic
Type	Smooth	Irregular
Length	Usually long	Usually short
Shouldering	Absent	Present
Mucosal fold destruction	Usually absent	Present
Age-group	Early childhood, young adults up to middle age	Middle age and above
Proximal dilatation	More pronounced	Less pronounced
Causes	Peptic, corrosives, achalasia, scleroderma, iatrogenic	Carcinoma, leiomyosarcoma post-radiotherapy

Causes of Smooth Esophageal Strictures

- *Inflammatory*:
  - *Peptic:* Usually lower esophagus.
  - *Scleroderma*—lower 2/3 esophagus; *poor* functioning LES, hypoperistalsis produces reflux esophagitis and stricture.
  - *Corrosives:* Strictures at sites of potential hold-up as aortic arch, esophagogastric junction. Alkalis are more prone than acids.
  - *Iatrogenic:* Prolonged nasogastric intubation produces prolonged dilated LES with reflux and stricture formation in lower-third esophagus.
  - Infections as tuberculosis.
- *Neoplastic*:
  - Carcinoma with submucosal spread.
  - Benign tumors as leiomyoma may produce smooth, eccentric, polypoidal mass.
  - Extrinsic mass as mediastinal lymphadenopathy and carcinoma bronchus, etc.

Irregular Esophageal Strictures

- *Neoplastic:*
  - Carcinoma.
  - Leiomyosarcoma.
  - Carcinosarcoma.
  - Lymphoma.
- *Iatrogenic:*
  - Radiotherapy.
  - Postoperative: Fundoplication.

TERTIARY CONTRACTIONS IN ESOPHAGUS

These are non-coordinated, non-propulsive contractions in esophagus seen mainly in distal 2/3 esophagus 5–10% of normal adult in 4th–6th decade show these.

Causes include
- Presbyesophagus:
  - Elderly patients with severely disordered motility due to muscle atrophy.
  - May cause chest pain or dysphagia.
- Diffuse esophageal spasm.
- Hyperactive achalasia.
- Neuromuscular disease:
  - Diabetes.
  - Parkinsonism.
  - Multiple sclerosis.
  - Thyrotoxic myopathy.
  - Myotonic dystrophy.
- Obstruction at the cardia:
  - Neoplasm.
  - Distal esophageal stricture.
  - Benign lesion.
  - Surgery (repair of hiatus hernia).

Findings:
- Spontaneous repetitive non-propulsive contraction—"yo-yo" motion.
- Corkscrew appearance.
- Compartmentalization of barium ("Rosary bead", "Shish kebab").

GASTRIC MASSES AND FILLING DEFECTS

- *Primary malignant neoplasms:*
  - Carcinoma:
    - Usually polypoidal with granular/lobulated surface.
    - Sessile lesions are detected by alteration in pattern of area gastricae or rugal folds.
    - Usual site is pyloric region.
  - *Lymphoma*:
    - Mostly are NHL
    - May be polypoidal, ulcerating or infiltrative.
    - Multiple polypoidal, tumor especially with central ulceration giving "bulls-eye" appearance, is characteristic.
    - Giant cavitating lesions with pronounced thickening of folds is suggestive of diagnosis.
  - Leiomyosarcoma:
    - Large exophytic tumors with central necrosis.
    - Usual site is fundus and body.
    - Association with functional extra-adrenal paragangliomas and pulmonary chondromas.
  - Kaposi's sarcoma:
    - Frequently seen in AIDS.
    - Multifocal, submucosal and occasionally polypoidal tumors.
    - Associated duodenal and small bowel involvement may be present.
  - Carcinoid:
    - Arise in distal antrum and along lesser curvature.
    - Submucosal nodule, which may be sessile or pedunculated.
    - Highly vascular tumor with hypervascular metastases.
- *Metastases (Secondary malignancies):*
  - Frequently ulcerate producing bull's eye lesion.
  - Common primaries include melanoma, bronchus, breast, etc.
- *Benign lesions:*
  - Polyps.
    - Hyperplastic (local glandular hyperplasia).

  Features:
  - Usually less than 1 cm.
  - Multiple.

  Location:
  - Fundus and body.

  Comments:
  - Most common.
  - Associated with familial polyposis coli.
  - Associated with atrophic gastritis.
  - No premalignant potential.
- Adenomatous polyps (dysplastic)

  Features:
  - Usually more than 1 cm.
  - Often solitary with nodular surface.

  Location:
  - Antrum.

  Comments:
  - Associated with atrophic gastritis.
  - Premalignant.
  - May prolapse into pyloric canal to produce gastric outflow obstruction.
- Villous (Hamartomas).

  Features:
  - Usually more than 3 cm.
  - Reticular appearance.

  Location:
  - Antrum is spared.

  Comments:
  - Associated with Peutz-Jeghers syndrome and Cowden's disease.
    - Submucosal lesion.
- Produces smooth bulge into lumen with obtuse angle with the normal wall.
  - Leiomyoma

  Most common, difficult to separate from leiomyosarcoma.
  - Lipoma

  Soft; changes shape with gastric peristalsis.
  - Others

  Neurofibromas, hemangiomas, lymphangiomas, ectopic pancreatic rests, duplication cyst, etc.

- *Extrinsic indentation:*
  Pancreatic tumors.
  - Splenic enlargement.
  - Hepatic enlargement.
  - Other retroperitoneal tumors.
  - Sub-diaphragmatic masses/collection.
- *Miscellaneous*

Bezoars
- Mobile mass in lumen with no attachment to wall.
- Trichobezoars are commonly seen in psychiatric patients.
- Phytobezoars are the commonest.
- When large, these take the shape of stomach with contrast/barium entering into the interstices of the bezoar.

LINITIS PLASTICA

Linitis plastica or *"leather bottle" stomach* is a result of submucosal spread of pathological process, leaving in most cases an intact mucosa resulting in a negative endoscopy. There is intense desmoplastic reaction, which leads to a rigid stomach wall and narrow lumen. There is loss of normal mucosal pattern and reduced capacity. The stomach wall is thickened and there is loss of normal peristalsis.

Differential Diagnosis
- *Malignancy:*
  - Scirrhous gastric carcinoma.
  - Lymphomas, both Hodgkin's lymphoma and Non-Hodgkin's lymphoma (NHL).
  - Metastatic involvement.
- *Inflammation:*
  - Chronic gastric ulcer disease with intense spasm.
  - Crohn's disease.
  - Sarcoidosis.
  - Eosinophilic gastroenteritis.
  - Polyarteritis nodosa (PAN).
  - Stenosing antral gastritis.
- *Infection:*
  - Tertiary stage of syphilis.
  - Tuberculosis.
  - Histoplasmosis.
  - Actinomycosis.
  - Strongyloidiasis.
- *Trauma:*
  - Corrosive gastritis.
  - Radiation injury.
  - Gastric freezing.
- *Others:*
  - Amyloidosis
  - Pseudolymphoma.
  - Cystic fibrosis.

Radiological Appearance

Barium meal: There is generalized narrowing of gastric lumen (tubular shape of stomach), with reduced capacity, the mucosa is often nodular and fold pattern is lost. There is loss of peristalsis appreciated on fluoroscopy.

Ultrasound: There is evidence of wall thickening, usually more than 6 mm. No evidence of active peristalsis is seen.

CT scan: Water distension with gas effervescence is used to demonstrate the true thickness of gastric wall, which is usually more than 1 cm. The nodular mucosal pattern can be appreciated, and surrounding organs and areas can be examined for associated changes like infiltration and lymphadenopathy in cases of malignancy. One peculiar property of linitis plastica associated with malignancy is contrast enhancement on CECT. This helps identify infiltrative tumors less than 1 cm in thickness.

Common Etiologies

Scirrhous gastric carcinoma: There is intense desmoplastic reaction associated with this carcinoma. It usually involves the antrum of stomach, but may extend to involve the entire stomach. There is firmness, rigidity, reduced capacity and a peristalsis of involved areas. On double contrast barium studies and CECT, there is loss of normal mucosal fold features, with sometimes granular or polypoid folds, and encircling growth. There is intense enhancement on CECT and surrounding infiltration may be present.

Lymphoma: Both Hodgkin's lymphoma and NHL may involve the stomach either partially or diffusely. Stomach is the most common site of GI tract lymphoma, especially NHL or extranodal Hodgkin's lymphoma. The flexibility of gastric wall is preserved and mucosal folds and wall may be grossly thickened (4–5 cm). On CT, there is homogeneous overall attenuation and minimal enhancement after contrast administration. There may be diffuse retroperitoneal and mesenteric adenopathy.

Metastatic involvement: There is usually a history of primary malignancy elsewhere, like malignant melanoma, breast, lung, colon, prostate, leukemia, secondary lymphoma. Breast carcinoma is the most common malignancy producing linitis plastica-like appearance.

Radiation injury: There is a positive history of radiotherapy received for primary malignancy in the nearby organs. There is intense desmoplastic reaction produced by radiotherapy leading to effacement of gastric folds. There is a latent period of one month to two years.

Acids: A positive history of acid ingestion can usually be elicited and is usually found in female patients. There are associated changes in esophagus.

Granulomatous diseases (Tuberculosis, Sarcoidosis): These may cause changes like linitis plastica. Usually associated changes are seen in the lungs. In cases of tuberculosis, changes may be seen in small intestines, and abdominal lymphadenopathy may be present with or without ascites.

Eosinophilic gastroenteritis: The patients may have a positive history of atopy and peripheral blood eosinophilia may be seen in 50% of the cases. Ascites may or may not be present.

Diseases, Features and Additional Points of Linitis Plastica

Diseases	Features	Additional Points
Gastric carcinoma	Loss of wall pliability	Irregular mucosal folds with destruction. Commonest cause
Lymphoma	Wall pliability pre-served, multifocal submucosal nodules	Folds architecture preserved
	Disease extent crosses the GE junction and/or pylorus	Massive associated lymphadenopathy
Metastases, especially breast	Wall pliability preserved	Fold architecture pre-served. Known primary
Local invasion as pancreatic carcinoma	Localized mucosal destruction	Pancreatic mass with evidence of invasion into stomach
Corrosives	Associated with strictures. Non-specific findings	H/o ingestion
Radiation therapy	Mucosal fold effacement. Large antral ulcers may be associated	H/o radiation exposure
Granulomatous disease as Crohn's disease, syphilis, tuberculosis	Nonspecific findings. Wall pliability preserved	Other stigmata elsewhere
Eosinophilic gastritis	Evidence of peripheral eosinophilia. History of allergy. Nonspecific features	Diagnosis by biopsy

GASTROCOLIC FISTULA

- *Inflammatory:*
  - Peptic disease with ulcer and perforation.
  - Crohn's disease with multiple fistulas and mucosal involvement and skip areas.
  - Chronic pancreatitis with enzyme leakage or duct rupture.
  - Granulomatous infections such as tuberculosis and actinomycosis.
- *Neoplastic:*
  - Carcinomas of stomach, pancreas or colon.
  - Metastases with perforation and fistulation.

RETROPERITONEAL FIBROSIS

Also known *as Ormond's disease* or *chronic periaortitis.*

It is a rare fibrotic process frequently involving the caudal aspect of retroperitoneum without effects on ureter, great vessels, lymphatic and even CBD, caused by proliferation of fibroblasts, acute infective cells and capillaries, all of which are surrounded by collagen fibers.

In 15%—associated with fibrotic process elsewhere in the body.

Differential Diagnosis (D/D)

Causes

Primary—2/3rd: Autoimmune with antibodies to 'CEROID' (insoluble lipid) systemic vasculitis associated with fibrosis outside retroperitoneum in 8–15%.

Age—Middle-aged to elderly
Sex—M:F = 2:1
Usually responsive to steroids.

Secondary: It includes
- Benign:
  - Medication 12%—most common is methysergide, but β blocker, methyldopa, hydralazine, antibiotics and other analgesics. Prolonged use causes abdominal, pulmonary and endocardial fibrosis. Early withdrawal often results in regression of the disease.
  - Retroperitoneal hemorrhage—because of trauma, ruptured aneurysm or retroperitoneal surgery like translumbar aortography and percutaneous renal biopsy.
    Aneurysm rupture—on CT-acute extraluminal blood is of soft tissue attenuation with vermiform finger-like extension in the retroperitoneum.
  - Post-traumatic chronic hematoma—decreased mass with a thick dense rim-peripheral calcification may also be seen.
- Infection: Like tuberculosis, syphilis, actinomycosis, brucellosis and fungal infection, etc. can lead to retroperitoneal fibrosis.
- Miscellaneous: Variety of intra-abdominal inflammatory conditions (diverticulitis, appendicitis, extravasation from the urinary tract, aneurysm of aorta and iliac artery).
- Malignant: 8–10%.
  Primary neoplasm or metastatic disease or lymphoma can provoke an extensive desmoplastic reaction.

Primary Retroperitoneal Tumor

Majority are malignant.
- Liposarcoma is most common.
  On CT—is an attenuation of fat density.
- Leiomyosarcoma—large heterogeneous masses.
  Low attenuation component—necrosis.
  No fat or calcification.
- MFH—heterogeneous soft tissue, necrosis positive.

Metastasis

Metastasis from colon and breast, soft tissue, lung, kidney, prostatic tumor incites a fibrotic reaction around itself.

Lymphoma

HL (Hodgkin's lymphoma)>NHL (Non-Hodgkin's lymphoma).

Enlarged lymph node may appear as discrete masses or confluent- soft tissue obliterating the retroperitoneal fat—loss of definition of fat plane but not involving aorta and IVC.

- *Excretory urography*—ureteric obstruction.
- Bilateral in 75%.
- Tapering lumen or complete obstruction—usually at L4-L5.
- Medial deviation of ureter which is obstructed and dilated.
- Other causes—normal in 18%.
  - Pelvic lipomatosis.
  - Following abdominoperineal resection.
  - Retrocaval ureter—right ureter passes behind the IVC at the level of L4.
  - Hypertrophy of psoas muscle of L3.
- USG—hypoechoic smoothly marginated mass that often appears as plaque around the distal aorta due to medial deviation of ureter.

CT: From minimal periureteral stranding to large lobulated masses obliterating the fat plane but not involving the aorta and IVC, indistinguishable from bulky lymphadenopathy.

D/D features of retroperitoneal fibrosis from primary RPF tumor.

RPF: Usually located at the level of L4 and plaque-like and infiltrating rather than nodular RPF usually surrounds the anterior and lateral aspect of great vessels, whereas marked displacement of aorta or IVC is seen in primary retroperitoneal tumor or in malignant LAP.

LAP in lymphoma is often-centered more cephalad in RP and may be bulkier at the level of renal hila.
- Malignant or infective may invade and destroy adjacent bones or organ.

NCCT: RPF—similar to that of muscle/focal or uniform hyper- density—increase collagen.

CECT: Exuberant enhancement.

MRI: Non-malignant RPF
- Homogeneous decrease signal intensity (similar to psoas muscle) on both T1 and T2—reflects mature and quiescent phase.
- Acute benign RPF—intermediate or increase on T2—increase cellularity and fluid.

Malignant

Heterogeneous on T2 WI.

Both malignant and non-malignant enhancement after IV gadolinium.

MRA and GRE are effective—to see the vascular involvement and collateral vessel formation.
- Radionuclide—Ga67 uptake during active infection.

MASS OF ILIOPSOAS COMPARTMENT

- Iliacus and psoas major muscles are chief flexors of lower limb.
- Due to their common *origin* and *insertion*, both are considered together.
- Structurally, they are structures located in posterior abdominal wall.
- Psoas minor is a small muscle absent in up to 70%.
- CT—isoattenuating; minimal/nil enhancement.

MRI—intermediate (T1, T2, PD).

USG—hypoechoic to liver/Iso—to renal medulla with linear echogenic fascial strips.

Plain X-ray—soft tissue density.
- Maximally thick at L3-L4. A linear area within fat about lumbar plexus.

Pathologies/Masses.
Inflammatory.
Neoplastic.
Pseudoaneurysm of lumbar artery.
Hemorrhage.
Iliopsoas bursitis.

Imaging

- Plain X-ray.
- Retroperitoneal air insufflation and tomography.
- CT.
- MRI.
- USG.
- Indirect—IVP, aortography, IVC inferior venocavography.

Salient Features

- *Inflammatory*—most common.
  - Pyogenic/tubercular.
  - Mostly secondaries—surgery, spine, kidney, pancreas, bowel, sometimes primary, also aortic bed.

- On CT and MRI:
  - Diffuse bulkiness.
  - Focal masses.
  - Iso to hypo on CT and with homogeneous/rim enhancement.
  - T1—iso/hypo; T2—hyper; PD—hyper.
  - Gas ±.
  - Calcification ±—tuberculosis.
  - Destruction and sclerosis of adjacent bone.
  - ± a phlegmon or an abscess.
- On USG:
  - Hypoechoic collection.
  - Bulky muscle.
- Plain X-ray—loss of psoas silhouette.
- Apart from imaging, radiologist helps in diagnosis and intervention. We should also try and find out the source of infection.

- *Neoplastic:*
  - 1/3-1/4 the causes of illiopsoas masses.
  - Sometimes, primary soft tissue tumor or sometimes secondarily by invading lesion as lipoma, liposarcoma, rhabdomyoma and sarcomas, teratoma, dermoid, etc.
  - Presence of fat is a sign of fat containing mass.
  - Difficult to differentiate from the above.
- *Hemorrhage:*
  - Due to trauma, iatrogenic, graft, VWD, hemophilia.
  - Expansile mass of various appearances, dual phase of resolution is seen.
  - Bone destruction is not seen.
  - Slowly it resolves forming a level or low density area. Calcifications and rim enhancement confuse it to infection. Superinfection is rarely a problem.
- *Bursitis:*
  - Presents as a flocculent mass in inguinal area with invagination towards hip.
  - Communication to hip is seen in early 15% by arthrography.
  - Due to rheumatoid arthritis, osteoarthritis. It is seen as areas of fluid in all modalities.

- *Pseudoaneurysm of lumbar arteries:*
  - Due to trauma/surgery.
  - Doppler USG/MRA gives good demonstration.

ANATOMY OF LIVER, BILE DUCTS AND PANCREAS

Left Portal Vein

- Absence of horizontal segment (0.2%).

Right Portal Vein

- Trifurcation of main portal vein (11%).
- Origin of RP segment from main portal vein (5%).
- Origin of RA segment from left portal vein (4%).
- Absence of main right, RA and RP portal segments.

RAS = right anterior segment	RPI = right posterior inferior	LMI = left median inferior
RAI = right anterior inferior	RPS = right posterior superior	LMS = left median superior
RAS = right anterior superior	C = caudate lobe	LLI = left lateral inferior
RP = right posterior segment	L = left portal vein	LLS = left lateral superior

Functional Segmental Liver Anatomy

(Goldsmith and Woodburne)		(Couinaud and Bismuth)
Caudate lobe		
Left lobe	Left lateral segment	Left lateral superior subsegment
		Left lateral inferior subsegment
	Left medial segment	Left medial superior subsegment
		Left medial inferior subsegment

Right lobe	Right anterior segment	Right anterior inferior subsegment
		Right anterior superior subsegment
	Right posterior segment	Right posterior inferior subsegment
		Right posterior superior subsegment

Functional Segmental Liver Anatomy

- Based on distribution of three major hepatic veins:
  - *Middle hepatic vein:*
    Divides liver into right and left lobe. Also separated by main portal vein scissura (Cantlie line) passing through IVC + long-axis of gallbladder).
  - *Left hepatic vein:*
    Divides left lobe into medial + lateral sectors.
  - *Right hepatic vein:*
    Divides right lobe into medial + lateral sectors.

Each of the four sections is further divided by an imaginary transverse line drawn through the right + left portal vein into anterior + posterior segments; the segments are numbered counter-clockwise from IVC.

Hepatic Arterial Anatomy (Michel's Classification)

Type I (55%)
- Celiac trunk trifurcates into left (LT) gastric artery + splenic artery + common hepatic artery.
- Common hepatic artery divides into gastro-duodenal artery + proper hepatic artery.
- Right (RT) hepatic artery + LT hepatic artery arise from proper hepatic artery.
- Middle hepatic artery (supplying caudate lobe) arises from:
  - LT/RT hepatic artery.
  - Proper hepatic artery (in 10%).

Type II (10%)
- Common hepatic artery divides into gastroduodenal + RT hepatic artery.
- LT hepatic artery replaced to LT gastric artery.
- Middle hepatic artery from RT hepatic artery.

Type III (11%)
- Common hepatic artery divides into gastroduodenal + LT hepatic artery.
- RT hepatic artery replaced to superior mesenteric artery.
- Middle hepatic artery from LT hepatic artery.

Type IV (1%)
- Common hepatic artery divides into middle hepatic artery + gastro-duodenal artery.
- RT hepatic artery + LT hepatic artery are both replaced.

Type V (8%)
- Accessory LT hepatic artery arises from LT gastric artery.

Type VI (7%)
- Accessory RT hepatic artery arises from superior mesenteric artery.

Type VII (1%)
- Accessory RT + LT hepatic artery.

Type VIII (2%)
- Combinations of accessory + replaced hepatic artery.

Type IX (4.5%)
- Hepatic trunk replaced to superior mesenteric artery.

Type X (0.5%)
- Hepatic trunk replaced to LT gastric artery.

Hepatic Fissures

- Fissure for ligamentum teres—umbilical fissure—invagination of ligamentum teres—embryologic remnant of obliterated umbilical vein connecting placental venous blood with left portal vein.
  - Located at dorsal-free margin of falciform ligament.
  - Runs into liver with visceral peritoneum.
  - Divides left hepatic lobe into medial + lateral segments (divides subsegment 3 from 4).

- Fissure for ligamentum venosum
  - Invagination of obliterated ductus venosus.
  - Embryologic connection of left portal vein with left hepatic vein.
    * Separates caudate lobe from left lobe of liver.
    * Lesser omentum within fissure separates the greater sac anteriorly from lesser sac posteriorly.
- Fissure for gallbladder
  - Shallow peritoneal invagination containing the gallbladder.
    * Divides right from left lobe of liver.
- Transverse fissure
  - Invagination of hepatic pedicle into the liver.
    * Contains horizontal portion of left + right portal veins.
- Accessory fissures
  - Right inferior accessory fissure.
    * From gallbladder fossa/just inferior to it to lateroinferior margin of liver.
  - Others (rare).

Normal Size of Liver

Sonographic measurements along vertical (craniocaudal) axis:
- Mid-clavicular line
  Less than 13 cm   = normal
  13.0–15.5 cm   = indeterminate (in 25% of patients)
  Less than 15.5 cm = hepatomegaly (87% accuracy)
- Preaortic line more than 10 cm.
- Prerenal line more than 14 cm.

Normal Hemodynamics Parameters of Liver

Portal vein velocity: more than 11 cm/sec.
Congestion index (= cross-sectional area of portal vein divided by average velocity): 0.070 ± 0.09.
Hepatic artery resistive index: 0.60–0.64 ± 0.06.

Liver Function Tests

- Alkaline phosphatase (AP)
  - *Formation:* Bone, liver, intestine and placenta.
  - *High increase*: Cholestasis with extra-hepatic biliary obstruction (confirmed by rise in GT drugs, granulomatous disease, sarcoidosis, primary biliary cirrhosis, primary + secondary malignancy of liver.
  - *Mild increase*: All forms of liver disease, heart failure.
- γ-glutamyl transpeptidase (GGT)
  - Very sensitive in almost all forms of liver disease.
  - *Utility*: Confirms hepatic source of elevated AP, may indicate significant alcohol use.
- Transaminases
  - *High increase:* Viral/toxin-induced acute hepatitis
    * Aspartate transaminase (AST); formerly serum glutamic oxaloacetic transaminase (SGOT).
  - *Formation*: Liver, muscle, kidney, pancreas, RBCs.
    * Alanine aminotransferase (ALT); formerly serum glutamic pyruvic transaminase (SGPT).
  - *Formation*: Primarily in liver.
    * Rather specific elevation in liver disease.
- *Bilirubin:* Helps differentiate between various causes of jaundice.
  - Unconjugated/indirect bilirubin—insoluble in water.
    * Formation: Breakdown of senescent RBCs.
    * Metabolism: Tightly bound to albumin in vessels actively taken up by liver, cannot be excreted by kidneys.
  - Conjugated/direct bilirubin—water-soluble.
    * Formation: Conjugation in liver cells.
    * Metabolism: Excretion into bile; not reabsorbed by intestinal mucosa + excreted in feces.
    Elevation:
    - Overproduction: Hemolytic anemia, resorption hematoma, multiple transfusions.

- Decreased hepatic uptake: Drugs, sepsis.
- Decreased conjugation: Gilbert syndrome, neonatal jaundice, hepatitis, cirrhosis and sepsis.
- Decreased excretion into bile: Hepatitis cirrhosis, drug-induced cholestasis, sepsis, extrahepatic biliary obstruction.
- Lactic dehydrogenase (LDH)
  – Nonspecific and, therefore, not helpful.
  – High increase: Primary or metastatic liver involvement.
- Alpha fetoprotein (AFP)
  – More than 400 ng/mL: Strongly suggests that focal mass represents a hepatocellular carcinoma.

Normal Size of Bile Ducts

- CBD at point of maximum diameter: ≤ 5 mm = normal; 6–7 mm = equivocal; ≥ 8 mm = dilated.
- CHD at porta hepatis + CBD in head of pancreas: 5 mm.
- Right intrahepatic duct just proximal to CHD: 2–3 mm.
- Cystic duct diameter: 1.8 mm.
  Average length of 1–2 cm.
  Distal cystic duct posterior to CBD (in 95%), anterior to CBD (in 5%).

Bile Duct Variants

Incidence

2.4% of autopsies;
13% of operative cholangiograms.
- Aberrant intrahepatic duct:
  May join CHD, CBD, cystic duct, right hepatic duct and gallbladder.
  – Anomalous right hepatic duct entering CHD/cystic duct (4–5%).
  Complications:
  – Postoperative bile leak, if severed.
  – Segmental biliary obstruction, if ligated.
- Cystic duct entering right hepatic duct.
- Ducts of luschka
  – Small ducts from hepatic bed draining directly into the gallbladder.
- Duplication of cystic duct/CBD.
- Congenital tracheobiliary fistula.
  – Fistulous communication between carina and left hepatic duct.
  – Infants with respiratory distress.
  – Productive cough with bilious sputum.
  √ Pneumobilia.

Pancreaticobiliary Junction Variants

- Angle between CBD + pancreatic duct:
  – Usually acute at 5°–30°.
  – Occasionally abnormal at up to 90°.
- Sphincter of Oddi
  – Muscle fibers encircling the CBD + pancreatic duct at choledochoduodenal junction.
    ◆ Choledochal sphincter—encircles distal CBD.
    ◆ Pancreatic duct sphincter (in 33% separate).
- Types of union between CBD + pancreatic duct:
  – 2–10 (mean 5) mm short common channel (85%) with a diameter of 3–5 mm.
  – Separate entrances into duodenum.
  – 8–15 mm long common channel.
  – Pancreatic duct inserting into CBD more than 15 mm from entrance into duodenum.
  – CBD inserting into pancreatic duct.

CONGENITAL GALLBLADDER ANOMALIES

Agenesis of Gallbladder

Incidence

0.04–0.07% (autopsy)

Associated with:
Common: Rectovaginal fistula, imperforate anus, hypoplasia of scapula + radius, intracardiac shunt.

Rare: Absence of corpus callosum, microcephaly, atresia of external auditory canal, tricuspid atresia, TE fistula, dextroposition of pancreas + esophagus, absent spleen, high position of cecum and polycystic kidney.

Hypoplastic Gallbladder

- Congenital.
- Associated with cystic fibrosis.

Septations of Gallbladder

- Longitudinal septa
  - Duplication of gallbladder
    - Two separate lumens + two cystic ducts.
    Incidence: 1:3,000 to 1:12,000
  - Bifid gallbladder—double gallbladder
    - Two separate lumens with one cystic duct.
  - Triple gallbladder (extremely rare).
- Transverse septa
  - Isolated transverse septum.
  - Phrygian cap (2–6% of population).
    - Kinking/folding of fundus ± septum.
    - Multiseptated gallbladder (rare).
    - Multiple cyst-like compartments connected by small pores.
  Cx: Stasis + stone formation.
- Gallbladder diverticulum
  - Persistence of cystohepatic duct.

Gallbladder Ectopia

Most frequent locations
(1) beneath the left lobe of the liver > (2) intrahepatic > (3) retrohepatic.

Rare locations:
1. Within falciform ligament.
2. Within interlobar fissure.
2. Suprahepatic (lodged between superior surface of right hepatic lobe + anterior chest wall).
4. Within anterior abdominal wall.
5. Transverse mesocolon.
6. Retrorenal.
7. Near posterior spine +inferior vena cava (IVC).
8. Intrathoracic gallbladder (inversion of liver).

Associated with: Eventration of diaphragm.
"Floating GB"
- Gallbladder with loose peritoneal reflections, may herniate through foramen of Winslow into lesser sac.

"Torqued GB"
- Results in hydrops.

Pancreas

Pancreatic development and anatomy:
- Dorsal anlage (in mesoduodenum).
  Origin: Arises from dorsal wall of duodenum.
  - Forms cranial portion of head + isthmus + body + tail of pancreas.
  - Prone to atrophy (poor in polypeptides).
  √ Drains to the minor papilla through accessory duct of Santorini.
- Ventral anlage (below primordial liver bud):
  Origin: Ventral bud arises from ventral wall of duodenum and is composed of right + left lobes (the left ventral bud regresses completely), migrates to opposite side of duodenum + fuses with dorsal anlage during sixth week GA.
  - Forms caudal portion of the pancreatic head + uncinate process + CBD.
  - Not prone to atrophy (rich in polypeptides).
  √ The ventral duct of Wirsung drains with the CBD through ampulla of Vater and becomes the major drainage pathway for the entire pancreas after fusion with the duct of Santorini.
- Main pancreatic duct of Wirsung distal portion of dorsal duct connects with ventral duct; proximal portion of dorsal duct may disappear.
- Accessory pancreatic duct of Santorini
  - Proximal portion of dorsal duct which has not atrophied.
- Ampulla of Vater
  - Space within medial wall of second portion of duodenum below surface of papilla of Vater.

- Major duodenal papilla—papilla of Vater
  - Drainage of common bile duct in 100%.
  - Drainage of main pancreatic duct of Wirsung in 90%.
- Minor duodenal papilla (Present in 60%)
  - Drainage of accessory pancreatic duct of Santorini.
  - Drainage of main pancreatic duct in 10%.
  - Located a few cm orad to papilla of Vater.

Spleen

- *Normal size:*
  - In adults: 12 cm length, 7–8 cm anteroposterior diameter, 3–4 cm thick; splenic index (L× W × H) of less than 480.
  - In children: Formula for length = 5.7 + 0.31 × age (in years).
- *Normal weight:* 150 (100–265) g. Estimated weight—splenic index × 0.55
- *CT attenuation*
  - Without enhancement: 40–60 HU; 5–10 HU less than liver.
  - With enhancement: Normal heterogeneous enhancement during parenchymal phase after bolus injection (due to varying blood flow rates through the cords of the red pulp).
- *MR signal intensity:*
  - On T1WI: liver > spleen > muscle.
  - On T2WI: spleen > liver.

Iron Metabolism

Total body iron: 5 g
- Functional iron: 4 g
- Location: Hemoglobin of RBCs, myoglobin of muscle, various enzymes
- Stored iron: 1 g
  Location: Hepatocytes, reticuloendothelial cells of liver Kupffer cells) + spleen + bone marrow
  Absorption: 1–2 mg/day through gut
  Transport: Bound to transferrin intravascularly

Deposition
- Transferrin-transfer to: Hepatocytes, RBC precursors in erythron, parenchymal tissues (e.g. muscle).
- Phagocytosis by:
  Reticuloendothelial cells phagocytize senescent erythrocytes (= extravascular hemolysis); RBC iron stored as ferritin/released and bound to transferrin.

INFLAMMATORY BOWEL DISEASE (IBD)

- The term IBD encompasses two forms of chronic, idiopathic, intestinal inflammation—ulcerative colitis and Crohn's disease.
- Unknown etiology.
- Ulcerative colitis.
  - Diffuse inflammatory disease of unknown etiology.
  - Involves primarily the colorectal mucosa.

Epidemiology

- More common than Crohn's disease.
- Steady incidence (2–10/100,000).
- Bimodal age distribution
  Peak – 15–25 years
       – 50–80 years (smaller).
- Risk factors
  - White –2–5 *risk.
  - Jewish –2–4 *risk.
  - Developed country.
  - Urban dweller.
  - Family H/o –30–100 *risk.
  - Sibling –(8.8% incidence).
  - Single.
  - Non-smoker.
  - Unknown.

Etiology and Pathogenesis

- Speculations.
- Genetic and familial factors:
  - Familial aggregation, increased frequency in monozygotic twins.
- Polygenes.
- HLA—B5, BW—52, DR2.

- Association with autoimmune disorder—sacroiliitis, ankylosing spondylitis, enteropathic oligoarthritis, anterior uveitis.
- Anatomic and physiological factors: Abnormal mucin production.
- Infectious factors: Chlamydia, mycobacteria, gut anaerobes, CMV, Yersinia and bacterial cell wall components have all been proposed.
- Enteric nervous system and gut hormones: sub P and VIP— increased release.
- Psychological and stress factors: Personality (neurotic, introverts).
- Chemical mediators: Pro-inflammatory cytokines—IL-1 increased.
- Environmental factors:
  - Smoking: Protective.
  - Oral contraceptives: Increased incidence.

Diet

Cow's milk protein, lactose intolerance, chemical food additives— carrageenan.

Clinical findings:

Variable in clinical course; waxes and wanes.
- Acute exacerbations of bloody diarrhea.
- M/C clinical features—diarrhea, abdominal pain, rectal bleeding, weight loss, tenesmus.
- Vomiting, fever, constipation, arthralgias— less common.

Radiologic findings:
- Plain film
  - Colonic fecal residue: distal extent of fecal residue gives an indication of the proximal extent of the colitis.
  - Mucosa
    - Smooth.
    - Granular irregular fuzzy, if ulceration—disrupted.
    - Intramural gas/pneumatosis.
  - Haustrations
    - Widening of haustral cleft with loss of parallel line.
  - Diameter
    - Upper limit of N— 5.5 cm
      - Other associated abnormalities like—renal calculi, sacroilitis, ankylosing spondylitis, AVN of femoral head.
  - Mural thickness
    - More than 3 mm.
      - Barium enema.
    - To confirm clinical diagnosis.
    - To assess the extent and severity of disease.
    - To differentiate ulcerative colitis from Crohn's disease and other colitides.
    - To follow the course of disease.
    - To detect complications.

Findings

Acute Changes

- Mucosal granularity
  - Hyperemia and accumulation of inflammatory cells in mucosa and gradual transition.

  Abnormality in quality and quantity of mucus.
- Mucosal stippling
  - Due to crypt microabscesses which rupture into lumen, cause ulcers and barium flecks to adhere.
- Collar button ulcers—crypt abscess breach the lamina propria and muscularis mucosae and undermine submucosa.
- Haustral thickening or loss—edema.
- Inflammatory polyps.
- Contiguous, confluent, circumferential disease.

Chronic Changes

- Haustral loss:
  - Alteration in tone of the taeniae, which are relaxed.
  - Colonic shortening due to massive hypertrophy and fixed shortening of muscularis mucosae (contraction) foreshortening of the colon.

- Luminal narrowing:
  - Benign strictures seen in 10% of patients.
  - Smooth tapering, rarely cause obstruction.
- Sometimes reversible, usually in distal colon.
- If irreversible, and located in proximal colon—suspicion of malignancy.
- Widening of presacral space
  - 1–1.5 cm moderate increase
    - Mural thickening due to proliferation, inflammation and infiltration of perirectal fat.
  - More than 1.5 cm definitely abnormal.
- Rectal value abnormality: N < 5 mm, S3–S4 level.

Proctitis
- Fold thickness > 6.5 mm with or without increased presacral space.
- Absent fold with increased presacral space—absent fold with normal presacral space—normal variant.
- Backlash ilitis:
  - Patulous and fixed ileocecal value that easily refluxes with persistent dilatation of terminal ileum.
  - Absent normal fold pattern with granular mucosa.
- Postinflammatory pseudopolyps.

Ultrasound
- Moderately thick hypoechoic wall.
- Typical wall stratification maintained.
- If extensive pseudopolyposis—wall stratification may be lost.
- Loss of haustra.

Computed Tomography
- Mural thickening.
- Target appearance of wall.
  - Due to submucosal edema (acute).
  - Due to fat proliferation (chronic).
- Rectal narrowing and widening of presacral space are hallmarks of chronic UC.
- When sufficiently large, pseudopolyps can be identified on CT.
- Mural thickening, unsuspected perforations and pneumatosis can be identified on CT in patients with toxic megacolon.

MRI
- Can identify mural stratification.
- Thickening and abnormal hypointensity of mucosa on T1 and T2 WI.
- Degree of mural enhancement correlates well with disease severity (on fat suppressed gradient echo).

Scintigraphy
- Ga-67 citrate.
- Indium-labeled leukocytes.
- Useful when there is danger of bowel perforation and extent and degree of disease activity must be assessed.
- FDG-PET.

Prognosis
- Most patients—mild to moderate disease.
- 15% to 25% require colectomy.
- Mortality
  - In first 2 years of disease in > 40 years old patients
  - 1/3rd   colonic disease
  - 1/3rd   complication
  - 1/3rd   unrelated cause

Crohn's Disease
- Chronic cicatrizing disorders of the alimentary tract, characterized by granulomatous inflammation of the mucosa, bowel wall and surrounding mesentery.
- Any part of alimentary tract.
- Terminal ileum and proximal colon most common site.

Epidemiology
- Uncommon disorder.
- Increasing in incidence.
- Bimodal age distribution—
  Peak—15–25 years.
  Smaller peak—50–80 years.

Risk Factors
- White race.
- Jewish (8-fold increase).
- Urban.
- Family history positive.
- Sibling with disease (30-fold increase).
- Single.
- Oral contraceptive use.
- Smoking (4-fold increase).
- Season (highest relapse rate autumn and winter, lowest in summer).

Pathogenesis and Etiology
- Unknown etiology.
- Genetic, environmental, infection, immunological and psychological factors.
- Increased PAF, PG and LT.
- Failure of suppressor T-cell generation, coupled with hyperactive state of helper T-cells.
- Defect in mucosal permeability—absorption of complex sugars and macromolecules.
- Increased deposition of type-5 collagen.

Clinical Features
Rectal bleeding, diarrhea, abdominal pain.
- Two type—colicky pain in lower abdomen relieved by defecation, severe pain in right lower quadrant simulating appendicitis.
- Abscess, fistula, perianal lesion.
  O/E—pallor, dehydration, anemia, weight loss, clubbing, abdominal distension, tachycardia and fever.
- Abdominal, tenderness, profound wasting and emaciation.
- Palpable intra-abdominal mass.

Radiologic Findings

Plain Film
- When confined to colon—plain film features are similar to ulcerative colitis.
- An extended gas-filled stricture is suggestive of granulomatous colitis.
- Small bowel obstruction.
- Evidence of—nephrolithiasis, gallstones, ankylosing spondylitis, sacroiliitis, avascular necrosis of femoral head.

Barium Examination
For evaluation of small bowel, enteroclysis should be the method of choice for the following indications:
- To demonstrate early changes.
- To demonstrate the full extent and possible presence of skip lesions, if surgery is contemplated.
- To determine the cause of any clinical deterioration in previously stable patient.
- To distinguish between spasm, active stenotic disease and a fibrous stricture.
- To investigate postoperative complications of Crohn's disease
- To definitively rule out the presence of Crohn's disease in small bowel.
- A fluoroscopic small bowel barium meal followthrough is adequate.
- As a follow-up study in clinically stable patients with known small bowel Crohn's disease.
- To investigate patients with Crohn's disease know to involve predominantly terminal ileum (with pneumocolon).
- To investigate possible recurrence of Crohn's disease in the neoterminal ileum after ileocecal resection.
- In patients with ileostomy—retrograde small bowel enema is recommended for the demonstration of more distal small bowel loops.

Early disease:
- Smooth symmetric fold thickening (obstructive lymphedema of submucosa).
- Coarse villous pattern (thickened adherent villi).
- Hyperplasia of lymphoid follicles with aphthoid ulcers.
- Shallow mucosal erosions, 1–3 mm, surrounded by small halo of edema.

Intermediate disease
- Progressive submucosal edema with widening of base of fold with partial or complete obliteration.
- Variable submucosal infiltrate with patchy fibrosis—distortion and interruption of fold.

- Enlargement and deepening of aphthoid ulcers.
- Stellate or rose-thorn appearance.
- May fuse—crescenteric or linear.
- Typical—long linear ulcer on mesenteric border.
- Thickening, sclerosis and retraction of mesentery—straightened mesenteric border, with redundant antimesenteric border.
- Localized mucosal thickening or inflammatory polyps, Nodular pattern of Crohn's disease. (Inflammatory infiltrate with patchy profound edema and granulation tissue).

Advanced disease
- Deep linear clefts of ulcers or fissures, axial and transaxial fissuring.
- Pseudopolyps ulceronodular or cobblestone pattern.
- Antimesenteric redundancy of bowel wall disappears with transaxial extension of ulceration.
- Bowel wall thickening with inflammation and fibrosis.
- Fat wrapping—hypertrophied sub-peritoneum is tethered towards the bowel wall by mesenteric perivascular fibrosis— spiral CT may show parallel thickened vessels traversing this (comb sign).

Barium enema

Early findings
- Nodular lymphoid hyperplasia
- Aphthoid ulceration
- Deep ulceration/confluent ulceration
- Cobblestone appearance
- Asymmetric, involvement
- Segmental distribution
- Skip lesions
- Inflammatory pseudopolyps

Late findings
- Fissures
- Fibrosis
- Haustral loss
- Sacculations
- Postinflammatory
- Pseudopolyps
- Intramural abscess stricture

Anorectal disease
Fissures ulcer, abscess, fistulae, hemorrhoids.

Computed Tomography (CT)
- Bowel wall thickening.
- During acute non-cicatrizing phase—stratification is maintained —with target or double halo appearance.
- With long-standing disease—transmural fibrosis—loss of stratification.
- CT may reveal—fibrofatty proliferation with creeping fat of mesentery. Stranding of fat, lymph node in mesentery, hypervascularity with perivascular fibrosis—comb sign (vascular jejunization of the ileum).
- Phlegmon, abscess.

Ultrasonography (USG)
TRUS (Transrectal ultrasound)
- Mural thickening is more than 4 mm—loss of stratification.
- Perianal and perirectal abscesses, fistulas.
- Heterogeneity of the anal sphincter.

Transabdominal Ultrasound
- Thickening of colonic and small bowel wall (target or bull's eye appearance).
- Loss of haustrations.
- Absent peristalsis.
- Increase blood flow in SMA with decreased RI.
- Diminished compressibility.

Magnetic Resonance Imaging (MRI)
- Can show extent and severity of inflammatory change.
- Detection of perianal and perirectal fistula, sinus tracts and abscesses.

Extraintestinal Complications of Inflammatory Bowel Disease (IBD)

- Hepatobiliary
  - Steatosis.
  - Cholelithiasis—impaired enterohepatic circulation of bile salts.

- Sclerosing cholangitis
  - Fibrous mural thickening of bile ducts.
  - Focal clustering of intrahepatic (IH) ducts.
  - Discontinuous areas of intrahepatic (IH) biliary dilatation without hepatic, porta hepatis or pancreatic masses.
    - Cholangiography—beading, pruning.
    - Cholangiocarcinoma.
    - Secondary biliary cirrhosis.
    - Liver abscess.
    - Pancreatitis.

Urinary tract complications
- Nephrolithiasis—oxalate calculi.
- Hydronephrosis.
- Fistulas—enterovesical.
- Musculoskeletal.
  - Arthropathy
    - Ankylosing spondylitis.
    - Sacroiliitis.
    - Avascular necrosis of femoral head.
    - Osteomyelitis, septic arthritis.
    - Osteoporosis.
    - Psoas abscess.
    - Pulmonary complication.
    - Serositis.
    - Interstitial lung disease (ILD).
    - Bronchiolitis/bronchiectasis/chronic bronchitis.
    - Necrobiotic nodules.

Chapter 6

Skeletal System and Joints

ABNORMAL SKELETAL MATURATION

Skeletal Maturation Disorders

Retarded
- *Chronic ill health:*
  - Congenital cardiac disorders.
  - Chronic renal failure.
  - Inflammatory bowel disease.
  - Malnutrition including rickets.
  - Maternal deprivation.
- *Chromosomal disorders:*
  - Down syndrome.
  - Turner syndrome.
  - Trisomy 18, etc.
  - Noonan syndrome.
  - Prader–Willi syndrome.
- *Endocrinal disorders:*
  - Hypothyroidism.
  - Hypogonadism.
  - Hypopituitarism.
  - Cushing's disease and steroid therapy.
- *Congenital syndromes:*
  - Bone dysplasias.
  - Malformation syndromes.
- *Miscellaneous:*
  - Extreme emotional deprivation.

Accelerated
- *Localized:*
  - Local hyperemia secondary to inflammation/infection.
  - Trauma.
  - Vascular malformations [hemangioma/arteriovenous malformation (AVM)].
  - Klippel-Trenaunay-Weber syndrome.
  - Maffucci syndrome.
  - Neurofibromatosis.
  - Macrodystrophia lipomatosa (Fig. 6.1).
- *Generalized:*
  - *Endocrinal:*
    - Idiopathic sexual precocity.
    - Hypothalamic masses.
    - Adrenal and gonadal tumors.
    - Hyperthyroidism.
  - *Congenital:*
    - McCune–Albright syndrome.
    - Cerebral gigantism.
    - Lipodystrophy.
    - Pseudohypoparathyroidism.
    - Weaver–Smith syndrome.
    - Marshall–Smith syndrome.
  - *Miscellaneous:*
    - Obesity in children.

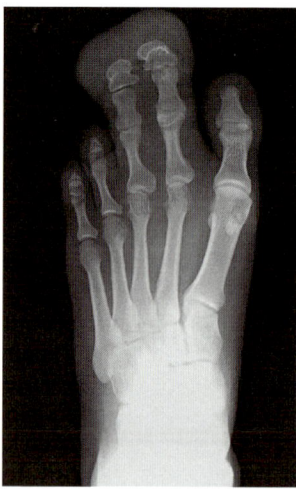

Fig. 6.1: Anteroposterior radiograph of foot shows macrodystrophia lipomatosa involving 2nd and 3rd digits.

Asymmetric

- *Localized gigantism:* Causes similar to localized accelerated maturation.
- *Localized atrophy:*
  - Paralysis.
  - Radiation treatment in childhood.

Premature Closure of Growth Plate

- Localized hyperemia due to chronic inflammation as in arthritides or infection, hemophilia.
- *Vascular malformation*—AVM.
- Trauma.
- Radiation treatment during childhood.
- *Thermal injury*—burns and frostbite.
- Multiple exostoses and enchondromatosis (Ollier's disease).

SHORT LIMB SKELETAL DYSPLASIA

Rhizomelic (Proximal Limb Shortening)

- *Achondroplasia:*
  - Large skull with small base and sella and a small foramen magnum.
  - Short ribs with deep concavities to anterior ends.
  - Decreased interpedicular distance caudally in lumbar spine.
  - Short pedicles with narrow lumbar canal.
  - Posterior scalloping with anterior vertebral body beaking.
  - Square iliac wings with champagne glass pelvic cavity.
  - Rhizomelic micromelic with bowing of long bones (Fig. 6.2).
  - Trident hands.
- *Hypochondroplasia:*
  - Similar to achondroplasia except skull never affected.
  - Height normal or mildly reduced.
- *Pseudochondroplasia:*
  - Similar to achondroplasia.
  - Except that skull is normal.
  - No changes seen in 1st year of life.
- *Chondrodysplasia punctata:*
  - Stippling in long bone epiphysis, spine, or larynx.

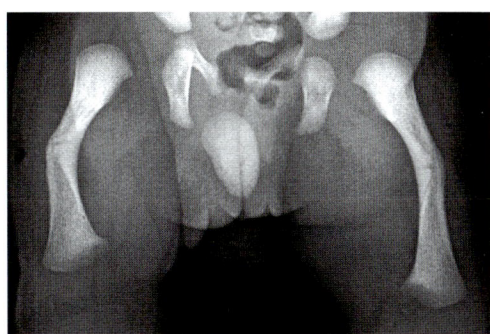

Fig. 6.2: Anteroposterior radiograph shows bowing of both femurs with right relatively shorter than left.

Mesomelic (Middle Segment Shortening)

- *Dyschondrosteosis:*
  - Also known as Léri–Weill disease.
  - Usually affects females.
  - Madelung's deformity.
  - Medial aspect of proximal/distal tibia defective with or without hypoplastic fibula.
- *Mesomelic dysplasia:*
  - Type Langer.
  - Type Reinhardt-Pfeiffer.

Acromesomelic (Middle and Distal Segment Shortening)

- *Chondroectodermal dysplasia:*
  - Also known as Ellis–van Creveld syndrome.
  - Paired long bones are short with dome-shaped metaphyses.
  - Abnormal medial tibial plateau with defective epiphyses laterally.
  - Postaxial polysyndactyly.
  - Carpal fusions seen especially capitate and hamate with delayed development of carpal bones.
  - Partial/total absence of teeth.
  - Abnormal hair and nails.
  - Rib cage similar to asphyxiating thoracic dystrophy.
- *Acromesomelic dysplasia*
- *Mesomelic dysplasia:*
  - Type Nievergelt.
  - Type Robinow.
  - Type Werner.

Acromelic (Distal Segment Shortening)

- *Asphyxiating thoracic dystrophy:*
  - Also known as Jeune's disease.
  - Thorax is stenotic.
  - Ribs are short and horizontal and clavicles are highly placed.
  - Polydactyly (Fig. 6.3).
- *Peripheral dysostoses.*

SHORT SPINE SKELETAL DYSPLASIA

Disease

- *Pseudoachondroplasia:*
  - *Spinal abnormality besides short spine*:
    - Platyspondyly with exaggerated grooves for ring apophyses.
    - C_1 and C_2 dislocation.

Other features:
- Short limbs.
- Marked joints laxity.
- Spondylometaphyseal dysplasia like type Kozowski.
  - Limb abnormalities besides spine involvement.
- *Spondyloepiphyseal dysplasia:*
  - Dominant variety.
  - Congenita.
  - Platyspondyly, maximal in thoracic spine.

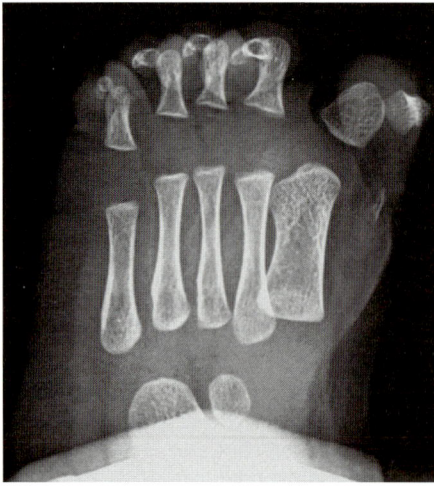

Fig. 6.3: Anteroposterior radiograph of foot shows polydactyly.

Other features:
- Severe tubular bone involvement.
- *Retinal detachment common:*
  - X-linked tarda.

Spinal abnormality besides short spine:
- Mounds of dense bone are found on superior and inferior surfaces of the posterior part of vertebral endplates.

Other features:
- Tubular bones minimally affected.
- Iliac wings are small.
- *Hip degeneration frequently occurs prematurely:*
  - Recessive.

Spinal abnormality besides short limbs:
- Generalized platyspondyly of least severity.

Other features:
- Nil.
- *Diastrophic dwarfism:*
  - Spinal abnormality besides other limb abnormalities:
    - Interpedicular narrowing in lumbar spine.
    - Progressive kyphoscoliosis.

Other features:
- Delta-shaped epiphyses.
- Hitchhiker thumb.
- *Metatrophic dwarfism:*
  - Spinal abnormality besides limb abnormalities:
    - Hypoplastic odontoid.
    - Severe progressive scoliosis.

Other features:
- Short limbs.
- Dumbbell-shaped long bones.
- *Kniest syndrome:*
  - Spinal abnormality besides limb abnormalities:
    - Platyspondyly.
    - Kyphoscoliosis.
    - Interpedicular narrowing of lumbar spine.

Other features:
- Dumbbell-shaped long bones.
- Irregular epiphyses.
- Limited and painful joint movements.

LETHAL NEONATAL DYSPLASIA

- *Osteogenesis imperfecta type II:*
  - Lethal *in utero*/early infancy.
  - Sclerae are dark blue.
  - Bones are grossly demineralized with thin cortices.
  - Numerous healed or healing rib fractures.
  - Type IIA:
    - Long bones are short, broad, and bowed.
    - Ribs are broad with continuous beading.
  - Type IIB:
    - Long bones as in Type IIA.
    - Ribs show less or no beading.
  - Type IIC:
    - Long bones are thinned and show multiple fractures.
    - Ribs are too thin and beaded.
  - Skull is enlarged with numerous wormian bones; mineralization may be retarded.
- *Thanatophoric dwarfism:*
  - Infants are stillborn or die immediately after birth.
  - Rhizomelic dwarfism with bowing of long bones.
  - Metaphyses are irregular.
  - Epiphyses of knee absent.
  - Short, wide, metacarpals and phalanges.
  - Marked platyspondyly with "H-shaped" vertebra on anteroposterior (AP) view of spine.
  - Poor mineralization of pelvic bones with small square iliac blades.
  - Cloverleaf skull.
  - Ribs are short and flared anteriorly.
- *Chondrodysplasia punctata:*
  - Rhizomelic type (recessive) is lethal.
  - Stippling or punctate calcification of tarsus and carpus, long bone epiphyses, vertebral transverse processes, and pubic bones.
  - Long bones show gross asymmetric shortening and metaphyseal irregularity.
- *Asphyxiating thoracic dystrophy*—patients die in infancy from respiratory distress.
  - Thorax is stenotic.
  - Ribs are short and horizontal.
  - Clavicles are highly placed.
- *Campomelic dwarfism:*
  - Long bones are bowed.
- *Achondrogenesis type I and II.*
- *Short rib syndromes with or without polydactyly (type I, II, and III).*
- *Homozygous achondroplasia.*
- *Hypophosphatasia*—gross general failure of ossification of skeleton.

DUMBBELL-SHAPED LONG BONES

- *Metatropic dwarfism*—short spine and short limb dwarfism.
- *Pseudochondroplasia*—short limb (rhizomelic dwarfism).
- *Kniest syndrome*—short spine and short limb dwarfism.
- *Diastrophic dwarfism*—short spine and short limb dwarfism.
- *Osteogenesis imperfecta:*
  - Type III—sclera blue at birth but usually normal in adolescence.
    - Bones are demineralized.
    - Vertebral compression and kyphoscoliosis.
    - Long bone show multiple fracture and bowing.
    - Sutures are wide with multiple wormian bones.
    - Dentinogenesis imperfecta.
- *Chondroectodermal dysplasia*—acromesomelic dwarfism with ectodermal dysplasia.

MUCOPOLYSACCHARIDOSES AND MUCOLIPIDOSIS (FIG. 6.4)

They are characterized by constellation of radiological signs related to skeletal system and share some common characteristics as:
- Abnormal bone texture.
- Widening of diaphyses.
- Tilting of distal radius and ulna toward each other.
- Pointing of proximal ends of metacarpals.
- Large skull with calvarial thickening.
- Anterior beaking of upper lumbar vertebrae.
- J-shaped sella.

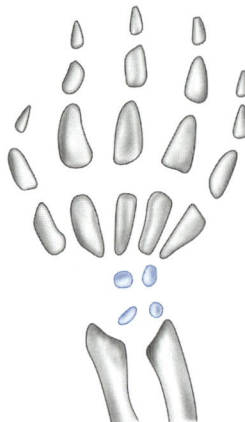

Fig. 6.4: Appendicular skeleton.

- Flared ilia.
- Fragmented femoral ossific nucleus.

MUCOLIPIDOSES

- Type I (neuraminidase deficiency).
- Type II (I-cell disease).
- Type III (pseudopolydystrophy of Maroteaux).

GENERALIZED OSTEOSCLEROSIS

Children

- *Dysplasias:*
  - Osteopetrosis.
  - Pyknodysostosis.
  - Craniotubular dysplasia.
  - Craniotubular hyperostoses.
- *Metabolic:*
  - Renal osteodystrophy.
- *Poisoning:*
  - Lead: Dense metaphyseal bands.
  - Flask-shaped femora.
  - Fluorosis: Thickened cortex with narrow medulla.
  - Ossification of tendons, ligaments, and interosseous membranes.
  - Hyper/Dense metaphyseal bands.
  - Vitaminosis D: Widened zone of provisional calcification.
  - Soft tissue calcification.
  - Hyper/Subperiosteal new bone vitaminosis A formation.
  - Reduced metaphyseal density.

- *Idiopathic:*
  - Caffey's disease.
  - Idiopathic hypercalcemia of infancy.

Adults

- *Myeloproliferative:*
  - Myelosclerosis.
  - Marrow cavity narrowed by endosteal reaction.
  - Patchy lucencies due to fibrous tissue.
- *Metabolic:*
  - Renal osteodystrophy.
- *Poisoning:*
  - Fluorosis.
  - Similar as in children.
- *Neoplastic:*
  - Osteoblastic metastases (Figs. 6.5A and B).
  - Lymphoma.
  - Mastocytosis.
  - Sclerosis of marrow with patchy areas of lucency.
- *Idiopathic:*
  - Paget's disease (Figs. 6.6 to 6.8).
  - Coarsened trabeculae.
  - Bone expansion.

SCLEROTIC BONE LESIONS

Developmental

- *Single:*
  - Fibrous dysplasia.

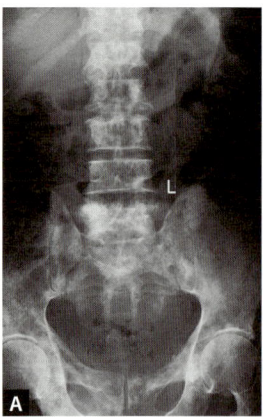
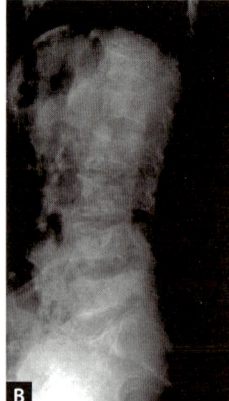

Figs. 6.5A and B: Anteroposterior and lateral radiographs of lumbosacral (LS) spine show osteoblastic metastases.

– Bone islands (enostosis):
  • Round/oval dense lesion in medullary location with radiating thorn-like spicules.
  • Usually less than 15 mm.
  • Grow up to skeletal maturity.

• Multiple:
  – Bone islands.
  – Fibrous dysplasia:
    • Cyst-like lesion in diaphysis or metaphysis with endosteal scalloping ± bone expansion with thick sclerotic border (rind sign)
    • Age = 3–15 years.
  – Osteopoikilosis/osteopathia condensans disseminata:
    • Dense round/oval/lanceolate lesion arranged parallel to long-axis of bone.
    • Seen usually at ends of long bones and around joints; in the carpus and tarsus.
    • No interval change.

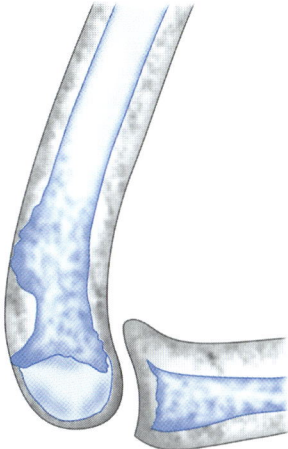

Fig. 6.6: Paget's disease: Early long bone changes. Lateral view of the humerus in a middle-aged man shows an "advancing wedge" (*blade of grass* or *flame shadow*) appearance at the end of the bone, characteristic of early Paget's disease. Since the disease process generally proceeds from one articular end of the long bone to the other, all three phases—(1) Early, (2) Intermediate, and (3) Late—may be seen in the same bone.

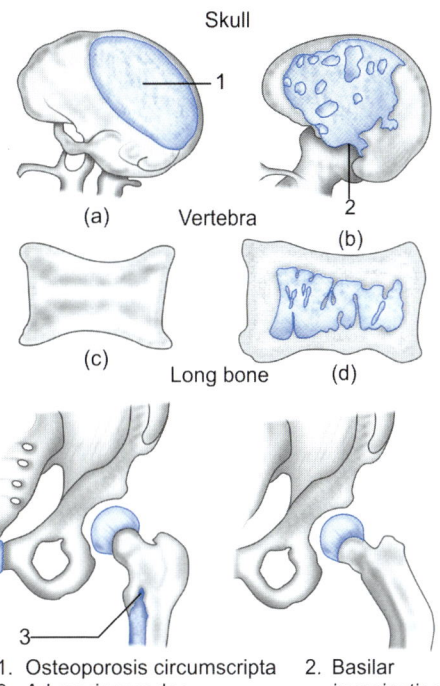

1. Osteoporosis circumscripta
2. Basilar invagination
3. Advancing wedge

Fig. 6.8: Progression of Paget's disease: a, c, and e early (osteolytic) "hot" phase and b, d, and f late (osteoblastic) "cold" phase manifestations of Paget's disease in (a, b) the skull, (c, d) vertebrae, and (e, f) long bones. a. Osteoporosis circumscripta, b. "Cotton-wool" appearance, c. Biconcave vertebra, d. "Picture frame" ivory vertebra, e. "Flame", "blade of grass" deformities, and f. Dense, larger diameter deformities.

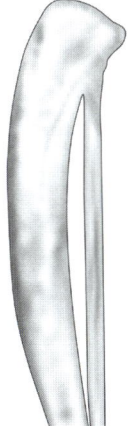

Fig. 6.7: Paget's disease: Late long bone changes. Lateral view of the tibia shows anterior bowing secondary to late phase.

– *Osteopathia striata/Voorhoeve's disease:*
  • Sclerotic striations in long bones parallel to long axis affecting both diaphysis and metaphyses.
– *Tuberous sclerosis:*
  • Patchy, sclerotic lesions in skull, vertebrae, pelvis, and long bones with irregular periosteal new bone formation.

Vascular
- Bone infarcts (single/multiple).
- *In sickle cell anemia:*
  – Sclerotic lesions in femoral or humeral head in medullary bone.
  – Sharply defined or ill-defined diffuse sclerosis.

Traumatic
- Callus (Single/multiple fracture sites).

Infective
- *Sclerosing osteomyelitis of Garré:*
  – Localized gross sclerosis in absence of apparent bone destruction.

Idiopathic
- *Paget's disease (single/multiple):*
  – Coarsened trabeculae, cortical thickening, and bone expansion.
  – Encroachment of medullary cavity with epiphyseal involvement as well.
  – "Cotton-wool spots" in skull.

Neoplastic
- *Single:*
  – Metastases.
  – Lymphoma (*De novo* or after RT of a lytic lesion).
  – Osteoma:
    • Usually skull, perineural spread (PNS), and mandible.
  – Ivory or dense type; spongy or trabeculated type. Broad-based with smooth well-defined margins.
  – Osteoid osteoma (Figs. 6.9 and 6.10):
    • Round/oval radiolucent lesion with dense surrounding sclerosis with a central nidus less than 1 cm.
    • Lesion sited in relation to cortical bone with dense scleroses extending into medullary cavity as well.
  – *Osteoblastoma:*
    • Similar to osteoid osteoma but central radiolucency is larger, approximately 2–10 cm in diameter.
  – *Primary bone sarcoma:*
    • Most common being osteosarcoma.
    • Wide zone of transition with periosteal reaction and soft tissue extension.

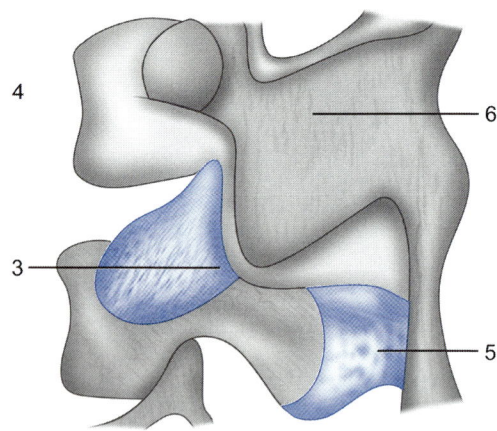

Fig. 6.9: Osteoid osteoma. The frontal projection shows an enlarged, dense right pedicle (3) and pars interarticularis (5), characteristic of osteoid osteoma [compare with normal pedicle on left (4 and 6)].

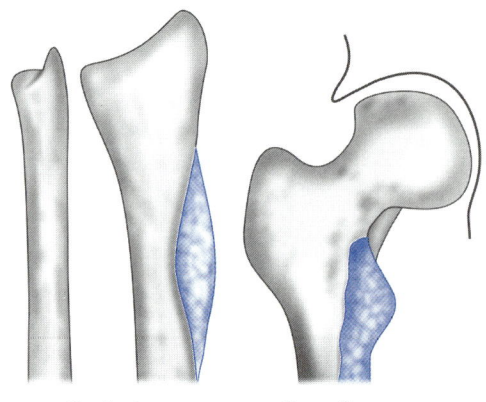

Cortical   Cancellous
Fig. 6.10: Osteoid osteoma.

Skeletal System and Joints

- Healed/healing benign or malignant bone lesions as lytic areas following RT on computed tomography (CT), bone cyst, fibrous cortical defect, etc.
- *Multiple*:
  - Metastases.
  - Lymphoma.
  - Osteomas.
  - Gardner's syndrome.
  - Osteomas, soft-tissue tumors, and polyposis coli.
- *Mastocytosis*:
  - Circumscribed areas of increased density due to thickening of medullary trabeculae (Figs. 6.11A and B).
  - Coarsened appearance of bone with indistinct endosteum.
- *Multifocal osteosarcomas*:
  - Multiple myeloma.
  - In 2–3%.
- *Multiple healed/healing benign or malignant bone lesions.*

BONE SCLEROSIS ASSOCIATED WITH PERIOSTEAL REACTION

Traumatic
- Healing fractures with callus formation.

Neoplastic
- Metastases.
- Lymphoma.
- Osteoid osteoma/osteoblastoma.
- Osteosarcoma.
- Ewing's sarcoma (Fig. 6.12).
- Chondrosarcoma.

Infective
- Osteomyelitis.
- Syphilis.

Idiopathic
- *Infantile cortical hyperostoses (Caffey's disease)*:
  - Age of onset is 9 weeks.
  - Marked periosteal proliferation and cortical thickening beneath soft tissue swellings.
  - Bones affected are mandible, ribs, scapula, ulna, and any other bone except phalanges and spine.
  - In long bones, diaphysis is only involved.

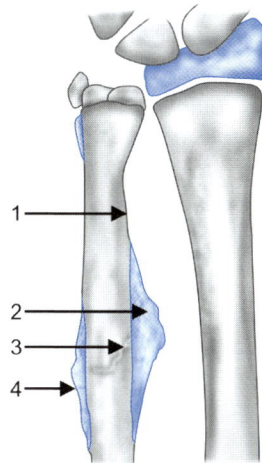

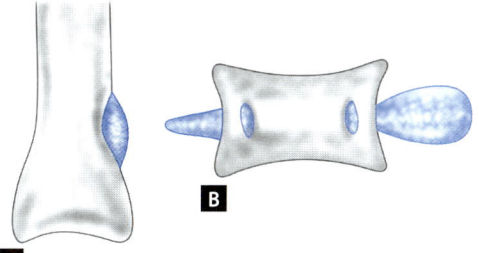

Figs. 6.11A and B: (A) Nonossifying fibroma; and (B) Osteoblastoma.

Fig. 6.12: Ewing's sarcoma. A permeative destructive lesion can be observed in the diaphysis of the distal ulna. Fracture callus merges with a "sunburst" periosteal reaction. The cortex on the radial aspect of the ulna is destroyed by a soft-tissue mass growing out into the soft tissue. A short, oblique pathologic fracture is also evident. Ewing's sarcoma cannot be differentiated radiologically from a non-Hodgkin's lymphoma. The latter occurs in an older age group (3rd and 4th decades). Differentiation from osteomyelitis can be difficult. However, unlike Ewing's sarcoma, metaphyseal involvement is usually a prominent feature of childhood osteomyelitis (see labeling in Figure 6.13).

- *Melorheostosis/Leri's disease:*
  - Dense irregular bone running along cortex of long bone, both externally and internally (dripping candle wax appearance).
  - Lower limbs are commonly involved.
  - Lesions are segmental and unilateral in distribution.

SOLITARY SCLEROTIC LESION WITH LUCENT CENTER

Neoplastic

- *Osteoid osteoma:*
  - Central lucent center less than 1 cm.
- *Osteoblastoma:*
  - Central lucency.
  - 2–10 cm in diameter.

Infective

- *Brodie's abscess:*
  - Metaphyseal lytic lesion with surrounding sclerosis.
  - Tunneling toward epiphyseal plate is pathognomonic.
- Granulomatous (syphilis, tuberculosis).

COARSE TRABECULAR PATTERN OF BONE

- *Paget's disease:*
  - Expansion of bone is associated.
- Osteoporosis.
- Osteomalacia.
- *Hemoglobinopathies:*
  - Especially thalassemia.
  - Expansion of marrow cavity destroys medullary trabeculae.
- *Hemangioma:*
  - Of vertebral bodies produces vertical coarse trabecular pattern with slight expansion (caudry cloth appearance).
- *Renal osteodystrophy:*
  - Associated sclerosis and subperiosteal bone formation is evident.
- *Osteonecrosis:*
  - Cystic defects with coarse trabecular pattern; periostitis and increased bone density may be seen if infection is the causative factor.
- *Fibrogenesis imperfecta ossium:*
  - Obliteration of trabecular architecture with coarsening of remaining trabeculae.
- *Gaucher's disease:*
  - Associated with hypoplasia of vertebral bodies, thinning of cortices of tubular bones, and subperiosteal new bone formation.
- Neoplasms as chondromyxoid fibroma where new bone is laid in pattern of coarse trabeculae.

CHARACTERISTICS OF METASTATIC LESIONS TO THE PRIMARY TUMORS

The characteristics of metastatic lesions to the primary tumors is given in Table 6.1.

CHILDHOOD TUMORS METASTASIZING TO BONE

- Neuroblastoma.
- Leukemias and lymphoma.
- Clear cell sarcoma (variant of Wilms' tumor).
- Rhabdomyosarcoma.
- Retinoblastoma.
- Ewing's sarcoma (Figs. 6.12 and 6.13).
- Osteosarcoma.

BUBBLY BONE LESIONS

Neoplastic

Benign

- Giant cell tumor (GCT).
- Angiomas.
- Chondromyxoid fibroma (Figs. 6.14 and 6.15).
- Enchondroma (Fig. 6.16).

Malignant

- Giant cell tumor.
- Osteoblastoma.
- Multiple myeloma.
- Metastases (kidney and thyroid).

Skeletal System and Joints

Table 6.1: Characteristics of metastatic lesions to the primary tumors.

Location of primary tumor/variety of primary tumor		Characteristic of metastatic lesions			
		Lytic	Blastic	Mixed	Expansile
1.	Bronchogenic carcinoma	✓			
2.	Bronchogenic carcinoid		✓		
3.	Breast	✓		✓	
4.	Gastric carcinoma		✓	✓	
5.	Colon	✓	Occasionally		
6.	Rectum	✓			
7.	Renal cell carcinoma	✓			
8.	Wilms' tumor	✓			
9.	Bladder		✓	✓	
10.	Prostate		✓		
11.	Thyroid	✓			
12.	Pheochromocytoma				
13.	Adrenal carcinoma	✓			
14.	Neuroblastoma	✓			
15.	Cervix	✓		✓ (rarely)	
16.	Uterus	✓			
17.	Ovary	✓			
18.	Testes	✓		✓ (rarely)	
19.	Squamous cell carcinoma of skin	✓			
20.	Melanoma	✓			

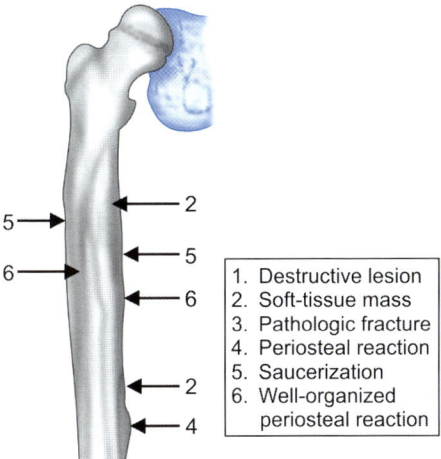

1. Destructive lesion
2. Soft-tissue mass
3. Pathologic fracture
4. Periosteal reaction
5. Saucerization
6. Well-organized periosteal reaction

Fig. 6.13: Ewing's tumor.

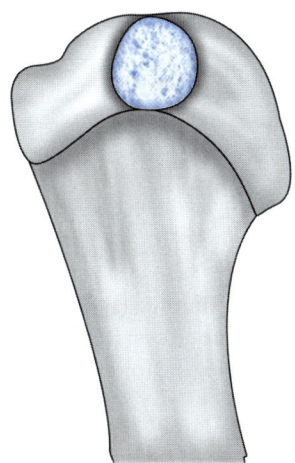

Fig. 6.14: Chondroblastoma.

Differential Diagnosis in Radiology

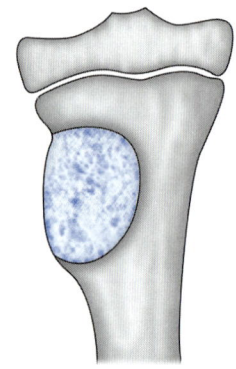

Fig. 6.15: Chondromyxoid fibroma.

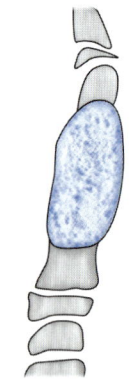

Fig. 6.16: Enchondroma.

Infection
- Brodie's abscess.
- Coccidioidomycosis.
- Echinococcus.

Endocrinal
- Hyperparathyroidism.

Tumor-like Lesions
- Nonossifying fibroma (*see* Fig. 6.11).
- Aneurysmal bone cyst (Fig. 6.17).
- Simple cyst (Fig. 6.18).

Idiopathic
- Histiocytosis X.
- Fibrous dysplasia.

PRIMARY BONE TUMORS: CLINICAL FEATURES, SITE OF PREDILECTION, AND RADIOLOGIC PRESENTATION (FIGS. 6.19 TO 6.24)

The clinical features, site of predilection, and radiologic presentation of primary bone tumors are shown in Figures 6.19 to 6.24.

RADIOLOGIC CHARACTERISTICS OF BENIGN AND MALIGNANT BONE LESIONS

The radiologic characteristics of benign and malignant bone lesions are illustrated in Table 6.2.

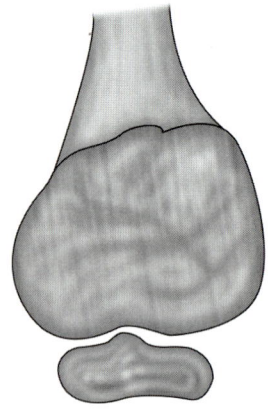

Fig. 6.17: Aneurysmal bone cyst.

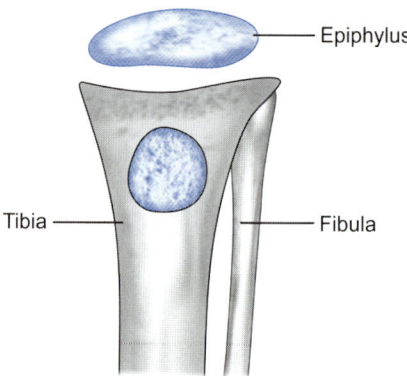

Fig. 6.18: Schematic diagram showing simple bone cyst.

SUBARTICULAR LYTIC BONE LESION
Arthritides (Figs. 6.25 to 6.35)

- *Osteoarthritis:*
    - Marginal osteophytes.
    - Subchondral sclerosis.
    - Reduced joint space.
    - Multiple cysts in load-bearing regions.
- *Rheumatoid arthritis:*
    - Cysts at/near the regions of capsular insertion.
    - Joint space narrowing.
    - Juxta-articular osteoporosis.
    - No sclerosis.
- *Calcium pyrophosphate arthropathy:*
    - More collapsed and fragmented articular surface.
    - Cysts larger than osteoarthritis.
    - Rest similar changes as in osteoarthritis.
- *Gout:*
    - Punched-out erosions with overhanging edge with adjacent soft tissue masses.
- *Hemophilia:*
    - Erosions and subchondral cyst with periarticular osteoporosis with preserved joint space until late in disease.

Neoplastic

- Metastases/multiple myeloma.
- Aneurysmal bone cyst.
- Giant cell tumor.
- Chondroblastoma.

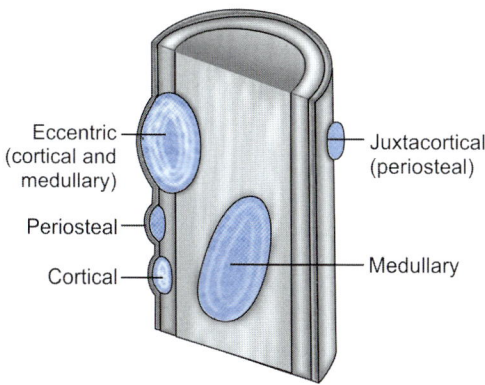

Fig. 6.19: Locations of tumors within a bone.

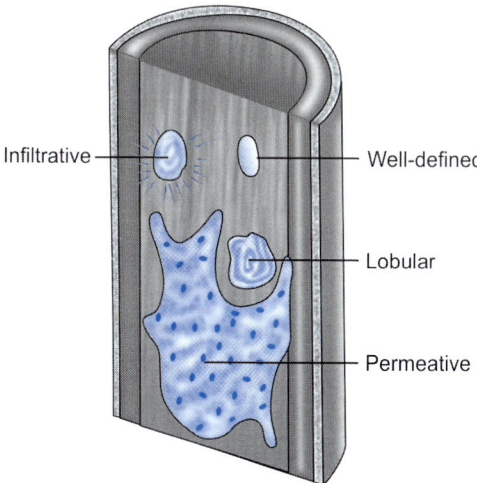

Fig. 6.20: Patterns of bone destruction.

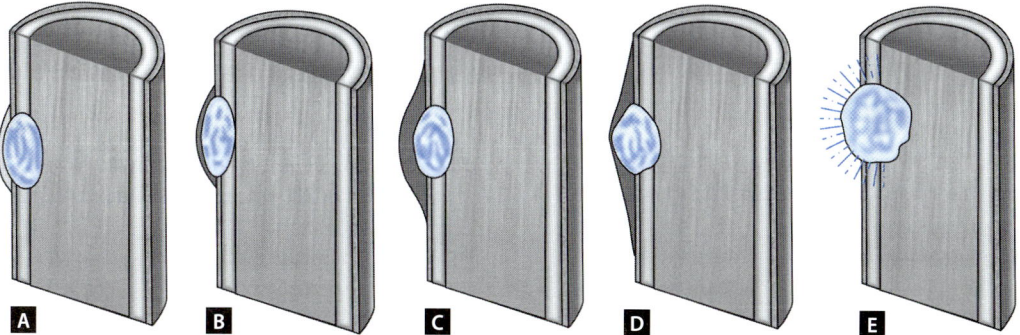

Figs. 6.21A to E: Types of periosteal reaction. (A) Well-organized; (B) Buttress; (C) Onion skin; (D) Codman's triangle; and (E) Sunburst.

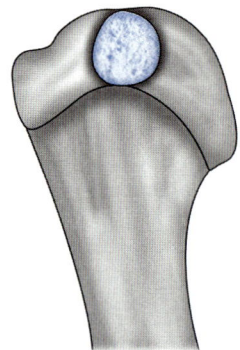

Fig. 6.22: Nonossifying fibroma (fibrous cortical defect).

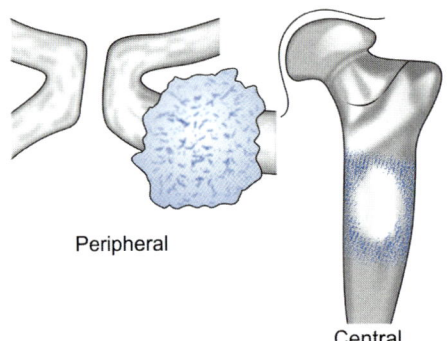

Fig. 6.23: Chondrosarcoma.

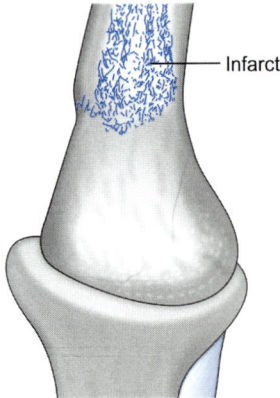

Fig. 6.24: Diaphyseal infarct. Lateral view of the distal femur in a 50-year-old man shows a typical diaphyseal infarct. This lesion, which is remote from the knee joint, was asymptomatic. The absence of punctate calcifications and lobular margins differentiates a bone infarct from an enchondroma.

Table 6.2: Radiologic characteristics of benign and malignant bone lesions.

		Benign	Malignant
1.	Margination	Well-defined	Destructive, poorly-defined
2.	Border	Sclerotic	Infiltrating
3.	Periosteal reaction	Less aggressive	More aggressive
4.	Zone of transition	Narrow	Wide
5.	Soft tissue mass	Absent	Present

- *Pigmented villonodular synovitis:*
  - Mainly lower limbs especially knees.
  - Soft tissue mass.
  - Cyst-like defects with sharp sclerotic margins.
  - Joint space destruction.

Miscellaneous

- *Post-traumatic:*
  - Especially in carpal bones.
- *Osteonecrosis:*
  - Associated sclerosis, collapse, and fragmentation of trabeculae.
  - Preserved joint space.
- *Tuberculosis:*
  - Completely or partially epiphyseal or partly metaphyseal.
  - No sclerosis.

OSTEOLYTIC DEFECTS IN THE MEDULLA

Well Defined

- *Nonexpansile:*
  - Marginal sclerosis:
    - Unilocular:
      - Geode (associated with arthritis).
      - Healing benign/malignant osseous lesion.
      - Brodie's abscess.
      - Simple bone cyst.
      - Enchondroma.
      - Chondroblastoma.
      - Fibrous dysplasia.

Skeletal System and Joints

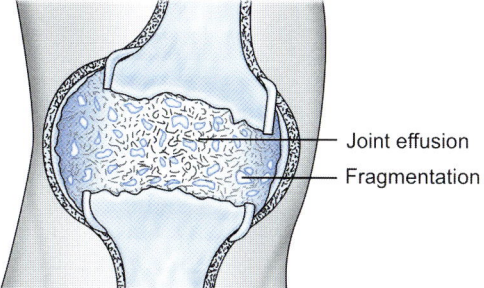

Fig. 6.25: Diarthrodial joint with neuropathic arthritis.

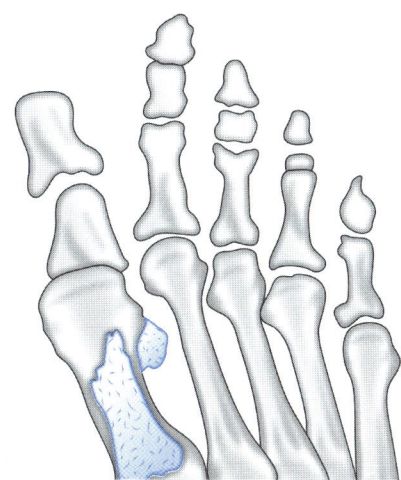

Fig. 6.27: Reiter's syndrome. Dorsiplantar projection of the foot shows marked resorption of the proximal side of the interphalangeal joint of the great toe resulting in a "mortar-and-pestle" or "pencil-in-cup" deformity. Also note the resorption at the distal interphalangeal joint of the fourth toe, fusion of the distal interphalangeal joint of the fifth toe, and marginal erosion at the proximal interphalangeal joint of the fifth toe. Involvement of the distal interphalangeal joints is not uncommon in the arthritis of Reiter's syndrome.

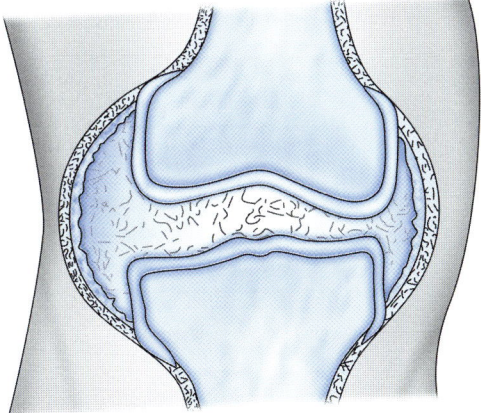

Fig. 6.26: Diarthrodial joint in lupus erythematosus.

- *Multilocular:*
  - Fibrous dysplasia.
  - Simple bone cyst.
- *No marginal sclerosis*:
  - Metastases.
  - Multiple myeloma.
  - Eosinophilic granuloma.
  - Brown tumor of hyperparathyroidism.
  - Enchondroma.
  - Chondroblastoma.
- *Expansile:*
  - *Eccentric expansile*
    - Giant cell tumor.
    - Aneurysmal bone cyst.
    - Enchondroma.
    - Nonossifying fibroma.
    - Chondromyxoid fibroma.

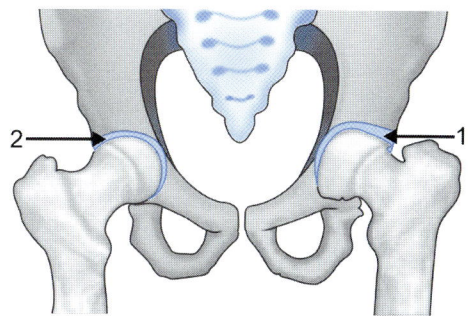

1. Medial wall of acetabulum 2. Iliopubic line

Fig. 6.28: Rheumatoid arthritis. Anteroposterior projection of the hips shows concentric narrowing of both the hip joints with axial migration of the femoral heads resulting in protrusio acetabulum (i.e. the medial wall of the acetabulum is medial to the iliopubic line). The intense sclerosis of the left femoral head and left acetabulum indicates secondary osteoarthritis; however, osteophytes are absent.

  - *Grossly expansile:*
    - Malignant lesions.
    - Metastases.

Differential Diagnosis in Radiology

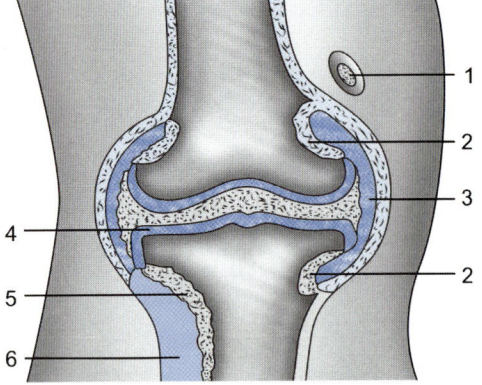

1. Subcutaneous nodule
2. Marginal erosion
3. Synovial hypertrophy
4. Diffuse articular loss
5. Enthesopathy
6. Tendon insertion

Fig. 6.29: Diarthrodial joint with rheumatoid arthritis.

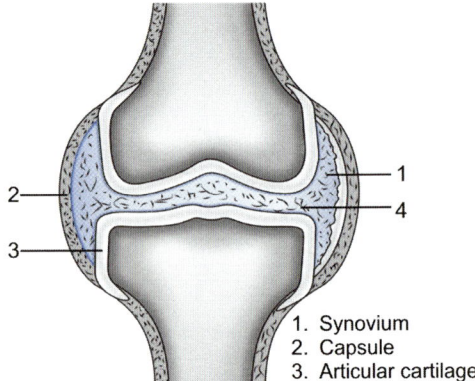

1. Synovium
2. Capsule
3. Articular cartilage
4. Synovial fluid

Fig. 6.31: Normal diarthrodial joint.

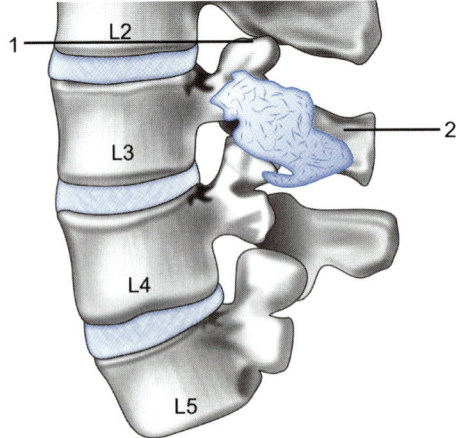

1. Posterior apophyseal joint   2. Hypertrophic bone

Fig. 6.30: Osteoarthritis of spine. Lateral tomogram of an old woman shows advanced degenerative change in the posterior apophyseal (facet) joints of the lumbar spine. Hypertrophic bone encroaches on the central spinal canal. Also note the spondylolisthesis at L4–L5, with calcification in the outer fibers of the annulus fibrosus at this level. The intervertebral disks are relatively well maintained. Note that the spinal apophyseal (facet) joints are synovial joints which may undergo degenerative change. The resulting sclerosis and hypertrophic bone may encroach upon the central spinal canal and produce a secondary form of spinal stenosis, as in this patient.

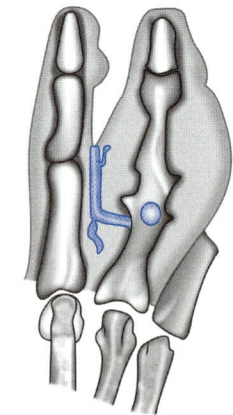

Fig. 6.32: Chronic tophaceous gout.

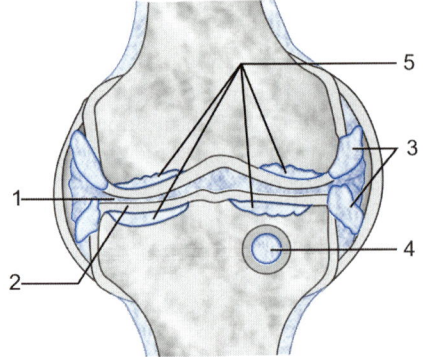

1. Joint-space narrowing
2. Diffuse articular loss
3. Osteophytes
4. Subchondral cyst
5. Subchondral sclerosis

Fig. 6.33: Osteoarthritis of diarthrodial joint.

- Plasmacytoma.
- Central chondrosarcoma.
- Telangiectatic osteosarcoma.

- Benign lesions:
  - Aneurysmal bone cyst.
  - Giant cell tumor.
  - Enchondroma.
- Nonneoplastic:
  - Fibrous dysplasia.
  - Hemophilic pseudotumor.
  - Brown tumor of hyperparathyroidism.
  - Hydatid disease.

Ill Defined

- Without periosteal reaction:
  - Nonexpansile (see Figs. 6.35A and B):
    - Metastases.
    - Multiple myeloma.
    - Hemangioma.
    - Lymphoma.
    - Malignant fibrous histiocytoma.
  - Expansile:
    - Chondrosarcoma
    - Giant cell tumor
    - Metastases from kidney/thyroid
    - Fibrosarcoma.
- With periosteal reaction:
  - Osteomyelitis (Fig. 6.36).
  - Ewing's sarcoma.
  - Osteosarcoma.

LUCENT BONE LESION CONTAINING BONE/CALCIUM

Neoplastic

- Metastases, especially breast.
- Chondroid lesions:
  - Benign:
    - Enchondroma.
    - Chondroblastoma.
    - Chondromyxoid fibroma.
  - Malignant:
    - Chondrosarcoma.
- Osteoid lesions:
  - Benign:
    - Osteoid osteoma
    - Osteoblastoma.
  - Malignant:
    - Osteosarcoma.
- Fibrous tissue lesions:
  - Malignant:
    - Fibrosarcoma
    - Malignant fibrous histiocytoma.

Miscellaneous

- Fibrous dysplasia.
- Osteoporosis circumscripta (Paget's disease).
- Avascular necrosis/infarction of bone.
- Osteomyelitis with sequestrum (Fig. 6.36).
- Eosinophilic granuloma.
- Intraosseous lipoma.

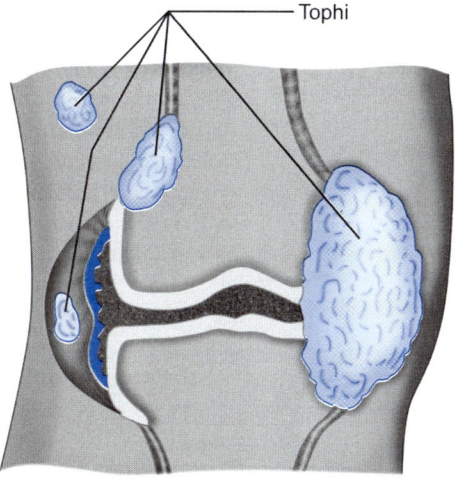

Fig. 6.34: Diarthrodial joint with chronic tophaceous gout.

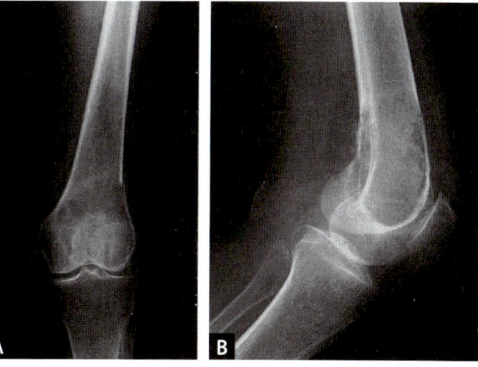

Figs. 6.35A and B: Anteroposterior and lateral radiographs of lower thigh shows non-Hodgkin's lymphoma of femur.

COMMON LYTIC BONE LESIONS

With Marked Sclerosis

- Brodie's abscess.
- Osteoblastoma.
- Osteoid osteoma.
- Stress fracture.
- Tuberculosis.

Multiple

- Fibrous dysplasia.
- Enchondroma.
- Eosinophilic granuloma.
- Metastases.
- Multiple myeloma.
- Brown tumors in hyperparathyroidism.

Seen in Less than 30 Years of Age

- Chondroblastoma.
- Aneurysmal bone cyst.
- Infection.
- Nonossifying fibroma (Fig. 6.37).
- Eosinophilic granuloma.
- Solitary bone cyst.

Seen on Both Sides of Joint

- Synovioma.
- Angioma.
- Chondroid lesion.

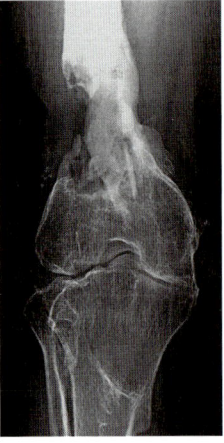

Fig. 6.36: Anteroposterior radiograph of knee joint region shows chronic osteomyelitis of lower end of femur with sequestrum formation.

LOCATION OF SOME COMMON NEOPLASMS/LESIONS

Epiphysis

- Chondroblastoma.
- Giant cell tumor (Fig. 6.38).
- Intraosseous ganglion.

Metaphysis

- Nonossifying fibroma.
- Chondromyxoid fibroma.

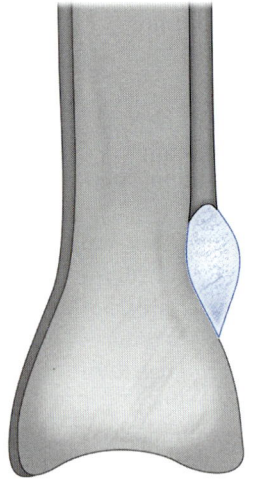

Fig. 6.37: Nonossifying fibroma.

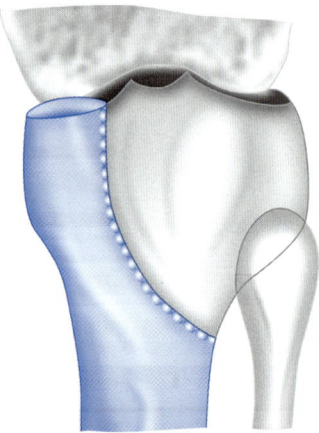

Fig. 6.38: Giant cell tumor.

- Simple bone cyst.
- Osteochondroma (Fig. 6.39).
- Brodie's abscess.
- Giant cell tumor.
- Osteosarcoma (Fig. 6.40).
- Chondrosarcoma.

Diaphysis

- Ewing's sarcoma.
- Nonossifying fibroma.
- Simple bone cyst.

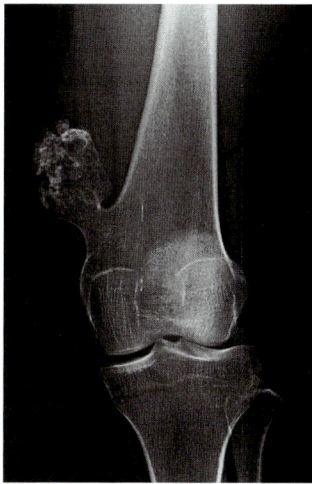

Fig. 6.39: Anteroposterior radiograph of lower thigh shows osteochondroma arising from the lower end of femur.

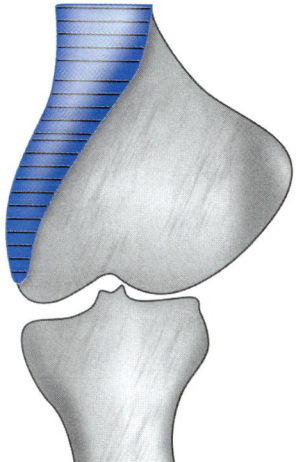

Fig. 6.40: Osteosarcoma.

- Enchondroma.
- Fibrous dysplasia.
- Osteochondroma (Fig. 6.41).

SEPTATED BONE LESIONS

The septated bone lesions are given in Table 6.3.

MOTH-EATEN BONE

Characterized by multiple, scattered lytic lesions of varying sizes with no major central lesion, and less well-defined/demarcated lesional margin with larger zones of transition.

- *Neoplastic:*
    - Metastasis/multiple myeloma—including neuroblastoma in child.
    - Leukemias/lymphomas.
    - Ewing's sarcoma.

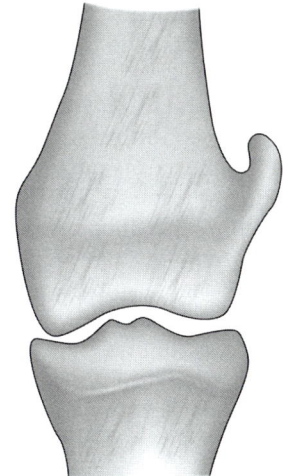

Fig. 6.41: Osteochondroma (exostosis).

Table 6.3: Septated bone lesions.

	Lesions	Type of septations
1.	Aneurysmal bone cysts	Delicate, horizontally-oriented
2.	Chondromyxoid fibroma	Coarse, thick
3.	Giant cell tumor	Delicate, thin
4.	Hemangioma (Fig. 6.42)	Striated, radiating
5.	Nonossifying fibroma	Lobulated

- Osteosarcoma/chondrosarcoma.
- Fibrosarcoma and malignant fibrous histiocytoma.
- Histiocytosis X/Langerhans cell histiocytosis.
- *Infective:*
  - Osteomyelitis.

OSTEOPENIA

Generalized (Figs. 6.43 and 6.44)

- *Osteoporosis (diminished osteoid production):*
  - In axial skeleton and appendicular skeleton:
    * Decreased number and thickness of trabeculae.
    * Cortical thinning.
    * Juxta-articular osteopenia with trabecular bone predominance.
    * Delayed fracture healing with poor callus formation.
  - In spine only:
    * Diminished radiographic density.
    * Increased vertical striations.
    * Prominence of endplates.
    * Picture framing and compression deformities with protrusion of disks.
  - Congenital:
    * Osteogenesis imperfecta.
    * Turner syndrome.
    * Homocystinuria.
    * Neuromuscular disease.
    * Mucopolysaccharidosis.
    * Trisomy 13 and 18.
    * Pseudo- and pseudohypoparathyroidism.
    * Glycogen storage disease.
    * Progeria.
  - Idiopathic:
    * *Juvenile:* Less than 20 years
    * *Adult:* 20–40 years
    * *Postmenopausal:* More than 50 years
    * *Senile:* More than 60 years.
  - Miscellaneous:
    * Renal osteodystrophy.
    * Disuse: Immobilization.
    * Collagen disease and rheumatoid arthritis.
    * Bone marrow replacement by leukemia/lymphoma, multiple myeloma/metastases.
    * Drugs (heparin, steroids, methotrexate, and vitamin A).
    * Radiation therapy.
  - Nutritional deficiency:
    * Scurvy (Fig. 6.45).
    * Protein-energy malnutrition (PEM).
    * Calcium deficiency (Fig. 6.46).
  - Endocrinopathy:
    * Hypogonadism.
    * Cushing's syndrome.

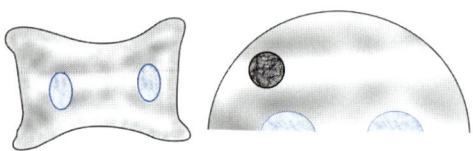

Fig. 6.42: Hemangioma of bone.

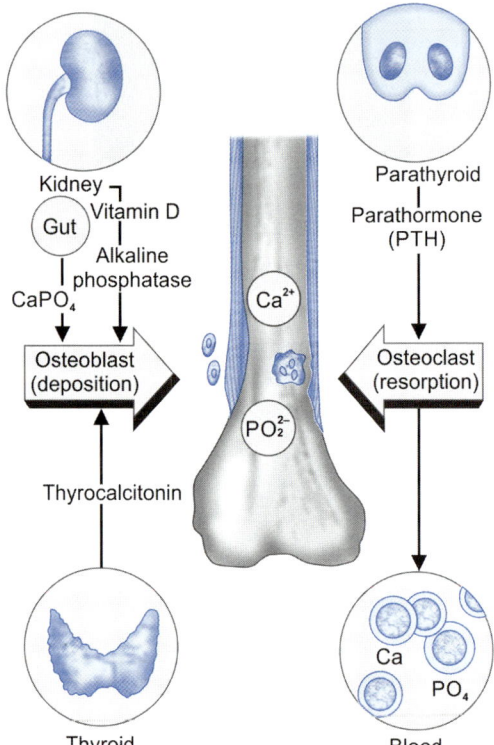

Fig. 6.43: Factors affecting resorption (osteoclastic activity) and deposition (osteoblastic activity) of calcium and phosphorus.

Skeletal System and Joints

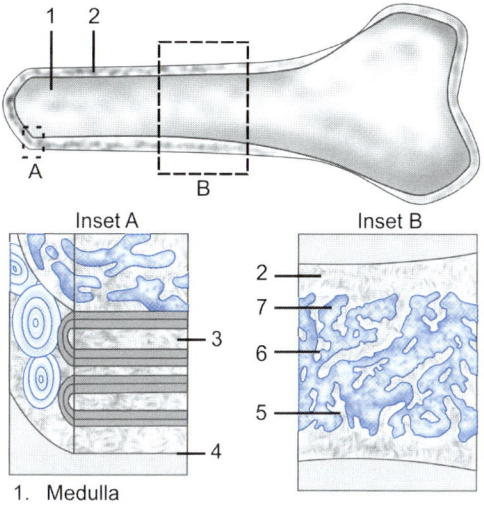

1. Medulla
2. Cortex
3. Haversian canal
4. Lacunae with osteocytes
5. Spongiosa
6. Osteocytes
7. Marrow

Fig. 6.44: Normal bone. Cross-sectional anatomy of normal adult bone indicating osteocytes and their effect on bone metabolism. Inset A: Location of osteocytes within the bone cortex. Inset B: Location of osteocytes within the bone spongiosa. *Note:* The conduits of metabolite transport within each area: Haversian canals in the cortex and vascular marrow in the medulla.

- Addison's disease.
- Diabetes mellitus.
- Pregnancy.
- Mastocytosis.

- *Osteomalacia*—accumulation of excessive amounts of uncalcified osteoid with bone softening (Fig. 6.47).
    – Uniform osteopenia.
    – Fuzzy indistinct trabecular detail of endosteal surface.
    – Thin cortices of long bone.
    – Coarsened, frayed trabeculae decreased in number and size.
    – Bone deformity from softening.

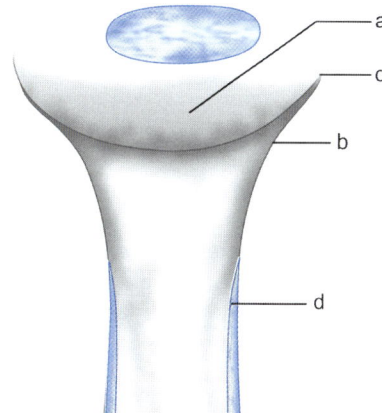

Fig. 6.46: Rickets. a. Widened growth plate; b. Fraying, splaying, and cupping of metaphysis; c. Thin bony spur; and d. Indistinct cortex.

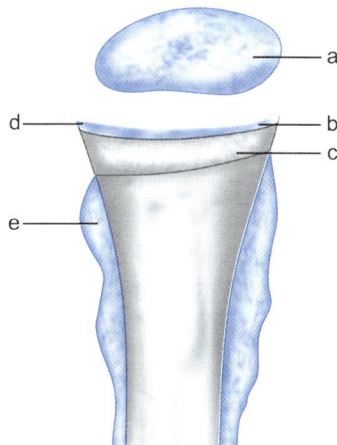

Fig. 6.45: Scurvy. a. Loss of epiphyseal density with pencil-thin cortex; b. Dense zone of provisional calcification; c. Metaphyseal lucency; d. Pelken spur; and e. Subperiosteal hematoma.

- Hyperthyroidism.
- Hyperparathyroidism.
- Acromegaly.

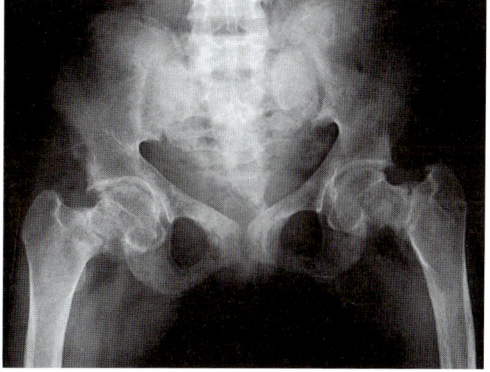

Fig. 6.47: Anteroposterior radiograph of pelvis shows pseudofracture through ischiopubic rami and femoral neck on both sides in a case of osteomalacia.

- Hourglass thorax.
- Bowing of long bones.
- Buckled/compressed pelvis.
- Increased incidence of fractures, biconcave vertical bodies.
- Mottled skull and pseudofracture.

Causes of osteomalacia:
- Dietary deficiency of vitamin D3 and lack of solar irradiation.
- *Deficiency of metabolism of vitamin D:*
  - Chronic renal tubular disease.
  - Chronic administration of phenobarbitone.
  - Diphenylhydantoin.
- *Decreased absorption of vitamin D:*
  - Malabsorption syndrome.
  - Partial gastrectomy.
- *Decreased deposition of calcium in bone:*
  - Diphosphonates (used for treatment of Paget's disease).
- *Hyperparathyroidism*—increased bone resorption by osteoblasts.
  Causes: Adenoma (most common), hyperplasia, carcinoma, ectopic hormone production, etc.
  - Loss of fine trabeculae with ground-glass appearance.
  - Subperiosteal bone resorption affecting radial side of middle phalanx of middle finger, medial proximal tibia, lateral end of clavicle, symphysis pubis, ischial tuberosity, medial femoral neck, dorsum sellae, superior surface of ribs, and proximal humerus.
  - Cortical tunneling producing "basketwork" appearance and "pepper-pot" skull.
  - Brown tumors in mandible, ribs, pelvis, and femora.
  - Bone softening leading to basilar invagination, wedged or codfish vertebra, triradiate pelvis, and pathological fracture.
  - Soft tissue calcification.
  - Marginal erosion at distal interphalangeal (DIP), ulnar side of base of little finger metacarpal, and hamate with normal joint space.
  - Chondrocalcinosis and periarticular calcification (capsular and tendinous).
- *Diffusely infiltrating bone disease:*
  - *For example:* Multiple myeloma, leukemia, and metastases.

Localized/Regional

- *Disuse* due to local immobilization secondary to fractures and neuromuscular paralysis.
- *Patterns of bone loss:*
  - Uniform (most common).
  - Spotty (periarticular).
  - Band-like (metaphyseal or subchondral).
  - Endosteal cortical scalloping.
  - Linear cortical lucencies.
- *Sudeck's atrophy (reflex sympathetic dystrophy):*
  - Associated with posttraumatic/postinfective states, myocardial infarction, calcific tendinitis, and cervical spondylosis.
  - Affects shoulder and hands.
  - Disuse osteoporosis.
  - Subperiosteal bone erosion.
  - Small periarticular erosions.
- *Transient osteoporosis of hip:*
  - Severe, progressive, osteoporosis of femoral head, neck, and acetabulum.
  - Full recovery in 6 months.
- *Regional migratory osteoporosis:*
  - Swelling and osteoporosis of joints of lower limbs.
  - Migratory nature differentiates it from other causes.
- Osteolytic tumor.
- Lytic phase of Paget's disease.
- *Inflammation*—rheumatoid arthritis, osteomyelitis, and tuberculosis.
- Early phase of bone infarct and hemorrhage.
- Burns and frostbite.

PERIOSTEAL REACTIONS: TYPES AND CONDITIONS

Continuous

- *Cortex destroyed:*
  - Simple shell like or expanded cortex.
  - Lobulated shell like.
  - *Ridged shell*—trabeculated or soap-bubble like.

Causes:
- Giant cell tumor.
- Aneurysmal bone cyst.
- Enchondroma.
- Nonossifying fibroma.
- Chondromyxoid fibroma.
- Expansile metastases.
- Plasmacytoma.
- Central chondrosarcoma.
- Telangiectatic osteosarcoma.
- Fibrous dysplasia.
- Hemophilic pseudotumor.
- Brown tumor of hyperparathyroidism.
- Hydatid.
- Intact cortex:
  – Solid—even, uniform thickness more than 1 mm, persistent, and unchanged for weeks.

Patterns:
- *Thin*—eosinophilic granuloma, osteoid osteoma.
- *Dense undulating*—vascular disease.
- *Thin undulating*—pulmonary osteoarthropathy.
- *Dense elliptical*—osteoid osteoma, long-standing malignant disease.
- *Cloaking*—storage disease, chronic infection.
  – *Unilamellar:*
    • Osteomyelitis.
    • Histiocytosis.
    • Benign tumors.
    • Healing fractures.
  – *Multilamellar:*
    • Osteomyelitis.
    • Histiocytosis.
    • Aneurysmal bone cyst.
    • Ewing's sarcoma.
    • Osteosarcoma.
  – *Parallel spiculated—hair on end:*
    • Ewing's sarcoma.
    • Osteosarcoma.
    • Metastases.
    • Thalassemia.
    • Syphilis.
    • Infantile cortical hyperostoses.

Interrupted
- *Buttressing:*
  – Solid periosteal bone is formed at lateral extraosseous margin of growing bone lesion, e.g. Ewing's sarcoma.
- *Codman's triangle*—angular periosteal configuration with underlying cortex.
  For example:
  – Hemorrhage.
  – Malignancy (osteosarcoma, Ewing's sarcoma).
  – Acute osteomyelitis.
  – Fracture.
  – Hemangioma.
- *Parallel or spiculated:*
  – Osteosarcoma.
  – Ewing's sarcoma.
  – Chondrosarcoma.
  – Fibrosarcoma.
  – Leukemia.
  – Metastases.
  – Acute osteomyelitis.

Complex
- *Divergent spiculated. "Sunray" appearance:*
  – Osteosarcoma.
  – Metastases (Colorectal).
  – Ewing's sarcoma.
  – Hemangioma.
  – Meningioma.
  – Tuberculosis.
  – Tropical ulcer.
- *Combination types:*
  – Ewing's sarcoma.
  – Osteosarcoma.

TYPES OF PERIOSTEAL REACTIONS
Solitary and Localized
- Traumatic.
- Inflammatory/infective.
- *Neoplastic:*
  – Benign.
  – Malignant.

Bilateral Involvement
- *Symmetrical:*

- *Vascular insufficiency (venous, lymphatic, and arterial):*
    - Usually confined to lower limbs.
    - Soft tissue swelling is seen.
    - Solid, undulating periosteal reaction.
    - Phleboliths seen in venous causes.
- *Hypertrophic osteoarthropathy:*
    - Periosteal reaction seen in metaphysis and diaphysis of radius, ulna, tibia, fibula, less commonly femur and humerus, and bones of hands and feet.
    - Thickness of periosteal reaction corresponds to the duration of disease.
    - Periarticular osteoporosis, soft tissue swelling, and joint effusions seen.
- *Pachydermoperiostosis (Fig. 6.48):*
    - Self limited, familial condition, and affecting boys at puberty with predilection for blacks.
    - Bones affected are radius and ulna, tibia, fibula mainly followed by bones of hands and feet.
    - Periosteal reaction is solid and spiculated and also involves the epiphysis in addition to metaphysis and diaphysis.
- *Thyroid acropachy:*
    - Solid, spiculated, and lace-like periosteal reaction affecting diaphysis of metacarpals and phalanges of hands and less commonly of feet.
- *Fluorosis:*
    - Solid undulating periosteal reaction in long bones, flat bone with osteosclerosis, ligamentous, and interosseous membranous calcification.

- *Asymmetrical:*
    - Arthritides:
        - Rheumatoid arthritis.
        - Psoriatic arthropathy.
    - Metastases.
    - Disseminated osteomyelitis.
    - *Osteoporosis/osteomalacia*:
        - Multiple fractures.
    - Nonaccidental injuries.
    - Bleeding diathesis.
    - Hand-foot syndrome (sickle cell dactylitis).
    - *Idiopathic:*
        - Degenerative.

PERIOSTEAL REACTION IN CHILDHOOD (FIGS. 6.49A TO D)
Benign
- *Physiological:*
    - Symmetrical involvement of diaphysis during the first 6 months of life.
- Battered child syndrome.
- Infantile cortical hyperostoses (<6 months of age).
    - Mandible, clavicles, and ribs usually affected.
- Hypervitaminosis A.
- Scurvy/rickets.
- Osteogenesis imperfecta.
- *Congenital syphilis:*
    - Usually diaphyseal.
- Drugs like prostaglandins E1 to treat ductus-dependent congenital heart disease (CHD).
- Eosinophilic granuloma.
- Osteomyelitis/trauma.
- Sickle cell disease.
- Kinky hair syndrome.
- *Juvenile chronic arthritis:*

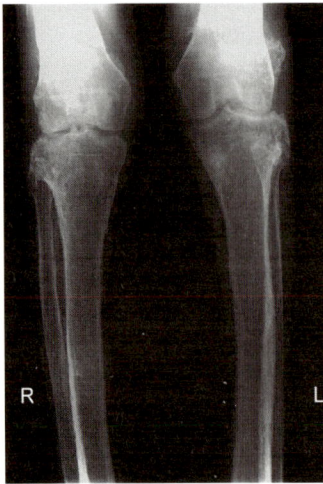

Fig. 6.48: Anteroposterior radiograph of both the legs showing features of pachydermoperiostosis.

Skeletal System and Joints

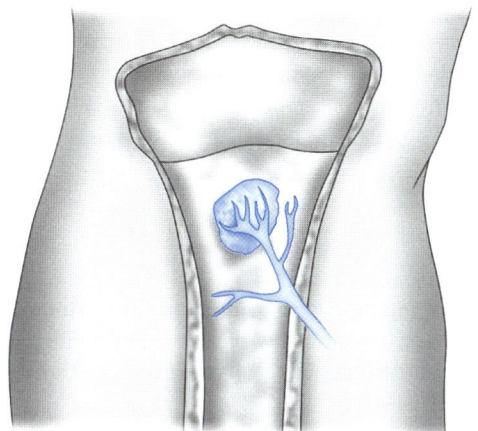

Fig. 6.49A: Routes of bone invasion: In hematogenous osteomyelitis, organisms gain access to bone via the nutrient arteries, which are most numerous in the metaphysis of a growing bone.

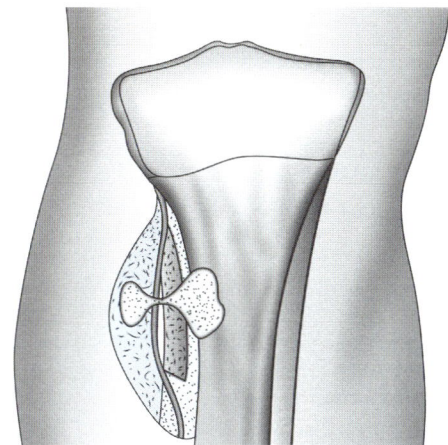

Fig. 6.49C: A missile wound enables organisms and debris to gain entry via a traumatic break in the skin and bone.

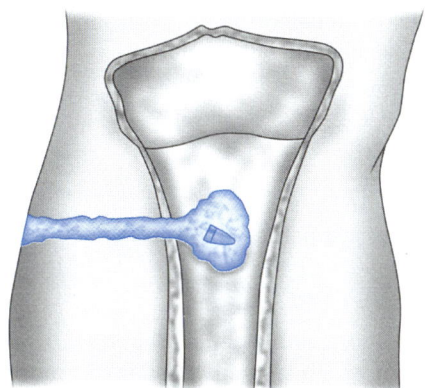

Fig. 6.49B: Contiguous spread from a soft tissue infection allows the organisms to penetrate the periosteal lining and the underlying cortex, gaining access to the medullary cavity. Pus elevates the periosteum, stimulating the formation of new bone (periosteal reaction).

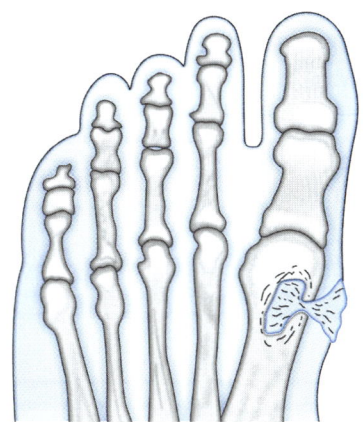

Fig. 6.49D: In diabetic osteomyelitis, fissures and ulcers form in the overlying skin secondary to diabetic vascular disease and organisms enter via these openings. As a consequence of vascular obstruction, leukocytes, antibodies, and antibiotics fail to reach the infected focus in the bone.

– Bilaterally symmetrical in the periarticular regions of phalanges, metacarpals, and metatarsals.

Malignant
- Multicentric osteosarcoma.
- Metastases from neuroblastoma and retinoblastoma.
- Acute leukemia.
- Ewing's sarcoma.

HYPERTROPHIC OSTEOARTHROPATHY
Pulmonary
- Carcinoma bronchus, especially oat cell carcinoma.
- Lymphoma.
- Abscess.
- Bronchiectasis.
- Metastases.

Pleural
- Pleural fibroma.
- Mesothelioma.

Cardiovascular
- Cyanotic CHD.

Gastrointestinal
- Ulcerative colitis/Crohn's disease.
- Dysentery.
- Lymphoma.
- Whipple's disease.
- Celiac disease.
- Cirrhosis.
- Nasopharyngeal carcinomas.
- Juvenile polyposis.

BONE DYSPLASIAS: ASSOCIATED WITH MULTIPLE FRACTURES

Reduced Density
- Osteogenesis imperfecta.
- Achondrogenesis.
- Hypophosphatasia.
- Mucolipidosis II.
- Cushing's syndrome.

Normal Osseous Density
- Cleidocranial dysplasia.
- Enchondromatosis.
- Fibrous dysplasia.

Increased Density
- Osteopetrosis.
- Pyknodysostosis.

EXCESSIVE CALLUS FORMATION

Causes
- Steroid therapy and Cushing's syndrome.
- Neuropathic arthropathy.
- Osteogenesis imperfecta.
- Nonaccidental injury.
- Paralytic states.
- Renal osteodystrophy.
- Multiple myeloma.

BONE WITHIN BONE APPEARANCE

It results from endosteal new bone formation.

Causes
- *Normal:*
  - In thoracic and lumbar spine (in infants).
  - Growth recovery lines (after infancy).
- Infantile cortical hyperostosis (Caffey's disease).
- Sickle cell disease/thalassemia.
- Congenital syphilis.
- Osteopetrosis/oxalosis.
- Radiation.
- Acromegaly.
- Paget's disease.
- Heavy metal poisoning (Bi, Pb, and Th).
- Prostaglandin E therapy.
- Leukemia.
- Tuberculosis.
- Rickets.
- Scurvy.
- Vitamin D toxicity.
- Reflex sympathetic dystrophy.

FATIGUE FRACTURES

Normal bone subjected to repetitive stresses (none of which is alone capable of producing a fracture) leads to mechanical failure over a period of time (Fig. 6.50).

Radiographic Signs
- *Cancellous bone:*
  - Subtle blurring of trabecular margins.
  - Faint sclerotic area due to peritrabecular callus.
  - Sclerotic band (due to trabecular compression and peritrabecular callus) perpendicular to cortex.
- *Compact bone:*
  - Subtle ill-defined cortex.
  - Intracortical lucent striations.
  - Solid thick lamellar periosteal new bone formation.

Skeletal System and Joints

- Endosteal thickening.
- Associated with fracture and its related activity are shown in Table 6.4.

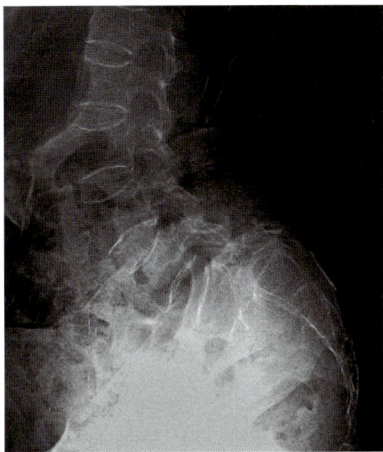

Fig. 6.50: Lateral radiograph of LS spine shows fracture through pars interarticularis with Grade III listhesis of L5 over S1.

PSEUDOARTHROSIS

Causes

- Nonunited fracture.
- Congenital in tibia and fibula—usually in neurofibromatosis.
- Fibrous dysplasia.
- Idiopathic juvenile osteoporosis.
- Osteogenesis imperfecta.
- Cleidocranial dysplasia—in femur.
- Ankylosing spondylitis.

IRREGULAR/STIPPLED EPIPHYSIS (FIG. 6.51)

Causes

- *Normal variant:*
  - In distal femur.
- *Avascular necrosis:*
  - Single in Perthes disease.
  - Multiple in sickle cell anemia.

Table 6.4: Endosteal thickening associated with fracture and its related activity.

	Fracture	Related activity
1.	Clay Shoveler's fracture (fracture spinous process of lower cervical/upper thoracic spine)	Clay shovelling
2.	Coracoid process of scapula	Trap shooting
3.	Ribs	Carrying heavy pack, golf, coughing
4.	Distal shaft of humerus	Throwing ball
5.	Coronoid process of ulna	Pitching ball, throwing javelin, propelling wheelchair
6.	Hook of hamate	Swinging golf stick/tennis racquet/baseball bat
7.	Spondylolysis (pars interarticularis fracture)	Ballet, lifting heavy weights, scrubbing floor
8.	Femoral neck	Ballet, long distance running
9.	Femoral shaft	Ballet, long distance running, gymnastics, marching
10.	Obturator ring of pelvis	Stooping, bowling, gymnastics
11.	Patella	Hurdling
12.	Tibial shaft	Ballet, jogging
13.	Fibula	Long distance running, jumping, parachuting
14.	Calcaneus	Jumping, parachuting, prolonged standing, etc.
15.	Navicular	Stooping on ground, marching, prolonged standing, ballet
16.	Metatarsal (commonly 2nd)	Marching, prolonged standing, stamping on ground
17.	Sesamoids of metatarsals	Prolonged standing

- *Hypothyroidism:*
  - Delayed appearance and growth of ossification centers.
  - Femoral capital epiphysis divided into inner and outer half.
- *Chondrodysplasia punctata:*
  - Stippling in long bones epiphyses, spine, and larynx which disappear by 2 years of age.
  - Asymmetrical shortening of limbs.
- *Multiple epiphyseal dysplasia:*
  - Delayed appearance and growth of epiphysis.
  - With or without metaphyseal irregularity.
- Spondyloepiphyseal dysplasia.
- Hypoparathyroidism.
- Down syndrome.
- Trisomy 18.
- *Fetal warfarin syndrome:*
  - Stippling of uncalcified epiphysis, particularly axial skeleton, proximal femora, and calcanei.
  - Disappears after 1st year.
- *Homocystinuria:*
  - Distal ulnar and radial epiphysis—pathognomonic.
- Zellweger's cerebrohepatorenal syndrome.
- *Fetal alcohol syndrome:*
  - Mostly calcaneus and lower extremities.
- *Meyer dysplasia:*
  - Confined to femoral heads.
- *Morquio's syndrome:*
  - Irregular ossification of femoral capital epiphysis.

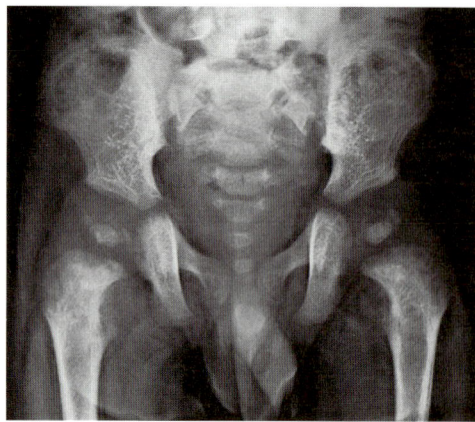

Fig. 6.51: Anteroposterior radiograph of pelvis shows bilateral stippled femoral head epiphysis in a patient of rickets.

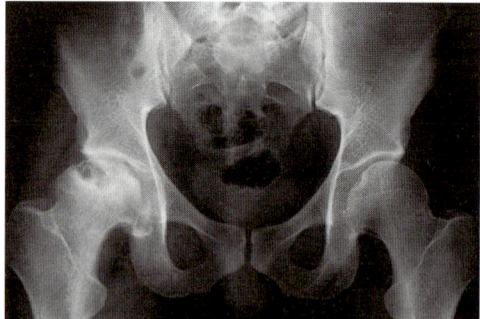

Fig. 6.52A: Anteroposterior radiograph of pelvis shows secondary degenerative changes following avascular necrosis (AVN) in both the hips.

AVASCULAR NECROSIS/ OSTEONECROSIS/ASEPTIC NECROSIS

This is the consequence of interrupted blood supply to bone with death of cellular elements (Figs. 6.52A and B).

Causes

- *Toxic:*
  - Steroids (>2 years of treatment).
  - *Nonsteroidal anti-inflammatory drug*—indomethacin.

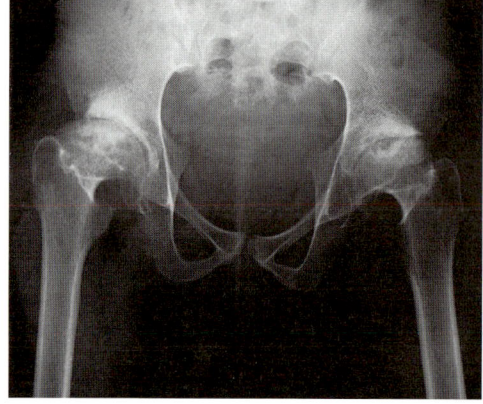

Fig. 6.52B: Anteroposterior radiograph of pelvis shows AVN of right hip.

- Alcohol.
- Immunosuppressives.
- *Traumatic:*
  - *Idiopathic*—Perthes disease (Fig. 6.53).
  - *Fractures*—femoral neck, talus, and scaphoid.
  - Radiotherapy.
  - Heat burns, electrical.
  - Fat embolism.
  - Frostbite.
- *Inflammatory:*
  - Rheumatoid arthritis.
  - Psoriasis.
  - Systemic lupus erythematosus.
  - Scleroderma.
  - Neuropathic arthropathy.
  - Osteoarthrosis.
  - Infection.
  - Pancreatitis.
- *Metabolic/endocrinal:*
  - Pregnancy.
  - Diabetes.
  - Cushing's syndrome.
  - Hyperlipidemia.
  - Gout.
  - Hypercholesterolemia.
  - Hyperuricemia.
- *Hematopoietic disorders:* Hemoglobinopathies as sickle cell anemia.
  - Hemophilia.
  - Gaucher's disease.
  - Histiocytosis.
  - Polycythemia.
- *Thrombotic/embolic:*
  - Dysbaric osteonecrosis.
  - Giant cell arteritis.
  - Endocarditis.
  - Polyarteritis nodosa.
  - Peripheral vascular disease.

Steinberg Classification for Avascular Necrosis of Hip

Stage 0 – Normal.
Stage 1 – Normal—barely abnormal trabecular pattern, abnormal bone scan/magnetic resonance imaging (MRI).
Stage 2A – Focal sclerosis and osteopenia.
2B – Distinct sclerosis with osteoporosis and early crescent sign.
Stage 3A – Subchondral undermining (Crescent sign) and cyst formation.
3B – Mild alteration in femoral head contour and subchondral fracture with normal joint space.
Stage 4 – Marked collapse of femoral head with significant acetabular involvement.
Stage 5 – Joint space narrowing with significant acetabular changes.

Magnetic Resonance Changes in Avascular Necrosis (Mitchell Staging)

The magnetic resonance changes in avascular necrosis (Mitchell staging) are given in Table 6.5.

SOLITARY RADIOLUCENT METAPHYSEAL BANDS

It represents a period of poor endochondral bone formation.

Causes

- Normal variant.
- Any severe systemic illness.
- Healing rickets.
- Scurvy.
- Leukemia, lymphoma.
- Metastatic neuroblastoma.

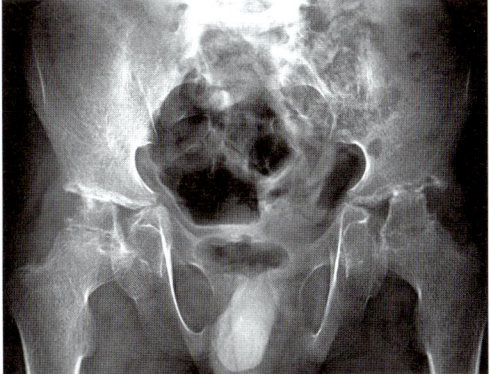

Fig. 6.53: Anteroposterior radiograph of pelvis shows bony ankylosis following Perthes disease in both hips.

Table 6.5: Magnetic resonance changes in avascular necrosis (Mitchell staging).

Stage	T1WI	T2WI	Comments
A	Increase	Intermediate	Fat
B	Increase	Increase	Subacute blood
C	Decrease	Increase	Fluid/edema
D	Decrease	Decrease	Fibrosis

(T1WI: T1-weighted image; T2WI: T2-weighted image)

- Congenital infection as syphilis.
- Growth lines.
- Metaphyseal fracture, especially in nonaccidental injuries.

SOLITARY DENSE METAPHYSEAL BAND

- Normal variant.
- Heavy metal poisoning (lead, bismuth, and phosphorus, etc.).
- Systemic illness.
- Rickets (healed).
- Scurvy.
- Sickle cell disease.
- Vitamin D intoxication.
- Cretinism.
- Congenital syphilis.
- Estrogen to mother during pregnancy.
- Leukemia.
- TORCH infection.
- Idiopathic hypercalcemia.
- Radiation.
- Osteopetrosis.

ALTERNATING RADIOLUCENT/DENSE METAPHYSEAL BANDS

- Growth arrest or Park's lines.
- Rickets, especially vitamin D resistant.
- Osteopetrosis.
- Chemotherapy.
- *Chronic anemias:*
  - Sickle cell type/thalassemias.
- Treated leukemia.

DENSE VERTICAL METAPHYSEAL LINES

- *Congenital rubella:*
  - Produces a characteristic "celery stalk" appearance.
- Congenital cytomegalovirus (CMV) infection.
- Hypophosphatasia.
- Localized metaphyseal injury.
- *Osteopathia striata:*
  - Bony exostosis may be associated.

FRAYED METAPHYSIS

- Achondroplasia.
- Congenital infections (rubella, syphilis).
- Copper deficiency.
- Chronic stress, e.g. wrists of gymnasts.
- Hypophosphatasia.
- Metaphyseal dysostosis.
- Rickets.
- Scurvy.

CUPPING OF METAPHYSIS

- Normal variant especially distal end of ulna and proximal end of fibula.
- Bone, dysplasias as achondroplasia, pseudoachondroplasia, etc.
- *Rickets:*
  - Associated with metaphyseal blurring and fraying.
- *Scurvy:*
  - Usually follows fracture.
- *Trauma:*
  - To growth plate; the changes will be asymmetrical.

ERLENMEYER FLASK DEFORMITY

This deformity is characterized by expansion of distal ends of long bones, especially femora.

Causes

It includes:
- Storage disorders as Gaucher's disease, Niemann–Pick disease.
- Rickets.
- Anemias, e.g. thalassemia with coarse trabecular pattern.
- Fibrous dysplasia.
- Osteopetrosis.
- Heavy metal poisoning, e.g. lead with thick transverse dense metaphyseal bands.

- *Metaphyseal dysplasia (Pyle's disease):*
  - Rare autosomal recessive disease. Characterized by sclerosis of skull vault and base, widening of medial ends of clavicle, and expansion of pubic and ischial bones.
- Down syndrome.
- Achondroplasia.
- Rheumatoid arthritis.
- Hypophosphatasia.
- Diaphyseal aclasis.
- Ollier's disease.
- *Craniometaphyseal dysplasia:*
  - Common, autosomal dominant condition.
- *Osteodysplasty (Melnick–Needles syndrome):*
  - Seen in females. Characterized by distorted irregular ribs and sigmoid-shaped clavicles; cortical irregularity, patchy sclerosis, and bowing of bones are also seen.

EROSION OF MEDIAL METAPHYSES OF PROXIMAL HUMERUS

- Normal variant.
- *Neoplastic:*
  - Leukemia.
  - Metastatic neuroblastoma.
- *Storage disorders:*
  - Gaucher's disease.
  - Hurler's syndrome.
  - Niemann–Pick disease.
- *Endocrinal:*
  - Hyperparathyroidism.
- *Arthropathies:*
  - Rheumatoid arthritis.

ABNORMALITY RELATED TO CLAVICLES

Erosion or Absence of Outer End of Clavicle

- Rheumatoid arthritis.
- Hyperparathyroidism.
- Posttraumatic osteolysis.
- Metastasis.
- Multiple myeloma.
- Cleidocranial dysplasia.
- Pyknodysostosis.

Penciled Distal End of Clavicle

- Scleroderma.
- Hyperparathyroidism.
- Infection.
- Rheumatoid arthritis.
- Trauma.
- Progeria.

Destruction of Medial End of Clavicle

- Metastasis.
- Infection.
- Lymphoma.
- Eosinophilic granuloma.
- Rheumatoid arthritis.
- Sarcoma.
- Rarely cleidocranial dysplasia.

RIB LESIONS

Neoplastic

- *Benign:*
  - Fibrous dysplasia (most common).
  - Eosinophilic granuloma.
  - Benign cortical defect.
  - Hemangioma.
  - Enchondroma (at costochondral/costovertebral junction).
  - Osteochondroma.
  - Giant cell tumor.
  - Aneurysmal bone cyst.
  - Langerhans cell histiocytosis.
- *Malignant:*
  - *Primary:*
    - Chondrosarcoma.
    - Osteosarcoma.
    - Fibrosarcoma.
    - Ewing's sarcoma.
    - Multiple myeloma/plasmacytoma.
  - *Secondary:*
    - *Adults:*
      - Metastases.
      - Desmoid tumor.
    - *Child:*
      - Metastatic neuroblastoma.

Non-neoplastic

- Healing fractures.
- Radiation osteitis.
- Paget's disease.
- Brown tumor of hyperparathyroidism.
- Osteomyelitis.

RIB NOTCHING

Superior Margin

- *Connective tissue disorders:*
  - Rheumatoid arthritis.
  - Scleroderma.
  - Systemic lupus erythematosus.
  - Sjögren's syndrome.
- *Metabolic:*
  - Hyperparathyroidism.
- *Miscellaneous:*
  - Marfan syndrome.
  - Restrictive lung disease.
  - Neurofibromatosis.
  - Poliomyelitis.
  - Osteogenesis imperfecta.
  - Progeria.

Inferior Margin

- *Arterial:*
  - Coarctation of aorta (CoA) (4th–8th ribs bilaterally).
  - Unilateral (U/L) and right-sided if coarctation is proximal to left subclavian artery.
  - Unilateral and left sided if associated with anomalous right subclavian artery distal to coarctation.
  - Aortic thrombosis.
  - Pulmonary stenosis, Fallot's tetralogy, or absent pulmonary artery (all causes of pulmonary oligemia).
  - Subclavian obstruction (post Blalock–Taussig shunt).
  - Upper three or four ribs ipsilateral to operation side.
- *Venous:*
  - Atrioventricular (AV) chest wall malformation.
  - Superior vena cava (SVC) obstruction.
  - Pulmonary AV malformation.
- *Neurogenic:*
  - Neurofibromatosis.
  - Intercostal neuroma.
  - Poliomyelitis/quadriplegia.
- *Osseous:*
  - Hyperparathyroidism.
  - Thalassemia.
  - Melnick–Needles syndrome.

ABNORMAL SHAPE, SIZE, AND DENSITY OF RIBS

- *Ribbon ribs:*
  - Osteogenesis imperfecta.
  - Neurofibromatosis.
- *Wide/thick ribs:*
  - Chronic anemias.
  - Fibrous dysplasia.
  - Paget's disease.
  - Achondroplasia.
  - Mucopolysaccharidosis.
  - Healed fracture with callus.
- *Bullous costochondral ends:*
  - Rachitic rosary.
  - Scurvy.
  - Achondroplasia.
- *Short ribs:*
  - Achondroplasia.
  - Achondrogenesis.
  - Thanatophoric dysplasia.
  - Asphyxiating thoracic dysplasia.
  - Mesomelic dwarfism.
  - Short rib polydactyly syndrome.
  - Spondyloepiphyseal dysplasia.
  - Enchondromatosis.
  - Chondroectodermal dysplasia.
- *Dense ribs:*
  - Osteopetrosis.
  - Fluorosis.
  - Mastocytosis.
- *Hyperlucent ribs:*
  - Osteopetrosis.
  - Cushing's disease.
  - Acromegaly.
  - Scurvy.

MADELUNG DEFORMITY

Characterized by shortening of distal radius with posterior subluxation of distal ulna.

Causes

- *Isolated congenital:*
  - Usually bilateral and common in females.
- Leri–Weill syndrome (dyschondrosteosis).
- Turner syndrome.
- Post-traumatic.
- Postinfectious.

CARPAL FUSION

Isolated

- *Congenital:*
  - Triquetral-lunate (most common).
  - Capitate-hamate.
  - Trapezium.
  - Trapezoid.
- *Acquired:*
  - Inflammatory arthritides as rheumatoid arthritis.
  - Pyogenic arthritis.
  - Posttraumatic.
  - Postsurgical.

Syndrome Related

- Acrocephalosyndactyly (Apert's syndrome).
- Arthrogryposis multiplex congenita.
- Ellis–van Creveld syndrome.
- Holt–Oram syndrome.
- Turner syndrome.
- Symphalangism.

ABNORMAL DIGITS

- *Brachydactyly (shortening/broadening of metacarpal ± phalanges):*
  - Idiopathic.
  - Post-traumatic.
  - Osteomyelitis.
  - Postinfarction as sickle cell disease.
  - Turner syndrome (4th ± 3rd and 5th).
  - Arthritis.
  - Osteochondrodysplasia.
  - Pseudo and pseudopseudohypoparathyroidism (4th and 5th).
  - Mucopolysaccharidosis.
  - Hereditary multiple exostoses.
  - Basal cell nevus syndrome.
- *Arachnodactyly (elongated/slender):*
  - Marfan's syndrome (metacarpal index = 8.4–10.4).
  - Homocystinuria.
- *Syndactyly (Fig. 6.54) (osseous ± cutaneous fusion of digits):*
  - Apert's syndrome.
  - Carpenter syndrome.
  - Down syndrome.
  - Neurofibromatosis.
  - Poland syndrome.
- *Polydactyly:*
  - Carpenter syndrome.
  - Ellis–van Creveld syndrome.
  - Meckel–Gruber syndrome.
  - Polysyndactyly syndrome.
  - Short rib polydactyly syndrome.
  - Trisomy 13.
- *Clinodactyly (curvature of fingers in mediolateral plane):*
  - Normal variant.
  - Clinodactyly.
  - Multiple dysplasias.
  - Trauma.
  - Arthritis.
  - Contractures (Fig. 6.55).

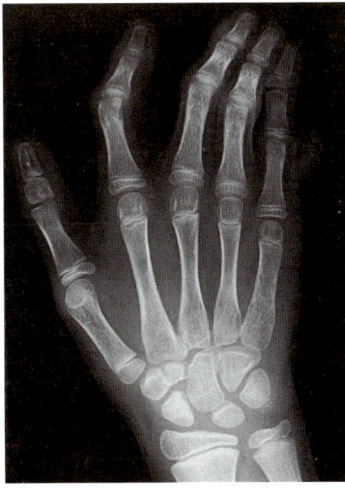

Fig. 6.54: Anteroposterior radiograph of hand shows syndactyly with polydactyly.

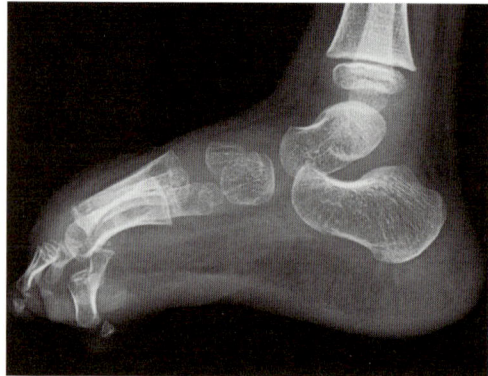

Fig. 6.55: Lateral radiograph of foot shows postburn contracture.

ABNORMAL THUMB

- *Broad:*
  - Acrocephalopolysyndactyly.
  - Acrocephalosyndactyly (Mitten hand and sock foot deformity).
  - Rubinstein–Taybi syndrome.
  - Oropalatodigital syndrome (large cone epiphysis of distal phalanx).
- *Large:*
  - Klippel–Trenaunay–Weber syndrome.
  - Maffucci syndrome.
  - Neurofibromatosis.
  - Macrodystrophia lipomatosa.
- *Short/small:*
  - Fanconi's anemia.
  - Holt–Oram syndrome.
  - Brachydactyly.
  - Cornelia de Lange syndrome.
  - Fetal hydantoin.
- *Absent:*
  - Fanconi's anemia.
  - Poland syndrome.
  - Thalidomide.
  - Trisomy 18.
- *Triphalangeal:*
  - Fanconi's anemia.
  - Holt–Oram syndrome.
  - Blackfan–Diamond syndrome.
  - Poland syndrome.
  - Trisomy 13 and 21.
  - Thalidomide.

- *Abnormal position:*
  - Proximal placed (Cornelia de Lange syndrome).
  - Diastrophic dysplasia and Rubinstein–Taybi syndrome.

LYTIC LESION IN DIGITS

Well Defined

- *Neoplastic:*
  - *Benign*:
    - Implantation dermoid.
    - Enchondroma.
    - Glomus tumor.
    - Osteoid osteoma.

Malignant

- Osteoblastoma.
- *Non-neoplastic:*
  - Sarcoid.
  - Solitary bone cyst.
  - Fibrous dysplasia.

Poorly Defined

- *Neoplastic:*
  - *Benign:*
    - Aneurysmal bone cyst.
    - Giant cell tumor.
  - *Malignant:*
    - Metastases.
    - Multiple myeloma.
    - Osteosarcoma.
    - Fibrosarcoma.
- *Non-neoplastic:*
  - Osteomyelitis.
  - Brown tumors of hyperparathyroidism.
  - Hemophilic pseudotumor.
  - Leprosy.

ACRO-OSTEAL CHANGES

Acro-Osteolysis (Fig. 6.56)

- Familial.
- Massive osteolysis.
- Essential osteolysis.
- Ainhum disease.
- *Acquired:*
  - Psoriasis.
  - Porphyria.

Skeletal System and Joints

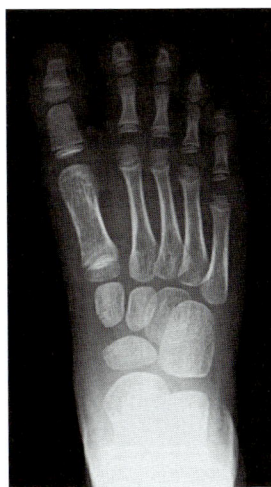

Fig. 6.56: Anteroposterior radiograph of foot shows acro-osteolysis.

- Ehlers–Danlos syndrome.
- Thromboangiitis obliterans.
- Ergot therapy.
- Raynaud's disease.
- Diabetes.
- Arteriosclerosis.
- Dermatomyositis.
- Polyvinyl chloride (PVC) workers.
- Rheumatoid arthritis.
- Scleroderma.
- Leprosy.
- Syringomyelia.
- Hyperparathyroidism.

Acro-osteosclerosis

- Patchy in nature.
  - Incidental (middle-aged and females).
  - Rheumatoid arthritis.
  - Sarcoidosis.
  - Scleroderma.
  - Systemic lupus erythematosus.
  - Hodgkin's disorders.
  - Hematological disorders.

Resorption of Distal Phalanges

- *Congenital*
- *Dysplasia:*
  - Cleidocranial.
  - Pyknodysostosis.
  - Acro-osteolysis of Hajdu and Cheney syndrome.
  - Pachydermoperiostosis.
- *Infective:*
  - Osteomyelitis.
  - Leprosy.
  - Sarcoid.
- *Trauma:*
  - Frostbite.
  - Thermal injuries.
  - Electrical injury.
  - Amputation.
- *Poisons:*
  - Ergot.
  - Polyvinyl chloride.
  - Phenytoin.
  - Snake/scorpion venom.
- *Metabolic:*
  - Hyperparathyroidism and porphyria.
- *Vascular:*
  - Scleroderma.
  - Pseudoxanthoma elasticum.
  - Occlusive vascular disease.
- *Neurotrophic:*
  - Tabes dorsalis.
  - Diabetes.
  - Congenital in difference to pain.
  - Myelomeningocele.
- *Neoplastic:*
  - Kaposi sarcoma.
- *Miscellaneous:*
  - Psoriasis.
  - Pityriasis rubra.
  - Epidermolysis bullosa.
  - Reticulohistiocytosis.
  - Ainhum.
  - Progeria.
  - Neurofibromatosis.

MONOARTHRITIS

- *Traumatic:*
  - Associated fracture.
  - Joint effusion especially lipohemarthrosis includes:
    - Secondary osteoarthritis.
    - Neurotrophic arthritis.
    - Pigmented villonodular synovitis (PVNS).

- *Septic arthritis (Figs. 6.57A to C) (tuberculous, pyogenic):*
    - Periarticular erosions.
    - Joint space narrowing.
    - Periosteal reaction.
    - Bony/fibrous ankylosis.
- *Collagen-like disease:*
    - Rheumatoid arthritis, especially chronic juvenile arthritis.
    - Rheumatic fever.

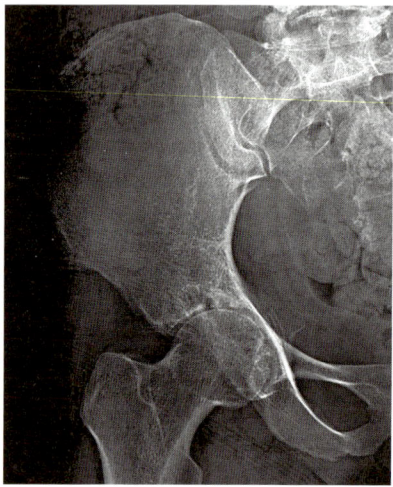

Fig. 6.57A: Anteroposterior radiograph of right hip shows early phase of tubercular arthritis.

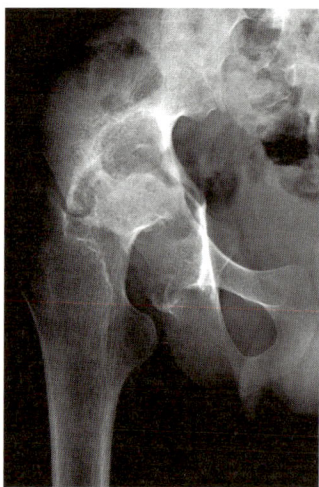

Fig. 6.57B: Anteroposterior radiograph of right hip shows late phase of tubercular arthritis with dislocation.

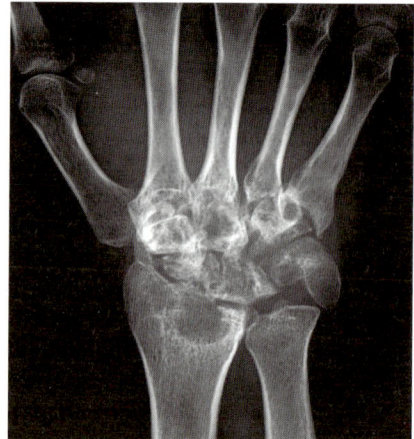

Fig. 6.57C: Anteroposterior radiograph of wrist shows tubercular arthritis.

- *Sarcoidosis:*
    - Psoriatic arthritis.
    - Ankylosing arthritis.
- *Biochemical arthritis:*
    - Gout.
    - Calcium pyrophosphate deposition (CPPD) disease.
    - Chondrocalcinosis.
    - Ochronosis.
    - Hemophilic arthritis.
- *Degenerative:*
    - Osteoarthritis.
- *Sympathetic:*
    - In response to, e.g. tumor.
- *Neuropathic arthropathy.*

ARTHRITIS WITH PERIOSTITIS

Causes

- Juvenile rheumatoid arthritis.
- Psoriatic arthritis.
- Reiter's syndrome.
- Infectious arthritis.
- Hypertrophic osteoarthropathy.
- Hemophilia.
- Uncommonly, rheumatoid arthritis.

ARTHRITIS WITH DEMINERALIZATION

Causes

- Hemophilia.
- Osteomyelitis.

- Rheumatoid arthritis, juvenile chronic arthritis.
- Reiter's syndrome.
- Scleroderma.
- Systemic lupus erythematosus.

ARTHRITIS WITHOUT DEMINERALIZATION

Causes

- Psoriatic arthritis.
- Osteoarthritis.
- Neuropathic arthropathy (Fig. 6.58).
- Gout.
- Sarcoidosis.
- Reiter's disease.
- Pigmented villonodular synovitis.
- Ankylosing spondylitis.
- Calcium pyrophosphate arthropathy.

ARTHRITIS WITH PRESERVED/WIDENED JOINT SPACE

Causes

- *Infective/inflammatory arthritis:*
  – Early stage due to joint effusion.
- *Psoriatic arthropathy:*
  – Due to fibrous tissue deposition.
- Gout.

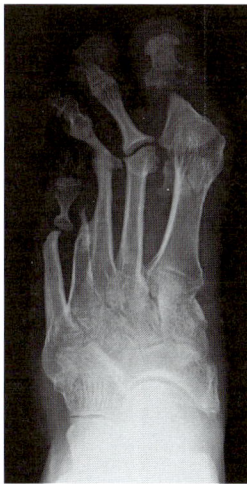

Fig. 6.58: Anteroposterior radiograph of foot shows neuropathic foot.

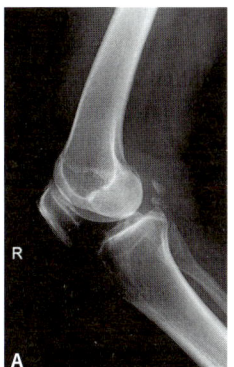 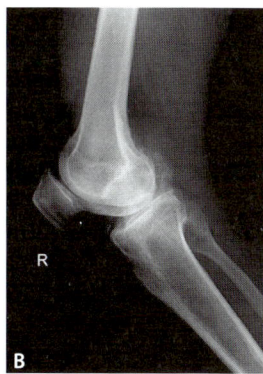

Figs. 6.59A and B: (A) Lateral radiograph of knee joint shows intra-articular loose bodies; and (B) Lateral radiograph of knee joint shows synovial osteochondromatosis in posterior part of joint.

- Pigmented villonodular synovitis.
- *Acromegaly:*
  – Due to cartilage overgrowth.

Arthritis with Soft Tissue Nodules

- Gout.
- Rheumatoid arthritis.
- Pigmented villonodular synovitis.
- Reticulohistiocytosis.
- Sarcoidosis.
- Amyloidosis.

Loose Intra-articular Bodies (Figs. 6.59A and B)

- Osteochondritis dissecans.
- Synovial osteochondromatosis.
- Chip fracture from trauma (osteochondral fracture).
- Severe degenerative joint disease (detached osteophyte).
- Neuropathic arthropathy.

Arthritis Mutilans

Characterized by telescoping joints due to resorption of bone ends secondary to destructive arthritis.

Causes

- Leprosy.
- Diabetes.

- Neuropathic arthropathy.
- Rheumatoid arthritis.
- Juvenile chronic arthritis.
- Psoriatic arthropathy.
- Reiter's syndrome.

ENLARGED FEMORAL INTERCONDYLAR NOTCH

Causes

- Hemophilia.
- Juvenile chronic arthritis.
- Psoriatic arthropathy.
- Rheumatoid arthropathy.
- Tuberculous arthritis.

PLANTAR CALCANEAL SPUR

Causes

- Idiopathic.
- Diffuse idiopathic skeletal hyperostosis.
- Ankylosing spondylitis.
- Psoriatic arthropathy.
- Reiter's syndrome.
- Rheumatoid arthritis.

CHONDROCALCINOSIS

Characterized by calcification of articular or hyaline cartilage.
- *Idiopathic*
- *Crystal deposition disease:*
    - Calcium pyrophosphate deposition.
    - Gout.
- *Metabolic:*
    - Wilson's disease.
    - Hemochromatosis.
    - Familial hypomagnesemia.
    - Ochronosis.
    - Diabetes.
    - Hypophosphatasia.
- *Endocrinal:*
    - Hypothyroidism.
    - Primary hyperparathyroidism.
    - Acromegaly.
- *Arthropathy associated:*
    - Rheumatoid arthritis.
    - Postinfectious arthritis.
    - Posttraumatic arthritis.
    - Degenerative arthritis.
- *Miscellaneous:*
    - Hemophilia.
    - Amyloidosis.

ANKYLOSIS OF INTERPHALANGEAL JOINTS

Causes

- Psoriatic arthritis.
- Ankylosing spondylitis.
- Still's disease.
- Erosive osteoarthritis (Figs. 6.60A and B).

ENTHESIOPATHY

Characterized by osseous attachment of tendon.

Causes

- Degenerative disorder.
- Seronegative arthropathies as ankylosing spondylitis, Reiter's disease, and psoriatic arthritis.
- Diffuse idiopathic skeletal hyperostosis (DISH) (Fig. 6.61).
- Acromegaly.
- Occasionally, rheumatoid arthritis.

SACROILIITIS

Unilateral

- *Infective:*
    - Pyogenic.
    - Tubercular.

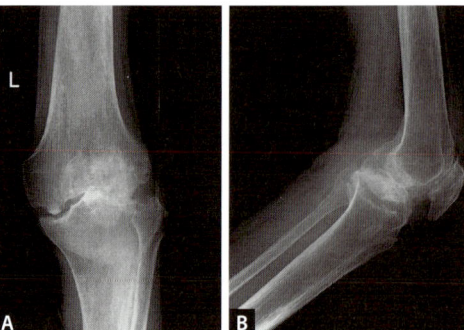

Figs. 6.60A and B: Anteroposterior and lateral radiographs of knee joint show features of erosive osteoarthritis.

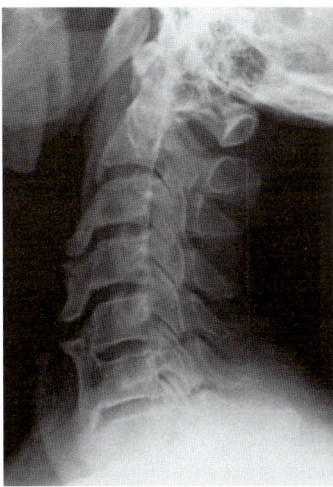

Fig. 6.61: Lateral radiograph of cervical spine showing features of diffuse idiopathic skeletal hyperostosis (DISH).

- *Degenerative:*
  – Osteoarthrosis secondary to abnormal mechanical stress.
  – Narrowing of joint space with subchondral sclerosis.
  – Osteophytosis.

Bilateral

- *Symmetrical:*
  – Ankylosing spondylitis.
  – Ankylosis of joint.
  – Ossification of ligaments.
  – Enteropathic arthropathy as in CD, UC, etc.
  – Osteitis condensans ilii.
  – Seen in young multiparous women.
  – Bone sclerosis with normal joint space.
  – Rheumatoid arthritis (in late stages).
  – Joint space narrowing.
  – Osteoporosis.
  – Deposition arthropathy (gout, CPPD, and ochronosis)
  – Slow loss of cartilage.
  – Subchondral sclerosis + osteophytosis.
  – Hyperparathyroidism.
  – Subchondral bone resorption.
  – Widening of joint space.
  – Paraplegia.

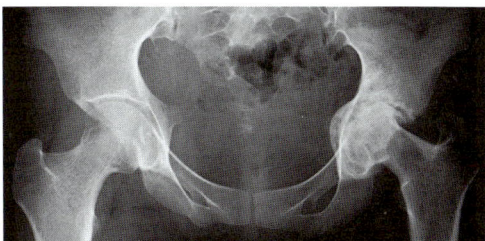

Fig. 6.62: Anteroposterior radiograph of pelvis shows protrusio acetabuli on left side.

  – Joint space narrowing.
  – Osteoporosis.
- *Asymmetrical:*
  – Psoriatic arthropathy.
  – Extensive erosion.
  – Ankylosis less common.
  – Reiter's syndrome.
  – Juvenile chronic arthritis.
  – Gouty arthritis.
  – Large well-defined erosion with adjacent sclerosis.
  – Osteoarthrosis.

PROTRUSIO ACETABULI

Characterized by acetabular floor bulging into pelvis. Criteria are acetabular line projecting medially to ilioischial line by more than 3 mm in males and more than 6 mm in females (Fig. 6.62).

Causes

Unilateral

- Tubercular arthritis.
- Trauma.
- Fibrous dysplasia.
- Marfan's syndrome.

Bilateral

- Rheumatoid arthritis and juvenile chronic arthritis.
- Paget's disease.
- Osteomalacia/osteoporosis.
- Ankylosing spondylitis.
- Idiopathic/familial.
- Marfan's syndrome.

WIDENING OF SYMPHYSIS PUBIS (DIASTASIS)

Normal Measurements
- Less than or equal to 10 mm in newborn.
- Less than or equal to 9 mm at 3 years of age.
- Less than or equal to 8 mm at 7 years of age and over.

Congenital
- *With normal ossification:*
  - Exstrophy of bladder.
  - Epispadias.
  - Hypospadias.
  - Imperforate anus with rectovaginal fistula.
  - Urethral duplication.
  - Prune belly syndrome.
  - Sjögren–Larsson syndrome.
  - Goltz syndrome.
- *With poorly ossified cartilage:*
  - Achondrogenesis/hypochondrogenesis.
  - Campomelic dysplasia.
  - Chondrodysplasia punctata.
  - Wolf's syndrome.
  - Trisomy 9.
  - Cleidocranial dysplasia.
  - Hypophosphatasia.
  - Hypothyroidism.
  - Pyknodysostosis.
  - Spondyloepiphyseal dysplasia.
  - Osteogenesis imperfecta.
  - Larson's syndrome.
  - Spondylometaphyseal dysplasia.

Acquired
- Pregnancy (resolves spontaneously by 3rd month postpartum).
- Trauma.
- Osteitis pubis (symmetrical bony irregularity with resorption and sclerosis).
- Osteolytic metastases.
- Osteomyelitis.
- Ankylosing spondylitis.
- Rheumatoid arthritis.
- Hyperparathyroidism (subperiosteal bone resorption).

FUSION OF SYMPHYSIS PUBIS

Causes
- Postinfective.
- Posttraumatic.
- Osteitis pubis.
- Osteoarthrosis.
- Ankylosing spondylitis.
- Alkaptonuria.
- Fluorosis.

RADIOGRAPHIC FINDINGS IN DEGENERATIVE, INFLAMMATORY, AND NEUROPATHIC ARTHRITIS

The radiographic findings in degenerative, inflammatory, and neuropathic arthritis are given in Table 6.6.

COMPARATIVE FEATURES OF SERONEGATIVE SPONDYLOARTHRITIDES D/D OF DWARFISM

Ankylosing Spondylitis

Sacroiliac Joints

- Sacriliitis is usually the first manifestation and is symmetrical and bilateral
  - The sacroiliac (SI) joints first widen before they narrow.
  - Subchondal erosion, sclerosis and proliferation on the iliac side of the SI joints.
  - At end-stage, the SI joint may be seen as a thin line or not visible.

See: Grading of sacroiliitis.

Spine

- Early spondylitis is characterized by small erosions at the corners of vertebral bodies with reactive sclerosis: Romanus lesions of the spine (shiny corner sign).
- Vertebral body squaring.
- Noninfectious spondylodiscitis: Andersson lesion.
- Diffuse syndesmophytic ankylosis can give a "bamboo spine" appearance.

Table 6.6: Radiographic findings in degenerative, inflammatory, and neuropathic arthritis.

	Degenerative	Inflammatory	Neuropathic
1. Soft tissue swelling/nodules	–	++	+
2. Soft tissue calcification	–	++	–
3. Joint effusion	+	+	++
4. Enthesopathies	–	++	–
5. Alignment deformities	+	++	++
6. Osteoporosis	–	++	–
7. Diffuse joint loss	+	++	+
8. Central/marginal erosions	–	++	–
9. Articular destruction	±	+	++
10. Subchondral cysts	++	±	–
11. Osteophytes	++	–	+
12. Subchondral sclerosis	++	–	±
13. Vacuum phenomena	++	–	±

++ occurs very commonly
± may or may not occur
+ occurs commonly
– does not occur.

- Interspinous ligament ossification can give a "dagger spine" appearance on frontal radiographs.
- Ossification of spinal ligaments, joints and disks (with fatty marrow within the ossified disc, best seen on MRI).
- Apophyseal and costovertebral arthritis and ankylosis.
- Enthesophyte formation from enthesopathy.
- Pseudoarthroses may from at fracture sites.
- Dural ectasia.

Osteochondrodysplasias—Short Limb Dysplasias

- *Rhizomelic (proximal limb shortening):*
  - Achondroplasia.
  - Hypochondroplasia.
  - Pseudoachondroplasia.
  - Chondrodysplasia punctata.
  - Thanatophoric dwarfism.
- *Mesomelic (middle segment limb shortening):*
  - Dyschondrosteosis.
  - Mesomelic dysplasia.
- *Acromesomelic (middle and distal limb shortening):*
  - Chondroectodermal dysplasia.
- *Acromelic (distal limb shortening):*
  - Asphyxiating thoracic dystrophy.

Short Spine Type

- Pseudoachondroplasia.
- Spondyloepiphyseal dysplasia.
- Diastrophic dwarfism.
- Metatropic dwarfism.
- Kniest syndrome.

Dysostosis Multiplex (Short Limb) + Short Trunk

- Hurler's syndrome.
- Morquio's syndrome.

Chromosomal Aberration

- Turner syndrome.

Endocrine Disease

- Hypopituitarism, cretinism.
- Hypergonadism.

Metabolic Disorder
- Hypophosphatasia, rickets.

Primordial Dwarfism
- Congenital growth disturbance, genetically transmitted.
- Appearance and fusion of ossification centers are normal.
- Bones are radiologically normal except that they are unusually small.
- These patients are dwarfs at birth and never attain normal stature.
- They are sexually normal and transmit dwarfism to their children.

Endocrine Disorders

Hypopituitarism
- Due to partial or complete lack of growth hormone.
- Typical hypopituitary dwarfism is known as Lorain–Lévi dwarfism.
- Patients present with short stature usually after 18 months of age, and are usually slender and well proportioned.
- Mentality is unaffected, delayed skeletal age, and sexual immaturity.
- Magnetic resonance imaging shows small sella and hypoplastic pituitary gland.

Cretinism
- Delayed skeletal maturation, i.e. delayed appearance and fusion of ossification centers.
- Dwarfism with delayed dentition, delayed closure of fontanelle, wormian bones, and fragmented epiphysis.
- Kyphosis with bullet-shaped vertebrae, usually L1 and L2.

Hypergonadism
- Ovarian granulosa cell tumor in females, pineal tumors in males, and hyperfunction of adrenal cortex.
- Sexual precocity with early appearance and rapid closure of epiphysis resulting in dwarfism.

Turner Syndrome
- XO chromosome pattern.
- Ovarian dysgenesis.
- Short stature with retarded epiphyseal development.
- Webbed neck, broad chest, pectus excavatum, cubitus valgus, and short fourth metacarpal.

Metabolic Disorders

Hypophosphatasia
- Severe forms result in dwarfism.
- Lack of calcification of metaphyseal ends of long bones.
- Decrease alkaline phosphatase activity.

Rickets
Causes delayed skeletal maturation, bowed legs and other deformities, and may result in short stature.

DYSPLASIAS

Rhizomelic

Achondroplasia
- Long bones are short and broad.
- Small square iliac blades, horizontal acetabuli.
- Lumbar canal stenosis due to decreased interpedicular distance.
- Large calvarium.
- Short stubby fingers.

Hypochondroplasia
- Short and broad femoral neck.
- Small iliac blades.
- Lumbar canal stenosis.
- Skull never affected.

Pseudoachondroplasia
- Long bones are short with broad metaphysis and irregular epiphysis.
- Ilia are large, platyspondyly with central anterior tongue.
- Skull normal.
- Short stubby fingers.

THANATOPHORIC DWARFISM

- Rhizomelic dwarfism with bowing of long bones known as telephone-handle long bones (Fig. 6.63).
- Severe platyspondyly, vertebrae resemble letter H.
- Short ribs, short wide metacarpals and phalanges.
- Skull shows lateral temporal bulging known as clover leaf skull.

Chondrodysplasia Punctata

- Rhizomelic.
- *Nonrhizomelic:*
  - Asymmetric shortening of long bones with metaphyseal irregularity.
  - Stippling of carpus, tarsus, and long bone epiphyses, around joints.

MESOMELIC DWARFISM

Dyschondrosteosis (Léri–Weill Disease)

- Bilateral Madelung's deformity.
- Shortening of radius with triangular distal epiphysis.
- Carpal bones wedged between radius and protruding ulna with lunate at apex.

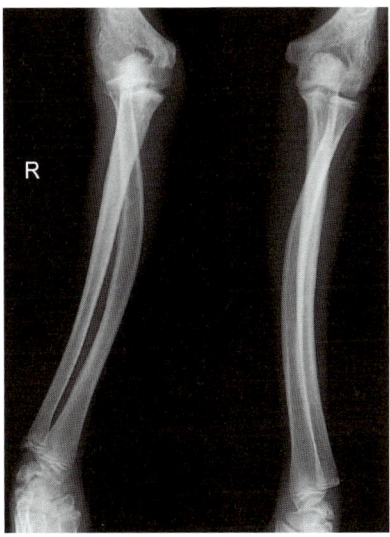

Fig. 6.63: Anteroposterior and lateral radiographs of forearm show bowing of both forearm bones.

ACROMESOMELIC DWARFISM

Chondroectodermal dysplasia (Ellis–van Creveld syndrome)
- Short stature with short limbs.
- Shortening of paired long bones and hypoplasia of fingers and nails.
- Hypoplastic lateral tibial plateau.
- Polydactyly is most characteristic.

ACROMELIC DWARFISM

Asphyxiating Thoracic Dystrophy

- Narrow thorax and short ribs causing respiratory distress.
- Polydactyly, clavicles are highly placed.

Short Spine Dysplasias

Spondyloepiphyseal dysplasia.
- Ovoid or pear-shaped vertebral bodies in infancy with severe platyspondyly in later life.
- Normal metaphysis.
- Retarded development of symphysis pubis and femoral heads, coxa vara.

Diastrophic Dwarfism

- Progressive kyphoscoliosis.
- Hypermobile and abducted thumbs known as hitchhiker's thumb.
- Delta-shaped epiphysis.
- First metacarpal is oval and hypoplastic—most distinctive feature.

Metatropic Dwarfism

- Progressive kyphoscoliosis.
- Dumbbell-shaped long bones.
- Tail-like appendage at distal end of gluteal cleft.

Short Limb + Short Trunk Dwarfs

- *Dysostosis multiplex*
- *Hurler's syndrome:*
  - Macrocephaly, J-shaped sella, and hook-shaped vertebral bodies.
  - Flaring of ilia, tapering of proximal ends of metacarpals.

- *Hunter's syndrome:*
  - Similar to Hurler's syndrome but less severe.
- *Brailsford–Morquio's syndrome:*
  - Severe platyspondyly with central protrusion.
  - Short and wide tubular bones.
  - Narrow pelvis.
- *Maroteaux–Lamy syndrome:* Dwarfism without mental impairment similar to Hurler's syndrome.

SCLEROTIC LESIONS OF BONE

Bone reaction can be:
- Offence.
- Defence.

It can also be classified as:
- Focal.
- Generalized.

Basically it is the role of osteoblasts.
- ↓→ Central reactive tumorogenic.
- Periosteal reactive tumorogenic.

Generic differential diagnosis of sclerotic lesion: "Vindicate"

Vascular	=	For example, hemangioma, infarcts.
Infections	=	For example, chronic osteomyelitis.
Neoplasm	=	For example, osteoma, osteoblastoma, secondaries.
Drugs/poisons	=	For example, vitamins A and D, fluorosis, oxalosis.
Idiopathic	=	For example, Caffey's, idiopathic hypercalcemia of infancy, Paget's.
Congenital	=	For example, bone island, osteopoikilosis, osteopetrosis, pyknodysostosis.
Autoimmune	=	For example, mastocytosis.
Trauma	=	For example, stress fracture.
Endocrine/ Metabolic	=	For example, hyperparathyroidism, Paget's disease, hypoparathyroidism, pseudohypoparathyroidism, and pseudopseudohypoparathyroidism.

Imaging

- Plain X-ray and tomography.
- Computed tomography scan.
- Magnetic resonance imaging.
- DEXA (i.e. densitometry).
- Bone scintigraphy.

Role of Radiologist

The role of radiologist is given in Table 6.7.

Salient Features

Osteopetrosis
- Primary fetal spongiosa—Not replaced properly by adult bone.

  ↓

  (high in calcium and brittle)
  —Grows in layers
  Prone to secondary infection
  Encroaches marrow
  ↓
  Extramedullary hematopoiesis
  Anemia

- Four types:
  1. AR; severe; fatal; diagnosed early.
  2. AD; mild; late diagnosed   A. Skull vault.

Table 6.7: Role of radiologist in preoperative and postoperative situations.

Preoperative	Postoperative
1. Soft tissue extent	1. Record site of operation
2. Description	2. Excision Biopsy specimen
3. Pathological fracture may be seen	3. Examination of adjacent normal bone
4. Aggressiveness	4. Correlation of microradiographic details to HPE
5. Specific diagnosis if possible	5. X-ray diffraction to matrix
6. Site of biopsy study	6. Decide whether bone seaking
7. Follow-up the cases	

3. AR; intermediate
4. Carbonic anhydrase deficiency with RTA and basal ganglia calcification.

B. Skull base + Rugger-Jersey spine.

- *Skull:* Thick, sclerotic bones (especially of base) with poorly pneumatized sinuses and encroached foramina. Dental abnormality.

Spine

Rugger-Jersey spine with listhesis.

Extremities: Bone within bone + Erlenmeyer flask + Cigar lucencies.

Pyknodysostosis:
- Autosomal-recessive, short stature, and multiple fractures with dense bones.

Skull

Brachycephaly, persistent fontanelle and wormian sutural bones, sclerotic skull (especially base) with facial hypoplasia, and obtuse mandible angle.

Spine

"Standing spool" vertebrae; listhesis, unfused neural arches and ribs, etc. clavicle defect—lateral ends.

Extremities: Normal modeling with patent medulla.

Fibrous dysplasia:
- Woman 10–30 years monostotic and is mostly asymmetrical, unilateral >> bilateral.
- Usually the lesion stops growing with age.
- Radiological appearance of a cyst, cotton wool, and ground glass depends upon the degree and distribution of calcium over the fibroid matrix. Basically it is a disease of medulla.
- Spinal involvement is rare while lesion is mainly metadiaphyseal and longitudinal with a thinned but preserved cortex.
- Deformities like "shepherd's crook", mask facies, and proptosis.
- Fractures, endocrinopathies, and fibrosarcomas (1%).

Renal Osteodystrophy and Hyperparathyroidism

- 9–34% patients of renal osteodystrophy (ROD) and rarely patients of primary and tertiary HP show e/o sclerosis, occur because of poor renal function (global).
- Predilection for axial skeleton and metaphysis of long bones.
- Other features are that of osteoporosis, osteomalacia.
- Osteitis cystica fibrosa, soft tissue changes.

Hypopseudohypo and Pseudopseudohypoparathyroidism

- Pelvis, inner skull table, proximal femur, and vertebral body are associated with abnormal dentition and basal ganglion calcification.
- Associated features in PHP are short 4th and 5th metacarpal, coxa vara or valga, cone epiphysis, bowing of bones, and soft tissue calcification.
- Pseudopseudohypoparathyroidism shows no radiological difference but has a normal blood chemistry.

Osteosclerotic Metastasis

- Prostate, pheochromocytoma, pancreas, carcinoid, cervix; colon, breast, stomach, TCC, testis, medulloblastoma, NP, neuroblastoma.
- Tumor new bone—osteosarcoma TCC, mucinous adenocarcinoma.

Carcinoma Prostate

- Cortical lung.

Caffey's Disease

- Idiopathic 9 weeks–5 months, sibling/cousin, presenting with fever—increase erythrocyte sedimentation rate (ESR)—pleural effusion.
- Triad of hyperirritability, soft tissue swelling, and bony cortical thickening.
- Patchy distribution, remission, and relapses.
- *Soft tissue swellings*—painful, deep, proceed bony change and unrelated to it.

- A/E fibula and spine purely diaphyseal:
  - Rickets
  - Scurvy
  - Congenital syphilis.
- Periosteal reaction is associated.

Idiopathic Hypercalcemia of Infancy

- Elfin facies, failure to thrive.
- Generalized bone density increased; sclerotic bands at metaphysis.
- Vitamin A excess.

Hypervitaminosis—A and D

- Basically periosteal reaction (painful), reversible, more than 1 year, bands.
- Soft tissue calcification (in vitamin D), normal mandible.

Fluorosis

- Usually due to excess fluorine in drinking water.
- Due to increased osteoclastic activity to fluorine.
- Adults >>, encroachment on medulla/foramina/spinal canal, etc.
- Membranes/ligament ossification.

Lead

- Again due to lead in water.
- Due to lead deposition + reactive changes.
- Increased density + metaphyseal bands + modeling deformity.

Paget's Disease

- Elderly; men; polyostotic (80%); fibula (rare).
- Three phases—(1) Lytic, (2) Mixed, and (3) Sclerotic; mosaic bone with lost corticomedullary differentiation.
- Bones are large, thick, deformed, and coarsened; joint deformities.
- Picture frame vertebra with collapse; lost lamina dura; hypercementosis.
- Skull has a cotton-wool appearance with the lytic lesions starting in outer while sclerosis in inner table.

Myeloma

- POEMS syndrome—seen in young men; spine, pelvis mostly involved.

Lymphoma

- Seen in low-grade NHL and in Hodgkin's lymphoma (HL).
- Sclerotic lesion may occur as a result of healing.

Myelosclerosis

A part of myeloid metaplasia.
- A group of conditions ranging from myeloid metaplasia, myelofibrosis to polycythemia rubra vera, and CML.
- Marrow—fibrous tissue—bone formation
- Has to be differentiated from osteopetrosis, fluorosis, and mastocytosis.

Mastocytosis

- One-third cases, presenting with urticaria pigmentosa, show bone changes.
- Coarsened trabecular pattern with focal lumpy/confluent areas of sclerosis. It may terminate as leukemia.

Bone Island and Osteopoikilosis

- Island is just a lump of bone (hamartoma). In osteopoikilosis, multiple islands are seen especially in periarticular areas and are well defined, lanceolate, along the trabecular.
- Familial and has to be differentiated from secondaries and tuberous sclerosis which shows ill-defined patchy, cotton-wool, flame-shaped opacities with islands.

Osteoma

Ivory spongy osteoid: Differentiation from neuroblastoma, osteomyelitis, granuloma; bleed; stress fracture.
- Small, well-defined tumor consisting primarily of well-differentiated bone; skull, PNS, mandible, and pressure symptoms.
- *Osteoid osteoma:* Diaphysis of long bone; neural arch; central nidus with surrounding sclerosis; periosteal reaction, if tumor is

near surface. Bone scintigraphy has an important role to play (Fig. 6.64).

Osteoblastoma

- Less than 30 years; flat bones and vertebral appendages; some call it a large irregular and aggressive osteoid osteoma.
- Large, irregular, well defined, expansile tumor with internal punctate calcification, differential diagnosis—GCT, aneurysmal bone cyst (ABC), osteoid osteoma, and osteosarcoma.

Osteosarcoma (Fig. 6.65)

- Most common primary malignant bone tumor; may be osteoblastic, chondroblastic, fibroblastic, or telangiectatic.
- Most common about the knee; 10–25 years; metadiaphyseal; medulla is the site of origin.
- Metastasis especially to lungs causing pneumatocele; Codman's triangle.
- A sclerotic destructive eccentrically growing mass showing good vascularity, differentiates other sarcomas, osteomyelitis; secondaries.

Rare Variants

Multifocal; diaphyseal; central; soft tissue osteosarcoma.
- Due to radiotherapy (3,000 rad for 7–10 years)—lytic aggressive: Radium ingestion known as secondary osteosarcoma.

- Other variants are parosteal and periosteal osteosarcoma.

Osteomyelitis

- Especially pyogenic, syphilitic, fungal, sarcoidosis, Garre's and Brodie's osteomyelitis.

Bone Infarcts (Fig. 6.66)

- Whether septic or aseptic, an infarct leads to an irregular sclerotic serpentine area in the medulla.

LYTIC LESIONS IN BONE

The lytic lesions in bone are described in Table 6.8.

Malignant

Healing benign or malignant.

Without marginal sclerosis:
- Eosinophilic granuloma (EG).
- Brown tumor.
- Multiple myeloma (MM).
- Metastasis.
- Enchondroma.
- Chondroblastoma.
- Metastatic neuroblastoma.

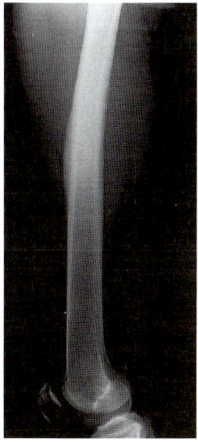

Fig. 6.64: Lateral radiograph of thigh shows osteoid osteoma of femur with small lucent nidus.

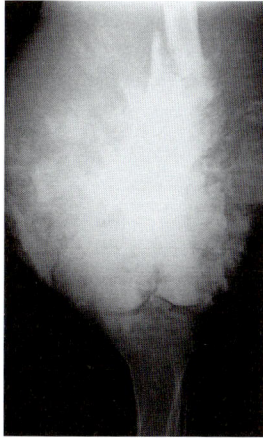

Fig. 6.65: Anteroposterior radiograph of thigh shows osteosarcoma of femur with pathological fracture.

Differential Diagnosis in Radiology

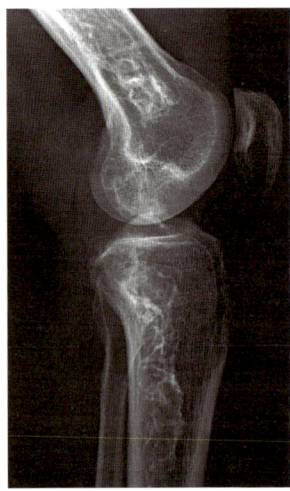

Fig. 6.66: Lateral radiograph of knee shows medullary infarcts in femur and tibia.

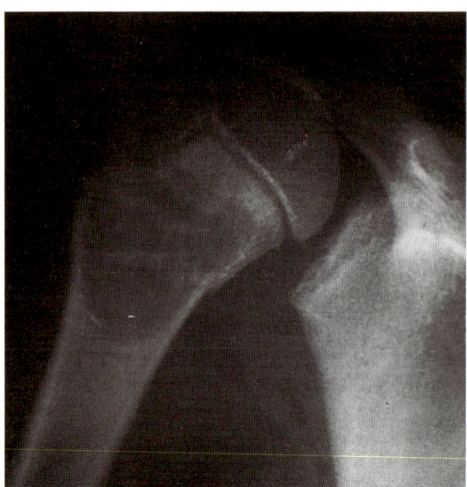

Fig. 6.67: Anteroposterior radiograph of shoulder shows simple bone cyst with pathological fracture.

Table 6.8: Lytic lesions in bone.

Single	Multiple
With marginal sclerosis	
• Geode/subarticular lucent cysts • Brodie's abscess • Fibrous dysplasia • Implantation dermoid • Neoplasm-benign-osteoid osteoma • Simple bone cyst (Fig. 6.67) • Geode (Multiple) • Chondroblastoma • Enchondroma • Adamantinoma	• Metastasis • Multiple myeloma • FD (Polyostotic) • Brown tumor • Eosinophilic granuloma • Metastatic neuroblastoma

Expansile Bone Lesion

- Giant cell tumor.
- Aneurysmal bone cyst.
- Enchondroma.
- Nonossifying fibroma (NOF).
- Chondromyxoid fibroma.

Geode

- Subarticular lucent bone lesion.
- Seen in osteoarthritis, rheumatoid arthritis (RA), and CPPD disease.
- Osteoarthritis and CPPD—multiple cysts in the load-bearing areas of multiple joints with surrounding sclerotic margin.
- Rheumatoid arthritis—no sclerosis.

Brodie's Abscess

- Localized bone infection presenting as subacute on chronic infection.
- Clinical presentation.
- Site—metaphysis—diaphysis.
- *Radiological features*—circumscribed area of bone destruction with a variable degree of surrounding bone reaction.

Tunneling

- Computed tomography and MR ovoid lesion with long-axis parallel to bone.
- *Scintigraphy*—enhances on the delayed isotope scan.
- Unknown etiology, M>F, 10–30 years.

Fibrous Dysplasia

Radiological Features

- Monostotic or polyostotic (multiple bones) (Fig. 6.68).
- *Location*—diametaphyseal, pelvis, femur, and rib, smooth, dense margin of varying width—"rind of an orange".

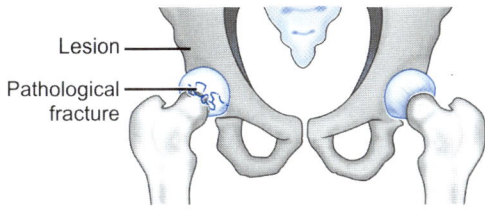

Fig. 6.68: Polyostotic fibrous dysplasia.

- *Cortex*—scalloped and thinned but intact.
- *Magnetic resonance imaging*—fluid-filled cyst.
- Mineralization/fibrous tissue.

Implantation Dermoid

- Cyst lined by epidermis.
- Previous history.
- R/F—well-defined round lytic lesion.
- Minimal sclerosis is seen surrounding the lesion.

Age

2nd and 3rd decades, M:F = 2.5:1.

Clinical Presentation

- Site—diaphysis or metaphysis of tubular bone.
- R/F—nidus—characteristic feature—10 mm or less surrounding, the nidus is a region of reactive sclerosis and periosteal new bone formation.
- Computed tomography—thin section—2 mm.
  - Scintigraphy—an intense focal abnormality and intense activity persistent on delayed image.

Solitary Bone Cyst

- *Unilocular:* Site—proximal humerus and femur—before epiphyseal closure calcaneum—mature skeleton.
- M > F.
- In metaphysis may extend into diaphysis.

Radiological Features

- Area of lucency is metadiaphysis.

- Overlying cortex is thinned out, sclerotic reaction around the margin, and no calcification.
- *Scintigraphy*—no abnormality in blood pool phase as in ABC.
- *Delayed image*—increased activity around the margin.

Chondroblastoma

- Second decade of age, epiphysis or apophysis.
- Frequently extend into metaphysis.
- Well defined, radiolucent, and oval lesion with thin rim of sclerosis and cortical expansion.
  Stippled calcification—25%
  Adjacent periosteal reaction
  Computed tomography and magnetic resonance—extension into soft tissue
  Bone scan—increased activity in blood pool phase.

Enchondroma

50% hands		20% = Femur, humerus, and tibia
		10% small bones feet
20% flat bones		
Age	—	2nd and 3rd decade, flecks of calcification within the tumor—popcorn appearance
Scintigraphy	—	Unremarkable
MRI	—	Hyperintense on T2WI (hyaline cartilage).

Adamantinoma of Long Bones

Midhalf of tibia (femur).
Age — 10–50 (average 35 years)
Sex — M:F = 5:4

Radiological Features

Multilocular appearance and satellite lesion are diagnostic.

Eosinophilic Granuloma

Age — 3–12 years
Site — Skull, pelvis, femur, and spine. Diaphysis in long bones two-thirds solitary.

R/F — Lucent lesion with sharply-defined margins active phase, no sclerosis
Healing phase — Peripheral sclerosis
Vertebra plana — Associated with paravertebral soft tissue mass.

Brown Tumor of Hyperparathyroidism

Site — Metaphysis and diaphysis unusually responsive to PTH solitary or multiple. Other associated feature is resorption of bones
- Chondrocalcinosis
- Pepper pot skull
- Renal lithiasis.

Multiple Myeloma (Plasmacytoma)

Solitary or multiple.
More than 40 years, M:F = 2:1.
- Persistent bone pain or pathological fracture.
- Radiological features—diffuse osteoporosis.
- Rounded or oval defects with sharp margin.
- No marginal sclerosis.
- Long bones, spine, clavicle, scapula, and skull.
- *Laboratory investigation*—increased total serum protein, Bence Jones proteinuria (abnormal urinary protein/hypercalcemia increase).

Metastases (Fig. 6.69)

Elderly age group : Spine, pelvis and ribs, proximal end of humerus and femur
Females : Most common is breast
Males : Prostate, lung, and kidney.
Majority are osteolytic.
- Soft tissue extension is uncommon without much periosteal reaction, lung, breast—lytic.
- Renal cell carcinoma—solitary lesion in pelvis and lumbar spine, if multiple less than six in number.
- *Thyroid*—expansile and lytic and often solitary.

- Laboratory alkaline phosphatase is increased.
- Serum carcinoma is increased.

Giant Cell Tumor (Osteoclastoma) (Fig. 6.70)

- *Age*—20–40 years, M>F.
- *Site*—Subarticular, bones adjacent to knee joint and wrist, and eccentric.
  - No calcification/ossification, no periosteal reaction.

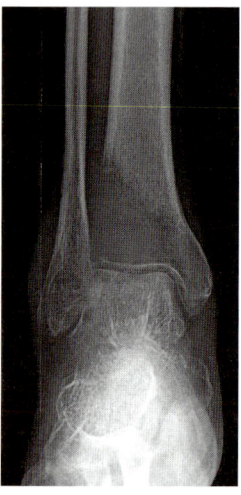

Fig. 6.69: Anteroposterior radiograph of ankle joint region shows osteolytic metastasis.

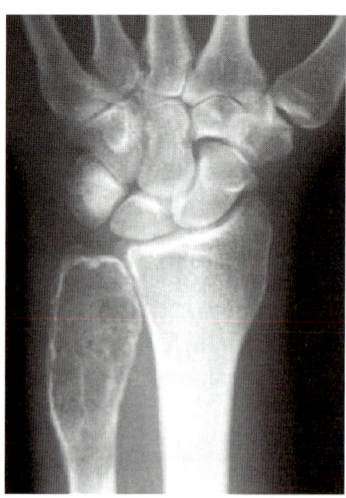

Fig. 6.70: Anteroposterior radiograph of wrist region shows giant cell tumor (GCT) of distal end of ulna.

- 40%—soap-bubble pattern or trabeculations. It may produce well-defined extension into soft tissue.
  - Blood pool phase of bone scan shows increased activity.

Aneurysmal Bone Cyst (Fig. 6.71)

- *Age:* Before epiphyseal fusion and usually central.
- *Site:* Long bones and lumbar spine. Neural arch increase.
- *RIF:* An area of bone resorption with expansion of overlying cortex thinned out and expanded.
- *Computed tomography and magnetic resonance:* Fluid levels in the extravascular space.

Chondromyxoid Fibroma

Peak — 20–30 years
Site — Metaphysis, around the knee joint

Radiological Features

- Eccentric space occupying lesion in metaphysis.
- Margins are well defined with surrounding sclerosis, no calcification.

Bone Scan

Increased activity localized to reactive sclerosis.

Metastatic Neuroblastoma (Fig. 6.72)

- Less than 5 years already known to have abdominal mass.
- R/F:
  - Multiple, often symmetric, lytic bone lesion.
  - Skull lesions are common.
- Cranial sutural margin may be infiltrated with widening of suture lines.
- Long bones and shaft may be penetrated.
- Diagnosis identification of primary tumor and raised blood level and urinary catecholamine.

Nonossifying Fibroma

10–20 years, around the knee joint.

Radiological Features

- Increased radiolucency with well-defined margin in metadiaphysis thin zone of reactive sclerosis.
- Cortex is expanded but remains intact and thinned.

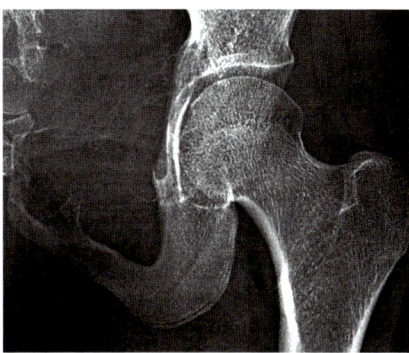

Fig. 6.71: Anteroposterior radiograph of left hip shows aneurysmal bone cyst (ABC) of pubic bone.

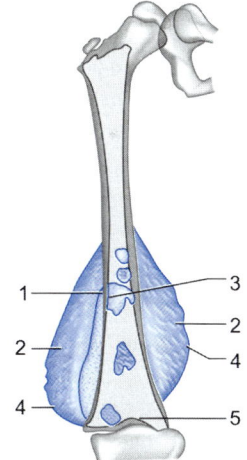

1. Areas of bone destruction
2. "Sunburst" periosteal reaction
3. "Codman triangle"
4. Circumferential soft-tissue mass
5. Pathologic fracture through growth plate

Fig. 6.72: Metastatic neuroblastoma. The permeative destructive lesion throughout the entire femoral shaft in a child with metastatic neuroblastoma. The tumor has penetrated into the soft tissues along the distal half of the shaft, resulting in a large, circumferential soft tissue mass. The presence of a "sunburst" periosteal reaction and Codman's triangles indicates the rapidity with which the tumor has broken through the periosteum. There is a pathologic fracture through the distal femoral growth plate.

DIFFERENTIAL DIAGNOSIS OF GENERALIZED OSTEOPOROSIS

Osteopenia

Generalized or regional rarefaction of the skeleton is decrease in bone density.

Causes of Diffuse Osteopenia

- *Osteoporosis*—diminished quantity of bone matrix but normal mineralization of remaining bones.
- *Osteomalacia*—normal quantity of bone but defective mineralization of osteoid.
- *Hyperparathyroidism*—increased bone resorption by osteoclasts.
- Diffuse infiltrative bone diseases, e.g.:
  - Multiple myeloma-leukemia.
  - Gaucher's disease.

Generalized Osteoporosis

- *Disorders of multiple/uncertain cause:*
  - Senile osteoporosis.
  - Juvenile osteoporosis.
  - Postmenopausal osteoporosis.
- *Endocrine:*
  - Cushing's disease.
  - Hypothyroidism.
  - Hyperthyroidism.
  - Hypogonadism.
  - Hypopituitarism.
  - Acromegaly.
  - Diabetes mellitus.
- *Congenital:*
  - Osteogenesis imperfecta.
  - Homocystinuria.
- *Nutritional disturbances:*
  - Scurvy.
  - Protein deficiency.
  - Calcium deficiency.
- *Drugs:*
  - Heparin
  - Steroids
  - Vitamin A.
- *Chronic diseases:*
  - Chronic renal disease—renal osteodystrophy
  - Hepatic insufficiency
  - Chronic inflammatory polyarthropathies
  - Gastrointestinal malabsorption syndromes
  - Chronic debility or immobilization.

Osteoporosis

- No evidence of hyperparathyroidism or osteomalacia.
- Evidence of conditions such as senility, immobilization, postmenopausal state, or other causes to explain it.

Roentgenological Changes

Most prominent in axial skeleton, proximal humerus, femur, wrist, and ribs.

- *Long bones:*
  - Cortical thinning with irregularity of endosteal surface.
  - The thin cortex maintains normal mineral content and appears dense.
  - Deossification of spongy bone.
  - Prominence of trabeculae in lines of stress.
  - Delayed fracture healing with poor callus.
- *Spine (Fig. 6.73):*
  - Diminished radiographic density.
  - Vertebral end plates are thin and dense with "pencilling in" of vertebrae.

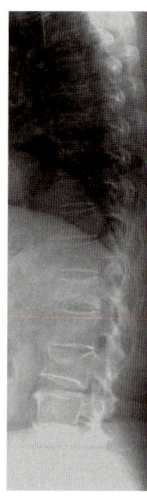

Fig. 6.73: Lateral radiograph of DL spine shows osteoporosis with collapse of vertebrae.

- Irregular endosteal surface of vertebral endplates.
- Vertical striations because of the loss of horizontal trabeculae and accentuation of vertical trabeculae along the lines of stress.
- Compression deformities with biconcave vertebral bodies—codfish vertebrae.
- Absence of osteophyte formation.

Senile Osteoporosis

Etiology:
- Reduced intestinal absorption
- Decreased adrenal function
- *Secondary hyperparathyroidism:*
  - There is proportionate loss of cortical and trabecular bone.
  - Fractures most commonly in femoral neck, proximal humerus, tibia, and pelvis.
  - F:M = 2:1.

Juvenile Osteoporosis

- Idiopathic self-limiting disorder
- Affects both sexes typically before puberty
- Clinically bone pain, backache, and limp
- Blood chemistry is normal
- Fracture of metaphysis of long bones with minimal trauma
- Vertebral collapse, wedging, and kyphosis.

Postmenopausal Osteoporosis

Affects women in 50–65 years age group.

Etiology:
- Reduced estrogen levels
- Nutritional status, level of activity, and genetic causes also influence
- There is disproportionate loss of trabecular bone with rapid bone loss
- Fractures commonly affect vertebrae with wedging fracture of distal radius.

Cushing's Syndrome

- Due to excess of adrenocortical steroids
- Negative calcium balance and hypercalciuria
- Decreased bone formation and increased resorption.

Imaging
- Osteoporosis.
- Exuberant callus formation causing increased density of endplates of compressed vertebral bodies.
- Multiple painless rib fractures.
- Osteonecrosis.

Hypothyroidism

- Cretinism in children, myxedema in adults.
- Retarded skeletal maturation, fragmented epiphysis.
- Bullet-shaped vertebrae.
- Osteoporosis.

Hyperthyroidism

- Increased metabolic activity with increase in bone formation and resorption
- Bone resorption causes generalized osteopenia in skull, pelvis, spine, and long bones
- Vertebral wedging, codfish vertebrae, and kyphosis
- Pretibial myxedema.

Hypogonadism

- Due to decreased production of gonadal hormones or luteinizing hormone (LH) and follicle-stimulating hormone (FSH) by pituitary.
  - *In males*—delayed closure of epiphysis with long limbs and short trunk.
  - *In females*—Turner syndrome—short stature, cubitus valgus, osteoporosis, short 4th metacarpal, webbed neck, and cardiovascular anomalies.

Hypopituitarism

- Deficiency of growth hormone results in cessation of endochondral ossification
- Retarded skeletal maturation and delayed skeletal growth
- Overall reduced bone density due to reduced bone formation.

Acromegaly

- Rarely causes osteoporosis
- Enlarged paranasal sinuses, prognathism, and frontal bossing

- Enlargement and scalloping of vertebral bodies
- Arrow head terminal phalanges and increased heel pad thickness.

Osteogenesis Imperfecta
- Inherited disorder of connective tissue with abnormal maturation of collagen
- *Classical clinical triad:* Fragile long bones, blue sclerae, and deafness
- Diffuse osteopenia with thin fragile long bones, multiple fractures, and bowed bones
- Exuberant callus.

Scurvy
- Long-term deficiency of vitamin C (>6 months)
- Children present with limb pain and irritability.

Imaging
- Epiphysis is small and sharply marginated by a sclerotic rim.
- Increased density of zone of provisional calcification.
- Transverse band of lucency in metaphysis known as Trümmerfeld zone.
- Metaphyseal spurs—Pelkan's spurs.

Protein Deficiency
Protein deficiency produces osteoporosis due to deficiency of matrix production, e.g. in malnutrition nephrosis, diabetes mellitus, Cushing's syndrome, and hyperthyroidism.

Heparin Toxicity
- Heparin has a direct local stimulating effect on bone resorption
- Large doses of heparin more than 15,000 units/day
- Hyperheparin states occur in Marfan's and Hurler's syndrome and mast cell disease.

Renal Osteodystrophy
Bony changes in patients suffering from chronic uremia due to long-standing renal disease.

Imaging Features
- *Secondary hyperparathyroidism*—bone resorption
- Osteoporosis
- Osteosclerosis—Rugger-Jersey spine
- Soft tissue calcifications.

Arthropathies (Rheumatoid Arthritis)
- May cause osteoporosis due to steroids or limitation of movement due to pain or muscle wasting
- Erosive changes, alignment deformities, and soft tissue swelling may be found.

Disuse Osteoporosis
- Results from lack of stress and strain on bone
- Frequently caused by paralysis or body cast
- Osteoblasts remain inactive and older bone is not replaced
- Relieved when the affected part is mobilized.

Osteomalacia
- Due to vitamin D deficiency in adults
- Defective mineralization of osteoid in mature cortical and cancellous bone
- *Pseudofractures or Looser's zones*—bilateral symmetrical focal accumulations of osteoid at right angles to long axis of bones
- Intracortical resorption, osteopenia with coarse trabecular pattern.

Hyperparathyroidism
- Affects mainly middle-aged women
- Increase in parathyroid hormone causes increase in osteoclastic bone resorption
- X-ray—subperiosteal, intracortical, subchondral, trabecular, and subligamentous bone resorption
  - Brown tumors, Pepper-pot skull
  - Osteopenia.

Diffuse Infiltrative Disorders
For example: Multiple myeloma, leukemia, and Gaucher's disease may cause extensive deossification because of proliferation of plasma cells, leukemic cells, or histiocytic cells in bone marrow.

SOLITARY DENSE VERTEBRA

Lymph

- Lymphoma
- Low-grade infection
- Metastasis
- Paget's disease
- Hemangioma.

Metastasis

- *Sclerotic metastasis*:
  - Medulloblastoma
  - Bronchus
  - Breast
  - Bladder
  - Bowel (especially carcinoids)
  - Lymphoma
  - Prostate.
- Lytic metastasis—after T/F.
- No alteration in vertebral body size.
- Disk spaces preserved.
- Multiple.
- Lower thoracic and lumbar spine—most common site.
- Sclerotic lesions are hypointense on both T1WI and T2WI.

Paget's Disease

- Usually a single vertebral body is affected—lumbar spine and sacrum
- Expanded body with thickened cortex and coarsened trabeculations and picture-frame vertebra
- Disk space involvement is uncommon
  - *Fish vertebra*—due to structural weakness (biconcave)
  - Involvement of posterior elements helps to differentiate from hemangioma.

Lymphoma

- HL>NHL—40–60 years
- Normal-sized vertebral body
- Disk spaces intact
- *Magnetic resonance*—focal or diffuse hypointensity than normal marrow on T1WI and iso or hyperintensity than normal marrow on T2WI

- Low-grade infection:
  - Endplate destruction
  - Disk space narrowing
  - Paraspinal soft tissue mass.

Hemangioma (Figs. 6.74A and B)

Prominence of the secondary bony trabeculae of the vertebral body causing a striate or honeycomb pattern.

- Expansion ±
- Lower thoracic and lumbar spine
- Multiple lesions in 25–30% cases
- *Nonenhanced computed tomography*—lucent lesion with typical "polka-dot" densities in medullary spaces

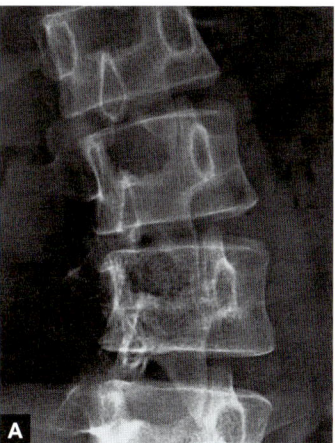

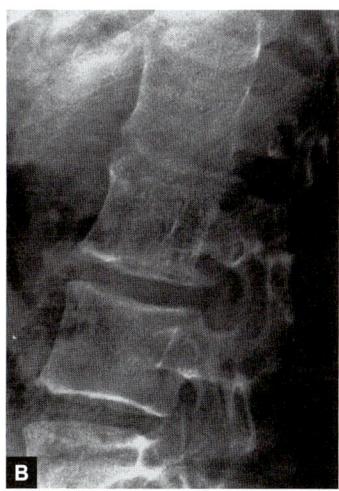

Figs. 6.74A and B: Anteroposterior and lateral radiographs of lumbar spine show hemangioma of vertebra.

- Hyperintense on both T1 and T2WI
- Disk space preserved.

ACRO-OSTEOLYSIS

- Loss of terminal tufts of digits
- Scleroderma/connective tissue disease
- Psoriatic arthritis
- Reiter's disease
- Frostbite (thumbs spared)/burns
- Leprosy
- Polyvinyl chloride exposure
- Hyperparathyroidism
- Cleidocranial dysostosis
- Progeria
- Pyknodysostosis
- Sarcoidosis.

Cleidocranial Dysostosis

Autosomal dominant, 33% sporadic.
- Skull
- Cranial dysplasia
- Wormian bones
- Basilar invagination.

Clavicles

Aplasia/hypoplasia usually lateral portion.

Other Skeletal Abnormalities

- Small, high scapula
- Wide symphysis pubis
- Acro-osteolysis.

Hajdu–Cheney Syndrome

An osteolytic syndrome with skull deformities, characteristic facies, osteoporosis, premature loss of teeth, joint laxity, short stature, dissolution of the terminal phalanges, hearing loss, and a hoarse voice.
- The changes in the terminal phalanges in this condition as well as in pyknodysostosis are pseudoosteolysis, that is the disorder of defective development rather than bone destruction of bone already formed.
- The patients show brachycephaly (projection of the occipital area and a deep groove at the lambdoid sutures, both in the occipital and parietal bones).

Progeria

An abnormal congenital condition associated with defect in the lamin type A gene, which is characterized by premature aging in children, where all the changes of cell structure occur.
- Normal at birth
- *Wizened old man:* Alopecia, atrophy of muscles, and skin
- *Atherosclerosis:* Coronary artery disease
- Dwarfism
- *Abnormal facies:* Receding chin, beaked nose, and exophthalmos.

Findings
- Acro-osteolysis
- Hypoplastic facial bones + sinuses
- Open cranial sutures + fontanelles, Wormian bone
- Coxa valga.

Pyknodysostosis

- Autosomal recessive
- Dense, sclerotic bones.

Features
- Open cranial sutures + fontanelles
- Wormian bones
- Dolichocephaly
- Sclerotic vertebrae
- Fractured long bones
- Short, stubby bones
- Partial agenesis/aplasia of terminal phalanges.

Psoriatic Arthritis

Types
- True psoriatic arthritis (one-third).
- Resembling RA (one-third).
- Combination of psoriatic and RA (one-third).

Findings
- No juxta-articular osteoporosis (unlike RA)
- Periosteal reaction—frequent
- Asymmetrical destruction of distal interphalangeal joints with ankylosis

- Resorption of terminal tufts with "pencil-in-cup" deformity
- Ivory phalanges
- Destruction of first toe interphalangeal joint with periosteal reaction and bony proliferation at distal phalangeal bone (pathognomonic)
- Asymmetrical syndesmophytes (lower cervical to upper lumbar spine)
- Squaring of vertebrae in lumbar spine
- Paravertebral soft tissue calcification
- Bilateral asymmetrical sacroiliitis.

Sarcoidosis

Noncaseating granulomatous disease.
- Unknown etiology
- Young adults, blacks more than whites
- Prognosis usually good
- May affect any organ
- Chest most often involved
- Diffuse pulmonary infiltrate, may resolve or progress to fibrosis
    - High-resolution computed tomography (HRCT) is the investigations of choice
    - Mediastinal adenopathy
    - *Early:* Septal thickening, peribronchovascular nodules, alveolar ground glass opacity
    - *Late:* Traction bronchiectasis, fibrosis, and honeycombing
    - Skeleton involved in 10%
    - *Differential diagnosis:* Bronchial/transbronchial biopsy (60–95% diagnostic), liver, or scalene biopsy.

Scleroderma/Progressive Systemic Sclerosis

- Hypertrophy than atrophy of collagen fibers
- 4–6th decades, M:F = 1:3
- *Bones:*
    - Punctate soft tissue calcification (fingertips, shoulder, and hips)
    - Acro-osteolysis (63%).
- Intercarpal joint space narrowing (late).
- *Chest:*
    - Evident in 10–25%
    - Pulmonary fibrosis with diffuse reticulate infiltrate
    - Predominantly in lower lungs.
- *Gastrointestinal:*
    - Esophageal dilatation and aperistalsis (>50%)
    - Hiatus hernia + GE reflux + Esophagitis.

Distal Esophageal Stricture

- Gastroparesis
- Dilation and dysmotility of small bowel
- Pseudosacculations and dysmotility of colon.

Reiter's Syndrome

- Males
- *Polyarthritis:*
    - Feet
    - Sacroiliac (SI) joint
    - Knee/ankles (joint effusion)
- Urethritis
- Uveitis/conjunctivitis.

Polyvinyl chloride may cause or feature the following:

Miscellaneous syndromes:
- Acro-osteolysis
- Carcinogenesis.

Symptoms and Signs

Raynaud's phenomenon.

Craniomandibular Dysostosis

- Acro-osteolysis
- Arthropathy
- Gastrointestinal bleeding
- Micrognathia
- Short stature.

SACROILIITIS

Only anteroinferior aspects of SI joint are covered with cartilage (1 mm hyaline cartilage on iliac side, 3–5 mm fibrous cartilage on sacral side, with normal joint width of 2–5 mm).
- *Erosions*—widening of joint space
- *Subchondral bone sclerosis*—bony ankylosis
- *Periarticular osteoporosis*—eventual return of normal bone density.

Differential Diagnosis of Sacroiliitis

- *Bilateral symmetrical:*
  - Ankylosing spondylitis
  - Psoriatic arthritis
  - *Intrabowel disease:* Crohn's, Whipple's
  - Rheumatoid arthritis
  - Deposition of arthropathy, gout, and CPPD
  - *Osteitis condensans ilii*—more common in females, young, and normal joint space (Fig. 6.75)
  - Hyperparathyroidism, subchondral bone resorption, and increased joint space
  - *Paraplegia*—decreased joint space and osteoporosis.
- *Bilateral asymmetrical:*
  - Psoriatic arthropathy—40% of cases.

Reiter's syndrome:
- Juvenile rheumatoid arthritis (JRA)
- *Osteoarthritis:* Smooth articular margins and well defined, decreased joint space, subchondral bone sclerosis, and anterior osteophytes (Fig. 6.76)
- *Usually unilateral involvement.*

Infection:
Osteoarthritis—abnormal mechanical stress.

ARTHRITIS INVOLVING SPINAL COLUMN

- Ankylosing spondylitis
- Rheumatoid arthritis

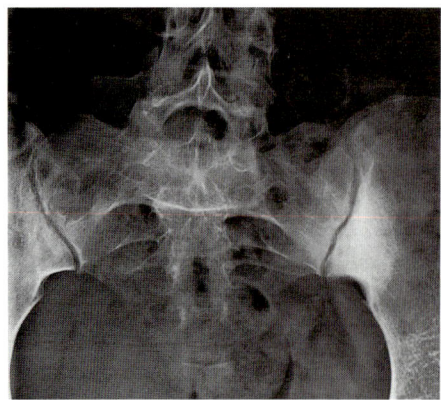

Fig. 6.75: Anteroposterior radiograph of sacroiliac (SI) joints shows idiopathic condensans ilii.

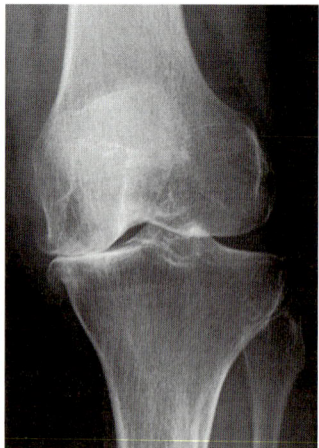

Fig. 6.76: Anteroposterior radiograph of knee joint shows osteoarthritis.

- Psoriatic arthritis
- Reiter's syndrome
- Osteoarthritis
- Diffuse idiopathic skeletal hyperostosis
- Juvenile rheumatoid arthritis.

Ankylosing Spondylitis (Figs. 6.77A and B)

- Seronegative
- 97% of patients for human leukocyte antigen (HLA) B27
- *Age:* Late teens and 20s sex—equal in both sexes, osteopenia
- *Sacroiliac joint*: Symmetrical, erosions (more on iliac side), joint widening heals by sclerosis—joint narrowing (whiskering), fusion.

Spinal Column

After the SI joint, begins at dorsolumbar or L-S region and then progresses to other areas.

Vertebral Body Squaring

- Osteitis and erosions adjacent to vertebral endplate margins— shiny or ivory corner.
- *All mineralization:*
  - Syndesmophytes—hallmark (annulus fibrosus calcification)—maturation leading to "bamboo spine", similar

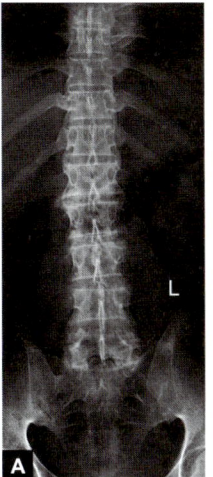 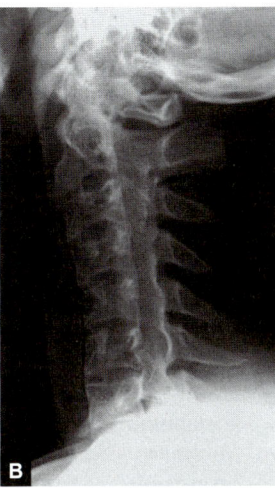

Figs. 6.77A and B: (A) Anteroposterior radiograph of lumbosacral (LS) spine with sacroiliac (SI) joints shows ankylosis of SI joints with bamboo spine in a case of ankylosing spondylitis; and (B) Lateral radiograph of cervical spine shows anterior and posterior longitudinal ligament ossification in a case of ankylosing spondylitis.

- *Spine*—segmental, asymmetrical, can involve any region
- *Paravertebral ossification*—common and characteristically symmetric, squaring of vertebral body. Atlantoaxial subluxation in some cases.

Other Features

- Frequently affection of hands
- Sausage digit
- Erosion at DIP and IP of great toe, cup and pencil appearance (because of osseous fusion of IP joint)
- Arthritis mutilans.

well-defined ossification seen in interspinous ligament and around minor and major joints.

Enthesitis

Shaggy or whiskered pattern at IT and GT.

Spinal Fusion

After the calcification of IV disk.

Psoriatic Arthropathy

- 10% patients develop arthritis before skin lesions appear
- In 25%—develops simultaneously
- 65%—psoriasis precedes arthritis.

Clinical Features

Normal bone, mineralization.

- *Sacroiliac joint*—seen in 50% of patients who have polyarthritis
- Bilateral symmetrical in 60%, asymmetrical in 40%
- *Erosion*—joint widening sclerosis. Fusion is less common than in ankylosing spondylitis
- *Enthesitis*—IT and calcaneum

Reiter's Syndrome

Young female, sexually-transmitted disease (STD), characteristic triad of arthritis, urethritis, and conjunctivitis associated with HLA-B27 skeletal involvement seen eventually in 80%.

- *Sacroiliac joint*—sacroiliitis—late in case of Reiter's disease, seen in 50% bilateral and asymmetrical. Fusion is less frequent than ankylosing spondylitis.
- *Spine*—similar to psoriatic arthritis, except paravertebral ossification which is asymmetrical segmental around the dorsolumbar junction. Another feature—affects the feet rather than hand, MTP and IP joints of great toe. Normal mineralization.
- Irregular erosion and enthesitis.
- Painful erosion and reactive spur very common around the calcaneum.

Rheumatoid Arthritis (Fig. 6.78)

- 20–55 years, female more than M<G, mainly affects the small joints
- *Sacroiliac joint*—sacroiliitis—seen in few patients, erosive process is not as aggressive as in other joints. Bone mineralization decreased
- *Spine*—most common site—upper cervical spine
- *Subluxation*—because of rupture of transverse ligament
- *Erosion of odontoid*—finally leading to fracture of odontoid leading to basilar invagination
- *Apophyseal joint and disk space*—rare eroded-fused
- Malalignment.

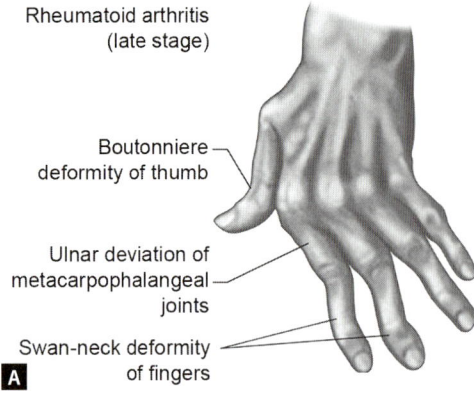

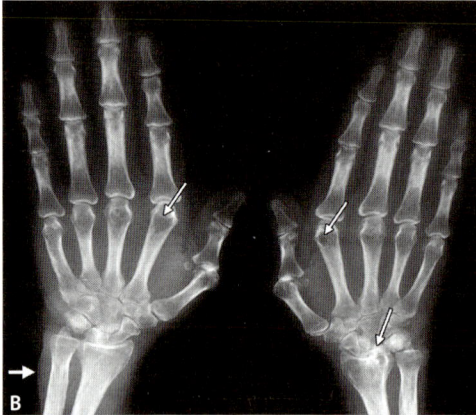

Figs. 6.78A and B: (A) Schematic diagram showing rheumatoid arthritis; (B) X-ray dorso-volar view of both wrists and hands in a known case of rheumatoid arthritis showing significant periarticular osteopenia, carpal crowding, bony deformity, erosions in multiple bones (thin arrows) and soft tissue swelling (thick arrow)

Osteoarthritis (Degenerative Changes)

- Degenerative arthritis of synovium—elderly.
- *Sacroiliac joint*—rarely involved—smooth anterior margins, joint space decreased, subchondral sclerosis, and anterior osteophytes.
- *Spine*—space bilateral and opposing bones become narrowed with marginal new bone formation—osteophyte—positive and horizontal.
- Most common sites are cervical and lumbar spine (lower cervical—C5–C6) and C6–C7.
- *Vertebrae (C3–C7) joints*—narrowing of these joints with osteophytic lipping.

Diffuse Idiopathic Skeletal Hyperostosis (Forestier's Disease)

- Elderly female, M:F = 3:1, HLA-B27 in some patients. Excessive ossification found at many sites.
- *Sacroiliac*—involved, the ligamentous part of joint fusion, less common.
- *Spine*—cervical and lower thoracic (on right side).
- Flowing ossification of spine involving four or more continuous vertebrae and hyperostosis of some ligamentous attachment and around the iliac crest, ischia, and above the acetabulum.
- *Normal vertebral and normal I/V disk space*—no erosion.

Enteropathic Spondyloarthropathies

- *Uncommon, Crohn's, Whipple's disease*—may be associated with joints, disease of secondary type.
- *Peripheral*—ST swelling and local periostitis patients are seronegative and HLA-B27 negative.
- *Sacroiliitis and spondylitis*—identical to ankylosing spondylitis. Do not correlate with gut disease activity. Patients are usually male and increase positivity for HLA-B27 antigen (approximately 60%).

Juvenile Rheumatoid Arthritis

- Less than 16 years, 10% Rh positive, 90% Rh negative, osteopenia
- *Sacroiliac joint*—bilateral asymmetrical, similar to ankylosing spondylitis
- *Spinal*—cervical spine under developed vertebral, increase IV disk space
- Atlantoaxial subluxation in seronegative patients. Other joint—metacarpophalangeal and intercarpal joints—usual site
- *Chronic synovitis and effusion*—increase of carpal bones and epiphysis.

BONE CYST

Cyst is a well-defined lucent lesion presenting in the bone. It can either be solitary or multiple and may be present in the epiphysis, metaphysis, or diaphysis. It can be expansile, nonexpansile, uniloculated, or multiloculated.

It may or may not have a sclerotic margin. The features, however, are not diagnostic and there is considerable overlap.

Nonexpansile Unilocular Cystic Lesions

- Fibrous cortical defect (Fig. 6.79)
- Nonossifying fibroma
- Simple unicameral bone cyst
- Brown tumor of HPT
- Eosinophilic granuloma
- Enchondroma
- Epidermoid inclusion cyst
- Post-traumatic/degenerative cyst
- Pseudotumor of hemophilia
- Interosseous ganglion
- Histiocytoma
- Arthritic lesion
- Endosteal PVNS
- Fibrous dysplasia
- Infectious lesions (Brodie's abscess)
- Metastasis.

Nonexpansile Multilocular Cystic Lesions

- Aneurysmal bone cyst
- Giant cell tumor
- Fibrous dysplasia.

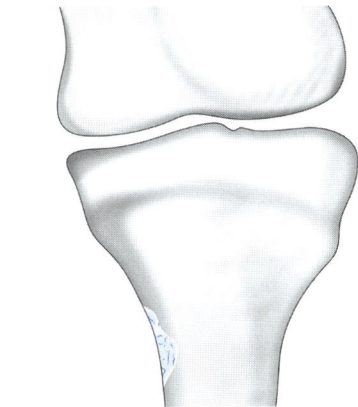

Fig. 6.79: Fibrous cortical defect. The most common benign bone tumor, it appears as a small oval lucency in the cortex of the posteromedial aspect of the proximal tibial shaft.

Expansile Unilocular Cystic Lesions

- Simple bone cyst
- Enchondroma
- Aneurysmal bone cyst
- Juxtacortical chondroma
- Nonossifying fibroma
- Eosinophilic granuloma
- Brown tumor of HPT
- Chondromyxoid fibroma
- Hydatid cyst
- Lipoma.

Lesions Surrounded by Marked Sclerosis

- Osteoid osteoma
- Brodie's abscess
- Chondroblastoma
- Plasmacytoma.

Multiple Cystic Lesions

- Fibrous dysplasia
- Enchondroma
- Eosinophilic granuloma
- Metastasis
- Multiple myeloma
- Brown tumors
- Cystic angiomatosis of bone
- Gaucher's disease.

Fibrous Cortical Defect

- Peak age 7–8 years, mostly before epiphyseal closure
- Present at metaphyseal cortex of long bones, most commonly posterior medial aspect of distal femur
- Round to oval, average diameter of 1–2 cm
- Extends parallel to long axis of the bone
- Cortical thinning and expansion may occur
- Smooth well-defined scalloped margins
- Involutes over 2–4 years.

Nonossifying Fibroma

- Much larger than fibrous cortical defect and present at an older age group of 10–20 years
- Majority are found near knee joint, distal end of femur being the most common site

- Sharply-defined radiolucent lesion at metadiaphysis and have a lobulated appearance with a thin zone of reactive sclerosis
- May cause cortical expansion but the cortex remains intact
- Lesions have a tendency to regress and multiple lesions may be associated with neurofibromatosis.

Simple Bone Cyst

- Also known as unicameral bone cyst
- Always unilocular and well defined
- Site of origin depends on the age of presentation, prior to epiphyseal fusion. They usually occur in the proximal humeri and femora. After epiphyseal fusion, some lesions may occur in bones, like calcaneum. By far, the most common site is proximal humerus
- During the stage of skeletal maturation, the lesion is carried from its usual metaphyseal location to diaphysis. The usual location is thus metadiaphyseal
- The overlying cortex is often thinned and slightly expanded with no periosteal reaction unless a fracture has occurred
- The lesions may be surrounded by a discrete sclerotic margin.

Brown Tumor of HPT

- Alike osteoclastoma and pathologically, it is due to replacement of bone by vascularized fibrous tissue and collection of osteoclasts
- Most common locations are jaw, pelvis, rib, and metaphysis of long bones
- Often eccentric and cortical in location and is most frequently solitary but may be multiple
- They are expansile, well marginated, and cyst-like with endosteal scalloping
- Other signs of hyperparathyroidism are present.

Eosinophilic Granuloma

- Most benign variety of histiocytosis X and, in 60–80% cases, it is localized to bone with age incidence of 2–30 years. Most common in 5–10 years of age. Solitary lesions are most common but they can be multiple
- Lesions arise within the medullary canal and skull is the site in 50% of cases and that too the diploic space of parietal bone being most frequent. The mono-ostotic involvement is most frequent
- These are round or ovoid punched-out lesions with beveled edges and with a sharply-marginated sclerotic rim is present
- Appearances may also be of hole within hole or that of button sequestrum
- There may be an overlying soft tissue mass.

Enchondroma (Fig. 6.80)

- Benign cartilaginous growth in the medullary cavity. Bones with enchondral calcification are affected, the skull is thus not affected
- Age of presentation is 10–30 years
- An oval or round lucency is present near epiphysis with fine marginal line with scalloped well-defined margins and ground-glass appearance
- Calcifications may be present in the lesion and there could be bulbous expansion of the bone with cortical thinning with no cortical breach or periosteal reaction
- Multiple enchondromas may be seen in Ollier's disease. In Maffucci's syndrome, multiple enchondroma are associated with soft tissue cavernous hemangiomas.

Epidermoid Inclusion Cyst

- Alike implantation cyst and is most commonly seen in the age group of 20–40 years

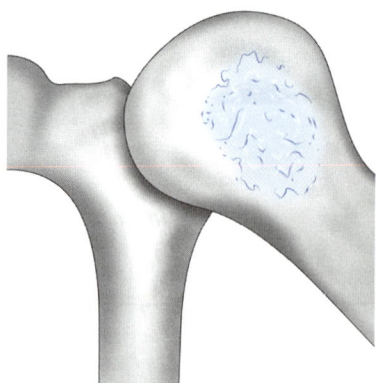

Fig. 6.80: Enchondroma.

- Seen in superficially located bones as in the calvarium, phalanx, and foot
- These are well-defined lesions with a sclerotic margin and cortex is frequently expanded and thinned
- No calcifications, soft tissue mass, or periosteal reaction are noted.

Geodes

These are cystic lesions, usually subarticular in location and are secondary to arthritis and osteonecrosis. The etiology is similar to post-traumatic cysts and is due to bone necrosis leading to intrusion of synovial fluid and a connection with the joint may be demonstrated.

Intraosseous Ganglion

- These are benign subchondral lesions without degenerative arthritis
- Usually presents in middle age with mild localized pain
- Most common at the epiphysis of long bones
- Well-demarcated solitary lesions with a sclerotic margin and with no communication to the joint.

Histiocytoma

- Benign fibrous histiocytoma of bone may mimic cystic lesions
- Usually presents in 23–60 years age group with localized pain and soft tissue swelling
- Long bone epiphyses are typically involved
- Presents as a well-defined lesion with or without a soap-bubble appearance and may have a sclerotic rim with no evident periosteal reaction. It may cause cortical expansion.

Fibrous Dysplasia (Fig. 6.81)

- Most common in the first 2 decades of life and the lesions are present in the medullary cavity
- Mono-ostotic variety is more common than polyostotic variety
- Patient may present with limb length discrepancy, shepherd's crook deformity of femur, facial asymmetry, tibial bowing, and rib deformity
- McCune–Albright syndrome is the association of polyostotic fibrous dysplasia with café-au-lait spots and endocrine dysfunctions like precocious puberty and is usually seen in girls
- Common locations are ribs, craniofacial bones, femoral neck, tibia, and pelvis
- Lesions have smooth dense margins which may be as thick as to resemble a rind of an orange
- The bone may be expanded and the cortex scalloped but intact
- They may be multilocular and are usually diametaphyseal
- In the skull, the sclerosis may cause encroachment of neural foramina
- There may be intralesional calcification so much, so that some lesions may have increased density.

Brodie's Abscess

- This is a type of subacute pyogenic osteomyelitis usually occurring at the metaphysis of long bones
- There is a central area of lucency surrounded by a dense rim of sclerosis
- Lucent channel-like tortuous configurations toward the growth plate are virtually pathognomonic
- There may be periosteal reaction and adjacent soft tissue swelling.

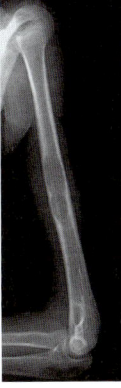

Fig. 6.81: Lateral radiograph of arm shows fibrous dysplasia of humerus.

Aneurysmal Bone Cyst (Fig. 6.82)

- Expansile lesion of bone containing thin-walled blood-filled cystic cavities, involving the vertebral neural arches and long bones more commonly
- Age range is 10–30 years and female patients are affected more often
- Purely lytic, expansile, and eccentric radiolucency with soap-bubble pattern of trabeculations is seen. There may be very slight sclerosis
- There may be rapid progression and the tumor may present with a pathological fracture
- The cortex may be thinned but is intact
- Three quarters of these cysts present before epiphyseal fusion are complete.

Osteoclastoma

- Usually occurs before epiphyseal fusion and most patients are less than 20 years of age
- May be associated with Paget's disease and usually present with pain swelling and tenderness at the affected site
- It is an expansile solitary large lucent bone lesion causing exquisite cortical thinning near the epiphysis, usually metaphyseal in location. The long bones are most frequently involved, usually around the knee joint

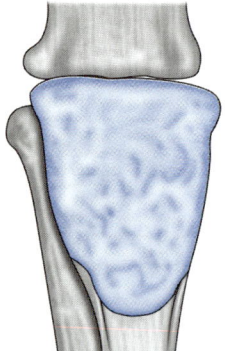

Fig. 6.82: Aneurysmal bone cyst. A large, medullary, and expansile (blow out) lucency is seen in the proximal tibial diaphysis, abutting the growth plate (physis). The marked attenuation of the cortices, the well-organized triangular periosteal reaction along the distal margin of the lesion, and the fact that the lesion is wider than the growth plate, are characteristic of an aneurysmal bone cyst.

- There is a soap-bubble appearance to the tumor with no evident sclerosis or periosteal reaction unless a fracture has occurred
- There may be a soft tissue extension that characteristically has no calcification
- When it involves vertebra, it may lead to collapse and may involve the adjacent disks and may cross the joints.

Chondromyxoid Fibroma

- Peak age incidence 20–30 years and usually presents at the metaphysis of long bones
- Expansile ovoid lesion with radiolucent center
- Well-defined sclerotic margin is present with no evident periosteal reaction.

Chondroblastoma

- Peak age incidence, 2nd decade, and is usually epiphyseal in location involving the long bones more often
- It is an oval-to-round eccentrically located lucent lesion with a well-defined sclerotic margin and may contain punctate calcification
- The cortex is intact; however, a thick periosteal reaction may be seen.

Plasmacytoma

- Solitary bubbly grossly expansile lesion
- Seen in 5th–7th decades of life, most commonly in thoracic or lumbar spine.

Multiple Myeloma

- Peak age is 5th–8th decades of life. There is an abnormal B-J protein in urine
- Generalized osteoporosis with multiple widespread punched-out lesions may be seen
- There may be an associated soft tissue mass in the regions where bone destruction has occurred
- May be associated with POEMS syndrome.

Metastasis

- Thyroid and kidney malignancies are the most common cause of metastasis that resemble bone cysts. However, lungs and breast carcinoma may also cause such appearance
- Usually a history of primary can be elicited.

Chapter 7

Urogenital System

Normal sectional anatomy of the kidney is illustrated diagrammatically in Figure 7.1.

ADULT AND NEONATAL KIDNEYS: DIFFERENCES

The differences between adult and neonatal kidneys are given in Table 7.1.

SMOOTH AND SMALL KIDNEYS

The features of smooth and small kidneys are described in Table 7.2.

SMALL, SMOOTH, AND UNILATERAL KIDNEYS

With a small-volume collecting system.

Ischemia due to Renal Artery Stenosis

Ureteric notching is due to enlarged collateral vessels and differentiates this from the other causes in this group.

Primary Uroradiologic Elements

Size: Normal to decreased (left 1.5 cm less than right and right 2 cm shorter than left; may have less than normal increase in renal surface area in response to contrast material or diuretics).

Contour: Smooth (global).

Table 7.1: Differences between adult and neonatal kidney.

	Adult	Neonatal
Contour	Smooth	Lobed
Medullary	Reflectivity, –ve	–ve
Cortex	Reflectivity, +ve	++
Collecting system	Echogenic inapparent	Echo-poor apparent

–ve: Negative; +ve: Positive

Table 7.2: Features of smooth and small kidneys.

Unilateral	Bilateral
• Ischemia due to focal arterial disease	Generalized arteriosclerosis
• Chronic infarction	Benign and malignant nephrosclerosis
• Radiation neoplasia	Atheroembolic renal disease
• Congenital hypoplasia	Chronic glomerulonephritis
• Postobstructive atrophy	Papillary necrosis
• Postinflammatory atrophy	Hereditary nephropathies
• Reflux atrophy	Hereditary chronic nephritis (Alport's syndrome) Medullary cystic disease Arterial hypotension Amyloidosis (late)

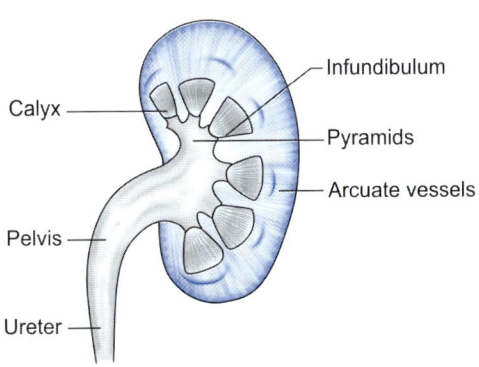

Fig. 7.1: Normal sectional anatomy of kidney.

Secondary Uroradiologic Elements
- *Pelvic-infundibulocalyceal system:* Attenuated (global)
- Notched proximal ureter (by ureteral arteries from lumbar branches of aorta), delayed opacification time.
- Increased density of contrast material [decreased glomerular filtration rate (GFR) allows increased salt and water absorption]
- Delayed washout of contrast material
- *Parenchymal thickness:* Wasted (global)
- *Calcification:* Linear (aneurysmal or atherosclerotic in renal hilus)
- *Arteries:* Stenotic, aneurysmal, and collateralized
- Angiography in atheromatous renal artery stenosis (RAS). There is an eccentric narrowing of the proximal third of the renal artery while in fibromuscular hyperplasia, there are segmental areas of stricturing and aneurysmal dilatation affecting the distal two-thirds of the renal arteries
- Color Doppler shows the increase in peak systolic velocities to greater than 1.5 m/s, spectral broadening, and increase in maximum diastolic flow velocities.

Chronic Renal Infarction

Primary Uroradiologic Elements
- *Size:* Normal to small
- *Contour:* Smooth (global).

Secondary Uroradiologic Elements
- Parenchymal thickness wasted (global, occasionally regional)
- *Nephrogram:* Diminished to absent contrast material density
- *Echogenicity:* Increased.

Radiation Nephritis

At least 23 Gy (2,300 rad) over 5 weeks. The collecting system may be normal or small. Depending on the size of the radiation field, both, one or just part of one kidney may be affected. There may be other sequelae of radiotherapy, e.g. scoliosis following radiotherapy in childhood.

Primary Uroradiologic Elements
- *Size:* Normal to small
- *Contour:* Smooth (global)
- *Lesion distribution:* Consistent with radiation field material.

Secondary Uroradiologic Elements
- *Parenchymal thickness:* Wasted (global, related to radiation field)
- *Nephrogram:* Diminished density of contrast.

End Result of Renal Infarction

Due to previous severe trauma involving the renal artery or renal vein thrombosis.
The collecting system does not usually opacify during excretion urography.

With Five or Less Calyces

Congenital Hypoplasia
- The pelvicalyceal system (PCS) is otherwise normal.

Primary uroradiologic elements:
- *Size:* Decreased
- *Contour:* Smooth (global).

Secondary uroradiologic elements:
- *Papillae:* Decreased number
- *Calyces:* Decreased number
- Small renal artery and a normal ureter.

With a Dilated Collecting System

Postobstructive atrophy: There is thinning of the renal cortex and if there is impaired renal function, this will be revealed by poor contrast medium density in the collecting system.

Primary uroradiologic elements:
- *Size:* Small (normal or enlarged in minority of cases)
- *Contour:* Smooth (global).

Secondary uroradiologic elements:
- *Papillae:* Effaced (global), may be normal in uncommon form

- *Pelvi-infundibulocalyceal system:* Calyces dilated (global, may be normal in uncommon form)
- *Parenchymal thickness:* Wasted (global).

Postinflammatory Atrophy

Primary uroradiologic elements:
- *Size:* Small
- *Contour:* Smooth (global).

Secondary uroradiologic elements:
- *Papillae:* Disrupted
- *Parenchymal thickness:* Wasted (global).

SMALL, SMOOTH, AND BILATERAL KIDNEYS

- Generalized arteriosclerosis

Primary uroradiologic elements:
- *Size:* Normal to small
- *Contour:* Smooth (global). May have random shallow scars.

Secondary uroradiologic elements:
- *Parenchymal thickness:* Wasted (global)
- *Attenuation value:* Sinus fat increased
- *Echogenicity:* May be increased in sinus and renal parenchyma.
- *Medullary cystic disease:*
  - Autosomal dominant disorder
  - Thin renal cortex
  - Variable number of small medullary cysts up to 2 cm on computed tomography (CT), ultrasound (US), or magnetic resonance imaging (MRI).
- *Amyloidosis, renal disease:*
  - No specific radiological findings
  - Bilateral enlargement in the presence of renal failure or nephrotic syndrome
  - The nephrogram is normal or diminished
  - Renal thrombosis
  - Angiography is abnormal, but findings are nonspecific
  - Gallium scans are extremely sensitive in the identification of renal amyloid.
- *Papillary necrosis:*
  - Thinning of the cortex
  - Partial sloughed papilla gives rise to density between papilla and pyramid.

A fissure forms which communicates with central irregular cavity. In total sloughing, the sloughed papillary tissue may (a) fragment and pass in urine; (b) cause ureteric obstruction; (c) remain free in calyx; and (d) remain in pelvis and form a ball calculus

– With complete detachment, loss of normal cupping of the calyx with filling defect in the collecting system.

A Analgesics, other causes are: Adipose
D Diabetes
I Infant at shock
P Pyelonephritis
O Obstruction
S Sickle cell disease
E Ethanol.

SMALL AND SMOOTH KIDNEYS

Smooth
- Uniform/undulating outline
- No focal indentation (especially against a calyx)
- Uniform cortical parenchymal thickness (1.5–2 cm)
- Uniform corticomedullary differentiation (CMD) (1:1/1:8)
- No focal variation in PT
- Vascularity adequate/mildly decreased
- Perirenal fascial planes uniform.

Small
- Anatomically
- *Radiography:* 9–11 cm right
- *Ultrasonography:* 11–13 cm right
- Computed tomography/magnetic resonance imaging
- *Age variation:* Young and old
- Normal impressions on body surface area and normal variation (Table 7.3).

Congenital
- *Quantitative decrease in renal tissue:* Quality N
- *Pelvis calyceal system:* Normal
- *Ureter:* Normal

Table 7.3: Normal impressions on body surface area and normal variation.

	Unilateral		Bilateral
1.	Congenital	1.	Generalized arteriosclerosis
2.	Postobstructive	2.	Chronic glomerulonephritis (CGN)
3.	Renal artery stenosis	3.	Chronic papillary necrosis
4.	Radiation nephritis	4.	Arterial hypotension
5.	Renal infarction	5.	U/L causes presenting B/L.

(B/L: Bilateral; U/L: Unilateral)

- *Opposite kidney:* Enlarged
- *Renal artery*: Small/normal
- Calyces less than five.

Postobstructive

- Early on the PCS ± dilated but later it is normal
- Parenchyma is thinned
- Obstruction Acute → Increased pressure in PCS

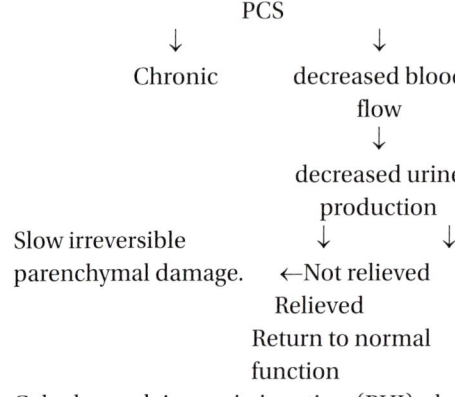

- Calculus, pelviureteric junction (PUJ) obstruction, retroperitoneal fibrosis, ureterocele, clot, FB, bladder mass, fungus ball, and stricture
- On imaging, PCSU dilated/N: Size N/decreased
- *Cortex:* N/decreased; nephrogram present/faint; poor
- *Pyelogram:* All depends upon level, severity duration.

Radiation Nephritis

- 2,300 Rad (23 Gy) for more than or equal to 5 weeks
- Due to small vessel disease
- *Pelvicalyceal system:* N/small
- Global cortical thinning
- Delayed but dense pyelogram with delayed washout.

End Result of Infarction

- Global decrease in size occurs when there is injury/avulsion to the main renal artery/segmental arteries
- Nonvisualization of kidney/PCS
- Kidney decreased in size and altered appearance on CT, MR, and US.

Renal Artery Stenosis

- Use of intravenous pyelogram (IVP) is nearly obsolete.
- *Doppler examination:*
  - AT more than 0.7 seconds
  - AT less than 2 cm/sec^2
  - PSV more than 180 cm/sec
  - AO:RA less than 1/25–3.
- *Captopril scintigraphy:* Proposed use for screening.
- *Magnetic resonance angiography/computed tomography angiography:* Useful corroborative.
- *Contrast invasive angiography:* Conventional
  ↓
  DSA → I/A
  → I/V.

Generalized Arteriosclerosis and Arterial Hypotension

- Systemic conditions are presenting with multisystem involvement
- Renal outline and PCS are normally seen
- Delayed appearing and increasingly dense pyelogram is seen
- Condition caused by AS is known as benign nephrosclerosis.

Chronic Glomerulonephritis

- Hallmark is immediate faint and persistent nephrogram

- On USG, CMD is lost with increased echogenicity
- Diagnosis by HPE.

Chronic Papillary Necrosis
- Usually bilateral with multiple papillae affected
- Different types of appearances depending upon stage and degree of papillary necrosis are seen
- Main causes are analgesics and diabetes.

SMALL AND SMOOTH KIDNEYS

Unilateral.

Dilated Pelvicalyceal System (Fig. 7.2)
- Postobstructive
- Normal/decreased function of other kidney
- Thinned cortex.

Hypovolemic Pelvicalyceal System
- RAS — Increased BP
- Radiation — H/O
- Infarction — H/O

Hypoplastic Pelvicalyceal System
- Congenital
- Patient asymptomatic.

Bilateral

Systemic
- Hypotension
- Arteriosclerosis.

These are systemic conditions with multisystem involvement.

Renal
- CGN — Normal calyx
- CPN — Abnormal calyx
- Unilateral causes.

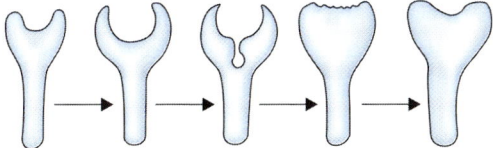

Fig. 7.2: Calyces showing grades of hydronephrosis.

SMALL AND IRREGULAR KIDNEYS
- Reflux nephropathy (chronic atrophic pyelonephritis)
- Lobar infarction
- Tuberculous
- Renal dysplasia.

Chronic Pyelonephritis/Reflux Nephropathy

A focal scar over a dilated calyx. Usually multifocal and may be bilateral. Scarring is most prominent at the upper and lower poles. Minimal scarring, especially at a pole, produces decreased cortical thickness with a normal papilla (Fig. 7.3).

Primary Uroradiologic Elements
- *Contour:* Normal (early, intermediate)
- Focal scar (late, may be multifocal)
- *Lesion distribution:* Unilateral (may be bilateral).

Secondary Uroradiologic Elements
- *Papillae:* Normal (early, intermediate)
- Retracted (late; focal)
- *Calyces:* Normal (early, intermediate)
- Widened (late; focal)
- *Parenchymal thickness:* Normal (early)
- Wasted (intermediate, late, and focal)
- Focal compensatory hypertrophy
- *Nephrogram:* Deficient enhancement (lobar, sublobar; full thickness; may be striated)
- *Echogenicity:* Increased (focal)
- Increased central sinus complex.

Lobar Infarction

A broad contour depression over a normal calyx. Normal interpapillary line.

Primary Uroradiologic Elements

Early (within 4 weeks)	Late (after 4 weeks)
Size—normal	Size—normal to small
Contour—normal	Contour—focal scar (may be multifocal)
Lesion distribution—unilateral (may be bilateral)	Lesion distribution—unilateral (may be bilateral)

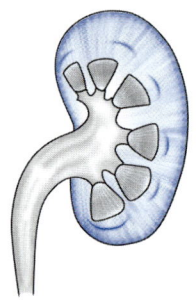
Normal cortex parallel to interpapillary line

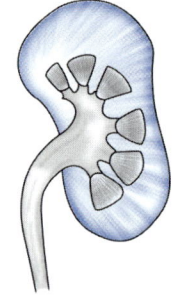
Lobar infarction
Broad depression over a normal calyx

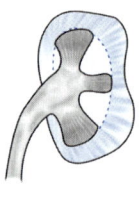
Reflux nephropathy focal scars over dilated calyces. Most prominent at upper and lower poles. May be bilateral

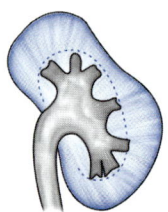
Spleen impression
Right kidney may show hepatic impression

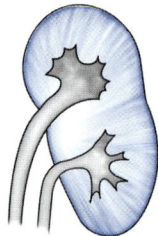
Duplex kidney
Renal size usually larger than normal

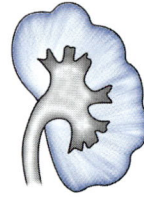
Fetal lobulation
Normal size
Cortical depressions between papillae

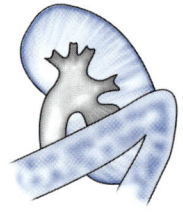
Overlying bowel
Spurious loss of cortex

Fig. 7.3: Unilateral scarred kidney.

Secondary Uroradiologic Elements

Early (within 4 weeks)
- Pelvic-infundiobulo-calyceal system—attenuated (focal, occasional)
- Nephrogram—absent (focal, occasional, global, rarely)

Late (after 4 weeks)
- Parenchymal thickness—wasted (focal) with normal interpapillary line
- Echogenicity—increased (focal)

Tuberculosis

- Calcification differentiates it from the other members
- Usually hematogenous from pulmonary disease, but sometimes secondary to tuberculous infection of the gastrointestinal tract or bone
- *Initial lesion in renal tuberculosis:* Small tubercles in the glandular and cortical arterioles progress to necrotizing lesions
- Tubercles enlarge and coalesce into necrotic irregular cavities

- Ultimately, there is ulceration into the adjacent calyx, with formation of fistulae and strictures
- The kidney becomes fibrotic and scarred
- Renal involvement is probably always bilateral; in 25% of cases, it is unilateral
- Imaging findings are typically asymmetrical
- Renal calcification in up to 50% of cases, dense punctate calcification associated with healed tuberculomas or renal calculi
- The classical urographic finding is multifocal caliectasis, due to irregular infundibular strictures. Parenchymal scars in advanced cases
- Ultimately, the kidney may become small, densely calcified, and nonfunctioning; the so-called autonephrectomy.

Renal Dysplasia

- Developmental parenchymal abnormalities resulting from abnormal development of the renal vasculature, renal tubules, collecting ducts, or drainage apparatus
- Biopsy may be necessary for diagnosis
- Multicystic dysplastic kidney is due to ureteric obstruction early in fetal life
- Usually unilateral, bilateral diseases are lethal
- Antenatal diagnosis is possible in the 3rd trimester
- Ultrasonography (USG) finding is of a multi-cystic mass without renal tissue
- One-third have contralateral urological abnormalities as PUJ obstruction or vesicoureteral reflux (VUR)
- Functional imaging with isotopes or IVU demonstrates lack of function
- Arteriography outlines a small thread-like renal artery.

LARGE AND SMOOTH KIDNEYS

Unilateral

- Renal vein thrombosis.
- Acute arterial infarction.
- Obstructive uropathy.
- Acute pyelonephritis.
- Xanthogranulomatous pyelonephritis.
- *Miscellaneous:* Compensatory hypertrophy.
    – Duplicated PCS.

Renal Vein Thrombosis

Common causes in children: Dehydration and shock, nephrotic syndrome, and cyanotic heart disease.

Adults:
- Renal cell carcinoma (RCC)
- Compression by tumor/lymph node or extension of thrombus from IVC, trauma.
- *Secondary to renal diseases:* Chronic glomerulonephritis, amyloidosis.
- *Sudden total occlusion:* Hemorrhagic infarct, permanent loss of function, and eventual shrinkage of kidney.
- *Partial obstruction:* Collaterals develop and the renal function is undisturbed.

Primary uroradiological elements:
- *Size:* Normal to large
- *Contour:* Smooth
- Unilateral.

Secondary uroradiologic elements:
- *Collecting system:* Attenuated, mucosal irregularity, nodularity, and notching. Abnormalities disappear on retrograde pyelography.
- *Parenchymal thickness:* Expanded.
- *Nephrogram:* Density varies from absent to normal, prolonged CMD.
- *Echogenicity:* Variable (initial 2 weeks—hypoechoic-after-hyperechoic).
- *Renal vein:* Dilated, intraluminal thrombus with diminished or absent flow.
- *Retroperitoneum:* Dilated collaterals—hemorrhage.

Acute Arterial Infarction

- Subtotal renal infarction is much common than infarction of the entire organ.
- *Most usual cause:* Embolus through thrombosis, superimposed on underlying arterial disease, may also lead to infarction.
    Primary uroradiological findings: Large, smooth, and unilateral.

Secondary uroradiological findings:
- *Collecting system:* Attenuated

- *Nephrogram:* Absent/diminished density, cortical rim enhancement; focal nephrographic defect occurs in early subtotal infarction
- *Echogenicity:* Normal/reduced
- Renal angiography defines the site of arterial block
- *Computed tomography:* Well-defined focal area of lower attenuation than that of adjacent, normally enhancing, parenchyma.

Obstructive Uropathy

Dilatation of PCS
  Obstructive
Nonobstructive
- Congenital (e.g. PUJ, PUV)
- VUR
- Acquired (stones, strictures, and tumors)
- Postobstructive dilatation
- Primary megaureter

IVU—features of acute obstruction:
- Increasingly dense nephrogram
- Modest kidney enlargement
- Delayed calyceal opacification
- Mild to moderate pelvicaliectasis
- Spontaneous pyelosinus extravasation.

Features of chronic obstruction:

Renal size:
- *Partial obstruction:* Increased complete obstruction—small nephrogram density: normal/decreased.
- *Parenchymal thickness:* Reduced (crescent, rim nephrogram).
- *Dilated pelvicalyceal system:* Ball pyelogram.
- *Ureters:* Dilated/tortuous
- *Ultrasound:* Excellent screening method.

Limitations:
- Miss one-third cases of acute obstruction
- Cannot differentiate extrarenal pelvis from PUJ obstruction
- Unenhanced helical CT of kidney, ureter, and bladder (KUB) is the most sensitive technique for diagnosing acute obstructive uropathy.

Acute Pyelonephritis

- Clinically acute pyelonephritis refers to symptom complex of pyrexia, bacteriuria, and flank pain.
- *IVU:* Diffuse renal enlargement.
  - Delayed/poor PCS filling of reduced density.
- *Severe acute pyelonephritis:* Nephrogram may be dense, persistent, or striated.
- *Ultrasound:* Focal/generalized renal swelling, iso-/hypoechoic.
- *Computed tomography:* Patchy enhancement with bands and wedge-shaped areas of reduced enhancement extending from papillae to the edge of the kidney.
- *Delayed scans (3–6 hours):* Increased enhancement in the prior areas.
- *Complication:* Abscess.

Xanthogranulomatous Pyelonephritis

- Chronic parenchymal inflammation caused by foamy histiocytes giving a yellowish appearance to the cut surface of the kidney.
- Usually associated with proteus infection in patients with calculus disease.

Radiological features:
- On IVU, the PCS fails to fill in the presence of good thickness of renal substance
- *Ultrasound:* Dilated PCS with low level echoes, renal parenchyma is of low echogenicity, and calculus is usually present
- *Computed tomography:* Multiple rounded low attenuation areas of soft tissue density surrounded by thick parenchyma
- Renal pelvis is contracted and contains calculus, associated perinephric, and psoas collection may be present.

Compensatory Hypertrophy

- Congenital absence of kidney
- Postnephrectomy
- Diseased, poorly functioning kidney
- Maximum size of contralateral kidney is usually reached in approximately 6 months.

Radiological features:
- Size of kidney increased
- Parenchymal thickness increased

- Pelvicalyceal system and ureter appear prominent (as urine flow rate becomes the normal from the functioning kidney).

BILATERAL LARGE SMOOTH KIDNEYS

- Proliferative/necrotizing disorders.
- *Abnormal protein deposition:*
  - Amyloidosis
  - Multiple myeloma.
- *Abnormal fluid accumulation*:
  - Acute tubular necrosis
  - Acute cortical necrosis.
- *Neoplastic cell infiltration:*
  - Leukemia.
- *Inflammatory cell infiltration:*
  - Acute interstitial nephritis.
- *Miscellaneous:*
  - Autosomal recessive (AR) polycystic kidney disease (PCKD)
  - Acute urate nephropathy
  - Nephromegaly associated with diabetes mellitus, hyperalimentation, and cirrhosis
  - Renal vein thrombosis
  - Bilateral hydronephrosis.

Proliferative/Necrotizing Disorders

- Only kidneys involved
  - Acute (poststreptococcal)
- Glomerulonephritis
  - (RPGN) Rapidly progressive
- Glomerulonephritis (GN)
  - Idiopathic membranous GN
  - Membranoproliferative GN
  - IgA nephropathy
- Renal involvement is part of multisystem disorder
  - Wegener's granulomatosis
  - Goodpasture's syndrome
  - Diabetic glomerulosclerosis
  - PAN
  - Allergic angiitis
  - Glomerulosclerosis associated with heroin abuse
  - Lobular GN
  - Hemolytic uremic syndrome
- Morphologic diagnosis of a specific disease within this group is dependent on integrating light, electron and immunofluorescent microscopic patterns of glomerular involvement with other clinical or laboratory abnormalities.

Radiological Features

- *Primary uroradiologic:* Large, smooth, and bilateral
- *Secondary uroradiological elements:* Collecting system is attenuated.
  - Parenchymal thickness is expanded. Echogenicity is increased.
  - HUS—selective hyperechogenicity of cortex relative to medulla.

Amyloidosis

- Caused by accumulation of extracellular eosinophilic protein substance in various organs.
- *Primary:* Renal involvement occurs is 35% cases.
- *Secondary:* Secondary to chronic suppurative/inflammatory disease.
- Renal involvement occurs in 80% cases.
  - Tuberculosis
  - Bronchiectasis
  - Osteomyelitis
  - Rheumatoid arthritis
  - Ulcerative colitis

Radiological Features

- *Primary urological elements:* Large, smooth, and bilateral
- *Secondary uroradiological elements:* Collecting system is attenuated.
  - Parenchymal thickness expanded, becomes wasted with time.
  - *Nephrogram:* Diminished density.
  - *Echogenicity:* Normal to increased.
  - Renal vein thrombosis (occasionally).

Multiple Myeloma

Multiple myeloma causes renal insult in 50% cases because of deposition of abnormal proteins in the tubule lumina.

Renal function is also compromised by:
- Increased blood viscosity.
- Nephrocalcinosis (because of hypercalcemia)
- Bence Jones toxicity on tubules.

Amyloidosis

Radiological Features
- *Primary:* Bilateral large smooth kidneys.
- *Secondary:* Collecting system is attenuated.
  – Parenchymal thickness is expanded.
  – *Nephrogram:* Diminished density.
  – *Echogenicity:* Increased.

Administration of contrast material in patients with multiple myeloma requires an awareness of potential hazards.

Dehydration should be avoided if the risk of complications is to be minimized.

Other Radiological Features
Osteopenia with well-defined lucencies of uniform size in spine, pelvis, skull, ribs, and shafts of long bones.
- Vertebral body collapse ± paravertebral shadow ±, intervertebral disk involvement
- Expansile ribs lesions
- Permeative mottled pattern of bone destruction present.

EXTRASKELETAL FEATURES

Hypercalcemia, hepatosplenomegaly, soft tissue tumors in sinuses, submucosa of pharynx, trachea, cervical lymph nodes, and GIT.

Acute Tubular Necrosis

State of reversible renal failure with or without oliguria that follows exposure of the kidney to certain toxic agents or to a period of prolonged, severe ischemia.

Toxic Agents

Bichloride of mercury, ethylene glycol, carbon tetrachloride, bismuth, arsenic, and urographic contrast in particular when administered to a patient of two preexisting renal diseases who has been dehydrated.

Ischemic Causes

Shock, crush injuries, burns, transfusion reaction, severe dehydration, and surgical procedures like renal transplantation or aortic resection.

Radiological Features

Contrast material enhanced imaging studies should not be performed knowingly in patients with ATN.

Collecting System

Attenuated, opacification is diminished/absent.
- *Nephrogram:*
  – 75% patients—immediate and persistently dense.
  – 25%—increasingly dense and persistent.
- *Echogenicity:*
  – Medulla—normal to diminished.
  – Cortex—normal to increased.

Acute Cortical Necrosis

Uncommon form of acute renal failure (ARF) in which there is death of the renal cortex and sparing of the medulla.
- A thin rim of subcapsular tissue on the external surface of the cortex and a thin rim of the juxtamedullary cortex are often preserved. This fine rim of viable cortex separate the necrotic cortex from the renal capsule externally and from the medulla internally
- Calcification occurs at this interface which is known as—*Tramline calcification*
- Calcification is detected microscopically at 6 days and radiologically at approximately 24 days (kidneys are still enlarged).

Radiological Features

- Bilateral enlarged smooth kidney
- *Collecting system:* Absent/faint opacification is effaced
- *Parenchymal thickness:* Expanded

- *Nephrogram:* Absent cortical nephrogram with selective enhancement of medulla
- *Calcification:* Cortical diffuse or tramline
- *Echogenicity:* Center hypoechoic (early phase)
  - Hyperechoic with acoustic shadow after calculus deposition.

Causes

- *Obstructive:* Premature separation of placenta, concealed hemorrhage, septic abortion, and placenta previa.
- *Adults:* Sepsis, dehydration, shock, burns, and snakebite.
- *Children:* Dehydration, infection, and transfusion reaction.

LEUKEMIA

Most common malignant cause of bilateral global renal enlargement (lymphoma occasionally produces such pattern but more commonly causes multifocal renal enlargement). Rarely, leukemia causes a unifocal renal mass due to chloroma, myeloblastoma, or a myeloblastic sarcoma. Enlarged kidneys can occur in leukemic patients without leukemic infiltration because of:
- Acute urate nephropathy
- Amphotericin-induced acute interstitial nephritis
- Renal candidiasis associated with intensive chemotherapy
- Lymphocytic rather than granulocytic tumors of leukemia are more frequently associated with renal enlargement
- Children with acute leukemia are more likely to develop nephromegaly as compared to adults
- Peripheral white blood cell (WBC) count can be normal or depleted at the time of renal involvement.

Radiological Features

- *Primary:* Bilateral smooth enlarged kidneys.
- *Secondary:* Collecting system—attenuated.
  - *Parenchymal thickness:* Expanded
  - *Nephrogram:* Diminished density
  - *Echogenicity:* Variable.
- Focal hemorrhage, subcapsular collections, obstructive clots in renal pelvis, and other R/F in children
- *Metaphyseal lucencies:* Distal femur, proximal tibia, and distal radius
- Permeative destruction of bone
- *Osteolytic lesions:* Diaphysis of long bone
- *Periosteal reaction:* Proliferation of leukemic deposits deep to periosteum leading to subperiosteal hemorrhage. MR will show the marrow involvement clearly.

ACUTE INTERSTITIAL NEPHRITIS

Characterized histologically by infiltration of the interstitium by lymphocytes, plasma cells, eosinophils, and a few polymorphonuclear leukocytes.

Usually results as a complication of exposure to certain drugs:
- *Antibiotics:* Methicillin, ampicillin, penicillin, amphotericin, and sulfonamides.
- *Nonsteroidal anti-inflammatory disorders:* Naproxen, ibuprofen.
- *Anticonvulsants:* Phenytoin.
- *Antihistaminics:* Cimetidine.

Cases usually evolve within a range of 5 days to 5 weeks after exposure.

Clinical Features

Fever, rash, eosinophilia, hematuria, proteinuria, and azotemia.

Radiological Features

- *Primary:* Bilateral smooth enlarged kidneys
- *Secondary:*
  - *Collecting system:* Attenuated
  - *Parenchymal thickness:* Expanded
  - *Nephrogram:* Diminished density
  - *Echogenicity:* Increased.

AUTOSOMAL RECESSIVE (INFANTILE) POLYCYSTIC KIDNEY DISEASE

Autosomal recessive PCKD is characterized by dilatation of renal collecting tubules, cystic dilatation of biliary radicles, and periportal fibrosis.

- *Autosomal recessive polycystic kidney disease neonatal:* Predominant renal and minimal hepatic involvement.
- *Juvenile:* Predominant hepatic and minimal renal involvement.

Radiological Features

- *Primary:* Bilateral smooth enlarged kidney
- *Secondary:* Neonatal form
  - Collecting system is attenuated.
  - Parenchymal thickness is expanded.
- *Nephrogram:* Diminished density: Striated.
- *Attenuation value:* Less than soft tissue (unenhanced CT).
- *Echogenicity:* Diffusely increased, loss of CMD.
- *Features of pulmonary hypoplasia:* Small malformed thorax, pneumothorax, and pneumomediastinum.

Juvenile Form

Nephrogram	:	Striated.
Calcification	:	Nephrocalcinosis (papillae).
Echogenicity	:	Increased.
Miscellaneous	:	Hepatosplenomegaly, varices, dilated bile ducts, and increased hepatic echogenicity.

Acute Urate Nephropathy

- Because of deposition of biurate crystals in the collecting tubules and interstitium leading to ARF
- Seen most commonly during therapy for cancer, particularly leukemia, malignant lymphoma.
- Myeloproliferative disorders and polycythemia vera.

Radiological Features

- Bilateral smooth enlarged kidneys
- Collecting system is normal
- *Nephrogram:* Progressively dense
- No opacification of PCS
- Alkaline diuresis
- Large fluid intake
- Use of allopurinol.

NEPHROMEGALY ASSOCIATED WITH CIRRHOSIS, HYPERALIMENTATION, AND DIABETES MELLITUS

- Nephromegaly associated with cirrhosis
- *Explanation:* Hyperplasia and hypertrophy of renal cells
- *Hyperalimentation:* Because of hyperalimentation, there is increase in fluid compartment of kidney related to hyperosmolality of the solution
- Renal enlargement reverses following cessation of therapy
- *Diabetes mellitus:* In the absence of diabetic glomerulosclerosis
- Renal enlargement is due to growth hormone effect, nephron hypertrophy and glycosuric osmotic diuresis.

NONVISUALIZATION OF A KIDNEY DURING EXCRETION UROGRAPHY

- *Absent kidney:* Congenital absence or postnephrectomy.
- Ectopic kidney.
- Chronic obstructive uropathy.
- *Infection:*
  - Pyonephrosis
  - Xanthogranulomatous pyelonephritis
  - Tuberculosis.
- *Tumor:* An avascular tumor completely replacing the kidney or preventing normal functions of residual renal tissue by occluding the renal vein or pelvis, e.g. RCC, Wilms' tumor.
- *Renal artery occlusion:* Including trauma.
- Renal vein occlusion.
- Multicystic kidney.

Salient Feature

- *Absent kidney:* Failure of the ureteric bud to reach the metanephron results in renal agenesis.

Associated Anomalies

- Failure of ipsilateral ureter and hemitrigone to develop
- Adrenal agenesis

- Absence of vas deferens, unicornuate uterus, and absence or cyst of seminal vesicle
- *VATER syndrome:* Vertebral and VSD
  - Anorectal atresia
  - Tracheal and esophageal lesions
  - Radial bone anomalies.
- *Contralateral renal anomalies:* Renal ectopia
  - Malrotation
  - *Plain film:* Absence of renal outline
  - Medial displacement of the splenic and hepatic flexure into renal bed
  - Compensatory hypertrophy of contralateral kidney
  - *Computed tomography or radionuclide imaging:* Definitive showing absence of unilateral absence of renal tissue.

  Other causes of atrophic kidney:
- Vesicoureteric reflux
- Infarct
- Bilateral renal agenesis associated with Potter's syndrome characterized by oligohydramnios, characteristic facies, and early death due to pulmonary hypoplasia.

Pyonephrosis

- Infection of an obstructed kidney may lead to pus developing within the renal pelvis or calyx
- Occurs in conjunction with the presence of calculi or undiagnosed PUJ obstruction
- *Imaging features:* Obstructed system with particularly early or severe loss of renal outline
- Cross-sectional imaging shows evidence of pus and inflammatory debris within the dilated PCS (e.g. echogenic areas are USG or increased density on CT with possible layering)
- *Xanthogranulomatous pyelonephritis*
- Chronic inflammatory process in which lipid laden histiocytes invade and replace normal renal parenchyma Seen in females, diabetics, and infecting organism is usually *Escherichia coli* and *Proteus mirabilis*
- *IVU:* Nonfunctioning kidney with calculi. 80% calculi is characteristically laminated or branched and fragmented
- Initially the kidney is enlarged and this may have a focal pattern simulating tumor but ultimately there is marked renal atrophy
- *Ultrasonography and computed tomography:* Loss of normal CMD and heterogeneity, which includes debris containing cystic areas and calculi.

Tuberculosis

- *IVU:* Stricture affecting the calyceal neck, with the formation of hydrocalyces.
- Strictures at the PUJ and at multiple levels in the ureter.
- Later the pelvis is affected and the entire kidney may become hydronephrotic and nonfunctioning (tuberculosis auto nephrectomy).
- Ultrasonography and CT demonstrates hydrocalyces and/or hydronephrosis which may contain a considerable amount of debris, areas of calcification, and parenchymal loss.
- In later stages, there is inflamed and contracted bladder.

Renal Artery Stenosis

Reduction of the internal diameter by at least 60%.
- Atheroma
- Fibromuscular dysplasia
- Polyarteritis nodosa
- Takayasu's arteritis
- Compression of the renal artery by retroperitoneal mass.
- *IVU:* The affected kidney may be initially small and smooth.

The reduced perfusion on the affected side produces a late nephrogram which is hyperdense.

Notching of the ureter due to compensatory hypertrophy of the ureteric artery.

- *Ultrasonography:* Excludes an obvious structural abnormality or coexistent condition that may relate to hypertension (renal scarring, hydronephrosis, calculus disease, or tumors).
- *Doppler:* Increase in the peak systolic velocity and renal: aortic velocity ratio of more than 3.5 or an absolute velocity of more than 180–200 cm/s.

Spectral Analysis of Intrarenal Arteries

- Renal artery stenosis of less than 75% is not detected by this technique
- More severe stenosis is characterized by reduction in the ascending slope of the systolic peak which can be measured as reduced acceleration (below 3 m/s/s), lengthened time to systolic peak (above 0.075), and increased resistive index (above 5%) and pulsatility index (above 0.012) of the affected kidney compared with the other side
- Computed tomography angiography
- Magnetic resonance angiography.

Renal Vein Thrombosis

- If thrombus is abrupt and complete, the imaging features are similar to an arterial infarct
- *Doppler ultrasonography:* It demonstrates loss of venous rather than arterial signal.
- *Subacute/partial thrombosis:* Smooth renal enlargement. The IVU will show a delayed but subsequently hyperdense nephrogram and pyelogram with either normal calyces or some evidence of compression due to parenchymal swelling.

  Notching of the ureter by dilated venous collaterals is occasionally seen.
- *Ultrasonography:* Loss of normal CMD. Diffuse reduction in echogenicity. Thrombosis of the renal vein.
- *Computed tomography:* Hypodense kidney.

Multicystic Kidney

- Ureter fails to develop and is atretic while the kidney is nonfunctioning
- *Ultrasonography or computed tomography:* The kidney is composed of noncommunicating cyst of varying size
- It is associated with an increased risk of contralateral PUJ obstruction.

Renal Tumors

Wilms' Tumor

- Present in first 3 years
- Bilateral in 5%
- *Associated abnormalities:* Cryptorchidism, hypospadias hemihypertrophy, sporadic aniridia, and Beckwith–Wiedemann syndrome
- *Secondaries in:* Liver and lung.
  - Tumor thrombus in IVC or right atrium
- *Plain film:* Bulging flank.
  - Loss of renal outline
  - Enlargement of renal outline
  - Displacement of bowel gas
  - Loss of psoas outline.

Calcification

- *Ultrasonography:* Large well-defined mass, increased echogenicity than liver. Solid with hemorrhage/necrosis. Lack of IVC narrowing on inspection suggests occlusion.
- *Computed tomography:* Large, well-defined, low attenuating, and heterogeneous with foci of even lower attenuation due to necrosis. Minimal enhancement compared with the residual rim of functioning renal tissue.
- *Magnetic resonance imaging:* Inhomogeneous, low signal (T1W), high signal (T2W). Inhomogeneous enhancement compared with residual renal tissue.

Renal Cell Carcinoma

- 90% of adult malignant tumors
- Bilateral in 10% and increased incidence of bilaterality in polycystic kidneys and von Hippel–Lindau disease. A mass lesion (showing irregular or amorphous calcification in 10% of cases). Calyces are obliterated, distorted, and/or displaced. Half shadow filling defect in a calyx or pelvis. Arteriography shows a pathological circulation.

DILATED CALYX AND DILATED URETER

With a Narrow Infundibulum
- Stricture.
- Extrinsic impression by an artery.
- *Hydrocalycosis:* Congenital.

With a Wide Infundibulum
- Megacalyces.
- Postobstructive atrophy.
- Polycalycosis.
- Pelviureteric junction obstruction.

DILATED URETER AND CALYCES (FIG. 7.4)

Vesicoureteric Reflux

Obstruction within lumen
1. Calculus
2. Blood clot
3. Sloughed papilla

No obstruction or reflux
1. Postpartum
2. Following relief of obstruction
3. Urinary tract infection
4. Primary nonobstructive ureter

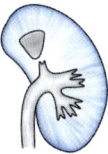
Dilatation of a single calyx
Most commonly due to extrinsic compression by an intrarenal artery (Fraley syndrome)

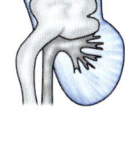
Duplex kidney with hydronephrotic upper moiety drooping flower appearance

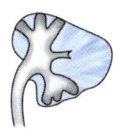
Pseudotumor in reflux nephropathy
Hypertrophy of unscarred renal parenchyma

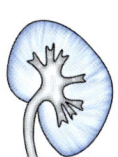
Hilar lip
Hyperplasia of parenchyma adjacent to the renal hilum

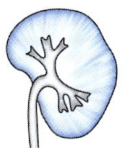
Prominent septum of bertin
Increased activity on Tc-DMSA scanning

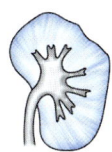
Renal cyst ultrasound
Confirms typical echo-free cyst

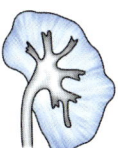
Multiple renal cysts' e.g. adult type polycystic disease spider leg deformity of calyces

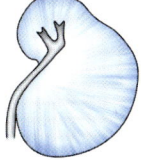
Tumor replacement of much of the normal renal tissues

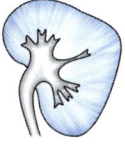
Dromedary hump left-sided variant

Fig. 7.4: Various anamolies of renal outlined calyces system of kidney.

In the Wall
- Edema or stricture due to calculus
- Tumor
- Tubercular stricture
- Schistosomiasis
- Postsurgical trauma
- Ureterocele
- Megaureter.

Outside the Wall
- Retroperitoneal fibrosis
- Carcinoma of cervix, bladder, or prostate
- Retrocaval ureter.

DILATED CALYX

Stricture
- *Tumor:* Usually a transitional cell carcinoma presenting as a mural growth. May be multiple
- Calculus
- *Tuberculosis:* Unilateral, collecting system—irregular margins, strictures, multifocal dilatation, and distinctive feature communicating parenchymal cavities
- Irregularity of papillary margin (earliest)
- Calcifications, variable parenchymal thickness.

Extrinsic Impression by an Artery
- Rarely cause symptoms
- *Fraley syndrome:* Infundibular obstruction
- Nephralgia
- Right upper pole calyx
- *IVP:* Early opacification and delayed emptying
- Angiography—also useful.

Congenital Hydrocalycosis
- Congenital dilatation of calyx
- Diagnosis is safely made only in childhood.

Postobstructive Atrophy
- Kidney is usually small, smooth
- Effaced papillae, dilated PCS
- Parenchymal wasting
- Compensatory hypertrophy
- Megacalyces and polycalycosis

- *Megacalyces:* Dilated calyces ± a slightly dilated pelvis
- *Polycalycosis:* Increased number of calyces—20–25
- Delayed visualization of calyceal system
- *Cortical thickness:* Normal
- Cause fetal obstruction, Boys > Girls.

Calculus
- Can cause mechanical obstruction, edema, or stricture
- Plain films, USG, CT—all help in diagnosis.

Blood Clot
- Volume of blood loss is large enough
- Trauma, tumors, AVM, and bleeding disorders predispose
- Usually asymptomatic, dissolve in 2 weeks
- *IVP:* Opaque urine, outlines the clot, and may dissect
- "Hand-in-glove" appearance
- *Ultrasonography:* Low-level echoes that separate sinus echoes
- *Computed tomography:* Appearance varies with time, does not enhance
- *Persistent clot:* May faintly calcify.

Sloughed Papilla
- When papillary necrosis evolves to the stage of flank necrosis, separation occurs between viable and dead parts
- Usually in analgesic nephropathy patients
- Obstruction at infundibulum, ureteropelvic junction, or ureter
- *IVP:* Triangle-shaped filling defect
- One or more calyces will dilate reflecting loss of papillary tip
- Calcium may deposit along the periphery
- *Occasionally very dense:* Indistinguishable from calculus.

Pelviureteric Junction Obstruction
- More common left side, 20% bilateral
- Cause neuromuscular incoordination, aberrant vessels

- *During acute episode-IVU:* Delayed, increasing dense nephrogram, and delayed appearance of PCS
- Calyces and dilated pelvis
- Contrast in collecting ducts—as crescents
- Ureters often not opacified
- *Milder cases:* Difficult to diagnose.

Tumors

- Tumors are very uncommon in ureter
- *TCC:* Renal pelvis > ureter (3:1)
- Seen in lower one-third of ureter, multicentricity and bilateral, if TCC
- Filling defects on IVU, never completely surrounded by opacified urine
- Polypoidal with smooth, irregular, or lobular surface
- *Squamous cell carcinoma:* Broad based and flat
- *Bergman's sign:* In ureteric carcinoma
  - Distinguishes from calculus
- *Ultrasonography:* Similar to renal parenchyma in echogenicity
- *Computed tomography:* Contrast enhancing mural mass projecting into lumen, circumferential, or eccentric thickening.

Tuberculous Stricture

- Marked irregularity of part or all of the collecting system or ureter because of both submucosal granulomas and mucosal ulceration
- Scars of healed tuberculous produce sharply-defined circumferential narrowing at one or several sites, often with irregular margins
- Fibrosis may progress during treatment of active tuberculous
- Pipe-stem ureter, thimble bladder.

Schistosomiasis

- Ureteral abnormalities are found in half of patients with bladder schistosomiasis
- *Early:* Minimal dilatation, slight mucosal irregularity, and diminished peristalsis
- *Then with time:* Calcification, mural thickening and straightening, beading, and multiple narrowing
- Some cases—bilharzial polyps—seen as filling defects
- No increased risk of TCC.

Ureterocele (Congenital)

- *Orthotopic ureterocele:* Best seen by IVU
- The distal ureter is dilated, projects into the lumen of bladder, opacified bladder urine surrounds the ureterocele separated by lucency, and cobra head deformity
- An ectopic ureterocele is seen on cystography as a smooth, nonopaque, and intravesicular mass
- Ectopic ureter causes—urinary tract infection (UTI), bladder neck destruction.

Primary Megaureter

- Ureter has a normally tapered distal segment but is otherwise dilated over a varying length, from a few centimeters proximal to tapered end including PCS
- Tapered segment is peristaltic.

Retroperitoneal Fibrosis

- Ureteric destruction of variable severity (75% bilateral)
- *Tapering lumen or complete obstruction—L4–L5*
- Medial deviation of ureters
- *Retroperitoneal, periaortic mass*—CT or US.

Retrocaval Ureter

- Ureter passes posterior to IVC and partially encircles it at L3–L4 with proximal dilatation
- Can cause flank pain, UTI.

Vesicoureteric Reflux

- Occurs when intramural segment of ureter in the UB is short and the angle of insertion is wide
- *VUR:* Decreases with age as lengthening of ureter occurs
- *Grading:*
  - Ureter only
  - Ureter, pelvis, and calyces
  - II + Mild dilatation of PCS, fornices normal

- Moderate dilatation of PCS + Unsharp fornices
- Gross distention + Effaced papilla
• Small, scarred kidney.

Postpartum
• More common on right side
• Urinary tract obstruction
• Effect of fimbriated *Escherichia coli* on urothelium.

GAS IN URINARY TRACT
Gas Inside the Bladder
• Vesicointestinal fistula.
• Cystitis.
• Following instrumentation.
• Penetrating wounds.

Gas in Bladder Wall
Emphysematous cystitis.

Gas in Kidneys and Ureters
• Any cause of gas in UB.
• Emphysematous pyelonephritis.
• Ureteric diversion.
• Fistula with bowel.

Gas Inside the Bladder
• *Vesicointestinal fistula:*
  – Can be due to diverticular disease, carcinoma colon or rectum, or Crohn's disease.
  – Pneumaturia is the presenting complaint.
  – Air visible in bladder lumen.
  – Fistulous communication can be demonstrated in 70% cases.
  – Focal thickening of bladder wall due to adjacent inflammation.
• Cystitis:
  – Due to gas-forming organisms.
  – Especially seen in diabetics and immunocompromised.
  – Usually *Escherichia coli* and rarely *Clostridium*.
• *Following instrumentation:*
  – Cystoscopy and catheterization may lead to air in bladder lumen.
• *Penetrating wounds:*
  – Trauma or any operative procedure may cause presence of gas in bladder lumen.

In Bladder Wall
Emphysematous Cystitis
• Uncommon complication of urinary tract infection by gas-forming organisms
• Almost pathognomonic of poorly-controlled diabetes
• Plain film shows translucent streaks or rings of air bubbles in bladder wall.
  Intraluminal air-fluid level may be positive.
  Ultrasound: Shows echogenic foci with distal shadowing in the area of bladder wall thickening.

Gas in Kidneys and Ureters
• Any cause of gas in urinary bladder.
• *Emphysematous pyelonephritis:*
  – Rare fulminating form of acute pyelonephritis.
  – Occurs usually in diabetics.
  – Radiologically there is gas in renal parenchyma and in perirenal tissues and PCS.
  – Gas may have streaky/mottled/loculated pattern.
  – Crescent of subcapsular or perinephric gas may also be seen.
  – Absent or decreased contrast excretion on IVP.
• *Ureteric diversion into the colon*
  – Ureterocolic anastomosis is performed after resection of bladder.
  – Air is seen in PCS and ureters.
• Fistula.

LOSS OF RENAL OUTLINE ON PLAIN FILM (*See* FIG. 7.4)
• Technical factors.
• *Absent kidney:*
  – Congenital
  – Postnephrectomy.

- Ectopic kidney.
- Perinephric hematoma.
- Perinephric abscess.
- Renal tumor.

Technical Factors
- Poor radiographic technique
- Overlying fecal matter, gas-filled bowel loops obscure renal shadows.

Congenital Absence of Kidney
- Can be unilateral or bilateral
- *Unilateral renal agenesis*—1:600 to 1:1,000 live births
- M:F = 1.8:1
- Often associated with other anomalies of the Vater anomalies, uterine anomalies
- *Radiologically:*
  - Visualization of single kidney
  - Colon occupies renal fossa
  - Compensatory hypertrophy of normal kidney.

Postnephrectomy
History of operation, scar in lumbar region. Surgical resection of 12th rib.

Ectopic Kidney
- Kidney is normally located opposite first to third lumbar vertebrae.
- Failure of ascent of kidney from pelvis may result in ectopic kidney.

There may be:
- *Longitudinal ectopia:* Pelvic, sacral, or intrathoracic kidney.
- *Crossed ectopia:*
  - *Pelvic kidney:* On IVU malrotated kidneys (Fig. 7.5) with short ureters.
- There may be associated contralateral renal agenesis, VUR, and hypospadias.

Intrathoracic kidney—is more common on the left.

Perinephric Hematoma
- Fills the entire perinephric space and displaces the kidney

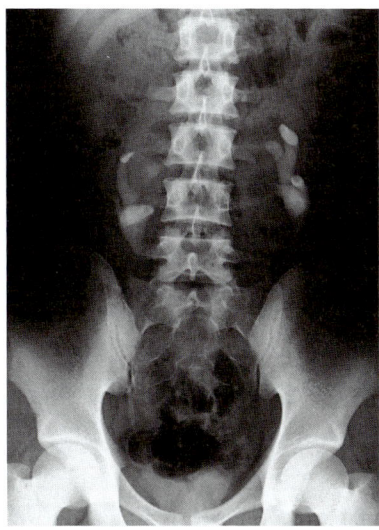

Fig. 7.5: An intravenous pyelogram (IVP) radiograph shows bilateral malrotated kidneys.

- Plain film shows loss of renal and psoas outline. Kidney is displaced anteromedially on IVU
- Ultrasound and CT show a perirenal collection
- Signs of trauma, e.g. fractured transverse process.

Perirenal Abscess
- Extension of acute pyelonephritis or renal abscess through the capsule
- Loss of psoas margin and obscuration of renal contour
- Scoliosis concave to the involved side
- Gas in perirenal tissue
- *IVU:* Shows unilateral impaired excretion; displacement of kidney
- *Ultrasound and computed tomography:* Show a complex, predominantly solid and hypoechoic mass with thick irregular wall, and perinephric collection and stranding gas within the lesion.

Renal Tumor
Tumor masses obliterate the perinephric fat planes and, therefore, cause loss of renal outlines on plain film.
- *Plain film:* May show soft tissue mass with calcification.

- *IVU:* Shows displacement and attenuation of PCS.
- *Ultrasound:* Shows heterogeneous mass displacing the collecting system and extending into perinephric fat planes.
- *Computed tomography:* Shows mass of heterogeneous attenuation with perinephric extension.

RENOVASCULAR HYPERTENSION

Renovascular hypertension is defined as hypertension that improves or resolves after correction of renal artery stenosis (RAS).

Signs of Unilateral Renal Artery Stenosis on IVU

- Unilateral delay of 1 minute or more in the appearance of opacified calyces.
- Small, smooth kidney:
  - Left more than 1.5 cm shorter than the right
  - Right more than 2 cm shorter than the left.
- Increased density of opacified calyces.
- Ureteric notching by collateral vessels.

Signs of Renal Artery Stenosis on Angiotensin-converting Enzyme Inhibitor Renal Scintigraphy

- Low probability suggested by a normal study
- Intermediate probability when:
  - Small kidney contributing less than 30% of total renal function.
  - Time for maximum activity (T_{max}) less than 2 minutes and shows no change following administration of angiotensin-converting enzyme (ACE) inhibitor.
  - Bilateral symmetrical cortical retention of tracer.
- High probability when unilateral parenchymal retention is indicated by:
  - A change in the 20-minute/peak uptake ratio more than 0.15, delayed excretion of tracer into the renal pelvis more than 2 minutes, or increase in the time to maximal activity Tmax of more than 2 minutes or 40% after administration of ACE inhibitor.
- Decreased sensitivity when bilateral RAS, impaired renal function, urinary obstruction, or long-term ACE therapy.

Signs of Renal Artery Stenosis on Doppler Sonography

- Peak velocity in the renal artery more than 100 cm/s.
- Renal artery velocity more than 3.5 × aortic velocity.
- Tardus parvus waveform-slope of the systolic upstroke less than 3 m/s² and acceleration time (time from onset of systole to peak systole) more than 0.075.
- Turbulent flow in the poststenotic renal artery.

Sign on Arteriography

- Reduction in luminal diameter more than 75%
- Systolic pressure gradient across the stenosis more than 15–25 mm Hg or more than 20% of aortic systolic pressure
- Evidence of collateral circulation into distal vessels
- Pharmacologic manipulation of collateral vessel flow (epinephrine restricts flow to the kidney and makes collaterals more apparent).

Computed Tomography Angiography

- Demonstrates both wall and lumen of the vessel
- Extent of plaque projecting into the vessel lumen
- Can demonstrate ostial stenosis
- Can be used to examine the patency of vessel that has been dilated by intravascular stents
- *Magnetic resonance angiography:* TOF MRA produced by unsaturated blood flowing into the plane of imaging.

PC Magnetic Resonance Angiography

Causes

- Atherosclerosis.
- Fibromuscular dysplasia.

- Thrombosis/embolism.
- *Arteritis*:
  - Polyarteritis nodosa (PAN)
  - TAO
  - Takayasu's disease
  - Syphilis
  - Congenital rubella.
- Neurofibromatosis.
- Trauma.
- Aneurysm.
- Arteriovenous (AV) fistula.
- Extrinsic compression.

Atherosclerosis:
- 66% of renovascular causes
- Stenosis of the proximal 2 cm of the renal artery
- Less frequently the distal artery or early branches at bifurcations
- More common in males.

Fibromuscular dysplasia:
- 33% of renovascular causes
- Stenosis ± dilatation which may give the characteristic "string of beads" appearance
- Mainly females less than 40 years
- Bilateral in 60% of the cases.

Takayasu's arteritis:
- Mainly young females less than 35 years of age
- Associated with fever and increased ESR
- Mainly involves the aorta or its major branches
- Luminal narrowing, occlusion, dilatation, or formation of aneurysms
- Causes stenosis of aorta or main renal artery.

Polyarteritis nodosa:
- Usually affect medium or small-sized vessels
- Characterized by multiple aneurysms which are sharply defined and 2–3 mm wide.

Neurofibromatosis:
- Coarctation of aorta
- ± stenosis of other arteries
- ± intrarenal arterial abnormalities.

RENAL CALCIFICATION

- Calculi
- *Dystrophic calcification due to localized disease:*
  - Infections.
  - Carcinomas.
  - Vascular.
  - Cysts.
- Nephrocalcinosis (Fig. 7.6):
  - Medullary.
  - Cortical.

Calculi

- Stones within the collecting system
- Usually sharp in outline
- Variable in size and number
- *IVP:* Shows hydronephrosis if obstructing
- *Ultrasonography:* Echogenic with acoustic shadow.

Dystrophic Calcification (Usually One Kidney or Part of One Kidney)

- *Infections:*
  - Tuberculosis:
    - Irregular, indefinite, and not dense as calculi
    - Usually nodular, curvilinear, or amorphous mottled calcification
    - More common in cortex, in various segments
    - *Multifocal:* Ureteric, UB, vas deferens, and seminal vesicles.
  - Hydatid:
    - Renal involvement in 3%
    - 50% of echinococcal cysts calcify
    - Usually polar
    - Curvilinear calcification.

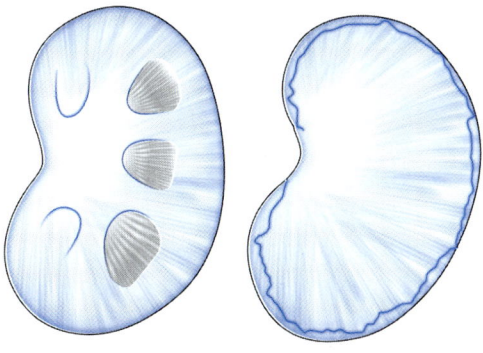

Fig. 7.6: Nephrocalcinosis.

- *Xanthogranulomatous pyelonephritis:*
  - Usually associated staghorn calculus in renal pelvis (Fig. 7.7)
  - *IVP:* Nonfunctioning/poorly functioning kidney.
    - Ill-defined renal outline
  - *Ultrasound:* Nephrolithiasis
    - Decreased echogenicity
    - Hydronephrosis.
  - *Computed tomography:*
    - Calculus with poorly-functioning kidney
    - Multiple nonenhancing masses (some with fat density)
    - Perinephric extension.
- *Abscess:*
  - Calcification in wall.
  - Or nodular calcification after resolution.
- *Tumors:*
  - *Renal cell carcinoma:*
    - 8–15% cases.
    - Generally nonperipheral, amorphous, and irregular.
  - *Wilms' tumor:*
    - Amorphous, irregular calcification in soft tissue mass.

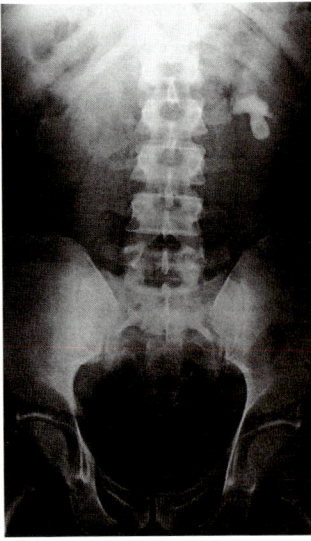

Fig. 7.7: KUB radiograph shows staghorn calculus in left renal area.

- *Cysts:*
  - Due to hemorrhage or infection.
  - May occur in:
    - Simple cyst
    - Multicystic dysplastic kidney
    - Adult PCKD.
- *Vascular:*
  - Subcapsular/perirenal hematoma.
  - *Aneurysm of renal artery:*
    - Curvilinear calcification or eggshell appearance.
  - Nephrocalcinosis.

Parenchymal Calcification

Medullary Nephrocalcinosis (Pyramidal)
- *Hyperparathyroidism:*
  - Primary >> secondary
  - Most common cause (16%)
  - Other signs of HPT such as bone erosions, brown tumors, and soft tissue calcifications.
- *Renal tubular acidosis:*
  - Most common cause in children
  - May be associated with rickets/osteomalacia
  - Calcification often dense than other causes.
- *Medullary sponge kidney:*
  - Not a true cause of nephrocalcinosis as calcification is within ectatic ducts rather than in parenchyma.
  - Numerous medullary cysts communicating with tubules which opacify during IVU.
  - Cysts contain small calculi giving bunch of grapes appearance.
- *Renal papillary necrosis (Fig. 7.8):* Calcification of shrunken necrotic papillae.
- *Causes of hypercalcemia or hypercalciuria:*
  - *Milk alkali syndrome:*
    - Due to long-standing calcium and alkali ingestion.
    - Severe hypercalcemia, hypercalcemia, irreversible renal failure, and ectopic calcification.

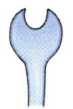 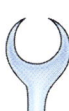 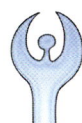 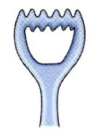 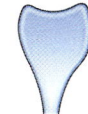

Normal   Swollen   Partial papillary necrosis   Total papillary necrosis   Necrosis in situ

Fig. 7.8: Grades of papillary necrosis.

- Sarcoidosis:
  - Renal involvement in 2–5% cases.
  - *Associated lung involvement:* Hilar LN, fibronodular infiltrate.
  - Bone lytic lesions.
- Hypervitaminosis D:
  - In excess of 50,000 U/day.
  - Deossification.
  - Widening of provisional zone of calcification.
  - Dense calvarium.
  - Metastatic calcification in arterial walls.
- *Primary hyperoxaluria:*
  - 65% less than 5 years.
  - Generally diffuse and homogeneous.
  - Recurrent nephrolithiasis.
  - Dense vascular calcification.

Cortical Nephrocalcinosis

Less than 5% of cases.

- *Acute cortical necrosis:*
  - Small kidney
  - Tramline/punctate calcification along margin of necrotic tissue
  - Ultrasonography shows hyperechoic cortex with shadowing.
- *Chronic glomerulonephritis:*
  - Small smooth kidneys with wasted parenchyma
  - Normal papillae and calices
  - Decreased density of contrast on IVU
  - *Ultrasonography:* Increased echogenicity with prominent sinus fat.
- *Hemolytic uremic syndrome:*
  - Common cause in children
  - Cortical necrosis fibrosis calcification
  - Clinically thrombocytopenia.

- *Alport's syndrome:*
  - Autosomal dominant
  - Polyuria, anemia, nerve deafness, congenital cataract, and nystagmus
  - Small smooth kidneys.
- *Rejected renal transplant:*
  - Small kidney
  - Cortical calcifications.

RENAL MASS

Adult

Unilateral

Solid

A. Tumors
   a. Malignant:
      Adenocarcinoma (RCC)
      - Lymphoma
      - TCC
      - Metastasis
      - Adult neuroblastoma
   b. Benign:
      - AML (Angiomyolipoma)
      - Oncocytoma
      - Adenoma
      - Mesenchymal tumors (lipoma, fibroma, myoma, hemangioma)

B. *Inflammatory masses:*
   - Acute focal pyelonephritis
   - Renal abscess
   - Xanthogranulomatous pyelonephritis
   - Malakoplakia
   - Tuberculoma.

Bilateral

A. Tumors
   Lymphoma

   Metastasis
   B/L malignant or benign
   Renal tumors

B. Cysts:
   - Adult polycystic kidney disease
   - Acquired cystic kidney disease.

Cystic

- Simple renal cysts
- *Inherited cystic disease:*
  - Multilocular cystic nephroma
  - Multicystic dysplastic kidney.
- Focal hydronephrosis.

Children (Pediatric)

Single
- Wilms' tumor
- Multilocular cystic nephroma
- Mesoblastic nephroma
- Focal hydronephrosis
- Traumatic cyst, abscess
- RCC
- Intrarenal neuroblastoma
- Malignant rhabdoid tumor

Multiple
- Multiple Wilms' tumors
- Angiomyolipoma
- Lymphoma
- Leukemia
- Nephroblastomatosis
- Adult polycystic kidney disease
- Abscesses

Renal Cell Carcinoma

- Most common urological malignant lesion in adults
- M:F = 2:1, 6th and 7th decades
- Unilateral, 2%—bilateral, and 9% multicentric (VHL, familial, dialysis)
- *Diagnostic triad:* Flank pain, gross hematuria, and palpable renal mass—4–9% of patients
- Usually solid
- *Less than 3 cm:* Homogeneous and smooth
- *Larger:* Necrosis and/or hemorrhage, dystrophic calcification
- *Plain X-ray:* Normal, soft tissue mass overlying/bulging renal outline, or loss of psoas outline
- *Calcification:* In 20% of RCC
- (nonperipheral or central)—87%—carcinomas
- *IVP:* 67% sensitive in detecting solid mass lesion of the kidney
- However, cannot determine the nature of a renal mass.

Primary Uroradiologic Elements

Size	– Large
Contour	– Unifocal mass
Lesion distribution	– U/L

Secondary Collecting System

Focal—dilatation, displacement, attenuation.

Nephrogram	:	Focal replaced, irregular margin.
Attenuation	:	Diminished, enhances less than normal parenchyma, unsharp parenchymal interface with ill-defined margin, a thick or irregular wall, enlargement of renal vein or IVC with or without filling defect.
Echogenicity	:	Variable
MR	:	SI similar to parenchyma on unenhanced T1 and T2WI, enhances with gadolinium.
Angio	:	Most RCC-hypervascular, presence of tumor vessels. Irregular tortuous, without normal tapering, randomly distributed, variable in caliber with unpredictable branching.
Lymphoma	:	Primary lymphoma—rare Usually – Secondary hematogenous – Direct extension. – NHL > HL – B/L > U/L – Multiple nodular, diffuse infiltration, bulky single tumor, solitary nodule, invasion from perirenal disease, and microscopic infiltration.

Earliest change: Metastatic nodules detected as nephrographic defects on contrast material enhanced imaging studies, at a time when kidneys may be normal in size and contour.

Primary Uroradiological Elements

Size	:	Large
Contour	:	Normal to multifocal masses
Lesion distribution	:	Bilateral.

Secondary Uroradiological Elements

Collecting system	:	Displaced, caliectasis without pelviectasis (from sinus spread)
Parenchymal thickness	:	Expanded (focal)
Nephrogram	:	Multifocal masses/attenuation value less than that of normal tissue: minimal enhancement with contrast material.
Echogenicity	:	Multifocal hypoechoic solid masses.

Transitional Cell Carcinoma

- Primary involvement of PCS and ureter.
- Focal, multifocal, or diffuse, transform the normally smooth mucosa into a surface, which is irregular or nodular.
- Twice as common in renal pelvis than as in the ureter.
- *Bilateral*—10%, multifocal 20–44%.
- M>F, 7th decade.
- Gross or microscopic hematuria flank pain.

IVP

- Primary investigative modality.
- Filling defect in renal pelvis, or calyx, calyceal cutoff, infundibular narrowing, poor or nonvisualization of one group of calyces, and nonfunctioning kidney, due to HDN.
  - HDN
  - Extensive destruction and replacement of renal parenchyma
  - Renal vein invasion.

Ultrasonography

- Iso or hypoechoic solid mass separating the central sinus echoes.
- Focal enlargement of renal cortex if seen suggests infiltration of renal parenchyma.

Computed Tomography

Pelvis or calyceal filling defect or a solid mass in renal sinus.

- Parapelvic fat line is initially compressed by the growing mass and, if disrupted, indicates invasion
- In large masses, a diagnosis of transitional cell carcinoma (TCC) is more likely if the mass is centrally located, with centrifugal extension, and preservation of renal shape
- Renal cell carcinoma tends to be eccentric, distorted renal outline, and shows relatively more enhancement.

Metastasis

Relatively common at autopsy—seen in 20% patients

- MC sites of primary: Lung, breast, colon, and malignant melanoma
- Multiple and bilateral
- *If single large:* Impossible to differentiate from primary (renal tumor—biopsy indicated)
- *Ultrasonography:* Hypoechoic
- *Computed tomography:* Small multiple solid renal lesion, less than 2 cm, and subcapsular in renal cortex.

Angiomyolipoma

- Radiologically most common, diagnosed benign renal neoplasm
- *Hamartoma:* Represents excessive growth of mature fat, smooth muscle and arteries normally present in the kidney
- F > M—most asymptomatic
- *Larger lesions:* Mass, flank pain, hematuria, and hypotension
- Association with tuberous sclerosis (TS)—80% of patients with TS have AML
- *X-ray:* In 10% of patients shows large soft tissue mass with fat radiolucency.

Typical Findings

Primary:
- *Size:* Large
- *Contour:* Unifocal mass
- *Distribution*: Unilateral
- *Secondary*: Collecting system—attenuated (focal); displaced (focal)
- *Nephrogram*: Replaced (focal)

- *Attenuation value:* Mixed (negative and positive values) (fat)
- *Echogenicity:* Heterogeneous, often hyperechoic
- *Magnetic resonance*: Signal intensity follows fat on T1 and T2WI and fat suppressed images.

Oncocytoma

- Uncommon benign tumor arise from PCT
- 4–7% of all renal tumors
- *Average size*—7 cm
- Often detected incidentally as they rarely bleed or cause pain unless extremely large.

USG	: Solid homogeneous mass with central stellate scar.
CT	: Well-defined solid mass with homogeneous central echo with central scar.
MR	: Homogeneous signal intensity. Low to moderate on T1 and relatively high on T2WI. Central stellate scar with well-defined capsule.
Angio	: Well-defined vascular renal tumor with a "spoke-wheel" pattern of vessels penetrating into the center of the tumor and homogeneous tumor blush.
Adenoma	: Seen in 15% kidneys at autopsy.
	: Usually as cortical subcapsular tumor.
	: Arise from tubular epithelium.
	: Difficult to distinguish from RCC. Natural history—unknown.
Wilms' tumor	: Most common abdominal and renal malignancy in children
	: 7–8/10 children/years
	: 80% in first 3 years
	: Association with cryptorchidism, hypospadias, and hemihypertrophy.

Sporadic Aniridia

- 10–15% bilateral
- *Plain film:* Abdominal mass displacing adjacent structures
- Calcification—in 5%
- *Ultrasonography:* Large well-defined mass, greater echogenicity than liver. Solid with hemorrhage and necrosis
- *Computed tomography:* Well defined, low attenuation with hemorrhage and necrosis
- *Magnetic resonance:* Inhomogeneous low signal on T1 and high on T2
- *Differentiation from neuroblastoma:* Second most common retroperitoneal tumor in children.

Wilms' Tumor	Neuroblastoma
• Intrarenal mass with distorted PCS anatomy	• Intraspinal extension
• Vascular structures (IVC, aorta) displaced	• Encased
• Heterogeneous with areas of necrosis.	• Solid homogeneous
• Ipsilateral IVC/renal thoracoabdominal sign	• Extend into chest
• Vein tumor thrombus (+)	• (–)
• Lung metastasis	• Bone metastases
• Usually does not cross midline	• Crosses midline
	• Calcification more common.

Congenital Mesoblastic Nephroma

- Most common solid renal tumor in newborn—can be diagnosed in utero on ultrasound
- *Mean age at diagnosis:* 3.5 months, associated polyhydramnios
- *Ultrasound/computed tomography:* Predominantly solid mass but even cystic and calcified component can be seen
- Does not extend into IVC.

Primary

Size	:	Large
Contour	:	Infiltrative bean-shaped mass
Lesion distribution	:	Unilateral
Secondary collecting system	:	Attenuated, caliectasis with

Attenuation value	:	pelviectasis nephrogram—replaced Soft tissue homogeneous (common)
Echogenicity	:	Soft tissue homogeneous (common)
Others	:	Polyhydramnios (in utero).

Multilocular Cystic Nephroma

- Uncommon neoplasm composed of multiple variable-sized cysts with prominent septa
- Arises as unilateral unifocal mass with the remaining portion of one kidney uninvolved or compressed by the tumors
- Surrounded by dense fibrous capsule
- Calcification of cyst wall uncommon
- Characteristically one or more of the cysts herniate into the renal pelvis to form filling defects.

Nephroblastomatosis

- Remnant of primitive blastoma as sheets or more discrete nodules in cortex
- Commonly associated with Wilms' tumor
- *IVP:* Multifocal distortion of PCS
- *Computed tomography:* Multiple nodules of varying sizes, situated in the peripheral portion of the kidney, with enlargement.
- *Surface:* Usually smooth
- Minimal contrast enhancement.

Simple Cysts/Localized Cystic Disease

Most common focal mass of the kidney.
- *Pathogenesis:* Not conclusively established
- Obstruction of renal tubule/blockage and expansion of calyceal diverticulum (Fig. 7.9)
- Cyst fluid is serous, not urine, lactate dehydrogenase (LDH) level—lower than serum

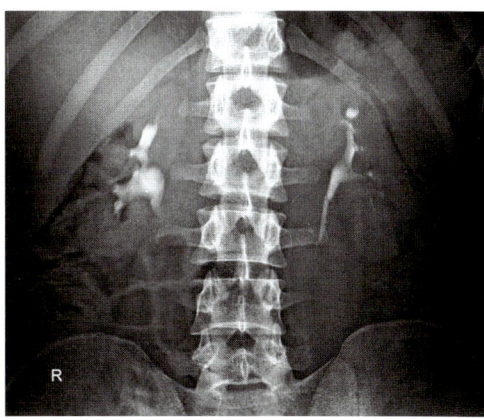

Fig. 7.9: An intravenous pyelogram (IVP) radiograph shows calyceal diverticulum in left kidney near the upper pole.

- Usually unilateral and single, most common site—polar (lower pole)
- Rarely numerous simple cysts completely replace the parenchyma of either the entire kidney or only a portion of one kidney—localized cystic disease composed of cluster of simple cysts that lacks a capsule and preserves the reniform shape of the enlarged kidney.

Cystic diseases to be distinguished from usually benign but sometimes malignant—multiloculated cystic neoplasms (grow by expansion and appear as ball-shaped encapsulated mass).

Simple Cyst Typical Findings

Primary:
Size	:	Variable.
Contour	:	Unifocal mass.
Lesion distribution	:	Variable.

Secondary:
Collecting system	:	Attenuated (focal), displace (focal)
Nephrogram	:	Displace (focal), replaced (focal), smooth margin, "thin-rim sign" when peripheral, "beak sign" when peripheral.
Calcification	:	Uncommon, curvilinear, peripheral.
Attenuation value	:	Water, no contrast enhancement.

Echogenicity	:	Anechoic, well-defined far walls, enhanced through sound transmission
MR	:	Signal intensity parallel's water.

Polycystic Kidney Disease

Multiple cysts in bilateral kidneys.

Primary

Size	:	Large
Contour	:	Multifocal masses.
Lesion distribution	:	Bilateral (may be asymmetric)

Secondary

Collecting system	:	Displaced, attenuated.
Nephrogram	:	Replaced (multiple masses with smooth margin, varying sizes, radiolucent with urography or angiography; water density/intensity, non-enhancing with CT/MRI).
Echogenicity	:	Multiple fluid-filled masses.
Cyst content	:	Serous with urea content equal to urine.

Acquired Cystic Kidney Disease

- Multiple renal cysts formation in patients with end-stage renal disease
- Seen in 40–50% of patients on long-term hemodialysis
- Multiple small bilateral cysts involving both renal cortex and medulla
- Increased incidence of renal neoplasms
- *Ultrasound:* Bilateral small kidneys with increased echogenicity with multiple cysts
- Solid or complex renal tumor may be present
- *Computed tomography:* Bilateral small kidney, with multiple cysts
- *Cyst wall calcification:* Common.

Acute Focal Bacterial Pyelonephritis and Renal Abscess

- Usually secondary to ascending inferior Gram-negative organism
- Most bacterial abscesses are associated with calculus in pelvis or ureter
- *IVP:* Reveals presence of focal renal mass
- *Ultrasonography:* Hypoechoic poorly-defined mass with internal echoes
- *Computed tomography:* Low density area with patchy enhancement
- Lack of well-defined wall and central low density differentiates it from renal abscess.

ABSCESS TYPICAL IMAGING FEATURES

Primary

Size	:	Large.
Contour	:	Unifocal mass.
Lesion distribution	:	Unilateral

Secondary

- *Collecting system:* Attenuated (focal), displaced (focal).
- *Nephrogram:* Normal (early), replaced (focal), irregular, and thick walls (late).
- *Attenuation value:* Normal to slightly diminished before contrast administration.
  – Enhances less than normal parenchyma (early) decreased and nonenhancing (late).
- *Echogenicity:* Variable hypoechoic (early) to anechoic (late).

CYSTIC DISEASE OF KIDNEYS

Renal cysts: Represent dilated nephrons or collecting ducts.

Cystic kidney	:	Is a kidney with 3–5 or more cysts.
Renal cystic disease	:	Refers to any disorder that results from the presence of multiple renal cysts.

- Simple cysts
- Atypical cysts

Cystic Neoplasams

Nongenetic conditions
- Cystic dysplasia or dysplasia
- Multicystic dysplastic kidney
- Multilocular cyst
- Localized cystic disease of the kidney
- Parapelvic cyst
- Simple cysts
- Calyceal cysts
- Medullary sponge kidney
- Acquired cystic disease of kidney (in CRF).

Imaging features
- Unilateral or bilateral
- Diffuse or localized
- Size of kidneys
- Extrarenal manifestations

Genetic Conditions

Autosomal Dominant
- Autosomal dominant, polycystic kidney disease
- Tuberous sclerosis, VHL
- Medullary cystic disease
- Glomerulocystic disease.

Autosomal Recessive
- Autosomal recessive polycystic kidney disease
- Juvenile nephronophthisis.

Cysts Associated with Syndromes
- Chromosomal disorders
- Autosomal recessive syndromes
- X-linked syndromes.

Classification of Renal Cysts

Renal Dysplasia
- Multicystic dysplastic kidney
- Focal segmental cystic dysplasia
- Multiple cysts associated with lower UT obstruction.

Polycystic Disease
- Childhood (AR)
- Adult (AD).

Cortical Cysts
- Simple cyst
- Multilocular cystic nephroma
- Syndromes associated with cysts
- Zellweger syndrome
- Tuberous sclerosis
- Turner syndrome
- VHL
- Trisomy 13
- Trisomy 18
- Hemodialysis.

Medullary Cysts
- Calyceal cyst (diverticulum) (Fig. 7.9)
- Medullary sponge kidney
- Papillary necrosis
- Juvenile nephronophthisis [medullary cystic disease (MCD)].

Miscellaneous
- Inflammatory
- Tuberculosis
- Hydatid.

Neoplastic
- Cystic degeneration of carcinoma.

Traumatic
- Intrarenal hematoma.

Extraparenchymal Renal Cysts
- Parapelvic
- Perinephric.

Simple Cysts

Ultrasonography Criteria

A renal fluid collection with the following features:
- No internal echoes
- Sharply-defined distal wall
- Posterior acoustic enhancement
- Round or oval shape.

Atypical Findings in a Cyst

- Internal echoes
- Septa
- Discernible wall
- Solid components within the cyst
- Calcification.

Differential Diagnosis

- Hydrocalyx
- Calyceal cyst
- Cavity
- Obstructed moiety of duplex system (upper pole)
- Hematoma
- Aneurysm or AVM.

Computed Tomography Criteria

- Sharp margination and demarcation.
- Smooth thin wall.
- Homogeneous attenuation (0–20 HU).
- No enhancement.

If CT findings are atypical or if patient has hematuria, nonenhanced scan should be obtained.

Magnetic Resonance Imaging Criteria

- Sharp margination and demarcation.
- Smooth thin wall.
- Homogeneous water-like signal intensity decreases T1WI, increases T2WI.
- No enhancement
  SS FSE sequences best suited.

Atypical Cysts

Bosniak classification of cystic renal masses according to CT criteria:
- *Category 1:* Classic simple cysts
- *Category 2:* Minimally complicated cysts, which do not require surgery.
  - Smooth, thin (<1 mm) septa
  - Small smooth plaques of fine linear calcification in cyst wall or septa
  - High density cysts (40–100 HU)
  - Can be followed with serial imaging, provided the following criteria are met:
    - Perfectly smooth, rounded, sharply-marginated homogeneous lesions.
    - No enhancement.
    - At least one-fourth of the lesion's circumference should extend outside the kidney so that the smoothness of the wall can be evaluated.
    - Size less than 4 cm.

Cystic Renal Cell Carcinoma may Rarely Show Similar Computed Tomography Features

- Hemorrhagic cysts on MRI—Increase T1WI, increase T2WI
  - Do not enhance fluid-iron levels.
- *Category 3:* Should undergo surgical exploration
  - Thick, irregular mural, or septal calcification
  - Numerous or thick (>1 mm) irregular septa
  - Uniform or slightly nodular wall thickening
  - Some category three lesions are benign, e.g. multilocular cystic nephromas, hemorrhagic renal cysts
  - Others are cystic RCCs.
- *Category 4:* Clearly malignant lesions with large cystic components which may show marginal irregularity or solid vascular elements.

Polycystic Kidney Disease

Autosomal Recessive Polycystic Kidney Disease (ARPKD—1980-81)

Presents in childhood.
- Bilateral large smooth kidneys with dense striated nephrogram.
- Markedly hyperechoic kidneys on USG with loss of CMD (small 1–2 mm cysts).
- Associated with congenital hepatic fibrosis and portal HT.
  - Dilated collecting ducts in renal medulla with relative preservation of the renal cortex.

Autosomal Dominant Polycystic Kidney Disease

Presents in 3rd–4th decades and terminal renal failure occurs in 10 years.
- Bilateral but asymmetrical lobulated enlargement of kidneys.

- Multiple smooth defects in the nephrogram, with elongation and deformity of calyces giving a "spider leg" appearance. Cysts may produce filling defects in the renal pelvis. Calcification in cyst walls.
- Associated with:
  - Liver and pancreatic cysts
  - Berry aneurysms (intracranial)
  - Colonic diverticulae
  - Increased incidence of RCC.

Diagnostic criteria	:	(Ravine et al. 1994)
<30 years	:	Two cysts unilateral or bilateral
30–59 years	:	Two cysts in each kidney
>60 years	:	> Four cysts

Unilateral (Localized) Renal Cystic Disease

- At the most one kidney is replaced by multiple cysts. However, the other kidney is normal
- No family history, no liver cysts, and no renal failure
- Affected kidney is enlarged and may show normal function.

Acquired Cystic Kidney Disease

It is characterized by the development of multiple renal cysts in patients without a history of hereditary renal cystic disease. Diagnosis is based on detection of at least 3–5 cysts in each kidney in a patient with CRF not due to hereditary renal cystic disease.
- Affected kidneys are usually small. However, nephromegaly eventually develops
- Hemorrhagic cysts occur in about 50% of these patients
- 40–100 HU on nonenhanced scans
- Increased incidence of small RCCs (<3 cm).

Extraparenchymal Renal Cysts

Parapelvic cyst: Lymphatic in origin.
- Located in or near the hilum
- Does not communicate with the renal pelvis
- Simple (multilocular; single/multiple: Unilateral or bilateral
- May compress renal pelvis and cause hydronephrosis.

Differential Diagnosis
Dilated or extrarenal pelvis.

Perinephric Cyst

- Secondary to trauma
- May compress the kidney, pelvis or ureter, leading to hydronephrosis or causing renal displacement.

Multilocular Cystic Nephroma

Cystic renal mass derived from metanephric blastoma, males less than 4 years; females 5th/6th decades; presents as abdominal mass.
- *Spectrum:* Benign (multilocular renal cyst)—malignant (multilocular cystic Wilms' tumor)
- No associated anomalies.
- *Ultrasonography:* Multilocular renal mass with multiple cysts and septations. Nonfunctioning on isotope imaging.
- Hallmark on imaging in presence of a capsule.

Multicystic Dysplastic Kidney

Two types:
1. Pelvico-infundibular atresia
2. Hydronephrotic type.

In the classic pelvico-infundibular type: No discernible renal pelvis. Seen on imaging, kidney may be small or normal in size, or enlarged containing multiple variably-sized noncommunicating renal cysts—No perfusion on renal scintigraphy.

In the hydronephrotic form of MDK: Dilatation of renal pelvis and calyces is seen with multiple noncommunicating cysts.

The affected kidney may remain unchanged, but it frequently undergoes spontaneous regression.

T2W pulse sequence can be used to diagnose MDK, especially in utero.

Medullary Cysts

- *Calyceal cyst (diverticulum):* Small, solitary cyst communicating via an isthmus with fornix of a calyx (*see* Fig. 7.8)
- *Medullary sponge kidney:* Bilateral in 60–80% cases.

Multiple, small, mainly pyramidal cysts which opacify during excretory urography and contain calculi.
- *Juvenile nephronophthisis (medullary cystic disease):* Normal or small kidneys, presents with polyuria. USG shows few medullary or corticomedullary cysts with loss of CMD and increased echogenicity.

CARCINOMA OF THE BLADDER

- Most common tumor of the gut
- TCC 90%; SCC 5%; adenocarcinoma 2%
- Peaks in the 7th decade
- Males predominate by 3:1
- Hematuria, most common clinical presentation
- Chemical agents such as aniline, biological agents (coffee, artificial sweeteners), radiation, chronic urothelial irritation, and nicotine are associated with bladder carcinogenesis. Bilharziasis is an independent risk factor
- Squamous cell carcinoma and adenocarcinoma have poor prognosis
- The lateral wall of the bladder and bladder diverticulae are more frequently involved
- Only 60% of known bladder tumors are detected on urograms
- Bladder tumors cause nonspecific intravesical filling defects
- The "Steeple sign" (contrast trapped within the interstices of tumor) suggests transitional cell carcinoma. Fungus balls or mycetoma may also occasionally entrap contrast material, but the pattern is lamellar and frequently associated with gas formation
- Computed tomography cannot accurately depict the depth of invasion of the bladder wall and cannot distinguish edema or inflammatory changes from tumor. CT can accurately evaluate perivesical and local pelvic extension
- Magnetic resonance imaging is superior to CT in determining local growth and detection of bone marrow infiltration
- *Stage of tumor:* Single most important prognostic parameter. Synchronous upper tract urothelial lesions must be excluded
- Clinical staging has an accuracy of 50% when compared with that with CT (32–80%) or MRI (73%)
- Overstaging commonly occurs as a result of edema after endoscopy and/or endoscopic resection and as a result of fibrosis from radiation therapy
- A staging classification that incorporates the TMN and Jewett-Strong-Marshall (JSM) system is useful:
  - *T1A*—indicates lesions involving the mucosa and submucosa
  - *T2B1*—invasion of the superficial muscle layer
  - *T3aB2*—invasion of the deep muscular wall
  - *T3bC*—invasion of perivesical fat
  - *T4aD1*—extension to perivesical organs
  - *T4b*—invasion of the pelvic and/or abdominal wall
  - *D2*—distant metastases
- Metastases occur in approximately 11% of cases, retroperitoneal nodes (34%); distant lymph nodes (17%); lumbar vertebrae (13%); lungs (9%); kidneys (8%); and adrenals (4%)
- Plain radiographic findings are nonspecific, particularly the presence of calcification. The calcification is on the surface in TCC. Intrinsic calcifications suggest an adenocarcinoma or the unusual cell type
- Irregular filling defects with broad base and fronds in the bladder are seen with IVU, CT and MRI. Increased thickness of the bladder wall in the region of the tumor should indicate infiltration. Unusually the tumor may present as diffuse thickening of the bladder wall
- Both CT and MRI have been shown to perform better than cystography in the diagnosis of tumors in the bladder diverticulae that are not depicted on cystograms because of obstruction at the diverticular orifice
- Ultrasonography is inaccurate for diagnosing early tumor, and it is useful in the diagnosis of obstructive uropathy. Vesical US can be performed endoscopically during

cystoscopy or suprapubically through suprapubic approach. Tumor is echo poor relative to the vesical wall. As the staging modality US is invasive
- On nonenhanced CT (NECT), the TCC is iso—to hyperattenuating relative to urine. TCCs demonstrate mild-to-moderate enhancement on contrast-enhanced CT (CECT), and they become hypoattenuating relative to opacified urine
- On MRI, the tumor is hyperintense than urine but hypointense than fat on both T1 and PDWI; the tumor is hypointense than urine on T2WI. Postgadolinium T1WI within the first 2 minutes can identify early tumors.

Differential Diagnosis

- *Nonneoplastic lesions:* Calculi, blood clot, fungus balls, inflammatory pseudosarcoma, and cystitis.

Primary

- *Epithelial tumors:* Papilloma, SCC, adenocarcinoma, carcinosarcoma, and undifferentiated tumors
- *Mesodermal tumors:* Smooth muscle—leiomyoma, leiomyoblastoma, leiomyosarcoma; neural tumors—neurofibroma, neurilemmoma; vascular—hemangioma, lymphangioma, hemangiosarcoma; fibrous—fibroepithelial polyp; mixed tumors—fibromyoma, fibrolipoma, fibromyxoma; lymphoma
- Metastases or direct invasion of the uroepithelium by tumors.

BLADDER OUTFLOW OBSTRUCTION

- *Prostate:*
  - Benign prostatic hyperplasia (BPH)
  - Prostate cancer
  - Other prostatic lesions—Wegener's granulomatosis
    - Lymphomatoid granulomatosis
    - Malignant lymphoma
- *Urethral:*
  - Congenital urethral valves
  - Urethral atresia
  - Urethral dysplasia
  - Anterior urethral diverticulum
  - Urethral stricture
  - Calculus
  - Meatal stenosis
- *Vesical:*
  - Acquired bladder neck stricture
  - Bladder calculi
  - Fungus ball
  - Bladder tumors
  - Neurogenic bladder
  - Bladder sphincter dyssynergia
- *Miscellaneous:*
  - Ectopic ureterocele
  - Prune-Belly syndrome
  - Hydrocolpos
  - Cervical/lower uterine segment leiomyoma
  - Vaginal carcinoma, rhabdomyosarcoma, phimosis.

Benign Prostatic Hyperplasia

Most common cause of vesical neck obstruction in adult males. On MCU the prostatic urethra appears elongated and compressed.
- *Cystogram:* Floor of urinary bladder is elevated with a rounded defect.
- Trabeculations and distention of urinary bladder with/without bladder diverticulae/bladder calculi.
- *IVU:* Hydronephrosis/hydroureter in advanced cases.
  - Distal ureters form a "J" (fish-hook) deformity.
- *US:* Diffusely altered inhomogeneous echo pattern. Demonstrate size and shape of gland.
  - Concomitant prostatic calculi + other features of obstruction.
- *CT:* Unequivocal enlargement—prostate is seen 2–3 cm or more above the symphysis and is surrounded by the bladder.
- *MR:* Appearance of prostate varies depending on the type of hyperplasia.
- *Nodular hyperplasia:* Enlarged gland with nodules of decreased signal intensity on T1WI and of varying intensity on T2WI.

- *Diffuse hypertrophy:* Enlarged gland with decreased signal intensity on T1WI and homo/inhomogeneous medium to high SI on T2WI.

Carcinoma of the Prostate

- 95% are adenocarcinoma; rarely squamous or TCC.
- *70% originates in periphery:* C zone; 20% in transitional zone and 10% in central zone.
- Screening for primary carcinoma is by digital rectal examination and serum PSA.
- *MCU:* Narrow prostatic urethra. Irregularity of urethra/floor of bladder laterosuperior of superolateral to urethra.
- *Seminal versiculogram:* Medial portion of seminal vesicles is reduced in size and the lateral portion may be dilated.
- *US:* Carcinoma is seen as hypoechoic area within the peripheral zone which warrants a TRUS-guided needle biopsy.
- *Feature of extracapsular invasion:* Contour deformity of capsule irregularity and duct tumor extension into periprostatic fat
- *CT:* Used for tumor staging (nodal, visceral, and bony)
- *Radionuclide bone scintigraphy:* Accurately detects small and early metastatic lesion.
- *MR:* Major role is in tumor staging, especially extracapsular extension seminal, vesicular, and bladder invasion.

Signal intensity of prostate carcinoma has been variously repeated as being of decreased, increased, and/or heterogeneous.

Congenital Urethral Valves

- Almost exclusively in males.
- *Anterior urethral valves:* Rare; Posterior urethral valves are more common.

Posturethral Valves

Types:
- Two mucosal folds extending from lower aspect of verumontanum to distal posterior urethra—most common.
- Two folds extending from cephalad aspect of verumontanum to bladder neck.
- Horizontal membrane in the region of verumontanum with central/eccentric opening.
- *Antenatal ultrasound:* Dilated bladder with thickened walls with dilated posterior urethra. Dilated PCS and ureter (50%).
- *Urinary tract rupture:* Urinary ascites, paranephric urinoma.
- Oligohydramnios and pulmonary hypoplasia.
- Cystic dysplasia
- *MCU:* Dilatation of prostatic urethra up to valves
- Valves may be seen as their crescenteric filling defect unilateral or bilateral VUR
- Ring-like constriction of vesical neck (detrusor muscle hypertrophy)
- *UB:* Thickened walls with trabeculations/sacculations.

Urethral Atresia

Exceedingly rare and is usually associated with renal dysplasia.

Urethral Dysplasia

- Entire urethra is dysplastic and this is associated with dysplasia of kidneys
- Suprapubic catheter is required to outline the urethra on MCU—thin line of contrast in the region of urethra but no normal anatomical landmarks can be distinguished.

Anterior Urethral Diverticulum

- Saccular, wide-necked ventral expansion of the anterior urethra, usually at the penoscrotal junction
- During micturition, the diverticulum expands with urine and obstructs the urethra.

Urethral Stricture

Causes: Infective, trauma, and instrumentation.
- Most common infective cause is gonorrhea. Postgonococcal strictures are several centimeter in length and involve bulbous urethra. Associated filling of glands of Littre and Cowper is seen during MCU.

Traumatic Stricture

Most common site is both prostatic and membranous urethra. Usually associated with pelvic fractures.

Urethral Calculus (Fig. 7.10)

- Rare and happens to be present in urethra during passage from the bladder
- Urethral calculus is so characteristic in position that the triangle is made from plain radiograph
- RGU and MCU provide definitive information as to the relationship of the radiopacity to urethra
- *Hourglass calculus:* Occupies bladder and prostatic urethra.

Acquired Bladder Neck Stricture

Formation of scar tissue at vesical neck can cause the following: Suprapubic/previous perineal/transurethral prostatectomy.

RGU: Shows dilatation of the distensible unscarred segments of the anterior and posterior urethra and visualization of contracted neck of bladder.

Bladder Calculi (Fig. 7.11)

- Arise as a result of stasis, infection, FB, or can descend from the kidney
- There are usually triple phosphate stones or uric acid mixed with urate

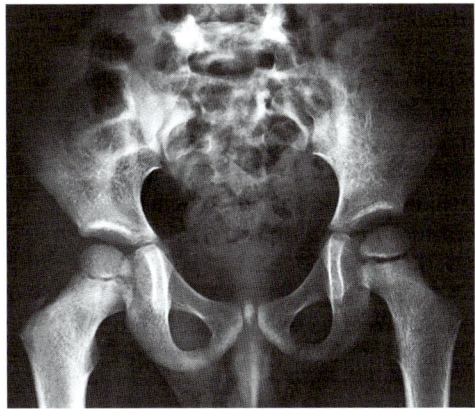

Fig. 7.10: Anteroposterior (AP) radiograph of pelvis shows calculus in posterior urethra.

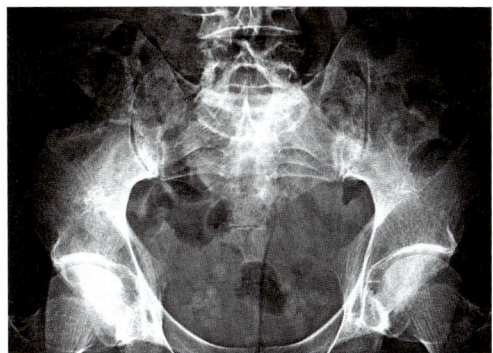

Fig. 7.11: Anteroposterior radiograph of pelvis shows vesical calculi.

- *X-ray:* Faceted/star-shaped/laminated calculus
- *US:* Echogenic focus with postacoustic shadowing.

  Feature of obstructive uropathy—thickened, trabeculated urinary bladder with hydroureteronephrosis.

Fungal Ball

In immunocompromised and diabetic patients, numerous hyphae within the urinary bladder unite to form a fungus ball, leading to bladder outlet obstruction.

- Fungus ball is associated with alternating lucent and opaque irregular laminations owing to gas formation
- It may be seen as mobile-filling defect during IVU or cystography.

Bladder Tumors

- *Epithelial:* Most common is TCC; squamous cell carcinoma and adenocarcinoma are rare.
- *Nonepithelial:*
  - *Benign:* Leiomyoma, fibroma
  - *Malignant:* Leiomyosarcoma, rhabdomyosarcoma.
  - *Most common site:* Around trigone and posterolateral wall of urinary bladder
  - *Cystogram:* Well-demarcated filling defect with lobulated margins
  - *US:* Nonmobile mass lesion/focal wall thickening.

- *CT:* Useful for detection of perivesical extension, invasion.
- *MRI:* Visceral and pelvic lymph node involvement.

Rhabdomyosarcoma

Constitutes about one-eighth of the childhood solid tumors.
- Peak period of incidence is 1–8 years
- Bladder is the most common site of rhabdomyosarcoma
- In males, tumor typically arises from the bladder wall or prostate; in females from vagina
- These tumors are quite large at the time of diagnosis and the exact site of origin of these tumors is difficult.

Radiological Features
- Lobulated soft tissue density mass in the bladder base or as echogenic soft tissue projecting into urinary bladder on US.
- Once diagnosed—chest X-ray, 99^m Tc-MDP bone scan and CT for staging.

Bladder-Sphincter Dyssynergia

Caused by asynchronous opening of the bladder neck with the detrusor contraction producing characteristic high-voiding pressure and low-flow rates.

Diagnosis Established by Videocystometrography
- Bladder neck opens slightly at first, but then widens further as the detrusor pressure falls
- Eventually patients develop hypertrophied bladder which is unable to overcome bladder outlet obstruction and decompensated obstruction.

Neuropathic Lesions of Bladder
- *Suprasacral cord lesion*:
  - Injuries to cerebral/pontine micturition area.
  - Loss of voluntary detrusor control and uncoordinated voiding. If bladder dysuria is also positive—detrusor contracts against a closed sphincter.
  - Diagnosis made by VCMG. On cystogram—UB is contracted, trabeculated, and thick-walled "pine cone bladder".
- *Damage to sacral/peripheral nerves:* Disrupts the vesical parasympathetic nerve supply
  - Underactive/non-acontractile bladder muscles
  - Large capacity bladder with smooth wall
  - Need to be evacuated by manual compression/abdominal straining and intermittent catheterization.

Complications

Vesicoureteral reflux (VUR), recurrent UTI, and stone formation.

Prune-Belly Syndrome

Caused by triad of deficient abdominal musculature, undescended testes, and urinary tract dysplasia.

Proposed Etiology
- Fetal urethral level obstruction which resolves in later gestation.
- Early mesenchymal developmental arrest.
- Protuberant abdomen.
- Small kidneys with minimal dilatation of PCS.
- Upper ureters are mildly dilated; lower ureters are tortuous and show disproportionate dilatation.
- Posterior urethra is markedly dilated prominently with a typical conical narrowing with poor stream in the distal urethra.
- Urinary bladder is of large volume, irregularly-shaped, thin walled, and with wide neck.

Ectopic Ureterocele

- This is a saccular dilatation of the intramural portion of the ureter as it passes through the bladder wall, which results because of the narrowed opening of the ectopic ureter
- Ectopic ureter most commonly occurs with the upper moiety of a kidney

- An ectopic ureterocele opening into the urethra, bladder neck, on vestibule—results in bladder outlet obstruction.

Radiological Features

Dilated ureter with small hydronephrotic upper pole moiety.
- Ureteroceles can be seen on ultrasound and on IVU show a characteristic "cobra head" sign—caused by contrast medium pooling in the ureterocele, which is surrounded by halo of radiolucent ureterocele wall of bladder mucosa.

TESTICULAR TUMORS

- Adult testes are ovoid glands measuring 3–5 cm in length, 2–4 cm in width, and 2–3 cm in anteroposterior diameter. Weight ranges from 12.5 grams to 19 grams
- Epididymis is posterolateral to testis, 6–7 cm in length divided into head (10–12 mm diameter), body (4 mm), and tail.

Differential Diagnosis of Testicular Tumors

- *Primary testicular tumors:*
  - *Germ cell tumors:* Seminoma
    - Nonseminomatous germ cell tumors (NSGCT)
  - *Embryonal carcinoma:* Choriocarcinoma
    - Teratoma
    - Yolk sac/Endodermal sinus tumor
    - Tumors of more than one histological type
    - Teratoma and embryonal cell carcinoma
    - Choriocarcinoma and any other type
  - *Tumors of gonadal stroma:*
    - Sertoli cell
    - Leydig cell
    - Granulosa cell
    - Undifferentiated
    - Combination
- *Secondary testicular tumors:*
  - Lymphoma
  - Leukemia
  - Nonlymphomatous metastasis (Lung and prostate)
- *Benign/miscellaneous lesions of testis:*
  - Tunica albuginea cyst
  - Intratesticular cyst
  - Tubular ectasia of rete testis
  - Cystic dysplasia
  - Epidermoid cyst
  - Abscess.

Germ Cell Tumors (95%)

Clinically patient presents with a palpable painless mass, chronic pain, or sense of heaviness. 15% cases have acute symptoms of pain following traumatic hematoma. Rarely patient presents with signs of distant metastasis (NSGCT).
- *Seminomas:* Accounts for 40% of testicular tumors. Peak prevalence is in the 4th decade
- *Ultrasound:* Well-circumscribed homogeneous hypoechoic mass
- *Multiple calcification (1–2 mm):* May be seen in one-third cases
- As tumor enlarges, it becomes heterogeneous (hemorrhage/necrosis)
- *Burnt-out seminoma:* Primary testicular tumor is not identified as a discrete mass despite a large tumor burden elsewhere in the body
- Seminomas are most common tumor type in cryptorchid testis
- *MR:* Lobulated homogeneous, intermediate SI on T2WI
- *NSGCT:* Peak prevalence is in the 2nd–3rd decades
- More likely to occur as combination of different histotypes rather than as isolated pure form
- More likely to be locally advanced and have a higher likelihood of metastases than seminomas
- *Ultrasound:* Heterogeneous and poorly defined
- *Calcification:* 50% cases
- *MR:* Heterogeneous with areas of high and low SI or T2WI

- Endodermal sinus tumor and teratomas are the most common tumors of infancy and early childhood.

Stromal Tumors (3–5%)

- 25% of these occur in children. Rest occurs between 20 years and 50 years
- It is not possible to differentiate between the different stromal or between stromal and germ cell tumors radiologically
- Most common stromal tumor is Leydig cell tumor
- Associated with gynecomastia (30%) (androgen/estrogen production)
  - Impotence
  - Loss of libido
  - Precocious puberty.

On ultrasound, these tumors are usually small, solid, and hypoechoic.

Spread of Testicular Tumors

- *Lymphatic:* Upper retroperitoneal, retrocrural, mediastinal, and supraclavicular lymph node
- Pelvic lymphadenopathy is less common and is suggestive of penetration of testicular capsule
- *Hematogeneous:* Lung, liver, brain, and bone.

Lymphomas

- Most common secondary testicular neoplasm. Peak age of diagnosis is 60–70 years
- Testicular involvement occurs in 0.3% cases of lymphoma (NHL)
- Most common cause of bilateral testicular tumor
- Majority of lymphomas are homogeneous, hypoechoic, and diffusely replace the testis. Focal hypoechoic lesions are rare.

Leukemia

- Second most common testicular metastatic tumor
- Testis acts as a sanctuary site for leukemic cells during chemotherapy because of blood gonadal barrier that inhibits concentration of chemotherapeutic agents. 64% cases of acute leukemia and 25% chronic leukemia show testicular involvement
- *Characterized by:* Diffuse infiltration producing diffusely enlarged hypoechoic testes.

Other Metastases

Uncommon occurs from lung and prostate and rarely kidney, stomach, colon, pancreas, and melanoma.
- Commonly multiple and bilateral (15%)
- Hypoechoic but may be echogenic/complex in appearance.

Cyst of Tunica Albuginea

- Located within the tunica; usually on anterior and lateral aspects of testes
- 5th and 6th decades
- Patient is asymptomatic, cystic lesion is 2–5 mm in size.

Intratesticular Cyst

- Simple cyst filled with clear serous fluid that varies in size between 2 mm and 18 mm.
- Probably originates from the rete testis possibly secondary to posttraumatic/postinflammatory stricture formation.

Tubular Ectasia of Rete Testes

- Usually associated with epididymal obstruction secondary to inflammation or traumatic lesions
- Characterized by variable-sized cystic lesion in the region of the mediastinum testis with no associated soft tissue abnormality and no flow on color flow Doppler imaging
- May be bilateral and associated with spermatocele.

Cystic Dysplasia

- Rare; seen in infants and young children
- Embryologic defect preventing connection of the tubules of the rete testes and efferent ductules
- Characterized by multiple interconnecting cyst of varying size and shape separated by fibrous stroma
- Renal agenesis/dysplasias frequently coexist with cystic dysplasias.

Urogenital System

Epidermoid Cyst
- Benign tumor of germ cell origin
- Occurs at any age, most frequently 2nd–4th decades
- Well-defined hypoechoic solid masses with echogenic capsule, internal echogenic contents may be present.

Abscess
- Results from complication of epididymo-orchitis, missed testicular torsion, gangrenous/infected tumor, and primary pyogenic orchitis
- Common infectious causes are mumps, smallpox, scarlet fever, influenza, typhoid, sinusitis, osteomyelitis, and appendicitis
- *Ultrasound:* Enlarged testicle containing a fluid-filled mass with hypoechoic/mixed echogenic areas
- *Complications:* Rupture pyocele/fistula to the skin.

SEMINAL VESICLE CALCIFICATION

Seminal vesicles are paired symmetric organs, present along the posterior aspect of prostate being separated from it by a fat plane.

These are accessory reproductive organs of males and there duct fuses with the vas to make the ejaculatory duct which opens on the verumontanum of posterior urethra.

Methods of Investigation
- *Plain X-ray:* These may sometimes show calcifications in the seminal vesicles, which may be confused to be of bladder origin. The calcifications may be seen as either specks of scattered calcification or mushroom shaped.
- *USG:* They appear as bilaterally symmetrical structure on the posterior and superior aspect of prostate and are normally heterogeneous in appearance.
- *CT:* They are seen as lobulated extraperitoneal pouches located superior to the prostate gland between the bladder and the rectum.
- *MRI:* They are seen as convoluted tubular structures. The seminal fluid within their lumen results in high-signal intensity on T2-weighted images; these lumens are surrounded by low-signal intensity of the tubular walls. MR imaging with endorectal coils provides excellent images.

Differential Diagnosis
- *Diabetes mellitus:* This is seen either as an incidental finding in a known case of diabetes mellitus (DM) or may masquerade as obstruction and with subsequent enlargement of the gland, leading either subfertility or infertility.
- *Chronic infections:* These include:
    - Tuberculosis.
    - Schistosomiasis.
    - Chronic UTI.
    - Syphilis.

  Calcification of seminal vesicle may be seen in either of the earlier diseases and is usually secondary to the involvement of either the urinary system, i.e. the kidneys, ureters, and bladder or secondary to prostatitis. The primary changes in the earlier organs give a clue to the real etiology of the calcification.
- Tubercular seminal vesicle calcifications may present with changes of renal tuberculosis (calcifications, calyceal cutoff sign, calyceal diverticulae, putty kidney, multiple ureteric strictures, and a small capacity thimble bladder). Changes of tubercular prostatitis may also be seen (abscesses, hypoechogenicity, and hemospermia calcifications)
- Schistosomiasis classically presents as bladder wall calcification, which may extend to involve the ureters but never the PCS. This calcification may secondarily also involve the prostate and seminal vesicle
- *Idiopathic:* This is by far the most common cause of seminal vesicle calcification, but may, however, present clinically as either hemospermia, ejaculatory duct obstruction, subfertility, or infertility. The diagnosis is that of exclusion.

DIFFERENTIAL DIAGNOSIS OF ABNORMAL NEPHROGRAMS

- *Dense persistent nephrogram with slow onset:*
    - Acute ureteral obstruction
    - Acute renal failure
    - Systemic hypotension
    - Renal vein thrombosis
    - Partial renal artery occlusion.
- *Dense persistent nephrogram with rapid onset:*
    - Acute renal failure
    - Hypotension secondary to contrast injection.
- *Persistent faint nephrogram:*
    - Acute renal failure
    - Chronic renal failure
    - Acute pyelonephritis.
- *Persistent dense nephrogram:*
    - Contrast nephropathy.
- *Rim nephrogram:*
    - Severe hydronephrosis
    - Acute complete arterial occlusion.
- *Striated urographic nephrogram:*
    - Acute ureteral obstruction
    - Infantile PCKD
    - Medullary sponge kidney
    - Medullary tubular ectasia.
- *Absent nephrogram:*
    - Sudden complete arterial occlusion
    - Sudden complete venous occlusion
    - Sudden complete long-standing ureteral occlusion
    - Acute renal failure
    - Acute cortical necrosis.
- *Inhomogeneous arteriographic nephrogram:*
    - Catheter-induced arteriospasm
    - *Small vessel disease:*
        - Nephrosclerosis
        - Necrotizing angiitis
        - Wegener's granulomatosis
        - PAN—polyarteritis nodosa.
- *Moth-eaten nephrogram:*
    - Scleroderma
    - Acute renal failure
    - Acute pyelonephritis
    - Early adult PCKD
    - Renal vein thrombosis.

FILLING DEFECT IN THE BLADDER

- *Neoplasm*: Majority are TCC. Other masses simulating carcinoma of bladder include:
    - Carcinoma prostate or rectum or seminal vesicle
    - Metastasis
    - Pheochromocytoma
    - Leiomyoma
    - Lymphoma
    - Malakoplakia.
- *Prostate*: Seen as impression on the floor of bladder.
- *Blood clot*:
    - Usually posttraumatic
    - Seen as filling defect.
- *Instrument*:
    - Urethral or suprapubic catheter
    - Can be confirmed sonographically.
- *Calculus*:
    - Many are nonopaque.
- *Ureterocele*:
    - It is the saccular dilatation of the intrarenal portion of a ureter as it passes through the bladder wall. Resulting from a narrowed opening of the ureteric orifice.
- *Schistosomiasis:*
    - There is calcification of the bladder wall which is about 1–3 mm wide.
- *Fungal ball*:
    - Appearance of a gas-filled, laminated rounded mass is diagnostic.
- *Malakoplakia*:
    - It is an inflammatory condition usually due to *Escherichia coli* infection. Radiographically a smooth, oval, or round filling defect is seen in the bladder.
- *Endometriosis*.

CARCINOMA PROSTATE

Anatomy

Prostate is a male accessory reproductive organ situated below the base of the bladder and surrounds the prostatic urethra, which runs through the peripheral zone. It is a pyramidal organ with its base directed upward. The normal

gland consists of glandular and nonglandular elements surrounded by a fibromuscular capsule. The basic architecture of prostate can be divided as follows:
- *Lobar anatomy:* The prostate is said to be composed of anterior, posterior, and median lobes
- *Zonal anatomy:* This is the anatomy revealed after anatomic dissection of prostate. It describes prostate to be composed of the following four glandular zones surrounding the prostatic urethra:
    1. *Peripheral zone* is the largest glandular zone containing approximately 70% of the prostatic glandular tissue and it is this zone that is the source of most prostatic cancers. It surrounds the distal urethral segment and is separated from the transition zone and central zone by the surgical capsule. It occupies the posterior, lateral, and apical region of the prostate.
    2. *Transition zone* contains approximately 5% of prostatic glandular tissue. It consists of two small glandular areas located adjacent to the proximal urethral segment. It is the site of origin of BPH. The verumontanum bounds the transition zone caudally.
    3. *Central zone* constitutes approximately 25% of the glandular tissue. It is located at the prostatic base. The ducts of the vas deferens and seminal vesicles enter the central zone, and the ejaculatory duct passes through it. It is relatively resistant to disease processes.
    4. The periurethral glands form about 1% of the glandular volume. They are embedded in the longitudinal smooth muscle of proximal urethra
- The prostaticovesical arteries arising from the internal iliac arteries supply the prostate. The prostate is a very vascular structure. The lymphatic drainage of the prostate is thus via the pelvic nodes to the internal iliac group
- *Incidence:* The prostate cancer is the second most common malignancy in males being superseded only by the carcinoma bronchus. It is said to be recognized in 35% of males above 45 years of age at autopsies. One out of 11 males will develop prostate cancer
- *Risk factors:* Advancing age, presence of testes, cadmium exposure, and animal fat intake.
- *Histopathology:* The prostatic carcinoma is usually an adenocarcinoma.

Premalignant Changes
- Prostatic intraepithelial neoplasia (PIN) is the lesion frequently associated with invasive carcinoma either next to it or elsewhere in the gland
- Atypical adenomatous hyperplasia leading to frank adenocarcinoma
- *Spread:* Mainly blood-borne along the neurovascular bundle.
- *Grading:* Gleason score 2–10. This is histopathological grading of prostatic carcinoma
    - 1, 2, and 3 glands surrounded by one row of epithelial cells.
    - 4 absence of complete gland formation.
    - 5 sheets of malignant cells.
- Low numbers on Gleason's score refer to well differentiated, high numbers to anaplastic tumors.

Categories
- *Latent:* Discovered at autopsy of a patient without signs or symptoms referable to the prostate (26–73%)
- *Incidental:* Discovered in 6–20% of specimens obtained during TURP for clinically benign BPH
- *Occult:* Found at biopsy of metastatically involved bone lesions/lymph nodes in a patient without symptoms of prostatic disease
- *Clinical:* Cancer detected by digital rectal examination based on induration, irregularity, or nodule
- *Prostate specific antigen:* Prostate specific antigen is a glycoprotein produced by

prostatic epithelium and it may be elevated in cases of carcinoma. Monoclonal radioimmunoassay is most commonly used and the normal values range from 0.1 ng/mL to 4 ng/mL.
- Cancers of less than 1 mL volume usually do not elevate PSA.
- Cancers with PSA levels of less than 10 ng/mL are usually confined to gland.
- 19% of prostate cancers do not elevate PSA.
- 16% of normal men have PSA more than 4 ng/mL.
- Benign conditions may also elevate PSA like BPH, prostatitis, and PIN.
- PSA levels may also be used in posttreatment screening of patients for disease recurrence.

Staging

American Urological Association system modified Jewett–Whitmore staging is used most commonly in the following cases:
- *No palpable lesion:*
  - A1 focal well-differentiated tumor less than 1.5 cm or less than 5% of resected tissue
  - A2 diffuse poorly-differentiated tumor more than 5% of chips from TURP specimen.
- *Palpable tumor confined to prostate:*
  - B1 lesion less than 1.5 cm in diameter confined to one lobe
  - B2 lesion more than 1.5 cm involving more than one lobe.
- *Localized tumor with capsular involvement:*
  - C1 capsular invasion
  - C2 capsular penetration
  - C3 seminal vesicle involvement.
- *Distant metastasis:*
  - D1 involvement of pelvic nodes
  - D2 distant nodes involved
  - D3 metastasis to bones, soft tissue, and organs.

American Joint Committee on Cancer Staging: AJCC or TNM Staging
- T0 No evidence of primary tumor
- T1 Clinically inapparent nonpalpable nonvisible tumor:
  - T1a less than three microscopic foci of cancer/less than 5% of resected tissue
  - T1b more than three microscopic foci of cancer/more than 5% of resected tissue
  - T1c tumor identified by needle biopsy.
- T2 Tumor clinically present + confined to prostate:
  - T2a tumor involves half of a lobe or less
  - T2b tumor involves more than half of one lobe
  - T2c tumor involves both lobes of any size but confined to prostate.
- T3 Extension through prostatic capsule:
  - T3a unilateral extracapsular extension
  - T3b bilateral extracapsular extension
  - T3c invasion of seminal vesicle.
- T4 Tumor fixed/invading adjacent structures other than seminal vesicles:
  - T4a invasion of bladder neck, external sphincter, and rectum
  - T4b invasion of levator ani muscle and/or fixed to pelvic wall.
- N Involvement of regional lymph nodes:
  - N1 metastasis in single lymph node less than 2 cm
  - N2 metastasis in single node more than 2 cm and less than 5 cm/multiple lymph nodes affected
  - N3 metastasis in lymph nodes more than 5 cm.
- M Distant metastasis:
  - M1a nonregional lymph nodes
  - M1b bone
  - M1c other sites.

Diagnostic Workup

Diagnosis is usually established by prostate biopsy guided by:
- Digital rectal examination
- Transrectal US.

In most cases, however, the diagnosis is established by histopathological examination of prostatic tissue obtained after TURP. After the establishment of the diagnosis, the standard staging workup includes:

- Digital rectal examination
- Serum acid phosphatase
- PSA levels
- Cell ploidy
- Bone scan
- *Cross-sectional imaging*: It includes US, CT, and MRI which are used to determine the local extent of the tumor and identify the operative candidates.

Prostate Imaging

Ultrasound

- With the advent of high frequency transducers (5–8 MHz) and transrectal approach, the zonal anatomy of the prostate can be identified
- On sonography, it is more useful to separate the prostate into a peripheral zone and inner gland which encompasses the transition and central zone and the periurethral glandular area
- A nonglandular region on the anterior surface of the prostate is termed as the anterior fibromuscular stroma
- The surgical capsule that separates the peripheral zone from the inner gland is identified as a hyperechoic band
- The seminal vesicles are identified as paired, relatively hypoechoic, and multiseptated structures surrounding the rectum cephalad to the base of the prostate gland
- The anterior urethra and its surrounding smooth muscle and glandular area appear relatively hypoechoic
- On coronal imaging, the junction of the hypoechoic periurethal area with the verumontanum creates an appearance resembling the Eiffel tower
- The peripheral zone has a uniform echogenicity
- The ejaculatory ducts are seen often coursing through the central zone from the seminal vesicles and joining the urethra at the verumontanum
- The prostate with the periprostatic fat is usually sharply defined. Hyperechoic structures within are most characteristic of fat, corpora amylacea, or calculi
- The sonographic appearance of most prostatic cancers is usually hypoechoic or mixed. Small cancers are usually hypoechoic
- The hypoechoic lesions have less stromal fibrosis and grade lower on the Gleason grades
- Hyperechogenicity in a cancer is the result of desmoplastic reaction; few extensive large cancers may also have hyperechoic appearance
- A significant number of prostatic cancers are isoechoic and thus difficult to detect and so the indirect signs like glandular asymmetry and capsular bulging may be indicative
- When the tumor replaces the entire peripheral zone, it will often be less echogenic than the inner gland which is the reversal of normal echo pattern
- When the entire gland affected by hyperplasia is replaced by tumor, the echogenicity becomes very inhomogeneous
- Sonographic staging allows for separation of those patients with macroscopic local extension into the periprostatic fat, seminal vesicle, or local lymph nodes from those with disease confined to the prostate gland
- Large tumors can be easily seen to extend to the outside of the capsule as a result of loss of symmetry and capsular irregularity
- Seminal vesicle extension is defined sonographically by enlargement, cystic dilatation, asymmetry, anterior displacement, hyperechogenicity, and loss of seminal vesicle beak
- Sonographic staging is more sensitive than CT for both local and periprostatic structures and lymph nodes.

Computed Tomography Scan

- Oral contrast opacification of small and large bowel is essential
- Positive contrast in the form of either 2% oral barium suspension or diluted water-soluble contrast media can be used
- Negative contrast in the form of plain water can also be used
- The oral contrast can be given the night before to opacify large bowel or an on-table contrast enema may also be used to opacify the rectum and large bowel

- Contrast is also given 45 minutes before examination to opacify small bowel. Both plain non-IV and post-IV contrast scans are taken in spiral mode
- Prostate is visualized as a musculoglandular organ situated between the bladder base above and the pelvic diaphragm below
- Computed tomography cannot reliably differentiate stage A tumors from stage B tumors. CT stage criteria are thus stage B or less, tumor confined to prostate; stage C, extracapsular tumor extension to involve the periprostatic fat, seminal vesicles, bladder, rectum, obturator internus muscle; stage D1, pelvic nodes greater than 1.5–2.0 cm in diameter; stage D2, enlarged lymph nodes above aortic bifurcation, bone metastasis, or extrapelvic metastases
- Computed tomography is also not an effective technique to differentiate stage B from stage C tumors. CT is most useful in evaluating advanced bulky disease (stage D1 to D2) with gross objective findings
- The most common signs of advanced disease are extraprostatic soft tissue masses invading the posterior bladder base or seminal vesicles (stage C). Associated pelvic (stage D1) and para-aortic (stage D2) lymph node metastases are usually easy to detect because they are large and multiple. Bone metastases should be evaluated on appropriate window and level settings.

Magnetic Resonance Imaging

- The prostate gland is best studied by using endorectal coils or by using pelvic multicoil arrangement
- T2-weighted images display the zonal anatomy of the prostate to the best advantage; acquisition in the axial and coronal or oblique coronal planes is usually most desirable
- T1-weighted images are important for the assessment of the integrity of the periprostatic fat and neurovascular bundle, and for the identification of sites of hemorrhage
- The normal prostate has a homogeneous low to intermediate signal on T1-weighted images
- Zonal anatomy can be demonstrated on T2 images comprising a low signal central zone and a higher signal peripheral zone
- The transition and central zone appear of similar signal intensity and are thus termed as central gland
- The periprostatic venous plexus can be visualized as a thin rim of higher signal intensity anterolateral to the peripheral zone
- Denonvilliers' fascia can be observed on sagittal images separating the prostate from the rectum
- The neurovascular bundle is sited posterolaterally at 5 and 7 o'clock positions on transverse section of prostate
- A normal appearing prostate gland on MRI does not exclude the presence of tumor and heterogeneity of the gland is a common nonspecific finding
- Magnetic resonance imaging is often undertaken for staging after a positive biopsy, which can lead to artifacts from hemorrhage and edema
- On T1-weighted images, a carcinoma is usually isointense to the normal gland
- On T2-weighted images (including fat suppressed), the majority of tumors appear low signal contrasted by the high signal from the peripheral zone, but this is not a specific finding
- Macroscopic capsular penetration can be assessed on MRI as focal thickening or bulging of capsule
- Periprostatic infiltration can be demonstrated on T1 images as a low signal within the periprostatic fat or as an intermediate signal using T2 fat suppressed scans
- Extension to seminal vesicles is best demonstrated on T2 transverse and coronal scans and to rectum and bladder on transverse and sagittal scans
- For the detection of adenopathy T1 images are required. MRI can detect bone metastases also

- Postcontrast (gadolinium-chelate) enhanced imaging shows prostatic cancer as enhancing more than the surrounding tissue but becoming isointense on delayed scans
- Magnetic resonance spectroscopy, also known as chemical shift imaging, is an emerging tool in the early detection of prostatic cancer. This relies on the changes in the emitted signal produced by a higher level of choline in carcinomas as compared to BPH
- *Bone scintigraphy:* This is the most sensitive method of detecting occult bone metastases
- *Screening:* It is postulated that all men above the age of 50 years should be screened yearly for the presence of carcinoma prostate by digital rectal examination and PSA levels.

Treatment

- Watchful waiting in patients with incidentally discovered carcinoma on TURP specimens and ages above 80 years
- Radical prostatectomy for disease confined to capsule + life expectancy of more than 15 years
- Radiation therapy either to patients with disease confined to capsule and life expectancy of less than 15 years or to disease outside capsule but with no spread
- Hormonal therapy (orchidectomy, diethylstilbestrol, and leuprolide acetate) for widely metastatic disease
- Cryosurgery
- Chemotherapy.

Conclusion

Prostatic carcinoma is the second most common carcinoma affecting males. It is thus desirable to have an effective screening program to identify the disease in its early stages. Digital rectal examination and PSA levels in the serum are currently used as screening procedures. Imaging only plays a secondary role in the management in deciding the correct line of treatment and identifying the cases fit for surgery. MRI currently is the imaging modality of choice for staging of carcinoma prostate with USG, especially TRUS being the second choice and CT only useful in advanced disease and for identifying bony metastasis.

THE PROSTATE

Normal Anatomy

Prostate gland is a flattened conical structure oriented in the coronal plane.
- Length of normal prostate is 2.5–3 cm
- Transverse diameter at base is 4–4.5 cm
- Thickness is 2–2.5 cm
- Normal weight is 20–25 g.

Prostatic Anatomy (Figs. 7.12A to E)

Lobar Anatomy

- Five lobular divisions
- The concept of median lobe is useful in evaluation of patients termed with BPH but this lobar anatomy is not useful for evaluating CA prostate.

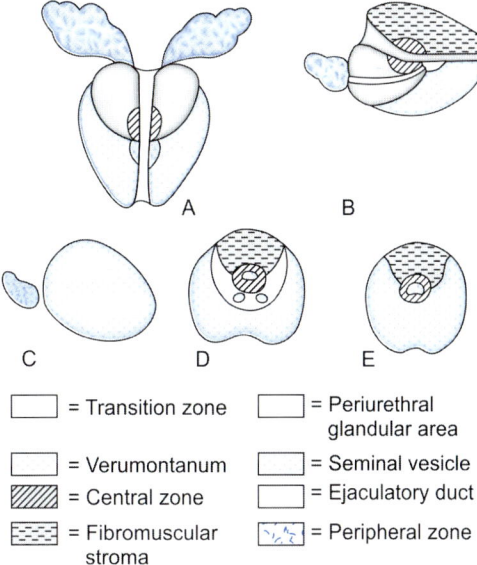

Figs. 7.12A to E: Diagram of prostate zonal anatomy. (A) Coronal section, midprostate; (B) Sagittal midline section; (C) Sagittal section, lateral prostate, and seminal vesicle; (D) Axial section, prostatic base. Paired ejaculatory ducts are seen posterior to urethra and periurethral glandular area. Peripheral zone encompasses most of posterior and lateral aspects of gland; and (E) Axial section, apex of gland showing mostly peripheral zone, and urethral and periurethral glandular area.

Zonal Anatomy
- Four glandular zones
  - One anterior lobe
  - Peripheral zone
  - One median lobe
  - Transition zone
  - One prostatic lobe
  - Central zone
  - Two lateral lobes
  - Periurethral glandular area
- A nonglandular region on anterior surface of prostate is anterior fibromuscular stroma.

Sonographic Anatomy
- Ultrasonography can differentiate prostate into a peripheral zone and inner gland comprising transition zone, central zone, and periurethral glandular area.

Peripheral Zone
- Contains 70% of prostatic glandular tissue
- Occupies posterior, lateral, and apical regions of prostate and surrounds distal urethral segments
- Ducts of peripheral zone drain in distal urethra
- It is the source of most prostate cancers
- It is separated from inner gland by the surgical capsule which is often hyperechoic due to corpora amylacea or calcifications.

Transition Zone
- Contains 5% of prostatic glandular tissue
- Located adjacent to proximal urethral segment
- Its ducts drain in proximal urethra at the level of verumontanum
- Site of origin of benign prostatic hyperplasia.

Central Zone
- Constitutes 25% of glandular tissue
- Located at prostatic base
- Its ducts drain in proximal urethra
- Relatively resistant to the disease process.

Periurethral Glands
- Form 1% of glandular tissue
- Also known as internal prostatic sphincter.

Adjacent Structures
- *Seminal vesicles*:
  - Seen in bow tie configuration on transaxial view.
  - Echogenicity is similar to or less than that of peripheral zone.
- *Vas deferens*:
  - Located anteromedial to seminal vesicle.

Volumetric measurement of prostate:

$V = \frac{1}{2} (L \times AP \times W)$ where V = Volume
L = Length
AP = Anteroposterior diameter
W = Width

Computed Tomography Anatomy
- Prostate gland is located just posterior to symphysis pubis and anterior to rectum
- Homogeneous soft tissue density on NCCT
- CECT: Peripheral zone may enhance to or lesser degree than central gland
- Zonal anatomy is more evident in older patients and in patients with enlarged gland.

Magnetic Resonance Anatomy
- On T1-weighted segments:
  - Prostate has homogeneous low signal intensity similar to skeletal muscle.
  - Neurovascular bundles are seen posterolateral to prostate gland at 5 o'clock and 7 o'clock positions.
  - Zonal anatomy is not well demonstrated on T1W segments.
  - In postgadolinium T1-weighted images, peripheral zone has a more uniform and cause intense enhancement than central gland.
- T2-weighted sequence:
  - Best for visualizing zonal anatomy.
  - Peripheral zone has a higher signal than central gland due to its more abundant glandular component and more loosely intervening muscle bundles.
  - Anterior fibromuscular band seen as low-signal structure.
  - True (anatomic) capsule of prostate and Denonvillers' fascia are seen as low-signal intensity bands.

- Surgical pseudocapsule can be seen in older patients at the interface between transition and peripheral zones.
- Periprostatic venous plexus seen as high-signal structure around prostate.
- Seminal vesicles look like grapes with high-signal intensity fluid and low-signal intensity walls.

Prostatic Lesions

Agenesis/Hypoplasia
Prostatic and seminal vesicle cysts.

Congenital
- Prostatic utricle cyst
- Müllerian duct cyst
- Seminal vesicle cyst.

Acquired
- Ejaculatory duct cyst
- Retention cyst.

Infection of Prostate
- Acute prostatitis
- Chronic prostatitis
- Prostatic abscess
- Granulomatous prostatitis.

Prostatic Calculi

Tumors of Prostate
- Benign
- BPH
- Malignancy
- Carcinoma.

Prostatic Agenesis/Hypoplasia
- Associated with hypospadias, epispadias, and exstrophy
- The only tissue visualized anterior to rectum is urethra with a thick periurethral muscle.

Prostate and Seminal Vesicle Cysts
- Well-defined smooth-walled anechoic structure with posterior acoustic enhancement
- Has septations/debris, if secondarily infected.

Prostatic Cyst

Prostatic Utricle Cyst
- Always present in midline
- Usually small
- Rarely contains spermatozoa
- May contain calculus
- Associated with other anomalies, e.g. Prune-Belly syndrome, hypospadias, and renal agenesis.

Müllerian Duct Cyst
- May extend from lateral to midline
- Can be large
- Never contain from spermatozoa
- Not associated with other anomalies.

Ejaculatory Cyst
- Usually small
- May contain spermatozoa
- Associated with infertility.

Retention Cyst
Secondary to benign prostatic hypoplasia.

Prostatic Infections

Acute Prostatitis
- Narrowing, elongation or straightening of prostatic urethra on MCU
- Enlarged hypoechoic gland with periprostatic inflammation and increased vascularity.

Chronic Prostatitis
- Reflux can be seen in prostatic ducts
- Focal areas of varying echogenicity are present with ejaculatory duct calcification.

Prostatic Abscess
- Localized hypoechoic in peripheral gland
- Peripheral rim enhancement present on CT.

Granulomatous Prostatitis
Nonspecific: Prostatic urethra elongated in infraverumontanum portion (cf. BPH) is widened (cf. CA prostate).

Specific (Tubercular):
- Features of associated genitourinary tuberculosis in other viscera
- Cavity formation in prostate with hypoechoic areas.

Prostatic Calculi
- Bright echogenic foci in prostate with ± posterior acoustic shadowing
- Corpora amylacea are thought to be precursor.

Types

True or endogenous	Urinary calculi	Exogenous calculi
↓	↓	↓
Develop from acini and ducts	Lodged in prostatic urethra	Form in preexisting abscess cavities of prostate gland

Benign Prostatic Hyperplasia
- *Criteria:* Prostate gland weighing more than 40 g in older men
  - Prostate is visualized in CT sections 2–3 cm or more above pubic symphysis
- Involves transition zone and periurethral glandular tissue
- Prostatic urethra elongated and slit like
- Enlarged prostate bulges in bladder floor with J (fish hook) deformity of ureters on IVU
- Secondary changes are:
  - Bladder trabeculations ± diverticulae and calculi
  - Hydronephrosis and hydroureter.

Carcinoma Prostate
- Involves peripheral zone in 70% cases
- Presents as hypoechoic area in peripheral zone of prostate
- *Criteria for extracapsular extension:*
  - Contour deformity of capsule
  - Irregularity
  - Obliteration of rectocapsular extension
  - Asymmetry or direct involvement of neurovascular bundle
  - Focal capsular retraction or thickening
  - Direct tumor extension in periprostatic fat.
- *Criteria for seminal vesicular invasion:*
  - Loss of angle between seminal vesicle and prostate
  - Direct tumor extension to seminal vesicle.
- Higher chlorine and lower citrate levels are seen in cancerous prostate tissue on proton MR spectroscopy
- Radionuclide bone seen is useful to detect skeletal metastases.

DIFFERENTIAL DIAGNOSIS OF ADRENAL MASS

A. *Neoplastic*
1. Cortical
   - Carcinoma
   - Adenoma
2. Medullary
   - Neuroblastoma
   - Ganglioneuroma
   - Pheochromocytoma
3. Stromal
   - Lipoma
   - Myelolipoma
4. Metastasis.

B. *Others*
1. Granulomas
   - Histoplasmosis
   - Tuberculosis
   - Blastomycosis
2. Bilateral hyperplasia
3. Cysts
4. Hematoma
5. Amyloid

Computed Tomography Features S/O Adrenal Mass
- Absence of normal adrenal gland.
- Mass at superior level of kidneys.
- Downward displacement of kidneys.
- Anterior displacement of IVC, pancreas, and splenic vessels. Positive biochemical test indicating hyperfunctioning of adrenal mass.

Structures Mimicking Left Adrenal Mass
- Upper pole of left kidney.
- *Gastric diverticulum:* Give oral contrast.
- Splenic lobulations/accessory spleen—on intravenous contrast, it enhances to the same level as body of spleen.
- Large mass in the tail of pancreas.
- Give intravenous contrast. Pancreatic mass usually displaces splenic vein posteriorly, whereas adrenal mass displaces it anteriorly.

Salient Features

- *Adrenal cortical carcinoma:*
  - Slow growing tumor
  - 50% nonfunctioning, 50% Cushing's, Conn's, or virilizing syndrome
  - Average size 8–10 cm at diagnosis
  - Average age at onset 45 years
  - *X-ray and IVP:* Show soft tissue shadow of mass, downward displacement of kidney calcifications
  - *USG:* Mixed echogenicity mass with calcifications
  - *CT:* Large mass with heterogeneous enhancement
  - Area of central necrosis
  - Thin capsule rim, calcifications
  - Liver and LN metastasis
  - *MRI:* Mixed intensity on T1 and hyperintense on T2.
- *Adrenal cortical adenoma:*
  - Usually nonfunctioning and symptomless
  - Unilateral, 2–5 cm
  - Variable density
  - Half have soft tissue density and half have low attenuation due to higher lipid content.

  Differential diagnosis with cysts which do not enhance.

Medullary Tumors

- *Neuroblastoma:*
  - Occur in children mostly less than 3 years
  - Present as abdominal mass or with secondaries
  - *X-ray and IVP:* Soft tissue mass with downward displacement of kidney
  - Downward drooping of pelvis and calyces
  - *USG:* Mixed density to echogenic tumor calcifications
  - Cystic areas of necrosis and hemorrhage
  - Encasement of aorta and IVC
  - *CT:* Irregularly-shaped solid mass
  - Soft tissue density with necrosis, calcifications, and hemorrhage
  - Local, distant invasion
  - Crossing of midline is highly suggestive
  - MIBG scan shows increased uptake by primary as well as metastatic tumors.
- *Ganglioneuroma:*
  - More mature form of neurogenic tumor
  - Children, 60% less than 20 years
  - Soft tissue mass with calcifications
  - May invade spinal canal.
- *Pheochromocytoma:*
  - Most common adrenal tumor in clinical practice
  - 90% arise in adrenal medulla
  - *10% ectopic:*
    - Hilum of kidney
    - Aortic bifurcation
    - Bladder wall
    - Mediastinum.
  - S/S—paroxysmal attacks of hypertension headache, sweating, palpitation, anxiety, and 50% have sustained hypertension
  - Elevated urinary VMA or metanephrine level
  - Usually solitary and located on the right side.
  - 10% cases are familial

  "RULE OF TEN"
  - Bilateral
  - Multiple
  - Extra-adrenal
  - Children
  - Malignant

  - Size 2–20 cm average—7 cm
  - *X-ray and IVP:* Soft tissue mass with renal displacement
  - *CT:* Unilateral homogeneous mass more than 2 cm and of soft tissue density
  - Solid with or without cystic areas or entirely cystic
  - Inhomogeneous with denser periphery with central necrosis
  - Enhance markedly to the point of becoming isodense with vascular structures
  - MIBG method of choice in ectopic or recurrent pheochromocytoma
  - Metastasis can occur in LN, bones, liver, and chest in malignant tumor.
    - *Stromal tumors:*
  - *Lipomas and myelolipomas:*
    - Rare nonfunctioning tumors
    - 1–2% incidence
    - Usually small
    - Highly echogenic on USG

- Varying proportion of myeloid and fat tissue
- Well-circumscribed mass with attenuation –30 to –140 HU with frequent foci of calcification.

- Metastasis:
  - Fourth most frequently involved site of blood-borne metastasis
  - Lung > Breast > Thyroid > Colon > metastasis
  - Bilateral adrenal masses in a patient with known primary in absence of hyperfunctioning suggests metastasis
  - In a patient with known malignancy unilateral adrenal mass could be metastasis, carcinoma, or adenoma. So, fine-needle aspiration cytology (FNAC) is a must
  - Metastasis produces unilateral or often bilateral circumscribed soft tissue density mass.

Granulomas

- Infections like tuberculosis, histoplasmosis, and blastomycosis result in solid or cystic mass with calcification
- Unilateral or bilateral.

Adrenal Cysts

- Endothelial
- Pseudocyst
- Epithelial
- Parasitic (hydatid)
- Smooth marginated, well-circumscribed usually U/L, low density mass, and non-enhancing
- Rim of calcification in 15%.

Adrenal Hemorrhage

- Abdominal mass or B/L masses
- Marginal calcification
- Bilateral adrenal hyperplasia
- Diffuse enlargement of adrenals.

PAINLESS HEMATURIA

Definition

Blood cells in urine, whether occult or frank constitute hematuria. *Hematuria* is mostly painless; pain is caused whenever there is obstruction to the outflow of urine (mainly by blood clot or stone, etc.).

To define hematuria more than three red blood cell (RBC)/HPF.

Etiology

- *Lesions in the urinary tract*:
  - Causes in kidney and pelvicalyceal system:
    - Polycystic kidney disease.
    - Acute nephritis; Tuberculosis; Filariasis
    - Angioma; Papilloma; TCC; RCC; Wilms' tumor
    - Essential hematuria.
  - Causes in ureters:
    - Papilloma
    - TCC
    - Pyeloureteritis cystica.
  - Causes in bladder:
    - TCC
    - Papilloma
    - Bilharziasis
    - Filariasis
- *Tuberculosis:*
  - Causes in prostate:
    - Varices caused by BPH
    - Malignancies.
  - Causes in urethra:
    - TCC
    - Angioma.
- *Lesions in adjacent organs*:
  - CA cervix invading the bladder
  - CA rectum
  - PID
  - Retroperitoneal masses pressing over renal vessels.
  - Several vesicle tumors.
- *Systemic causes with secondary renovascular effects*:
  - Hematopoietic causes: Hemophilia; scurvy; Malaria; Purpura; Sickle cell disease.
  - Congestive: Renal vein thrombosis; Right-heart failure.
  - Infarcts: Subacute infective Endocarditis. Myocardial infarction.
  - Collagen vascular diseases.

- Drugs:
  - Sulfonamides
  - Salicylates (in large doses)
  - Anticoagulants
  - Phenolphthalein
  - Urates
  - DFM
  - Chloroquine
  - Pyridium
- *Hematuria-like conditions:*
  - Porphyrinuria
  - Myoglobinuria.

Clinical Features

- Urine normal in appearance
  Known as microscopic hematuria, i.e. more than five RBC/HPF in 2–3 urinalysis.
- Urine of altered color.
- Fever.
- Lump and other signs and symptoms.
- Outflow obstruction.

Pathology

Hematuria

Medical (Renal/glomerular)	Urological (Surgical epithelial)
• Associated with cast	• Associated with no cast
• Associated with proteinuria	• No proteinuria
• Dysmorphic RBC (especially if glomerulus) IgA nephro-pathy—child MPGN—adult	• Rounded eumorphic • RBC • >1/HPF • Abnormal
• Eumorphic rounded RBC	• Eumorphic
• RBC if TID	
• Up to 10 6/24 hours—normal	• Round • Regular
• But >2/HPF—abnormal	• Smooth • Even hemoglobin distribution

- Dysmorphic:
  - Acanthocytes
  - Schistocytes
  - Amylocytes
  - Echinocytes
  - Somatocytes
  - Codocytes
  - Knizocytes
  - It is basically the urological hematuria which is more accessible to radiological diagnosis as the nephrological causes are usually evaluated by laboratory methods.

Radiological Evaluation

Always ask a small question:
- *Is the urine bright red:* Lower urinary tract origin—gross
- *Is the urine smoky:* Upper urinary tract origin—occult

Keep in mind the major causes:
- Malignancies
- Infections
- Stone
- BPH
- Renal parenchymal lesions
- Trauma
- Benign idiopathic.

Always try to reach to two or three possibilities before starting investigation.

X-ray abdomen—28
   CXR—1.4 MSV—28 weeks radiation
X-ray pelvis—24
   CXR—1.2 MSV—24 weeks
IVU—88
   CXR—4.4 MSV—88 weeks
CT abdomen—176
   CXR—8.8 MSV—176 weeks

Plain X-ray

Abdomen

- *Calcified nodes:* Tuberculosis.
- *Cyst wall calcification:* Polycystic kidney disease.
- Evidence of mass lesion.

Chest

- For cardiac evaluation as right heart failure is a cause.
- For looking at any tubercular foci.

Bones

To evaluate and correlate for hemophilia; sickle cell anemia; scurvy; cardiovascular disease; and renal osteodystrophy.

Intravenous Pyelography

- Is always the imaging modality of choice in any patient presenting with hematuria, whether painful or painless.
- Gives a gross global idea about the structure and function of urinary tract.
- Gives a baseline investigation for further comparison.
- Polycystic kidney disease—Swiss cheese nephrogram.
- Spider web pyelogram.
- *Renal cell carcinoma:* Distorted/destroyed/displaced/delayed
  - Pyelogram
  - Nephrogram.
- *Transitional cell carcinoma:* Role of IVP is to r/o multicentricity, to comment on function, and to evaluate back pressure.
- *Renal vein thrombosis:* Increasingly dense nephrogram with delayed pyelogram.
- *Tuberculosis:* Thimble bladder; corkscrew/pipestem ureter; renal cavities/perirenal collection/pyelonephritis.

Barium Examinations

- For example, tuberculosis
- For example, Ca rectum.

Ultrasonography ± CD

- For general survey of KUB even before IVP
- In renovascular diseases.

Computed Tomography Scan

- For retroperitoneal evaluation
- For land marking masses
- For renovascular evaluation.

Magnetic Resonance Imaging

Better imaging modality due to multiplanar capabilities.

Renal Scan

Has only minimal corroborative role.

Arteriovenography

Especially when intervention is contemplated.

Newer Modalities

- Magnetic resonance urography
- Computed tomography
- Endovesicle USG
- Sonourethrography
- Positron emission tomography (PET).

RGU/MCU

Definitive modality for evaluation of UB and urethral lesions.

Computed Tomography Urography

Perlman, 1966
- *Protocol:* Projectional technique
  - Conventional
  - Digital
  - Computed tomography scanned projectional images.
- *Protocol:* Reconstructional technique
  - Two-dimensional (2D)
  - Three-dimensional (3D).
    - Phases almost similar to liver
    - For urothelial lesions conventional > CT URO.

Magnetic Resonance Urography

- An MRCP-like technique—IC T2W single/multislice.
- Gadolinium + T1W.
- Fusion
  - At present reserved for patients who cannot undergo CT URO/IVP—pregnant, pediatric, allergy, and poor renal function
  - Calculus detection is a limitation
  - Fine-needle aspiration cytology
  - BX.

Conclusion

It is always essential to provide from randomizing modality, i.e. the sound followed by IUD/CTs.

Chapter 8

Head, Neck, and Spine

LUCENCY IN THE SKULL VAULT: WITHOUT SCLEROSIS

Neoplastic	Traumatic	Metabolic	Infective
• Multiple myeloma	• Burr hole • Lepto-meningeal cyst	• Hyper-parathy-roidism	• Tuber-culosis • Hydatid • Syphilis • Pyogenic osteomye-litis
• Metastasis			
• Hemangioma			
• Neurofibroma			
• Paget's sarcoma			

Idiopathic—Osteoporosis Circumscripta

Multiple Myeloma

More than 40 years, males:females 2:1, increase of total serum protein because of production of abnormal immunoglobulin. Leukopenia, anemia, abnormal urine protein—Bence Jones protein—50% of hypercalcemia, hypercalciuria, and amyloidosis.

Radiological Features:
- Generalized decrease in bone density, localized area of lucency in red marrow, lesion also seen in mandible, clavicle and scapula.
- Adjacent soft tissue mass.
- Spine—collapse with paravertebral soft tissue mass (IV disks are not affected).
- Pedicle and post-arches are less frequently affected, proximal end of humerus and femur are also affected.

Hemangioma
- Well-circumscribed area of punctate or stellate rare faction without expansion.
- Prominent vascular grooves may present in the vicinity and external carotid arteriography shows a blush.

Neurofibroma

Lucent defect in occipital bone (adjacent to it—lambdoid suture).

Paget's disease in males more than females, elderly.

Most common site—Sacrum and lumbar spine
↓
Skull → pelvis → femur

Osteoporosis circumscripta occurs in the active lytic phase of Paget's disease.
- It starts in the lower part of the frontal and occipital region and can cross suture line.
- Destructive process affecting the outer table and sparing the inner table.

Hyperparathyroidism

Usually pepper-pot skull. Rarely severe enough to cause overt lytic lesions.
- Mandible is a common site for "brown tumors". There may be a loss of lamina dura.
- "Basilar invagination" is a common finding.

Traumatic

"Burr hole"—history of surgery.

Leptomeningeal cyst: Develops after head injury. If dura is torn, the arachnoid membrane can prolapse and the pulsation of cerebrospinal fluid (CSF) can cause progressive widening and scalloping of the fracture line.

Langerhans' Cell Histiocytosis

Proliferation of histiocytic cells, particularly in the bone marrow, the spleen, liver, and lymphatic gland and lungs. Later, cells become swollen with lipid deposit.

Eosinophilic Granuloma

Most mild expression of histiocytosis.
  Age—3–12 years, especially boys.
  Site—any bone (one-fourth in skull)
  Two-thirds—pelvis, skull, and femur.
  RF—translucent areas of bone destruction with sharply defined margins—in active phase. Peripheral sclerosis seen in the healing phase.
  The lesion is having beveled edges difficult to differentiate between destruction of the inner and outer tables.

- Button sequestrum may be seen
- Other RF—spine—solitary lesion in spine, may collapse—leading to vertebra plana
- Most common site is thoracic spine
- Paravertebral soft tissue mass present
- Disk space—maintained
- Long bones—predilection for diaphysis
- Mandible and lamina dura—osteolytic lesion leading to "floating teeth" appearance.

Metastasis—In Adults

Most common site for metastasis—spine, pelvis, and ribs with proximal ends of humerus and femur and less often skull areas correspond to sites of persistent hematopoiesis.

- Primary tumors in male—carcinoma prostate, lung, and kidney.
- In female—breast—two-thirds of cases of bronchial carcinoma develop secondaries—laboratory finding.
- Serum alkaline phosphatase increase in metastasis but normal in multiple myeloma. Serum Ca^{++} increase.
- Ca prostate—prostate-specific antigen (PSA) and acid phosphatase increase.
- Radiological features (RF)—mainly osteolytic, develop in medulla and extended in all directions, destroying the cortex—not much periosteal reaction.
- Soft tissue extension uncommon, multiplicity in pediatric age—especially neuroblastoma and leukemia ± wide suture.
- *Infective*: Tuberculosis—osteomyelitis—skull is a rare site.
- *Pyogenic OM*: Usually direct infection from a frontal sinus or secondary to a compound fracture
- *Syphilis*: Moth-eaten appearance.

LUCENCY IN THE SKULL VAULT: WITH SURROUNDING SCLEROSIS (FLOWCHART 8.1)

- *Fibrous dysplasia (FD)*—unknown pathogenesis.
- Replacement of medullary bone by fibrous tissue.
- Age—3–15 years.
- Most common site—femur, pelvis, skull, mandible, and ribs.
- Two types—(1) monostotic, (2) polyostotic—lesions tend to be unilateral.

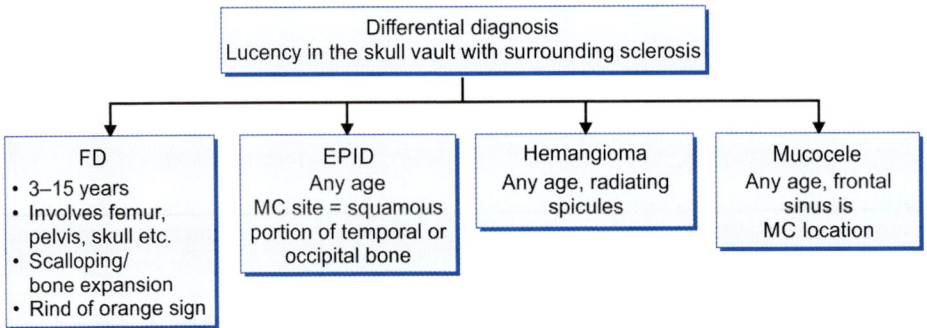

Flowchart 8.1: Lucency in skull vault with surrounding sclerosis.

- RF—cyst-like lesion in the diaphysis or metaphysis with endosteal scalloping ± bone expansion.
- No periosteal new bone.
- Rind sign—thick sclerotic border, ground glass appearance.
- Common site in skull—in skull, FD takes two main forms—sclerotic and cystic.

Sclerotic form: More common, involves the base or facial skeletons which are expanded and dense and sometimes showing ground glass appearance. Most common cause of leontiasis ossea.

Cystic form: Produces a small lesion in skull vault expanding the outer table and giving a blistered appearance.

Developmental

Epidermoid: Thin sclerotic margins with scalloping.

Most common site: Squamous portion of occipital or temporal, although can involve any region.

Intramedullary in origin, so can expand and involve both inner and outer bones. More homogeneous radiolucent center.
- *Meningocele*: Midline defect
- Smooth and sclerotic margins with an overlying soft tissue mass
- Most common site—occipital bone, may occur in the frontal, parietal or basal bones
- *Neoplastic hemangioma:* Rarely has sclerotic margin. Radiating spicules of bone within it
- *Langerhans' cell histiocytosis:* Only a sclerotic margin of it is in the healing phase
- *Infective:* Chronic osteomyelitis—Brodie's abscess—intraosseous abscess surrounded by intense sclerosis.

Mucocele of Frontal Sinus

If the ostium of sinus becomes blocked and infection does not supervene, the sinus fills with mucus—mucus acts as slow growing mass lesion, expanding the sinus and thinning the sinus wall—can give rise to proptosis.

THICKENING OF THE SKULL VAULT

Generalized
- Marble bone disease
- Dystrophia myotonica
- Acromegaly
- Paget's disease
- Cooley's anemia.

Localized
- Meningiomas
- Primary osteosarcoma
- Osteomas
- Ossifying fibromas
- Fibrous dysplasia
- Leontiasis ossea
- Hyperostosis frontalis interna.

Generalized Hyperostosis

Marble Bone Disease
- The bones of the skull base are mainly affected with sclerosis and thickening, mainly in the anterior cranial fossa.
- The cranium is affected to a lesser degree.
- The sphenoid and frontal sinuses and mastoids are under-pneumatized or not at all.
- Neural foramina may encroach upon and blindness results in serious cases.

Dystrophia Myotonica
- They show a thickened skull vault with a small pituitary fossa.

Acromegaly
- Thickened skull vault in association with the enlarged sinuses and prognathous jaw.
- The vault thickening involves both tables and the diploe is encroached upon and difficult to distinguish.

Paget's Disease
- Vault becomes widened and thickened, with alterations in its bony texture. There are also osteomalacic changes and the bones become softer and more pliable, giving rise to platybasia with basilar invagination.
- Skull shows a typical irregular mottled texture to the thickened bone.

Cooley's Anemia
- Generalized thickening of the skull with a characteristic and diagnostic appearance.

- Widening of the diploe.
- Its texture becomes abnormal with radiating linear spicules of the sunray or hairbrush type. Sometimes, the bone change in this type of anemia may be more localized, affecting mainly the frontal region.

Localized Hyperostosis of the Skull

Meningiomas

These commonly invade the bony skull and produce a localized hyperostotic reaction. The diagnosis is often suggested by the classic meningioma site, i.e. parasagittal or sphenoidal ridge.
- Originally the hyperostosis is confined to the inner table but later it may grow through the diploe and outer table and present as a palpable lump.
- When protruding externally, the lesion can sometimes show sunray spicules.
- Other radiological evidence of meningioma such as enlarged vascular markings leading to the lesion or signs of raised intracranial pressure may also be present.
- If the meningioma grows from the sphenoidal ridge into the orbit, it can present with proptosis.

Primary Osteosarcoma

It is very rare but can give rise to localized hyperostosis often with sun ray spicules. It is most common as a complication of Paget's disease.

Osteomas

These can occur in the skull vault when they appear as dense flat ivory nodules growing from the surface.
- More commonly they present as chance findings growing from the wall of the frontal sinus.
- They are usually small—under 1 cm in size.

Ossifying Fibroma

These are relatively rare.
- They most frequently commence in the paranasal sinuses, particularly the antrum.
- They can produce large density calcified masses.

Fibrous Dysplasia

- It is an important cause of localized hyperostosis involving the skull vault, facial bones or skull base.
- It may occur as an isolated lesion or in association with lesions in other bones (polyostotic fibrous dysplasia and Albright syndrome).

Leontiasis Ossea

It is a form of hyperostosis affecting the frontal bones and facial bones and giving rise to severe facial deformity.

Hyperostosis Frontalis Interna

- Mysterious condition frequently seen in adult skulls.
- Occurs almost exclusively in postmenopausal women.
- It is characterized by irregular nodular thickening of the inner table of the skull vault, mainly the frontal bone. The lesions are characteristically bilateral and symmetric and spare the midline.

GENERALIZED INCREASE IN DENSITY OF SKULL VAULT

Idiopathic	–	Paget's disease
		Fibrous dysplasia, myelosclerosis
Congenital	–	Osteopetrosis
		Pyknodysostosis
		Pyle's disease
Metabolic	–	Renal osteodystrophy
		Fluorosis
Neoplasm	–	Sclerotic metastases
		Meningioma
Endocrinal	–	Acromegaly
Hematological	–	Chronic hemolytic anemia, phenytoin therapy

- Idiopathic—myelosclerosis—peak age—6th decade, cause is unknown.
  Sex—both the sexes are equally affected.
  Pathologically—obliteration of marrow by fibrosis or bony sclerosis—leading to normochromic and normocytic anemia.

Hemopoiesis in spleen and liver, so they are enlarged.
RF—bone sclerosis in 40% of cases.
Most common pattern—diffuse but may be patchy.
- Marrow diameter decreased and blurred CMD.
- Lucent areas due to fibrous tissue.
- One-third cases show periosteal new bone.

Fibrous dysplasia—two forms—(1) sclerotic and (2) cystic form, sclerotic form—more common of the two, especially in the polyostotic version.

Site—base and facial skeleton which are expanded and dense.
Most common cause of leontiasis ossea.
Lower density areas (cyst or fibrotic masses) within the sclerotic bones—strong with evidence of fibrous dysplasia.

Paget's Disease

Male more than female, older than 40 years. Skull is involved in two-thirds of cases.
Mixed pattern of sclerosis and lysis is common. An early change is a spotty cotton wool. Increased density of bone and also thickening of vault.
Middle and outer tables are most affected and thickened with coarse trabeculations.

Meningioma

Sclerosis is more marked than expansion and extension from the sphenoid bone into the facial skeleton is much less common.

Metastasis

Irregular lysis or sclerosis and multiplicity prostate and breast are most common. Diffuse osteosclerosis is also seen occasionally in Hodgkin's lymphoma and leukemia and very rarely with multiple myeloma.

Congenital

Osteopetrosis—several types. More severe types are autosomal recessive.
- RF—generalized increased density.
- Skull base are initially affected with sclerosis and thickening.
- Cranium is affected to a lesser degree/sphenoid, frontal, and mastoid are under pneumatized or not at all.
- Neural foramina encroached upon and blindness result in serious cases.

Pyknodysostosis

Autosomal recessive in inheritance. Patients are usually short (<150 cm).
Skull—brachycephaly with wide suture and persistence of open fontanels into adult life.

Wormian Bones

Site—calvarium, base of skull and orbital rims are very dense. Facial bones are small and maxilla is hypoplastic.
Mandible has no angle, it is obtuse.

Other Features

Limbs	–	Increased density of bones Thorax lateral ends of clavicle are hypoplastic. Ribs are dense
Spine	–	Failure of fusion of neural arches, spondylolisthesis Spoon-shaped V bodies
Hand	–	Acro-osteolysis with irregular distal fragments of distal phalanges.

METABOLIC

Renal Osteodystrophy

Bony changes in patients suffering from chronic anemia due to long standing renal disease.
- Osteosclerosis occurs in 25%
- Skull and spine are commonly involved and can look similar to Paget's disease.

Other Features

Secondary hyperparathyroidism—subperiosteal resorption, subchondral resorption, and brown tumors.
- Osteomalacia/rickets
- Osteoporosis

- Aluminum toxicity
- Soft tissue calcification (vascular and periarticular)
- Fractures.

Fluorosis

Chronic ingestion of excessive amount of fluoride results in fluorosis.
- Osteosclerosis is seen with concentration of 8 PPM in drinking water, calvarium is rare site.

Other Features

Osteosclerosis predominantly in axial skeleton.
- Calcification or ossification of ligaments
- Enthesopathy.

Acromegaly

Enlarged frontal sinus, prognathism, enlarged sella, and thick vault.

LOCALIZED INCREASE IN DENSITY OF THE SKULL VAULT

In Bone

- *Neoplasm*:
  - Sclerotic metastases
    - Most common prostate and stomach.
  - Ivory osteoma
    - Commonly affects the peripheral nervous system (PNS). Slow growing dense lesion—well-defined spherical or hemispherical shape.

  Mostly less than 1 cm in diameter, rarely exceed 2–3 cm.

  Complication—large osteoma may interfere with drainage of the sinus, CSF rhinorrhea, pneumocephalus or even meningitis.
    - Treated lytic metastases—especially breast—primary.
    - Treated brain tumors.
- Paget's disease.
- Fibrous dysplasia.
- Depressed fracture due to overlapping bone fragments (Fig. 8.1).

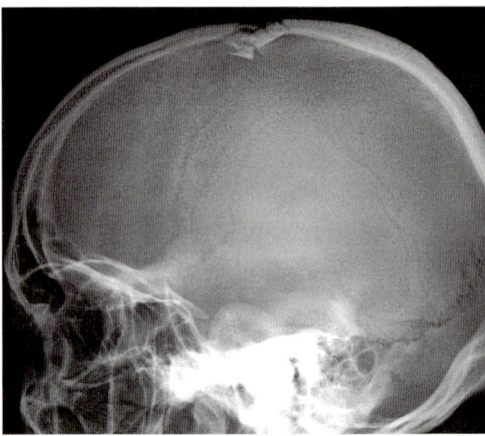

Fig. 8.1: Lateral radiograph of skull shows depressed fracture through the parietal bone at the level of vertex.

- Hyperostosis frontalis interna—seen in postmenopausal female, involves the frontal bone.

  Bilateral and symmetrical.

  Thickening of inner table—"choppy sea appearance". Adjacent to bone.
  - *Meningioma*: Mainly involves the inner table but if breaks through the outer table, it may cause a "hair-on-end" appearance. 15%—show calcification.

    Abnormal increase in vascular channel and signs of raised intracranial pressure.

    Common sites—parasagittal/olfactory grove, sphenoid ridge, and tentorium.
  - Calcified sebaceous cyst.
  - *Old cephalohematoma*—usually seen in the parietal region and may be bilateral in neonate (Figs. 8.2A and B).

    Caused by subperiosteal bleeding during birth, does not cross suture.
  - *Tumors*:
    - Gliomas are the most common tumors
    - 5% show calcification
    - Oligodendroglioma
    - 50% cases calcification
    - Craniopharyngioma—mainly in children, calcification in 75% cases
    - Position of calcification—midline and just above the sella.

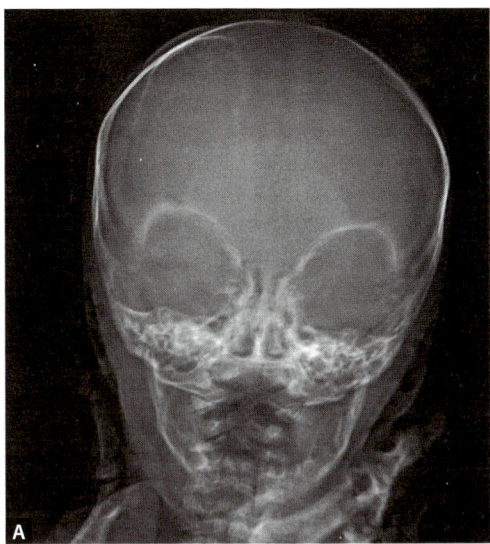

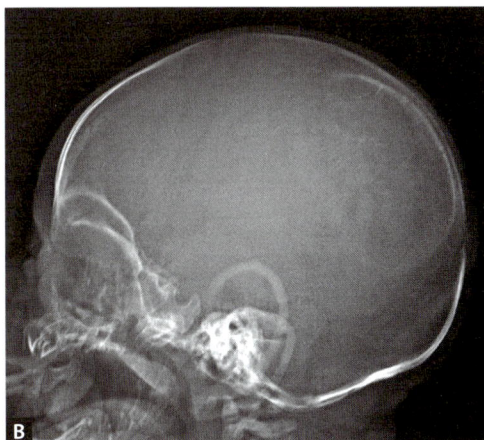

Figs. 8.2A and B: Anteroposterior (AP) and lateral radiographs of skull show calcified cephalohematoma along the right parietal convexity.

Chronic Subdural Hematoma

- Calcification in the membrane.
- Characteristic position adjacent to skull vault.

Basal Ganglia Calcification

Bilateral and symmetrical, seen in the region of basal ganglia, primary or idiopathic—related to age, secondary—hypoparathyroidism, pseudohypoparathyroidism, Fahr's syndrome.

Button Sequestra

Eosinophilic granuloma (EG) tends to erode both tables of skull. The outer table is more extensively destroyed at time producing a characteristic. Double contour, with radiodense focus within the lytic area termed as button sequestra.

DESTRUCTION OF PETROUS BONE (APEX)

Acoustic Neuroma

Arising from 8th nerve, increase in size of internal auditory meatus (>1 cm in diameter or > 2 cm asymmetric between the two sides (1 mm in height and 2 mm in length).

- Erosion of crista transversalis and apparent shortening of the internal auditory meatus may occur
  B/h Bilateral in NF 2
- CT—isodense to brain, CECT—more enhancement
  MR—fast spin-echo (FSE) T2 intermediate SI
- Congenital cholesteatoma—in the petrous apex, they form a well demarcated expanded cystic lesion, which may enlarge to erode the IOC and bony labyrinth.
  No IV contrast enhancement.
  MRI—T1—low signal, T2—high signal.
  Cholesteatoma tends to encase arteries without causing obstruction.
- *Cholesterol granuloma* is a cystic granulomatous lesion containing hemosiderin and cholesterol deposits.
  CT appearance—similar to congenital cholesteatomas.
  MRI—high signal on both T1 and T2 due to presence of meth-Hb and other Hb break down products and increase of protein content.
- *Meningioma*—tend to excite a bony proliferative response and produce narrowing of pons acusticus internus rather than erosion.
  CT—local hyperostosis and erosion of petrous bone.

- Density similar to brain tissue, often surrounding zone of low density.
  CECT and MR—contrast uptake in most cases. MR may show a "dural tail" adjacent to dural infiltrate.
  Typically a meningioma does not enter the IOC.
- Metastasis—particularly breast, kidney and lung. Irregular cystic defect.
  Pain and nerve paresis are common.
- 5th nerve neuroma—are rare.
  If arising from the intracanalicular or intracranial segments, cannot be distinguished radiologically from the acoustic neuroma.
  CT—expansion of facial nerve canal.
  CECT—enhancement.
  MR—sensitive.
- Nasopharyngeal angiofibroma.
  Usually large area of destruction in the floor of the middle cranial fossa.

BASILAR INVAGINATION

Elevation of the floor of the posterior cranial fossa.
- *Primary form:*
  - Less with narrow foramen magnum + occipitalization of atlas.
- *Secondary form:*
  Osteogenesis imperfecta.
  Paget's disease, osteomalacia.
  Craniometric line used to diagnose basilar invagination or platybasia (Fig. 8.3).
  - Wachenheim's line (clivus canal line)
    Line drawn along lines into cervical canal.
    Normal odontoid tip is ventral and tangential to this line. Odontoid tip transects the line in basilar invagination.
  - Chamberlain's line—joins post-pole of hard palate to opisthion.
    Tip of dens lies 3-6 mm below this line. Odontoid process bisects the line in basilar invagination.
  - MC Rae (FM line)—joint anterior and posterior edges of foramen magnum (basion to opisthion).

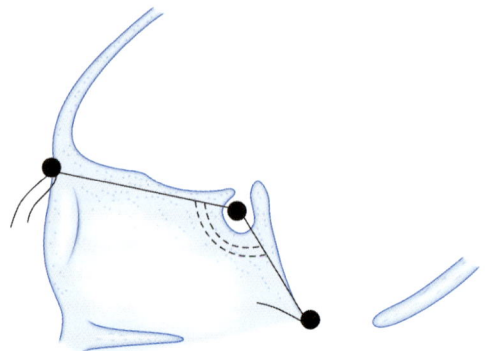

Fig. 8.3: Basal angle to measure platybasia.

Tip of dens does not exceed this line.
- Fishgold's bimastoid line—line connecting tip of mastoid process.
  Odontoid tip may be 10 mm above the line.

Osteogenesis Imperfecta

Due to disorder of collagen.

Four Types

Type 1 = Gracile, osteoporotic bones.
Rapid fracture healing ± exuberant callus.

Type 2 = Lethal perinatal.
Extremely severe osseous fragility.

Type 3 = Moderate to severe osseous fragility, severe deformity of long bones and spine results in severe dwarfing.
- Cystic expansion of ends of long bones.
- Wormian bones.

Type 4 = Osseous fragility with normal sclerae with severe deformity of long bones and spine.
- Paget's disease—caused by excessive abnormal remodeling of bones
  - Site—spine—75%, proximal femur—75%
  - Skull—65%
  - Pelvis—40%

Three stages of the disease are as follows:
1. Active (osteolytic)—skull—osteoporosis circumscripta.

2. Osteolytic and osteosclerotic areas.
3. Inactive (osteosclerotic).
- *Osteomalacia—increased uncalcified osteoid in the mature skeleton.*
  Decreased bone density.
  Looser's zone—common sites are the scapula, femoral neck and shafts, pubic rami and ribs.
   Bilateral symmetrical transverse lucent bands of uncalcified osteoid, which, later in disease, have sclerotic margin.
   – Coarsening of trabecular pattern.
   – Bone softening, protrusion acetabuli, bowing of long bones, biconcave vertebral bodies and basilar invagination.

Platybasia

Flattening of base of skull does not always accompany basilar invagination but occur in similar situation.
   The index is basal angle or sphenoid angle. Angle between roof of sphenoid and clivus more than 180°.

Causes

- Osteomalacia
- Rickets
- Hypoparathyroidism
- FD
- Paget's disease
- Arnold–Chiari malformation.

HAIR ON END SKULL VAULT

Hemolytic Anemia

Sickle cell anemia: Develops due to abnormal hemoglobin.
   RF – Deossification due to marrow hyperplasia.
   – Decrease in density of bones with thickening of trabeculae.
   – "Hair-on-end" skull vault (Fig. 8.4) seen in 5%, begins in the frontal region and can affect all the calvarium except that which is below the internal occipital protuberance since there is no marrow in this area.
   The diploic space is widened due to marrow hyperplasia.

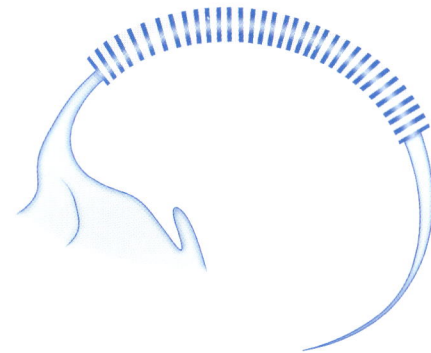

Fig. 8.4: Hair-on-end appearance on skull vault.

Other Features

- Thrombosis and infarction in diaphysis of small tubular bones in children and in metaphysis and subchondrium of long bones (adults).
- Secondary osteomyelitis.
- Abdomen—splenomegaly and splenic sequestration.

Thalassemia

- Marrow hyperplasia in thalassemia major is more marked than in any other anemia.
- Severe hair-on-end appearance.
- Impediment of pneumatization of maxillary antrum and mastoid sinus.
- Lateral displacement of orbit, rodent facies.

Other Features

Earliest changes in small bones of hands and feet, widened medullary spaces with thinning of cortices.
- Erlenmeyer flask deformity
- *Chest*:
  – Cardiac enlargement
  – Paravertebral masses
- *Abdomen*:
  – Hepatosplenomegaly
  – Gallstones
- *Others*:
  – Hereditary spherocytosis
  – Elliptocytosis
  – Pyruvate kinase deficiency
  – Glucose-6-phosphate dehydrogenase (G6PD) deficiency.

Neoplastic

- *Hemangioma*:
  - Mostly cavernous
  - *Age:* 4th or 5th decade. M:F = 1:2
  - *Location:* Vertebral body and calvarium.
  - RF: Less than 4 cm round osteolytic lesion. Sunburst or hair-on-end and without definite margin may occur in diploe, producing palpable lump secondary to widening of diploe.
- *Meningioma*: Only rarely, when it breaks through the outer table.
- *Metastasis*: Prostatic carcinoma, retinoblastoma, neuroblastoma (skull) and GI tract.

Cyanotic Heart Disease

- Due to erythroid hyperplasia. Hypertrophic pulmonary osteoarthropathy may occur
- Iron deficiency anemia—severe childhood cases.

MULTIPLE WORMIAN BONES

Common in infancy but only considered significant when 6 × 4 mm or larger in size, more than 10 in number and with a tendency to be arranged in a mosaic pattern (pork chops).

- *Pyknodysostosis*: Abnormal recessive.
  - Short limbed dwarf with some features of osteopetrosis and cleidocranial dysplasia.
- Osteogenesis imperfecta.
- Rickets in healing phase.
- Kinky hair syndrome.
- Cleidocranial dysplasia.
- Hypothyroidism/hypophosphatasia.
- Otopalatodigital syndrome.
- Primary acro-osteolysis/pachydermoperiostosis.
- Down syndrome.

Osteogenesis imperfecta—heterogeneous group of a generalized connective tissue disorder leading to a micromelic dwarfism, caused by bone fragility, blue sclera and dentinogenesis imperfecta.

Two types	< Congenita
	Tarda—4 types—1 to 4 (I to IV)
RF	Diffuse demineralization, cortical thickening, multiple fracture, and pseudoarthrosis with bowing

- Normal exuberant callus formation
- Rib thinning or notching
- Wormian bones persisting into adulthood
- Basilar impression
- Biconcave vertebral bodies with Schmorl's nodes
- Rickets in healing phase
  - Age group: 4–18 months
- Location metaphysis of long bones subjected to stress are particularly involved (wrists, knees, and ankles)
- RF cupping + fraying of metaphysis
- Poorly mineralized epiphyseal centers with delayed appearance
- Coarse trabeculations
- Deformities common
- Frontal bossing
- Multiple wormian bones.

Cleidocranial Dysplasia—AD

- Delayed ossification of midline structure.
  - Skull: Decreased ossification of skull.
    - Wormian bones
    - Widened fontanel + sutures
    - Large mandible
    - Hypoplastic PNS.
  - Chest and upper extremity:
    - Hypoplasia or absence of clavicle (10%)
    - Supernumerary ribs, short radius, and hemivertebrae
  - Pelvis and lower extremity:
    - Delayed ossification of bones at symphysis pubis and hypoplastic iliac bones.

Hypothyroidism

- Delayed skeletal maturation, fragmented stippled epiphysis
- Wide sutures/fontanel with delayed closure
- Delayed dentition
- Delayed pneumatization of sinuses
- Wedging of D-L vertebral bodies.

Hypophosphatasia

- Autosomal recessive
- Low activity of serum, bone, and liver alkaline-phosphatase resulting in poor mineralization

- Phosphoethanolamine as a precursor of alkaline phosphatase
- Normal serum Ca^{++} and phosphorus
- RF moderate to severe dwarfism
- Resembles rickets
- Separated cranial sutures.

POSTERIOR FOSSA CYSTS AND CYSTS-LIKE MASSES

- Dandy-Walker syndrome (DWS) malformation and variant
- Mega cisterna magna
- Posterior-fossa arachnoid cyst
- Enterogenous cyst
- Inflammatory
- Dermoid
- Epidermoid
- Cystic neoplasm.

Dandy-Walker Malformation

- Atresia of embryonic roof of 4th ventricle—caused by cystic dilatation of 4th ventricle and enlarged post-fossa with upward displacement of lateral sinuses, tentorium, and torcular herophili associated with varying degree of vermian hypoplasia or aplasia.
  Floor of 4th ventricle is present, cystically dilated 4th ventricle balloons posteriorly.
  Complete vermian absence in 25% and mild hypoplasia. The vermian remnant typically appears as rotated and elevated above the post-fossa cyst.
  Cerebellar hemisphere—varying degree of hypoplasia. Brainstem—hypoplastic or compressed.

Associated Features

- Corpus callosum agenesis (CCA)
- Gray matter heterotopia
- Clefts, polymicrogyria
- Occipital cephalocele
- Polydactyly and cardiac anomalies.

Mega Cisterna Magna

- Vermis and cerebral hemisphere, 4th ventricle normal
- Enlarged posterior fossa cyst can cause scalloping of occipital and squamous base.

Posterior Fossa Arachnoid Cyst

- CSF-filled masses enclosed within split layer of arachnoid
- 4th ventricle and vermis normal but displaced
- Non-enhancing mass, parallel in CSF attenuation.

Enterogenous Cyst

- Developmental cyst (the notochord and foregut may fail to separate during formation of definitive alimentary canal)
- Anterior to brainstem
- 4th ventricle and vermis normal
- Equal or slightly higher attenuation.

Inflammatory

- 4th ventricle—normal but may be distorted
- Enhancement after contrast administration
- Calcification common
- Slightly hyperdense to CSF.

Dermoid and Epidermoid

Both epidermoid and dermoid cysts are ectodermal inclusion cysts.
  Epidermoid—4th ventricle is most common intra-axial site.
  Dermoid—vermis and 4th ventricle most common infra-tentorial site.
  Calcification is common in dermoid.

Cystic Neoplasm

- Site—vermis and cerebellum
- Vermis and 4th ventricle—normal but distorted
- Calcification common
- Common tumors—cerebellar astrocytoma and ependymoma.

ENLARGED SYLVIAN FISSURE/MIDLINE CRANIAL FOSSA OF CSF DENSITY

- Schizencephaly open lip
- Arachnoid cyst
- Epidermoid

- Cystic neoplasm
- Infarct
- Loculated hygroma
- Porencephalic cyst.

Schizencephaly—(split-brain)—is a gray matter lined CSF-filled cleft that extends from the ependymal surface of the brain, through the white matter to the pia.

Closed lip - cleft walls are in apposition
Two types (Type I)
open lip—walls are separated (Type II).
clefts can be U/L, B/L or symmetrical/asymmetrical

- *Porencephalic cysts*—result from insults to otherwise normally developed brain
  CSF space is lined by gliotic white matter not by dysplastic heterotopic cortex
- Arachnoid cysts are benign, congenital, intra-arachnoidal space occupying lesions that are filled with clear CSF-like fluid.

  Age incidence—all ages, 75% occur in children; M:F = 3:1.

  Location: Supratentorial—50–60%—middle cranial fossa, 10% suprasellar and quadrigeminal region.

  CT—smoothly demarcated noncalcified extra-axial mass that does not enhance.
    - Pressure erosion of adjacent calvarium.
    - Ipsilateral pneumosinus dilatans.

  MR—sharply demarcated extra-axial mass. Displaces or deforms adjacent brain.
- Parallel to CSF signal intensity (SI) on all pulse sequence.

Epidermoid:
- Congenital non-neoplastic inclusion cyst.
- Acquired—result of trauma.
  Age and sex—peak—4th decade, no gender predilection.
  90%—intradural; 10%—intra-axial.
  Most common site—basal subarachnoid space
  40–50%—cerebellopontine (CP) angle cisterns.
  NECT—attenuation similar to CSF, lobulated margin.

Calcification—10–25%
Occasionally—appear hyperdense due to hemorrhage, high protein, etc.
CECT—most do not enhance.
MR—confined and insinuate along basilar CSF cistern, similar to CSF.
SSFP, MR, and DWMR—to differentiate from a cyst.
Engulf the main vessels and nerve while arachnoid cyst displaces.

Cystic neoplasm—contrast enhancement is common.

Infarct—old chronic infarct.
- At any age
- Lined by gliotic white matter
- Changes of volume loss present
- Loculated hygroma
  - CSF density.
  - Membrane can be seen on CE MR study.

SKULL BASE AND CAVERNOUS SINUS (FLOWCHART 8.2)

- Skull base is composed of the ethmoid, sphenoid, occipital bone, and paired frontal and temporal bones.
- Anterior skull base lesion consists of orbital plates of ethmoid bones.
- Cribriform plate of ethmoid bone.

Extracranial
Most arise from nose and PNS.

Benign
Mucocele: Accumulation of impacted mucus secondary to occluded draining sinus ostium.
- If a mucocele becomes infected, it is termed as mucopyocele.
- In descending order of frequency, mucocele are found in frontal, ethmoid, maxillary, and sphenoid sinus.

Imaging—they are usually of soft tissue density mass with bone expansion and remodeling.

Inverted papilloma (IP)—benign and slow growing.

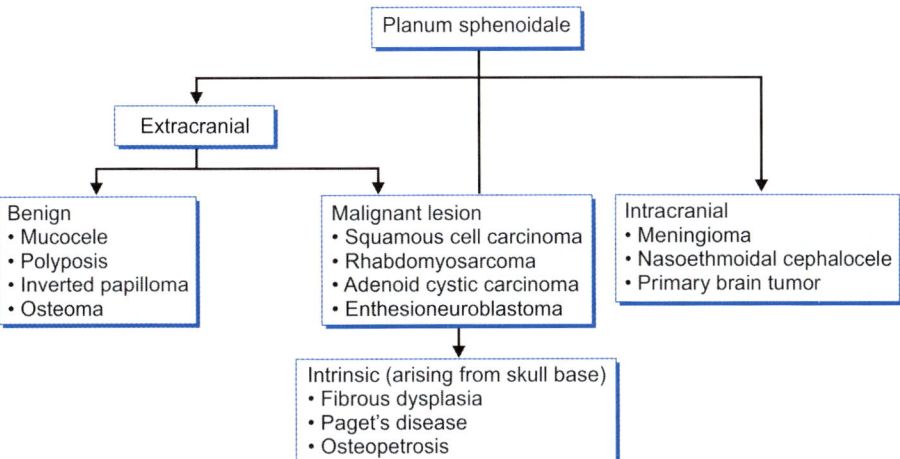

Flowchart 8.2: Planum sphenoidale.

Inverted papilloma arise in the nasal vault near the junction of ethmoid and maxillary sinuses, in the region of middle turbinate.

Imaging—a unilateral polypoidal nasal fossa soft tissue mass widens the nasal vault, sometimes destroying the bone and extending into the adjacent ethmoid and maxillary sinuses.
- Focal erosion of cribriform plate with cephalad extension sometimes.

Osteoma: Benign bone tumor made up of mature cortical bone. Frontal sinus is the most common site.

Osteoma can expand and erode the sinus wall. Malignant sinonasal masses can cause extradural intracranial extension.

In children—most common extracranial malignant that involves the skull base is rhabdomyosarcoma.

Most common soft tissue sarcoma in children.

Imaging—bulging soft tissue mass with areas of bone destruction, T1—similar to mass, T2—hyperintense meningeal and perineural spread are common.

Adult—98% of nasopharyngeal tumors in an adult are carcinoma.
- SCC—80%
- Adenocarcinoma—18%
- Nasopharyngeal Ca—spread directly into the skull base, as well as along muscle.
- They extend intracranially along neural and vascular bundles via osseous foramina.

Esthesioneuroblastoma (ENB)

Esthesioneuroblastoma or olfactory neuroblastoma (NB) arises from bipolar sensory receptor cells is the olfactory mucosa.
- Can occur at any age—Bimodal distribution
   2nd and
   4th decade
- ENB often confined to the nasal cavity but may extend to the PNS, orbit or brain through the cribriform plate.

Imaging—high nasal vault mass. MR—variable signal.

Moderate to inhomogeneous enhancement.
- Bacterial/fungal sinusitis
- Sarcoidosis
- Sinonasal lymphoma
- Wegener granulomatosis.

Intrinsic Lesion
- Fibrous dysplasia
- Paget's disease
- Osteopetrosis.

Intracranial
- Most common lesion that involves the anterior skull base is meningioma
- Planum sphenoidale or olfactory groove—site of origin
- Broad based, anterior basal subfrontal mass

- Strong and uniform enhancement
- Presence of tumor brain interface cleft
- Gray-white matter buckling
- Hyperostosis of adjacent bone
- Nasoethmoidal cephalocele—complex masses of mixed soft tissue and CSF and are contiguous with intracranial sutures, typically through a widened calvarial opening. Crista galli will be absent or eroded
- Peripherally located brain neoplasm like ganglioma causes pressure erosion of adjacent skull.

CENTRAL SKULL BASE LESIONS

Contents are:
Upper clivus, sella turcica, cavernous sinus, and sphenoid sinus.

- *Osteomyelitis*:
  - Predisposing factors—immunocompromised states, diabetes, chronic mastoiditis, PNS infection, and trauma.
  - Frontal sinusitis is very frequent leading to osteomyelitis.
  - RF loss of bone density, trabecular detail, sequestrum formation, blurring, and loss of sinus outline.
  - Complication—cerebral infarct, meningitis, subdural empyema, and brain abscess.
- *Fungal sinusitis*:
  Imaging CT—multisinus nodular mucoperiosteal thickening, high attenuation foci within the soft tissue masses.
  - Extensive lesion can produce skull base destruction.
    - MR—low signal on both T1 and T2, surrounded by a high signal rim on T2.
    - Complication—cavernous sinus thrombosis, blood, vessel invasion, and rapid intracranial dissemination.
- *Non-fungal granulomas*—also have intracranial extension like Wegener's granulomatosis, LMG (lethal midline granulomas—lymphoma variant).
  - CT—E/O mucosal ulceration and bone destruction in nasal cavity and PNS without the ST mass, thus distinguishing from simple malignancy.
  - MRI—decreased signal on both T1 and T2.
  - While simple inflammatory thickening will be bright on T2.
- *Primary neoplasm*—common tumors that affect the central skull base are:
  - Pituitary adenoma—slowly expanding that erodes the sella turcica.
  - Typically extend superiorly through the diaphragmatic sella and laterally into the cavernous sinus.
- Sometimes may expend inferiorly and cause destruction of central skull base
- *Meningiomas* of central skull base are located along the sphenoid wing, diaphragm, sella, clivus, and cavernous sinus.
  Focal lobulated or flat "En plaque" mass bony destruction or hyperostosis is occasional.
- *Nerve sheath tumors*—in central skull base, most often affect the cavernous sinus and Meckel's cave.
  Most common schwannoma to involve the central skull base and cavernous sinus is trigeminal and schwannoma.
  - They are encapsulated, well-delineated tumors.
  - They are quite vascular and hemorrhage and necrosis may occur.
- Juvenile angiofibroma (JNA)—highly vascular, locally invasive lesion that originates near the sphenopalatine foramen of adolescents.
  - Spread along neural foramina and fissure into the pterygopalatine fossa, orbit, middle cranial fossa, sphenoid sinus, and cavernous sinus.
  - CT—soft tissue density mass.
  - Highly vascular and strongly enhancing.
- *Chordoma*—slowly growing, destructive tumor, histologically benign but locally invasive.
  - One-third occurs in spheno-occipital region.
  - Mostly occur in midline and primarily involves the clivus.

- *Enchondroma*—most common benign osteocartilaginous tumor in this location
  An expansile, lobulated soft tissue mass with scalloped endosteal bone resorption, and curvilinear matrix mineralization.
  The characteristic findings.
  – MR—iso with muscle on T1, hyper on T2
  – Postcontrast T1 weighted (T1W)—enhancement of scalloped margin.
- *Metastasis*: It can arise via regional extension of head and neck malignancy or hematogenous spread from extracranial primary site.
  Prostate, lung, and breast = MC.

  ↓
  diffuse/focal cystic destructive lesion.
  Mixed hyperostosis
  and bone destruction ⎤ may resemble
  with an associated   ⎦ hemangioma
  ST mass.
  Lateral orbital wall is a favorite site for prostatic metastases.

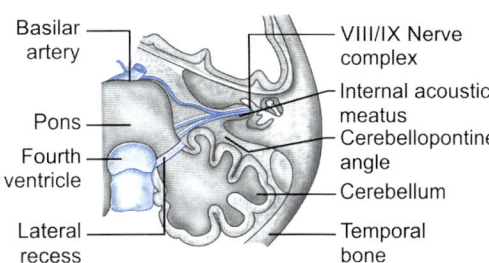

Fig. 8.5: Anatomic diagram depicts the cerebellopontine angle anatomy. Lesions that arise from each component are indicated.

CEREBELLOPONTINE ANGLE MASSES

Cerebellopontine angle cistern lies between anterolateral surface of the pons and cerebellum and the post surface of the petrous temporal bone (Fig. 8.5).

Important structures within the CP angle cistern—5th, 7th, and 8th cranial nerves.

Superior and anterior inferior cerebellar arteries.

Tributaries of superior petrosal veins.

Cerebellopontine angle masses—very common in adults.

Majority are extra-axial.
- Arising in CP angle cistern:
  – Schwannoma (acoustic)—75%
  – Meningioma—8–10%
  – Vascular ectasia/aneurysm—2–5%
  – Epidermoid—5%.
  Other schwannoma
  – Arachnoid cyst.
  4th ventricle/lateral recess
  – Ependymoma
  – CP papilloma.

Brainstem/cerebellum
  – Exophytic glioma metastasis
  – Hemangioblastoma.
Temporal bone
  – Cholesterol granuloma
  – Gradenigo syndrome
  – Paraganglioma
  – Metastasis.
- Acoustic schwannoma—usually solitary, multiple seen in 5% of cases and characteristic of NF-2
  Age: 5th–6th decade
  with NF-2 appear earlier
  Sex: M < F (1:1.5–2)
  Plain X-ray—widening of IOC
  Anteromedial petrous apex erosion may be enlarged foramen ovale/rotundum/SOF (superior orbital fissure) (CANAL).
  CT—NECT—iso to hypodense.
  CECT—almost all schwannoma enhances strongly, small tumors—uniform
  Large heterogeneous pattern
  Peripheral arachnoid cyst or pools of trapped CSF.
  MRI—characteristic findings of extra-axial mass.
- Distinct vascular/CSF cleft between tumor and brain
- Enlarged CP less than enlarged CP cistern.
- Corticomedullary junction of cerebellum appears displaced and brainstem rotated
- Ice-cream cone appearance due to intracanalicular component
  – T1—two-thirds are hypo
  – T2 and PD—hyper—foci of cystic degeneration in larger lesion

- All show enhancement
- Peritumoral edema seen in 37% cases.

Angio-hypo to avascular tumor.
- Draping, stretching of vessels
- Meningioma—posterior fossa meningioma accounts for approximately 10% meningioma—site—post surface of petrous temporal bone and clivus.
  - Arise from arachnoid cap cells
  - Associated with NF-2
  - Sex = F > M peak—4th-6th decades.

Plain Film
- Bone erosion and hyperostosis
- Enlarged vascular channel
- Tumoral calcification and expanded PNS (pneumosinus dilatans).

Angiography—vascular tumor
Dual supply—meningeal and cerebral artery giving a characteristic radial or sunburst appearance.

CT—sharply circumscribed round or lobulated mass that abuts dural surface, usually an obtuse angle.

70-75%—homogeneously hyperdense.
25%—isointense
Ca^{++}—20-25%
Cystic changes or necrosis—8-23%
Peripheral edema—60%
CECT—intense and homogeneous enhancement—in 90%.

MR—gray-white interface "buckling" or displacement cleft or pseudo-capsule of CSF and vessels that surround the mass.
- T1—iso or slightly hypointense.
- T2—variable.
- *Epidermoid tumor*—intracranial epidermoid is cystic lesion that insinuates along CSF cistern.

Age—20-60 years.
No gender predilection.
Location—40-50% occurs at CP angle cistern.

Imaging—plain film—round on lobulated well-delineated focal bone erosion with sclerotic margins.

Angio—avascular mass effect.
NECT—well-delineated lucent appearing lobulated masses with attenuation similar to CSF.
Ca^{++}—10-25%
Occasionally hyperdense on NECT.
CECT—most do not enhance although enhancement at the tumor margin. Epidermoid tumors encase vessel and engulf the intracranial nerves.

MRI—most are confined to, and insinuate along, the basilar CSF cisterns.
Signal intensity similar to CSF.
White epidermoid—iso or hyper to brain on T1 because of increased lipid content.
Steady-state free precession (SSFP) and diffusion weight MR are helpful in differentiating the lesion with arachnoid cyst.
- *VB dolichoectasia*—on elongation and dilatation of vertebrobasilar artery
- *Elongation of basilar artery*—if any portion of it extends lateral to the margin of the clivus or dorsum sellae or if the artery bifurcates above the plane of suprasellar cistern.
- Ectasia is diagnosed if the diameter of the basilar artery is greater than 4-5 mL on CT.
  - Angiography—non-selective angiography demonstrates well
  - MRI and magnetic resonance angiography (MRA) give signal void on MR.
- Arachnoid cysts—are benign, congenital, intra-arachnoidal space occupying lesions that are filled with clear CSF-like fluid.

Age—75% occur in children. F:M = 3:1. Five to ten percent of arachnoid cysts occur in posterior fossa at much power percentage than CP angle and cistern magna.

NECT—CSF density extra-axial masses do not enhance on contrast administration.
Pressure erosion of adjacent calvarium.
Ipsilateral pneumosinus dilatans.
MRI—they parallel CSF SI on all sequences.
- Ependymomas—are slow growing lobulated neoplasms that are often partly cystic.

Age—6 times more common in children.
Peak—1-5 years and mid 30 years.
Location—rarely arise in C-P angle cistern.

Imaging—angiography—hypovascular to extremely hypervascular lesion.

CT—iso on NECT, 50% exhibit Ca^{++}

Mild to moderate enhancement.

MRI—lobulated ST mass hypo or iso on T1 and hyper on T2-weighted image (T2WI). Cystic portion—hypo on T1 and hyper to brain on T2WI.

- *Pilocystic astrocytoma*—(juvenile or cystic cerebellar)

  Age—children and young adults.

  Location around the 4th ventricle and cerebellar hemisphere.

  Angio—avascular.

  NECT—hypo or isodense mass/Ca^{++} seen in 10%.

  Variable but strong enhancement.

  Sometimes having mural nodule in a large cyst.

  MR—hypo or iso on T1 and hyper on T2.
- *Metastasis*—1–2% of CP mass

  Usually have multiple or B/L cranial nerve and leptomeningeal lesions coexisting parenchymal lesions are identified in 75% of these cases.

SUPRASELLAR MASS (FIG. 8.6)

Intrasellar Lesions (Pituitary)

- *Common*:
  - Pituitary hypertrophy
  - Microadenoma
  - Cyst (Rathke's cleft cyst and pars intermedia cyst).
- *Uncommon*:
  - Craniopharyngioma
  - Metastases
  - Aneurysm.

Infundibular Lesions

I. *Uncommon*
   a. Astrocytoma
   b. Germinoma
   c. Histiocytosis
   d. Lymphoma/leukemia
   e. Meningitis
   f. Metastasis
   g. Sarcoidosis

II. *Rare*
   a. Hypophysitis
   b. Choristoma
   c. Pituicytoma

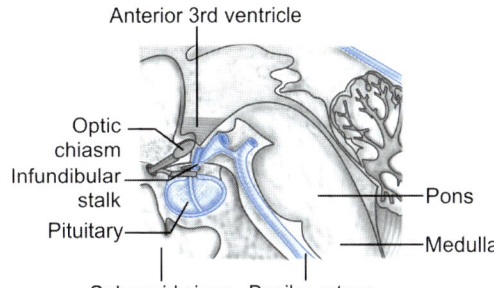

Fig. 8.6: Anatomic diagram depicts the sella turcica and suprasellar region as seen from the lateral view. Common lesions and their differential diagnosis by location are indicated.

Suprasellar Lesions

I. *Common*
   1. Aneurysm
   2. Cranio-
   3. Glioma
   4. Meningioma
   5. Macroadenoma

II. *Uncommon*
   1. Cyst (arachnoid, inflammatory)
   2. Dermoid/pharyngioma epidermoid
   3. Ectopic neurohypophysis
   4. Hamartoma
   5. Lipoma

Anterior Third Ventricle/Optic Chiasmatic Lesions

I. *Common*
   1. Glioma

II. *Uncommon*
   1. Colloid cyst
   2. Germinoma
   3. Glioependymal cyst
   4. Metastases

Sphenoid Sinus/Cavernous Sinus Lesions

I. *Common*
   1. Osteomyelitis
   2. Meningioma
   3. Metastasis

II. *Uncommon*
   1. Chordoma
   2. Histiocytosis
   3. Lymphoma
   4. Osteoma/osteosarcoma/osteochondrosarcoma
   5. Sarcoid
   6. Schwannoma
   7. Thrombus

Common Masses
- Macroadenoma (upward extension)
- Meningioma
- Aneurysm
- Craniopharyngioma
- Glioma (usually pilocystic astrocytoma).

Uncommon
- Lipoma
- Dermoid/epidermoid
- Cysts (arachnoid, Rathke's cleft)
- Focal meningitis
- Metastasis
- Ectopic neurohypophysis.

Macroadenoma—upward extension of pituitary adenoma through the diaphragmatic sella accounts for one-third to half of all suprasellar masses in adults.

Pituitary adenoma with suprasellar extension typically has a figure of eight appearance.

Mostly enhances strongly but inhomogeneously.

Calcification is rare.

MRI—similar to gray matter on T1 and T2 sequences.

Hemorrhage, cyst formation can complicate the MR appearance.

Meningioma
- Second most common suprasellar neoplasm in adults.
- Most parasellar meningioma originates from the sphenoid ridge, diaphragm or tuberculum sella.
- NECT slightly hyperdense.
- Strong uniform enhancement, but not as intense as adjacent pituitary gland and cavernous sinus, allowing most meningioma to distinguish from adjacent pituitary adenoma.

Craniopharyngioma
- Half of all suprasellar tumors in children.
- 2nd peak—4th-6th decades
- 90% of craniopharyngioma—exhibit calcification.
- Enhanced and at least partially cystic. MRI SI varies with cyst content on T1 sequence but majority of craniopharyngioma are hyperintense on T2WI.

- *Astrocytoma*—of the visual pathway, optic nerve, chiasma and optic tracts account for 25% of pediatric suprasellar neoplasm.
- CT—iso or hypodense mass and frequent enhancement following contrast administration.
- MRI—hypointense on T1 but hyper on T2WI.

Hypothalamoneurohypophyseal Axis Germinoma
- Most are both intra- and suprasellar.
- Age—most patients are less than 30 years. MR—an infiltrating mass isointense to brain on T1, moderately hyperintense on T2WIs.
  – Enhances strongly and homogeneously after contrast administration.
  – CSF dissemination throughout the ventricular system and subarachnoid space is common.

Epidermoid Tumor
Occasionally occurs in the suprasellar cistern.
On imaging—lobulated, irregular, frond-like surface. Appearance similar to CSF on imaging studies.

Dermoid Tumor
Well-delineated, lobulated masses that typically occur in or near the midline. Suprasellar dermoids are uncommon.
- On imaging—usually appear similar to fat.
- Ruptured dermoids may spill their contents throughout the CSF spaces and elicit severe chemical meningitis.

Metastasis—to the hypothalamic–pituitary axis represents approximately 1% of sellar–suprasellar masses. Breast cancer is the most common site in female followed by lung, stomach and uterus.

In men, common primary tumors are neoplasm of the lung, followed by prostate, bladder, stomach and pancreas.

MRI—Isointense on T1 and hyperintense on T2WI. Moderate enhancement following contrast administration.

Vascular Lesion
Vascular ectasias and supraclinoid ICA (internal carotid artery). Aneurysms are the most common suprasellar non-neoplastic masses in adults.

- Imaging appearance of aneurysm is variable, depending on the presence and age of thrombus and various flow parameters.

Congenital

- *Suprasellar arachnoid cyst (SSAC):*
  - Ten percent of arachnoid cysts occur in the suprasellar region.
  - On imaging, they appear as smoothly marginated masses that are similar to CSF density.
  - SSAC—neither calcify nor enhance.
  - A displaced, compressed 3rd ventricle can be seen on MR studies.
- *Rathke's cleft cyst (RCC)* is a benign epithelium lined cyst that probably arises from remnants of Rathke's pouch.
  - RCCs usually have both supra- and intrasellar components
  - CT and MR—vary with cyst content.
  - Calcification is absent.

SELLAR AND SUPRASELLAR MASSES

Common Causes	Rare Causes
1. Pituitary adenoma	1. Rathke's cleft cyst
2. Craniopharyngioma	2. Arachnoid cyst
3. Aneurysm	3. Visual pathway glioma (VPG)
4. Suprasellar meningioma	4. Chordoma
	5. Metastasis
	6. Epidermoid and dermoid
	7. Teratoma
	8. Germinoma

Pituitary Adenoma

- Fifteen percent of all intracranial tumors.
- Microadenoma—less than 10 mm in height.
- Macroadenoma—10 or more than 10 mm.

Classification

- Endocrine active—80% (like prolactinoma, acromegaly/gigantism, hepatosplenomegaly).
- Endocrine inactive—20%.

Plain X-ray (Fig. 8.7)

Macroadenoma

Pituitary fossa increases in size, expands and erodes. In classic case, give "ballooned sella" appearance with backward bowing of dorsum, under cutting of anterior clinoid and downward protrusion of floor and extension to sphenoid sinus.

Microadenoma

It produces local bulging of sellar floor or Double floor' appearance.

In case of acromegaly—other features like thickening of skull vault, grossly enlarged sinuses and prognathous jaw seen.

CT

The most common microadenoma and prolactinoma typically produce some enlargement of pituitary and a discrete hypodense region within the enhanced gland on CECT.

Other imaging findings are thinning or asymmetry of the sellar floor, displacement of infundibulum from the midline (infundibulum sign) and displacement of capillary tuft (tuft sign).

The macroadenoma are isodense or slightly hyperdense mass and enhance uniformly on CECT. Cystic or necrotic areas may be seen within it. In some cases, calcification is seen in the rim of the tumor or less commonly throughout the tumor matrix. The adenoma usually enlarges the sella, compresses the sphenoid sinuses or encroaches on the suprasellar cistern and may displace the chiasm or temporal lobes. Sometimes it extends into the anterior end of 3rd ventricle and causes hydrocephalus, rarely it destroys the skull base degenerated to carcinoma.

MRI

The normal pituitary yields a homogeneous brain-like signal in most pulse sequences and

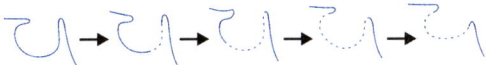

Fig. 8.7: Erosion and osteoporosis of the sella, with no expansion.

is best shown in sagittal and coronal images. The normal optic chiasm, carotid vessels, and sphenoid sinus are also highly conspicuous. Macroadenoma are usually of relatively lower signal than normal brain on T1WIs of higher signal or T2WIs. Regions of lower signal on T1 and higher signal on T2 are seen within the tumor and usually represent cyst when rounded and circumscribed and necrosis when more irregular. Areas of recent hemorrhage found frequently and are seen as high signal on T1WIs.
- Microadenoma on T1WIs with IV gadolinium showing delayed enhancement of the adenoma compared to the normal gland.

PITUITARY APOPLEXY

Pituitary tumor occasionally undergoes ischemic necrosis and hemorrhage if the blood supply to the tumor is impaired and leads to rapid expansion of tumor. This is known as pituitary apoplexy.
- It may also occur as a complication of pregnancy in postpartum period called Sheehan's syndrome.

CT

Shows hyperdensity due to hemorrhage or may show only hypodensity in the sella with a rim or enhancement.

MRI

It is more sensitive than CT. A subacute hemorrhage in the pituitary gland has hyperintensity on T1W and T2W images.

Empty Sella

A varying amount of CSF within the sella with the pituitary gland occupying less than 50% of the volume of sella is defined as empty sella.

Classification

1. *Primary (idiopathic)*: Common in females, patients are often obese, multiparous and hypertensive.
2. *Secondary*:
    I. After hypophysectomy or tumor removal.
    II. After radiation therapy of sellar contents.
    III. After infarction of pituitary gland.

X-ray

The sella often appears enlarged. The enlargement, however, is more globular and symmetric and the cortex of the sella remains intact.

CT (Empty Sella)

Pituitary fossa to be occupied largely by tissue of CSF or water density rather than a normal gland. The "infundibulum sign" can be used to differentiate an empty sella from other low density process, such as cystic tumor or an infrasellar 3rd ventricle which displaces the infundibulum.

Craniopharyngioma

It is the second most common sellar tumor and account for 3% of all intracranial tumors. Seventy percent of cases occur before 20 years of age.

X-rays

Shows suprasellar calcification, expansion of sella and/or erosion of dorsum sellae. Such findings in a child are highly suggestive of craniopharyngioma. However, there is often a typical deformity of the sella which can be helpful in cases without calcification—mostly in adults. The sella appears elongated and the dorsum may be short and bowed forward as if pressed on from above.

CT

Suprasellar calcification is more readily identified by CT and always suggests the diagnosis. The tumors are often cystic or partly cystic and the cyst may be multiple or single. Calcification occurs frequently in the wall or solid portion. After contrast injection, there is enhancement of the outer walled solid portion. The cystic component does not enhance.

MRI (Craniopharyngioma)

On MR with T1WI, the cystic contents are of variable SI, most often hypointense but occasionally hyperintense. On T2WI, the cystic contents may be slightly or markedly hyperintense. On CEMR, the solid portion and the wall enhance.

Suprasellar Meningioma

It arises on dural surface of the anterior clinoid process, diaphragm sella, tuberculum, dorsum sellae or cavernous sinus.

X-ray

Localized hyperostotic reaction seen. Other evidence such as enlarged vascular markings and sign of raised intracranial pressure seen. With meningioma arising in the region of anterior clinoid, a rare manifestation is local bone extension with pneumatization, so called "blistering" seen.

CT

Shows a well-defined and smoothly margined iso- to hyperdense mass which enhances homogeneously intensely on CECT. Perilesional edema may be present. Rarely meningiomas have cystic hypodense area within it. Globular calcification is seen in 10% of cases.

Hyperostotic bone adjacent to tumor is characteristic.

MRI

It is isointense with brain on T1WI. So, this can be missed unless a contrast enhanced study is done. After IV gadolinium, most meningioma are homogeneously enhancing on T1WI.

ANEURYSM

X-ray

Calcifications are rare and seen as characteristic arc-like or circular marginal calcification.

CT

It is seen as a high density suprasellar or parasellar mass and enhances strongly related to circles of Willis on CECT. They may have calcification in the rim, when an organized thrombus is present. The aneurysm appears non-homogeneous in CECT because the thrombus enhances less than as the lumen and the vessel wall.

MRI

In T1 and T2W serial images, flowing blood within the aneurysm has very low SI.

Turbulent flow may produce a heterogeneous signal. A thrombus within an aneurysm usually has SI higher than that of flowing blood.

In T1W gradient echo images, the lumen of an aneurysm typically has high SI. The vascular anatomy in the sellar region and the presence of suspected aneurysm can be confirmed with MRA.

RATHKE'S CLEFT CYST

CT

Shows a rounded mass in the suprasellar cisterns with no calcification. The values of density vary from that of CSF to more solid looking.

MRI

Shows a homogeneous high signal on both T1 and T2WIs possibly due to altered blood in the cyst fluid.

ARACHNOID CYST

CT

The characteristic CT appearance of the cyst is a mass with CSF density (5–15 HU) and no solid or enhancing component structure. In MRI, the cyst has an intensity similar to or slightly higher than the CSF in spin density and T2WIs.

EPIDERMOID AND DERMOID

CT

The tumors are usually of fatty density. But the density can be as high as that of CSF or higher, depending on the contents. The margin may be ill-defined and that does not enhance with contrast medium. The presence of calcification or fat in a predominantly cystic lesion suggests a dermoid rather than epidermoid.

MRI

They are usually isointense with CSF on T1W and isointense or slightly brighter on T2WIs.

TERATOMA

X-ray

- Calcification is present in 50% of mature teratoma.
- Very rarely presence of dental element seen and that is the true diagnostic feature.

CT

Shows cystic or multicystic tumor. The specific diagnosis will depend upon recognition of multiple tissues like fat, calcified element, and dental element.

GERMINOMA (ATYPICAL TERATOMA)

CT

On CT, germinoma may be hypodense or hyperdense, homogeneous or non-homogeneous, enhancing or non-enhancing and frequently calcified. Presence of a pineal as well as suprasellar mass, which enhances homogeneously when seen in a young male, is characteristic of germinoma.

MRI

Germinoma is typical isointense with brain in T1WI and sometimes hyperintense in T2WI. Fat within it has high and low signal intensities in T1WI and T2WI respectively. Intense enhancement is common after IV gadolinium.

VISUAL PATHWAY GLIOMA

Usually seen in first decade of life. About 6–45% of patients with visual pathway glioma (VPG) have neurofibromatosis type I.

CT

It appears as an expansile mass involving the optic nerve, chiasm and tract and/or a mass that infiltrate and expand the hypothalamus. They are isodense to hypodense before contrast and usually show enhancement. The optic nerve may be uniformly enlarged with peripheral enhancement.

CHORDOMA

Commonly occur between 4th and 6th decades of life. They are locally invasive, slow growing involving the clivus and the sphenoid bone.

CT

Characteristic findings are destruction of bone in skull base and a soft tissue mass that is often calcified and may extend to nasopharynx.

MRI

The tumor appears as a lobulated inhomogeneous mass, generally isointense with brain on T1W and of higher signal on T2WIs. Calcification is seen as focal areas of signal void.

Metastasis

Metastasis to sellar region most commonly arise from lung, breast, kidney, GI tract, lymphoma, leukemia, and nasopharyngeal tumor.

Imaging

Magnetic resonance imaging effectively demonstrates the mass that may be invading the pituitary fossa, cavernous sinus, sphenoid sinus, and sellar cortex. Bone destruction is better evaluated with CT.

NEUROSURGEON'S QUERIES

When a neurosurgeon preoperatively reviews a pituitary CT scan or MRI, his interest is focused on several anatomic features possible, considered insignificant to the radiologist. If trans-sphenoidal surgery is anticipated, imaging consideration includes the degree of pneumatization of sphenoid sinus, location of sinus, septa, and sinonasal inflammatory disease, bony dehiscence of the optic and carotid canals and vascular anomalies like anterior communicating artery aneurysms or the "kissing" carotids. So, the additional information is required from imaging to help plan surgery.

EXPANDED PITUITARY FOSSA (FIG. 8.8)

Size -N range is
- height = 6.5–11 mm
- length = 9–16 mm
- breadth = 9–19 mm.

Causes

1. Para/intrasellar mass
   - Pituitary adenoma
   - Craniopharyngioma
   - Prolactinoma
   - Meningioma
   - Aneurysm.
2. Raised intracranial pressure—due to dilated 3rd ventricle.
3. Empty sella.
   - Primary—defect in diaphragm sella allows pulsating CSF to expand the sella.
   - Patients are usually obese with hypertension and headache.
- Associated with benign intracranial hypertension.
- S × R—abnormal in 85%—shows symmetric expansion with no erosion.
- Secondary—pituitary tumor at treatment of a pituitary lesion may distort the diaphragmatic sellae.

Posterior Fossa Neoplasm in Childhood

Fifty to sixty percent of pediatric cerebral tumors.
- Cerebellar astrocytoma.
- Medulloblastoma.
- Ependymoma.
- Brainstem glioma.
- Choroid plexus papilloma.

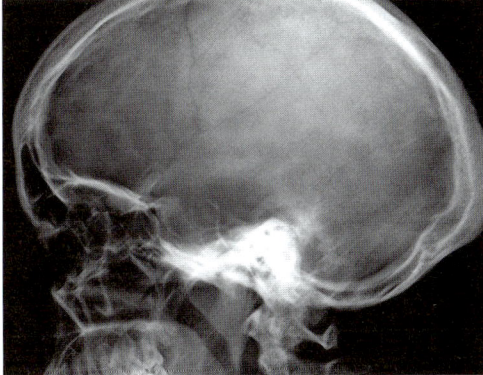

Fig. 8.8: Lateral radiograph of skull shows enlarged sella.

Cerebellar Astrocytoma

- Most common posterior fossa tumor in pediatric age group. Peak at age 10.
- Location—around the 3rd or 4th ventricles.
- Angiography—only an avascular mass effect.
  - Occasionally a mural module shows neovascularity.
  - CT—sharply demarcated and smoothly marginated hypo- or isodense masses.
  - Calcification in 10% obstructive hydrocephalus.
  - CECT—strong but variable.
  - Some show enhancing mural nodule in a large cyst.
  - MR—most cerebellar astrocytomas are cystic so, hypo- or iso- on T1 and hyper on T2.
  - Mural nodule and solid T—enhance.
  - Pontine and medullary gliomas—are usually diffusely infiltrating neoplasms that are inhomogeneously hypodense on T1 and hyperdense on T2-weighted image (T2WI).
  - Obstructive hydrocephalus is mild or absent.

Medulloblastoma

It is arise from bipotential embryologic cells located in the roof of the 4th ventricle.
- Incidence—15–25% of primary brain tumor in children, 75% occurs before 15 years and rest at age of 24–30 years.
- Site—75%—in vermis.
- Less common location—is lateral cerebellum seen in older children and adults.
- Extension—tends to metastasize early, widely and massively through cerebrospinal fluid (CSF).
- Brain parenchyma metastases through Virchow–Robin perivascular space.

Imaging

- Angio—hypo or avascular.
- CT—midline vermian mass that displaces the 4th ventricle anteriorly and cisterna magna posteriorly.
  - Hyperdense on NECT. Obstructive hydrocephalus. Calcification in 15%.

- CECT—strong and homogeneous enhancement
- Atypical changes—cystic changes—65%
- isodense to brain—3%
- absent CE—3%
- MRI—typical medulloblastoma fills the 4th ventricle and extending inferiorly through foramen of Magendie into the cisterna magna. Heterogeneous hypointense on T1WI. Heterogeneous postcontrast enhancement.

Ependymoma

- A rise from floor or roof of the 4th ventricle and protrude through the outlet foramina into adjacent cisterns.
- Incidence—15% of posterior fossa neoplasm is childhood.
- Peak age—1–5 years, second smaller peak—mid-30 years.
- Site—60% located below the tentorium. 40% above the tentorium.
- 90% of infratentorial occurs in 4th ventricle.

Angi	–	variable.
CT	–	iso to NECT
50%	–	calcification
CECT	–	mild to moderate inhomogeneous enhancement
MRI	–	solid component hypo- or isointense on T1WI and hyperintense on T2WI.

Choroid Plexus Papillomas

These are one of the most common brain tumors in children under 2 years of age.
- Location—most common location is lateral ventricle, trigone in children. 4th ventricle is most common site in adults.
- Imaging—angiography—highly vascular neoplasm.
- Enlarged choroidal artery.
- CT—75% are iso- or hyperdense to brain on NECT. Calcification in 25%.
- Tumor margins are irregular and frond-like CECT—intense and heterogeneous enhancement.
- MRI—lobulated mass isointense to brain on T1 and iso- and slightly hyper on T2WI.

RING ENHANCING LESIONS ON CONTRAST-ENHANCED COMPUTED TOMOGRAPHY

- Primary neoplasm—GBM, meningioma, leukemia, pituitary macroadenoma, and craniopharyngioma.
- Metastatic Ca and sarcoma.
- Abscess—bacterial, fungal, and parasitic.
- Empyema of epidural/subdural or intraventricular space.
- Resolving infarction.
- Aging hematoma.
- Thrombosed aneurysm.
- Radiation necrosis.

Primary Neoplasm

High grade astrocytoma
- *Anaplastic astrocytoma:*
  - Age—40-60 years
  - Location—cerebral white matter most common.
  - CT—inhomogeneous/mixed density tumors on NECT. After contrast injection, they enhance strongly but non-uniformly and irregular rim enhancement is common.
- Peripheral edema is present.
- GBM—most common of all primary intracranial CNS tumors; age—75 years.
  - Location—deep cerebral white matter of frontal and temporal lobes in most cases.
  - NECT—heterogeneous in appearance.
  - Ca^{++}—rare.
  - Peripheral edema.
- *Striking*:
  - Enhancement.
- Strong but very inhomogeneously thick, irregular rim enhancement.

Parenchymal Metastasis

Most common tumors to metastasize to brain are:
- Lung.

- Breast.
- Malignant melanoma.
- Age—more than 40 years.
- Location—anywhere, gray-white matter junction.
- NECT—most metastases are isodense to brain, hyperdense metastases occur in round cell tumor. Edema associated with metastasis is striking.
- CECT—both solid and ring-like enhancements with irregular wall.

Abscess

- Most abscesses are caused by pyogenic bacteria.
- But sometimes *Mycobacterium tuberculosis* and fungi, such as actinomycosis and parasites can cause abscess.
- Location—gray-white matter junction—most common location frontal and parietal lobes are most frequent. Multiple abscesses are uncommon except in immunocompromised.
- CT—in late cerebritis stage—an irregular enhancing rim surrounds a central low density area edema.
- Delayed scan shows contrast "ill in" in the central low density region. An abscess rim is typically thickened near the cortex and thinnest near the ependyma.
- ^{99m}Tc HMPAO—a new radionuclide imaging label for leukocytes and radiolabeled polyclonal.
- IgG (immunoglobulin G/antibodies may be helpful in selected cases.

Epidural or Subdural Empyema

- Fifty percent of cases are caused by sinusitis frontal sinusis the most common site.
- CT—crescentic or lentiform extra-axial fluid collections that increase density on CT, and mildly hyperintense to CSF on T2WIs.
- Location—the cerebral convexities and interhemispheric issue are common sites.
- CECT—a surrounding membrane that enhances intensely and uniformly following contrast administration.

Resolving Hematoma

- Between 1 week and 6 weeks subacute intracranial hemorrhage (ICH) become virtually isodense with adjacent brain parenchyma on NECT.
- Subacute ICH show peripheral enhancement after contrast administration because there is blood-brain barrier breakdown in the vascularized capsule that surrounds the hematoma.

Thrombosed Aneurysm

- Partially thrombosed aneurysm have a patent lumen inside a thickened, often partially, calcified wall that is lined with laminated clot.
- The residual lumen and outer rim of the aneurysm may enhance strongly following contrast administration.

Radiation Necrosis

- Extensive radionecrosis and recurrent or persistent neoplasm produce a similar picture, i.e. an expanding contrast-enhancing mass.
- PET may be helpful for determining the extent of cerebral gliomas as well as distinguishing radiation necrosis from residual neoplasm.

SUPERIOR ORBITAL FISSURE ENLARGEMENT

- It is large foramen, which connects orbit with the middle cranial fossa.
- Between greater and lesser wing of sphenoid bone approximately 22 mm long, comma-shaped.
- Inferomedial portion is wider, superolateral portion—thinner. Right muscle origin divides into superior and inferior parts.
  - Superior division—LFT (lacrimal, frontal, trochlear) nerves.
  - Inferior division—superior and inferior division of CN III.
- V, cranial nerve and nasociliary branch.
- Inferior and superior ophthalmic vein.
- Sympathetic nerve plexus.
- SOF is directed toward the cavernous sinus and a small amount of fat protrudes through the SOF into the region of anterior cavernous sinuses.

Causes

A. *Congenital/Developmental*
   - Neurofibromatosis
   - Hypoaplasia of greater wing (GW) of sphenoid
   - Spheno-orbital encephalocele
   - Orbital cysts — Enterogenous cyst Congenital
   - Dermoid/teratoma
   - Mandibular-facial dysostosis (MFD)
B. Infective
   Tolosa–Hunt syndrome/ophthalmoplegia
C. Trauma
D. Vascular causes
   - Aneurysm
   - AVM/CCF
   - CST (cavernous sinus thrombosis)
E. Neoplasm
   - Extraorbital—neurogenic tumor
   - Orbital—lymphoma
   - Capillary hemangiomas
     • Parasellar chordoma
     • Meningioma
     • Juvenile angiofibroma
     • Metastasis.
F. Neurofibromatosis-Phakomatoses
   NF-1
   NF-2

Skull and dural lesions are common in NF 1
- Hypoplasia of GW of sphenoid with spheno-orbital
- Encephalocele temporal lobe herniation
- Proptosis (often pulsatile).

Bare Orbit Sign

- Calvarial defect due to lambdoid suture.
- Dural ectasia.
- Enlargement of IOC.
- Plexiform neurofibromas—hallmark of NF and one-third of all patients with NF 1.
  - Multiple tortuous worm-like masses that arise along the axis of a muscle or nerve.
  - V1 most common site in head and neck.
- *Enterogenous cysts*—rare, congenital. Cyst lined by single layer of epithelial cells.
  - Cyst may be seen in anterior cranial fossa and orbit.
  - CT—homogeneous, well-circumscribed, hyperdense lobular, non-enhancing.
  - Extension through SOF may be seen.
  MR— hyper on T1
         variable on T2.

Dermoid/Teratoma

Dermoid and epidermoid—among the most common orbital tumors of childhood.
- Most frequent location—superior and temporal aspects.
- Although congenital, but may appear in two-thirds disease. Both have fibrous capsule.
- CT—well-circumscribed lesion with decreased diameter; larger one can extend through SOF.

Dermoid	*Epidermoid*
Calcification +ve characteristic	No Ca^{++}
signal of fat present +ve	-ve
Fat-fluid level	

- MR—decreased signal on T1 and increased on T2/FLAIR/DW. Teratoma—rare congenital germ cell tumor having all three elements.
- No bony invasion, but causes orbital enlargement.

Congenital Cystic Eye

- Present as complex cyst occupying the orbit. CT and MR—enlarged orbit containing a rounded/ovoid septated cyst. Ipsilateral SOF increased.
- MR—signal intensity (SI) of the cyst is the same as that of the normal vitreous.

A. *Rudimentary Connection to a Thinned Opposite Nerve*

- Primitive ectopic lens.
- In colobomatous orbital cyst—globe and optic nerve are seen on CT and MR.
- *MFD*—orbital defect.

Due to developmental defect affecting 1st and 2nd branchial arches.
- Maxilla and molar bones are poorly developed.
- Downward slopping floor of orbit.
- CT—defective lateral orbital floor.
- Greater wing of sphenoid may be hypoplastic.

B. Infective

- *Tolosa-Hunt syndrome:* Painful external ophthalmoplegia unilateral (U/L) immediate relief following steroid treatment. *Imaging*—occlusion of the superior ophthalmic vein on affected side with partial/complete obliteration of ipsilateral cavernous sinus.
- *Carotid angiography/MRA*—in excluding the aneurysm as a cause of syndrome.

C. Trauma

Greater wing of sphenoid bone—is a thinner bone—offers least resistance to fracture.
- Neural foramina—represent weak points in the bones and nerve within the foramen may be crushed, contused or lacerated.
- Severe trauma can result in SOF syndrome including a dilated pupil, ptosis with sometimes extraocular muscle dysfunctioning.

D. Vascular

1. Aneurysm of the intracavernous part of the ICA.
   - Spontaneous
   - Postsurgical (pseudo)
   - Sphenoid sinus infected—especially fungal, can extend into the cavernous sinus
   - Large aneurysm result in Widening of SOF—may erode into the floor of middle cranial fossa.
2. Pressure in nerves of cavernous sinus cause—ophthalmoplegia.
3. Can rupture into the sphenoidal sinus or SA space → erosion of anterior clinoid process.
   - MRA/CA—can be helpful in diagnosis.

AVM/CCF

Arteriovenous shunts in orbit are rare.
- CCF-proptosis, chemosis, venous engorgement, pulsatile exophthalmos, and an auscultable bruit.
- CT/MR—proptosis.
- Engorgement of SOV.
- Increase of ipsilateral EOM.
- Cavernous sinus thrombosis (CST)—arises from an infection in an area having venous drainage to the CS.

Source of infection:
- CST may develop from a septic thrombophlebitis arising in the ophthalmic vein.
- Proptosis and ophthalmoplegia, meningitis, B/L CN palsies.
- Thrombosed CS—decreased attenuation non-enhancing lateral border bow laterally.
- Carotid artery within the cavernous sinus.
- SOV—markedly enlarged and often thrombosed.
- MR—enlarged vein that appears less hyperintense than the vein on normal side.
- CST—causes—engorgement of cavernous sinus and ophthalmic veins and enlargement of EOM.

NEOPLASM

Orbital Tumors

Capillary Hemangioma

- Occur in infants, during the first year of life. Increases in size for 6–10 months and through them gradually involutes may extend.
- CT—poorly to well-marginated, irregular, enhancing lesions.
  - Most are extraconal.
- Dynamic CT—intense homogeneous enhancement.
- MR—hypointense on T1 and hyperintense on T2WI.

Lymphoma

Seventy-five percent of orbital lymphoma will have systemic lymphoma.
- Seen in adults.
- CT/MR—homogeneous areas of high density, having a sharp margin seen either in the anterior portion of orbit, retrobulbar area or superior orbital compartment
- *Extension of extracranial tumor*
- *Neurogenic tumor*:
  - Schwannoma (nerve sheath tumor) arise from nerve sheath. The nerve most commonly affected in the central skull base is the trigeminal nerve.
  - Tumor can extend through the SOF into the orbit.
  - CT—obliteration of fat of SOF—if small.

- Expanded foramen with smooth margin, if large.
- Enhances after contrast administration.
- Similarly neurofibroma can affect the mass.
- *Parasellar chordoma* arising from embryonic notochord, at any age between 30 years and 50 years.
- (Male > Female).
- CT—bone destruction as well as soft tissue mass.
  - Radiodense—present—represents remaining fragment of bones.
  - ST—enhances.
  - MR—T1W soft tissue mass—hypo- to isocystic isointense areas (hemorrhage/mucoid material)—increased signal on T1WI, bony fragment signal void.
  - T2—high SI.

Meningioma

- Can arise from any part of the sphenoid bone, from the initial site of origin, the tumor extends along the dural surface.
- Tumor grows into the orbit, causes widening of SOF—patient presents with proptosis.
- On CT—enhancement of the soft tissue component of tumor.
- Ca^{++} may be seen.
- Hyperostosis may be seen.
- Pneumosinus dilatans.
- MR—iso to brain parenchyma.
- GD-DTPA—enhances homogeneously.
- Dural tail.

Nasopharyngeal Angiofibroma—Benign Tumor

Arising adjacent to sphenopalatine foramen
- Adolescent male boy.
- Nasal obstruction/epistaxis.
- Very vascular.
  - CT/MR
  - Enhances intensively
  - MR—T1—intermediate SI, high SI on T2.

Metastasis

Direct Encroachment

Perineural spread: Tumor can selectively follow a nerve or the sheath of a nerve to reach and ultimately pass through a foramen.
- Adenoid cystic Ca
  - Lymphoma
  - Melanoma
  - SCC.
- Trigeminal nerve and its branches travel from the brainstem to many areas of the face, sinus and oral cavity. This nerve is primary route for peripheral spread of tumor of head and neck.
- Perineural spread along vein rare but lacrimal gland and skin malignancy can extend along with nerve through SOF
  - Enlargement of nerve and foramen.
- Effacement/obliteration of the fat plane.
- Enhancement of a normal-sized nerve on a gadolinium enhancement suggestive of tumor spread.
  - *Hematogenous metastases*—lung, bronchus, kidney, prostate usually causes lytic destruction.
  - If GW of sphenoid is affected—metastasis tends to grow in all directions.

TEMPORAL BONE SCLEROSIS

- Otospongiosis/otosclerosis.
- Fibrous dysplasia.
- Paget's disease.
- Osteogenesis imperfecta.
- Osteopetrosis.
- Progressive diaphyseal dysplasia.
- Endosteal hyperostosis.
- Osteopathia striata.
- Ossifying fibroma.
- Meningioma.
- Metastasis.
- Inflammatory lesion-chorionic mastoiditis.
- Hyperparathyroidism.
- Labyrinthine ossification.

Differential Diagnosis of Temporal Bone Sclerosis

- Otosclerosis/otospongiosis
  - Disorder of bony labyrinth—stapes.

- Adult male, peak is 2nd–3rd decades
- B/L in 80% cases
• Tinnitus and hearing loss (conductive).

Pathology

Type: Fenestral or retrofenestral (cochlear).

Fenestral: Progressive connective hearing loss.
   Normal tympanic membrane, no evidence of middle ear inflammation.
   HRCT: Early—small, demineralized focus anterior to oval window—protrudes slightly into the middle ear cavity.
• Narrowing of the oval window, thickening of the posterior piece of the stapes, small decreased density lesion in the lateral wall of the labyrinth.

Cochlear

Combined sensory nerve and conductive hearing loss.
CT: Demineralization of cochlear capsule and area just anterior to the oval window—B/L symmetrical.
• "Double ring" or 4th turn sign—low density demineralized endochondral defect around the cochlea.
• Chronic/sclerotic phase—these lesions can undergo remineralization and become indistinguishable from the normal dense cochlear capsule.
  - MR—both T1 and T2—very subtle signal changes in demineralized cochlear capsule.

Fibrous Dysplasia

• Unknown etiology. Females more than males in the ratio of 2:1.
• Pathologically: It basically involves the cancellous bone.
• Monostotic—at puberty.
• Oligo-ostotic.
• Polyostotic—unilateral—may be seen beyond the 3rd or 4th decade.
  - R/F—pagetoid—most common more than 30 years—bony expansion, area of opacity and lucency, sclerotic—temporal bone, younger, expansile, ground glass appearance.
  - Cystic—younger, cystic lesion with sclerotic border.
  - Present as conductive hearing loss, increased size of temporal bone, obstruction of external auditory canal, etc.
  - CT—increase in bone thickness and density.
  - Loss of trabecular pattern.
  - Obliteration of the mastoid air cells and external auditory canal, cochlear capsule may be involved.
  - MR—low to intermediate signal on both T1 and T2WIs moderate to marked enhancement.

Paget's Disease

Chronic inflammatory disorder that results in the eventual replacement of normal bone by thickened less dense weaker bone.
• More than 40 years.
• Temporal bone—most often B/L.
• Petrous pyramid, external auditory canal, middle ear, otic capsule ossicles are rarely involved.
• ± Hearing impairment—conductive or sensory nerve or mixed. HRCT—decreased density of bone areas may show mixed appearance of bone thickening and sclerosis.
• Mastoid process—bone thickening, demineralization or a mosaic pattern.
• MR—variable, T1—decreased SI.
• Heterogeneous high signal primary hemorrhage.

Osteogenesis Imperfecta (van der Hoeve's Syndrome)

Genetic disorder of connective tissue caused by an error in type I collagen formation.
• CT of temporal bone—proliferation of undermineralized, thickened bone around the otic capsule.
• Narrowing of middle ear cavity, obstruction of windows, facial canal narrowing.
• Demineralization is much more extensive; D/D—cochlear ossification.

Osteopetrosis

Defect in the mechanism of bone remodeling.
- Generalized increase in bone density.
- Temporal bone CT.
- Increased density of petrous pyramid and mastoid bone, lack of pneumatization of mastoid air cells.
- IOC shortened and trumpet-shaped, ossicles may be thickened and enlarged.

Progressive Diaphyseal Dysplasia

- Rare, autosomal dominant.
- Diagnosed in childhood.
- CT—middle ear may be completely encased by sclerotic bone with widespread neural foramen narrowing.

Endosteal Hyperostosis

- *Van Buchem's disease:* Autosomal recessive.
- Temporal bone shows a marked increase in overall size.
- Extensive sclerosis.
- Narrowing of EOC and IOC
- *Osteopathia striata (Voorhoeve's syndrome)*—autosomal dominant generalized temporal bone sclerosis.
- *Meningioma*—most meningioma arise outside the middle ear from the meninges covering the posterior petrous bone. Some meningioma may subsequently invade the temporal bone.
- C-P angle < meningioma—can cause temporal bone sclerosis.
- CT—semicircular dural base lesion.
- Partially calcified and usually enhances, hyperostosis of posterior margin of temporal bone is different but air space changes are very sensitive.
- MRI—isointense to brain (gray matter).

Metastasis

- Temporal bone is susceptible to any neoplasm that typically metastasizes to bone.
- Tumor of breast, lung, stomach, prostate, and kidney.
- Prostatic and stomach tumors—cause osteoblastic metastasis.
- CECT: Enhancement.

Chronic Mastoiditis and Chronic Suppurative Otitis Media (Fig. 8.9)

Following repeated bouts of osteomyelitis and accompanying mastoid infection.

Gradual reduction in the number of mastoid aircells with thickening of mastoid and reactive sclerosis of the bony septa.

Labyrinthine ossification: Ossification of the membranous labyrinth may occur as a result of a previous inflammatory process, trauma and surgery such as labyrinthectomy.

Ossification may be localized and limited to the basilar turn of cochlear or round window niche.

INTERVERTEBRAL DISK SPACE CALCIFICATION

1. *Degenerative spondylosis*
   - Seen in nucleus pulposus.
   - Confined to dorsal region.
   - Other signs of degenerative spondylosis:
     - Disk space narrowing
     - Osteophytosis
     - Vacuum sign.

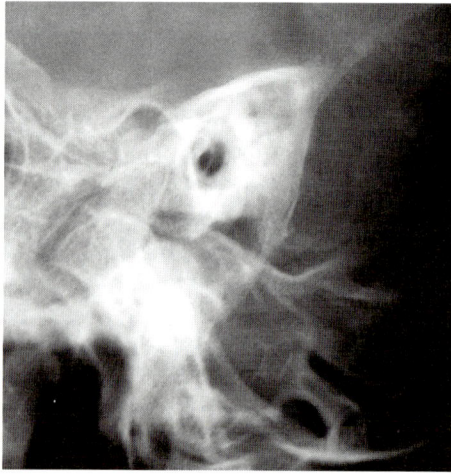

Fig. 8.9: Lateral oblique radiograph of mastoid shows chronic mastoiditis with cholesteatoma.

2. *Alkaptonuria*
   - Onset of arthropathy—4th decade.
     – Osteophytosis
     – Disk space narrowing
     – Osteoporosis.

Calcification is in the inner fibers of annulus fibrosus. Severe changes progress to ankylosis.

3. *CPPD*
   - Calcification seen in outer fibers of annulus fibrosus. Associated conditions:
     – Hyperparathyroidism.
     – Hemochromatosis, gout, Wilson's disease.
     – Osteophyte formation.
4. *Ankylosing spondylitis*
   - Calcification in outer fibers of annulus fibrosus
   - Square vertebral bodies
   - Syndesmophytes formation
   - Ankylosis.
5. *Juvenile chronic arthritis* may mimic anykylosing spondylitis.
6. *DISH (diffuse idiopathic skeletal hyperostosis).*
   - Elderly male.
     – Common location—cervical spine.
     – Anterior flowing osteophytes involving more than four contiguous vertebrae.
7. *Gout*
   - May show IVD calcification
   - Predilection of joints of lower extremity, especially 1st metatarsophalangeal joints.
8. Idiopathic—seen in children.
   - Cervical spine—most often affected, may be asymptomatic or associated with fever/neck pain persistent in adults.
9. Following spinal fusion.

IVORY VERTEBRAL BODY

Single or Multiple Very Dense Vertebrae

- Lymphoma
- Osteopetrosis
- Osteoblastic metastasis
- Paget's disease
- Low-grade infection
- Hemangioma
- Trauma
- Fluorosis
- Myelosclerosis
- Sickle cell disease.
- Lymphoma—MC is HD (Hodgkin's disease).
  – Normal size vertebral body.
  – Disk space intact.
  – Mediastinal, retroperitoneal (RP) and mesenteric lymphadenopathy.
- *Osteopetrosis*

Defective osteoclast function with failure of proper reabsorption.
  – Rugger-Jersey spine—sclerosis of both end plates of vertebra or sandwich spine
  – Diffuse osteosclerosis.
- *Osteoblastic metastasis*
  – Usually primary sites are prostate, stomach, and carcinoid
  – Initial lytic metastasis which after treatment has become sclerotic
  – Normal vertebral body size
  – IVD space preserved until late.
- *Paget's disease*
  – Usually a single vertebral body is affected.
  – Expanded vertebral body with a thickened cortex and coarsened trabeculations.
  – IVD space normal.
- *Low-grade infection*
  – End plate destruction
  – IVD space narrowing
  – Paraspinal soft tissue mass.
- *Hemangioma*
  – Sclerosis is accompanied by coarsened trabecular pattern with prominent vertical striation
  – Expansion may or may not be there
  – IVD space—normal.
- *Trauma*

With history of trauma
  – Vertebral height is usually decreased with anterior wedging
  – IVD space—normal.
- *Fluorosis:* Due to chronic fluoride poisoning.
  – Generalized increase in bone density
  – Characteristic feature is calcification in the interosseous membrane
  – Thorn spine.

- *Myelosclerosis*
  Hematologic disorder of unknown etiology with gradual replacement of bone marrow elements by fibrosis.
  – More than 50 years
  – Lumbar spine—most common spine to be involved
  – Rugger-jersey spine
  – Diffuse increase in density in almost all bones.
- *Sickle cell disorder*
  – Hematological disorder
  – Biconcave vertebral due to depression of the central portion of the vertebral end plate and "H"- shaped vertebrae
  – Due to infarction of vertebral body.

ATLANTOAXIAL SUBLUXATION

When the distance between the posterior aspect of anterior arch of atlas and anterior aspect of the odontoid process exceeds 3 mm in adults and older children or 5 mm in younger children.

Causes

1. *Trauma*
   – Usually associated with odontoid fracture.
2. *Congenital*
   Occipitalization of atlas—fusion of basion and anterior arch of atlas.
   – Congenital insufficiency of transverse ligament
   – OS odontoideum/aplasia of dens
   – Down's syndrome
   – Morquio's syndrome
   – Bone dysplasia.
3. *Arthritis:* Due to laxity of transverse ligament or erosion of dens.
   – Rheumatoid arthritis—associated erosion of odontoid
   – Psoriasis
   – Reiter's syndrome
   – AS—usually a late feature.
4. *Inflammatory process:* Pharyngeal infection in childhood, retropharyngeal abscess, coryza, otitis media, etc.
   – Destruction occurs after 8–10 days of onset of symptoms.

POSTERIOR SCALLOPING OF VERTEBRAL BODY (FIG. 8.10)

- *Tumors in the spinal canal*
  – Ependymoma—most common
  – Dermoid, lipoma/neurofibroma and less commonly meningioma. These lesions cause raised intraspinal pressure which leads to scalloping of vertebral body.
    • Ependymoma—usually site is lower spinal cord, conus medullaris well demarcated/diffusely infiltrating tumor.
    • Local mass with extensive areas of cystic degenerates, hemorrhagic and Ca^{++} calcification.
- *Chronic hydrocephalus* (communicating—also known as extraventricular hydrocephalus).
  R/F—symmetric enlargement of lateral 3rd and 4th ventricles.
  – Dilatation of subarachnoid cisterns.
  – Normal or effaced.
  – Transependymal flow of CSF.
- *Neurofibromatosis*—scalloping is due to mesodermal dysplasia and is associated with dural ectasia.
  There may be enlargement of an intervertebral foramen and flattening of one pedicle—"dumbbell" tumor.

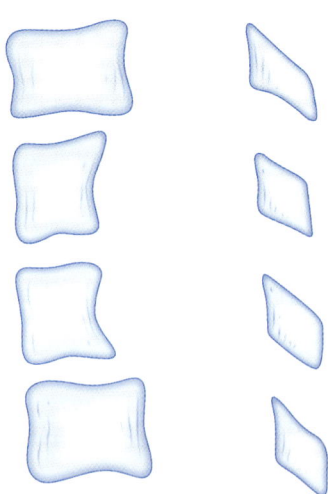

Fig. 8.10: Posterior scalloping of vertebral bodies.

- *Acromegaly*
  - Increased AP transverse diameter of vertebral body
  - Osteoporosis
  - Spur formation
  - Calcified disks
  - Increased heel pad thickness, prognathism, spade-like fingers.
- *Achondroplasia*
  - Spinal stenosis
  - Anterior vertebral body peaks in upper lumbar spine, wide intervertebral foramen
  - Lumbar angulation kyphosis + sacral lordosis.
- *Mucopolysaccharidoses*
  - In Hurler and Hunter disease
  - In Hurler—dorsolumbar kyphosis with lumbar gibbus
  - Anterior-beak at T12/L1/L2
  - Long slender pedicle
    - Spatulated rib configuration.
- *Morquio's syndrome*
  - Hypoplasia/absence of odontoid process of C1-C2 instability with anterior subluxation
  - Platyspondyly
  - Ovoid vertebral body with central anterior beak at lower thoracic and upper lumbar vertebrae
  - Widened intervertebral (IV) disk spaces.
- *Osteogenesis imperfecta*
  - Biconcave vertebral body.
    - Schmorl's nodes
    - Increased height of IV disk space.
- *Marfan's syndrome.*

ANTERIOR SCALLOPING OF VERTEBRAL BODIES (FIG. 8.11)

Aortic Aneurysm

- IVD space remains intact
- Well-defined anterior vertebral margin
- Calcification may or may not be seen
- Usually seen in elderly patients M:F = 5:1.
- Widening of aorta; twice the size of normal aorta.

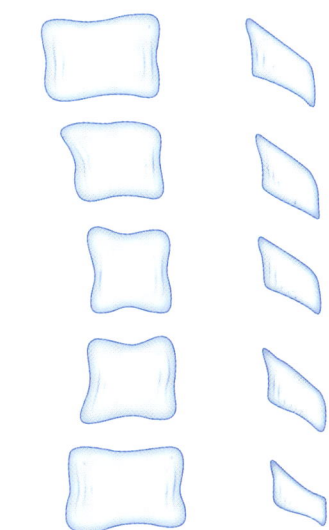

Fig. 8.11: Anterior scalloping of vertebral bodies.

Tubercular Spondylitis (Figs. 8.12A to D)

- Marginal erosion of effected vertebral bodies.
- Ivory vertebrae—reossification as healing response to osteonecrosis.
- IVD space destruction.
- Widening of paraspinal soft tissue mass.
- Calcification may or may not be seen.
- Usually seen in children and adults.
- Dorsolumbar region is the most common to be involved. Multiple contiguous involvement of multiple vertebral segments.
- Angular kyphotic deformity in adults.

Lymphadenopathy

- Pressure resorption of bones results in a well-defined anterior vertebral body margin unless there is a malignant infiltration of bones.
- IVD space maintained.

Delayed Motor Development

(*Down's Syndrome*)
Also k/a Mongolism—Trisomy-21.
- Atlantoaxial subluxation
- "Squared vertebral bodies"—center high and narrow
- Positive lateral lumbar index—(ratio of horizontal to vertical diameter of L2).

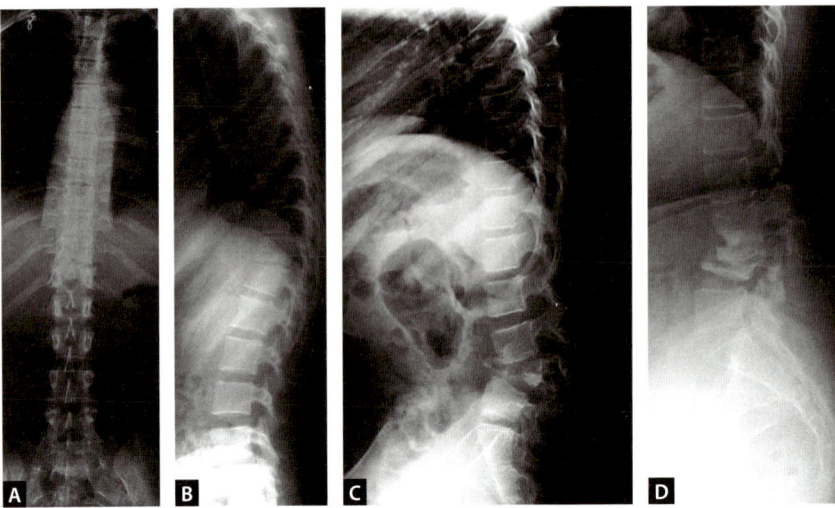

Figs. 8.12A to D: Anteroposterior (AP) and lateral radiographs of spine show tubercular spondylitis in varying stages; (A and B) Early stage (end plate with diskal involvement and paravertebral collection); (C) Intermediate stage (stage of sclerosis with collapse); and (D) Late stage (sclerosis with vertebral fusion).

ANTERIOR VERTEBRAL BODY BEAKS (FIG. 8.13)

Diagram—involves 1–3 vertebral bodies at the dorsolumbar junction and usually associated with kyphosis.

Hypotonia is probably the factor, which leads to an exaggerated dorsolumbar kyphosis, anterior herniation of the nucleus pulposus and subsequently an anterior vertebral body defect.
- *Central beaking*
    - Morquio's syndrome
    - Psuedoachondroplasia.
- *Lower one-third*
    - Hurler's syndrome
    - Achondroplasia
    - Cretinism
    - Down's syndrome
    - Neuromuscular disorder.

Mucopolysaccharidosis
- Morquio's—central beaking (Fig. 8.13A) at dorsolumbar vertebral body Hypoplasia/absence of odontoid process
- C1-C2 instability with anterior subluxation
- Platyspondyly
- Widened IVD space.

Hurler Syndrome
- Beaking in lower one-third of anterior vertebral body (Fig. 8.13B)
- Anterior beaking at T12/L1/L2
- Long slender pedicle
- IVD space—Normal
- Spatulated rib configuration.

Achondroplasia
- Beaking in the lower part of lumbar vertebral bodies, spinal stenosis
- Wide intervertebral foramen
- Lumbar angular kyphosis + sacral lordosis
- Pseudoachondroplasia
- Cretinism or hypothyroidism
    - Demineralization
    - Dense vertebral margins
    - Delayed skeletal maturation

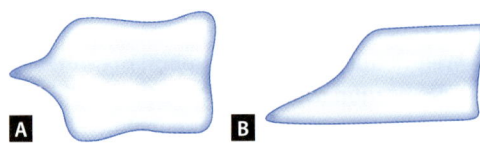

Figs. 8.13A and B: (A) Central beak of vertebral body; (B) Beaking of lower one-third of anterior vertebral body.

– Fragmented, stippled ossification
– Wide sinuses/fontanels with delayed closure.

Down's Syndrome

- Trisomy 21
- Atlantoaxial subluxation
- Squared vertebral bodies
- Positive lateral lumbar index (ratio of horizontal to vertical diameter of L2)
- IVD space N.

BLOCK VERTEBRA (FIG. 8.14)

- Congenital
- Klippel–Feil syndrome
- Rheumatoid arthritis
- Ankylosing spondylitis
- Tuberculosis
- Operative fusion
- Post-traumatic.

Congenital

- Segmentation failure.
- Most common site—lumbar and cervical spine.
- The ring epiphysis of adjacent vertebrae does not develop and thus the AP diameter of the vertebrae at the site of the segmentation defect is decreased.
- Anterior concavity.
- The articular facet, neural arches or spinous process may also be involved.
- A faint lucency can be seen, sometimes representing vestigial disk.

Klippel-Feil Syndrome

- Segmentation defect in cervical spine
- Feil's triad:
  – Low hairline
  – Short neck
  – Limited cervical movement
- C2-C3 and C5-C6 are most commonly involved
- Scoliosis more than 20 in more than 50% of patients
- Sprengel's shoulder—30%
  – ± omovertebral body
- Cervical ribs
- Facial asymmetry
- Genitourinary abnormality—66%
- Renal agenesis in 33%
- Deafness in 33%.

Rheumatoid Arthritis

Especially juvenile chronic arthritis, juvenile onset rheumatoid arthritis.
- Angulation at fusion site
- Posterior elements usually do not fuse.

Ankylosing Spondylitis

Middle-aged Patients

- Squaring of vertebral body because of fusion of anterior concavity of vertebral body.
- Calcification in IVD space and anterior and posterior longitudinal ligament.
- Syndesmophyte formation—extending from one vertebral margin to another.

Tuberculosis

- Usually affects young patients
- Vertebral body collapse
- Destruction of IVD space

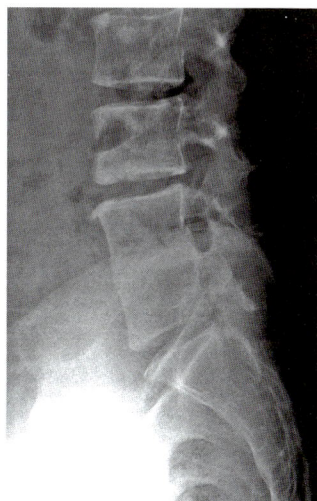

Fig. 8.14: Lateral radiograph of spine showing L4/L5 block vertebrae.

- Paraspinal soft tissue mass
- Paraspinal calcification
- May be angulation of spine.

Postoperative Fusion

History of operation.

Post-traumatic

Simulating a congenital block.

ENLARGED VERTEBRAL BODY

Generalized

- Gigantism
- Acromegaly.

Local—Single or Multiple

- Paget's disease.
- Benign bone tumor.
  – ABC
  – Hemangioma
  – GCT.
- Hydatid.

Gigantism—excess of growth hormone before skeletal maturity results in gigantism.

Acromegaly—results from excessive GH production by an eosinophilic adenoma after skeletal maturity.

- Enlargement of spine or vertebral bodies with characteristic posterior scalloping.

Other characteristic features are:
- Enlarged mastoid air cells and sinuses
- Pituitary fossa enlargement
- Spade-like fingers
- Increased thickness of heel pad.

Paget's Disease

- Especially involves the lumbar spine. Age >40 years.
- Enlargement and coarsened trabeculae.
- Cortical thickening producing picture framing.
- It can also involve the appendages and neural arch.

ABC

- Age—10–30 years.
  – Usually lytic and expansile lesion but cortex intact.
  – Involves both the anterior and posterior elements, more commonly shows rapid growth.
  – Thin internal strands of bone.
  – *Hemangioma*
    ◆ Most common benign tumor of vertebral body.
- Age—10–50 years
  – Site—dorsal or lumbar.
  – Usually affects the vertebral body, but rarely involves the posterior elements.
  – Prominent primary trabeculae with lytic vertebral body—"accordion sign".

GCT

Involvement of the body alone is most common. Expansion is minimal.

Hydatid

Over 40% of cases of hydatid disease in bones occur in vertebra.
- Thoracic region is most common site
- Disease tends to involve adjacent vertebrae and ribs and to spare the intervertebral disks
- Cysts cause bubble-like round or lobulated circumscribed lytic lesions in the bones with virtually no sclerotic reaction
- Adjacent soft tissue mass which tends to be extensive and causes extradural compression.

SOLITARY COLLAPSED VERTEBRA

Differential Diagnosis

- Langerhans' cell histiocytosis
- Neoplastic disease
  – Malignancy
    ◆ Metastasis
    ◆ Multiple myeloma/plasmacytoma
    ◆ Lymphoma
  – Benign
    ◆ Hemangioma
    ◆ GCT
    ◆ ABC
- Osteoporosis
- Trauma
- Infection
- Paget's disease.

Langerhans' Cell Histiocytosis

Eosinophilic granuloma is the most frequent cause of a solitary vertebral plana in childhood.
- Vertebral plana is osteochondritis of vertebral body causes increased density and collapse of vertebral body.
- Adjacent disk spaces are normal or increased.
- Posterior elements are usually spared.
- *Neoplastic disease.*

Benign

Hemangioma:
Most common benign tumor of spine.
Age—10-45 years
- Site—lumbar spine is the most common site.
- Fifty percent only in the vertebral body and half may extend into the post-element.
- Size of vertebral body—normal.
- Soft tissue mass is seen in small number of patients.
- R/F—increased translucency with a characteristic fine vertical striation.
- GCT—rarely seen in spine.

Age—20-40 years (mature skeleton)
- R/F—a zone of radiolucency without evidence of calcification or new bone formation.
- Site—neural arch is more commonly involved than body.

Age—10-20 years in immature skeleton.
- RF—area of bone resorption with slight or marked expansion.

Malignant Lesion

Metastasis: Breast, bronchus, prostate, kidney, and thyroid account for the majority of patients with a solitary spine metastasis.
- Focal areas of bone destruction
- Disk spaces are preserved until late
- Destruction of pedicle = +
- The bone may be lytic, sclerotic or mixed.

Multiple myeloma/plasmacytoma:
- Common site for plasmacytoma
- Age—elderly

- Osteopenia with discrete lucencies—the lucencies are usually widely disseminated at the time of diagnosis—seen in spine, pelvis, skull, ribs, and shafts of long bones uniform in size and are well-defined.
- Vertebral body collapse occasionally with disk destruction paravertebral shadows may or may not be seen.
- Involvement of pedicle is late
  Normal alkaline phosphatase level.
  - Osteoporosis
  Usually seen in older population.
  - Generalized osteopenia.
  - Coarse trabecular pattern due to resorption of secondary trabeculae.
  - Preserved intervertebral disk space.
- *Trauma*:
  - Intervertebral disk spaces are usually preserved.
- *Infection*:
  - Destruction of vertebral end plates and adjacent disk spaces.
  - Collapse is usually accompanied by soft tissue mass. Blurring or displacement of psoas shadows.
- *Eosinophilic granuloma:*
  - Most common cause of a solitary vertebral plana in childhood. Adjacent disk spaces are usually normal or increase in height. Post elements are usually spared.
- *Paget's disease*
  - Neural arch is affected in most cases, sclerosis and expansion is seen.
  - Width of body increases. Increase in interpedicular distance. Characteristic finding of picture framing is seen due to thickened vertebral end plates.
    Collapse is common and may cause spinal nerve compression. Vertebral enlargement distinguishes this from osteoporotic or malignant disease.

MULTIPLE COLLAPSED VERTEBRAE

- Osteoporosis
- Neoplastic disease
- Trauma
- Scheuermann's disease

- Infection
- Langerhans' cell histiocytosis
- Sickle cell anemia.

Osteoporosis

- Decrease in bone mass.
- Trabeculae loss →pencilling of vertebral bodies by the more radiographically dense plates.
- Biconcave vertebral bodies (codfish vertebrae).

Neoplastic Disease

- Usually wedge fractures are seen.
- Seen in osteolytic metastasis and osteolytic marrow tumors, e.g. multiple myeloma, leukemia, and lymphoma.
- RF—altered or obliterated normal trabeculae.
- Disk spaces are usually preserved till late.
- Paravertebral soft tissue mass is more common.

Trauma

- History of trauma, usually lower cervical, lower dorsal or upper lumbar.
- Discontinuity trabeculae.
- Sclerosis of fracture line due to compressed and overlapped trabeculae.
- Disk spaces are preserved.
- Usually without soft tissue mass.

Infection

- Usually starts anteriorly beneath the end plates.
- Extends beneath the anterior longitudinal ligament or into the disk which is rapidly destroyed and loses height.
- Vertebral destruction in the body above or below.
- In most cases, two vertebral bodies are involved.
- Collapse of vertebral body is usually accompanied by soft tissue masses.
- Blurring or displacement of psoas shadows.
- Kyphosis and cord compression may also be seen.

- Radiologically it is not possible to differentiate between pyogenic and tubercular but few signs are said to be helpful. Pyogenic is rapidly progressive while tuberculosis is slow in progress. Pyogenic infection shows marked osteoblastic response and tuberculosis is usually associated with large paravertebral abscess.

Scheuermann's Disease (Fig. 8.15)

- Age—onset at puberty.
- Location—LT or UL (lower thoracic or upper lumbar)
  - RF—anterior wedging of vertebral body of more than five
  - Increased AP diameter of vertebral body
  - Slight narrowing of intervertebral disk space
  - Schmorl's nodes—up to 30% of cases
  - End plate irregularity.

Infection

Both tubercular and pyogenic can cause collapse of vertebrae.
- In Indian setting, tuberculosis is more common than pyogenic.
- RF—destruction of end plates adjacent to a destroyed disks.

Paravertebral soft tissue abscess with or without calcification.

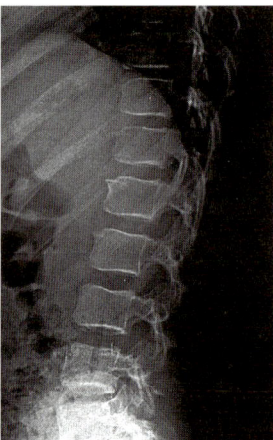

Fig. 8.15: Lateral radiograph of spine showing Scheuermann's disease.

Langerhans' Cell Histiocytosis

Most common site is thoracic.
- Disk spaces preserved
- Rare involvement of posterior elements
- No kyphosis.

Sickle Cell Anemia

Characteristic step-like depression in the central part of the end plate.

INTRASPINAL MASSES

It can be classified into three categories:
1. Extradural masses (Fig. 8.16).
2. Intradural extramedullary (Fig. 8.17).
3. Intramedullary masses (Fig. 8.18).

Extradural Masses

Prolapsed or Sequestered Intervertebral Disk
- Occur at all levels—Most common L4-L5, L5-S1 in cervical spine—C6-C7 is most common.
- Usually extradural but occasionally penetrates dura, especially in thoracic region.
    - NECT—soft tissue mass with effacement of the epidural fat and displacement of the thecal sac
    - MR—will delineate the extent of herniated nucleus pulposus.

Metastasis
Myeloma and lymphoma deposits are common.
- Associated vertebral infiltration.
- Destruction in body or neural arch may lead to collapse.
- Paravertebral mass.
- E/O primary tumor.

Neurofibroma (Fig. 8.19)
- Solitary or multiple in neurofibromatosis
- Lateral indentation of theca at the level of the intervertebral foramen.
    - Enlarged neural foramina (Fig. 8.19).

Tumors
- *Hemangioma*—most common benign tumor of vertebral body. Focal or diffuse.
    - Lytic lesion with prominent vertical striation.

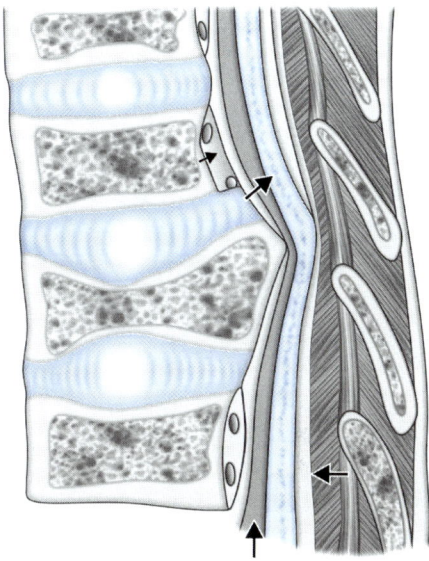

Fig. 8.16: Imaging features of an extradural mass—the dura (small arrow) and spinal cord (large arrows) are displaced.

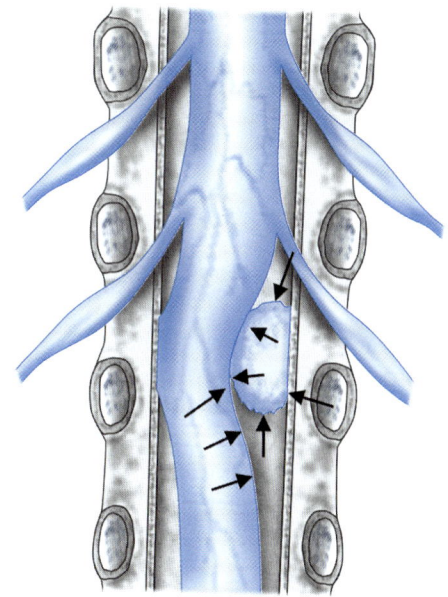

Fig. 8.17: Imaging findings of an extramedullary intradural mass—mass displaces the spinal cord and enlarges the lateral subarachnoid space. A sharp crescenteric interface formed between mass and contrast column.

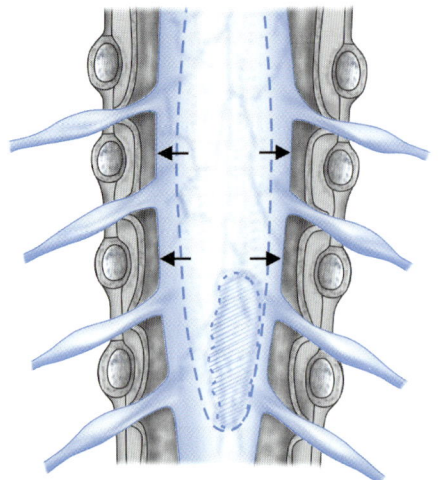

Fig. 8.18: Imaging features of an intramedullary mass—shows diffuse cord enlargement.

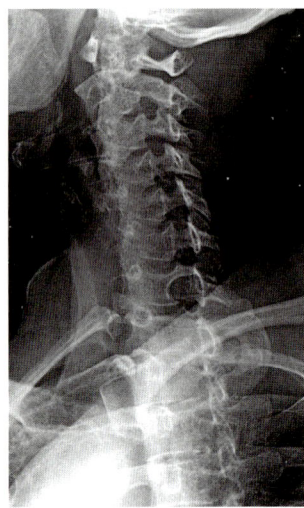

Fig. 8.19: Oblique radiograph of spine showing enlarged neural foramina in neurofibroma.

- *Neuroblastoma or ganglioneuroma:*
    - Common in pediatric population
    - Arising from sympathetic chain in paraspinal location.
- *Meningioma*:
    - In 85% cases, they are intradural
    - 15%—extradural
    - Sex—F > M, middle-aged
    - Site—thoracic spine.

Hematoma
- It may be due to trauma, dural AVM.
- Anticoagulant therapy.
- CT and MRI show signal characteristic of blood on MR—hyperintense on both T1 and T2WIs.

Abscess—Epidural abscess
- Secondary to disk or vertebral sepsis, long segment extradural mass with marginal enhancement (usually involves > 6 vertebrae).
- Plain film—osteomyelitis disk space narrowing. Myelogram, CT myelogram—extradural soft tissue mass.
- *MR:* Extradural soft tissue mass iso- to hypointense on T1 hyperintense on T2WI.
- *CEMR:* Diffuse homogeneous or slightly heterogeneous enhancement is seen in 70% cases—phlegmonous stage or thick thin enhancing rim that surrounds a liquefied low signal pus collection.

Extradural Arachnoid Cysts
- Extradural arachnoid cysts are CSF fluid outpouchings of arachnoid that protrude through a dural defect.
- Two-thirds in lower thoracic spine.
    - Long segment CSF density extradural mass
    - Widening of interpedicular distance
    - Scalloping of vertebral bodies
    - Pedicle thinning, erosion.

Intradural Extramedullary Masses

The common intradural extramedullary masses are meningiomas neuromas, ependymoma, metastasis, and lipoma. The tumors present either as extradural or as intramedullary masses.

Intramedullary Masses

Tumors

- *Ependymoma*—most common intramedullary tumor in adults:
    - Mean age—43 years.
    - Location—conus medullaris and filum terminale.
    - Plain film—wide canal or bone destruction.

- Myelography—nonspecific cord widening multisegmental lesion.
- CT—nonspecific canal widening.
- Scalloped postvertebral body.
- Enlarged neural foramina.
- MR—iso to cord on T1 and hyper on T2.
- *Astrocytoma*—low grade tumors:
  - Most common intramedullary tumor in children
  - Cervical spine is most common site
  - Multisegmental involvement is the rule
  - Plain film:
    - Widened interpedicular distance with mild scoliosis
  - NECT:
    - Widened canal, multisegmental cord enlargement
  - MR:
    - Iso or slightly hypo- on T1WIs
    - Hyperintense on T2WIs
    - Enhances following contrast administration.
- *Hemangioblastoma*:
  - 75% intramedullary
  - 50% occurs in thoracic cord
  - Imaging—dilated tortuous feeding artery and veins.
  - MR—diffuse cord expansion with high signal on T2WIs.
  - Cyst formation or syrinx—50–70% of cases.
- *Dermoid*—including lipoma, teratoma:
  - Most common site—conus medullaris
  - CT and MR signal—lipomatous tissue—decreased density signal on CT, bright signal on T1WI
  - Cystic space—decreased density on CT, increased SI on T2
  - Soft tissue—intermediate density and signal on CT and T1WI MRI
  - May enhance after contrast administration.
- *Cysts*:
  - Congenital and acquired hydrosyringomyelia
  - Inflammatory cysts
  - Hematomyelia

MRI—with contrast enhancement, it is helpful in differentiating these from cord neoplasm.

All cord neoplasms will enhance while cysts do not.

- *Hematoma/contusion*:
  - On CT—only E/O cord swelling
  - MR—blood signal—increased on T1 and T2.
- *Myelitis/cord edema*:
  - CT—nonspecific
  - MR—T1—isointense, T2—hyperintense.
- *Infarct*—expanding in acute phase.

DIFFERENTIAL DIAGNOSIS OF POSTERIOR FOSSA CYSTS

- Dandy–Walker malformation
- Dandy–Walker variant
- Mega cisterna magna
- Posterior fossa arachnoid cyst
- Enterogenous cyst
- Inflammatory cyst
- Cystic neoplasm
- Dermoid
- Epidermoid.

Dandy–Walker Malformation

Failure of development of the anterior medullary velum, atresia of the 4th ventricle outlet foramina.

Skull and Dura

- Large posterior fossa
- High tentorial insertion (lambdoid-torcular inversion)
- High transverse sinuses.

Ventricles and Cerebrospinal Fluid Spaces

- Fourth ventricle open dorsally to large posterior fossa cyst
- Hydrocephalus in 80%.

Cerebellum, Vermis, and Brainstem

- Vermian and cerebellar hemispheres hypoplasia
- Vermian remnant anterosuperiorly everted above cyst

- Cerebellar hemispheres winged antero-laterally in front of cyst
- Brainstem may be hypoplastic, compressed
- Heterotopias, cerebellar dysplasias common.
  - Associated CNS anomalies
  - Corpus callosum agenesis in 20–25%
  - Heterotopias, gyral anomalies, schizencephaly
  - Cephaloceles.

Dandy–Walker Variant

- Mild vermian hypoplasia with a variably-sized cystic space caused by open communication of the posterior 4th ventricle and cisterna magna through an enlarged vallecula (keyhole deformity).
- 4th ventricle is often enlarged but the posterior fossa is typically normal size.
- The inferior vermian lobules are variably hypoplastic.

Mega Cisterna Magna

- A large cisterna magna is present and may extend above the vermis to the straight sinus.
- Occasionally, posterior fossa appears enlarged with scalloping of occipital square.
- An enlarged normal cisterna magna is easily opacified following contrast instillation into the lumbar arachnoid space.

Arachnoid Cyst

- Benign, congenital, intra-arachnoidal, space occupying lesions that are filled with CSF-like fluid.
- Occur in all ages but 75% occur in children.
- 50–65%—in mid-cranial fossa.
- 5–10%—posterior fossa (cerebellopontine angle and cisterna magna).
- CT smoothly demarcated, noncalcified extra-axial mass that does not enhance
- Unless hemorrhage occurs, arachnoid cysts are similar to CSF in attenuation.
- Pressure erosion of the adjacent calvarium can occur.
- Cyst may displace vermis and 4th ventricle.

Enterogenous Cyst (Neurenteric Cyst)

- This is rare intraspinal mass and even less frequent intracranial lesion.
- Typically intradural extramedullary posterior fossa masses.
- Cerebellopontine angle and craniocervical junction.

CT—well-defined, non-calcified, nonenhancing lobulated mass and are typically hypodense compared to adjacent brain parenchyma.

MR—most lesions are iso- or mildly hyperintense compared to CSF on T1WIs and moderate hyperintense on proton density and T2WIs.

Pilocytic Astrocytoma

- 5–10% of all gliomas
- Children and young adults
- Located typically around 3rd and 4th ventricles
  - Optic chiasm and hypothalamus—most common.

Cerebellar vermis/hemispheres—next.

CT—round or oval sharply demarcated and smoothly marginated hypo-or isodense masses.

- Calcification occurs in 10%
- Some lesions enhance homogeneously and solidly others have a small enhancing mural nodule in large cyst.
- Wall does not show enhancement (non-neoplastic).
- In some, the cyst fluid enhances, with dependent layering that creates a contrast-fluid level, particularly if delayed scans are obtained.
- Hydrocephalus may occur relatively early and moderate. Severe if in vermis

MR:
  - Hypo- or isointense on T1
  - Hyperintense on T2

Mural nodules and solid tumors enhance strongly but somewhat inhomogeneously.

ENLARGED OPTIC FORAMEN

- Normal size—4.4–6 mm
- Increased size, if diameter more than 7 mm
- A difference of more than 1 mm is diagnostic.

Concentric Enlargement

- Optic nerve glioma
- Neurofibroma
- Extension of retinoblastoma
- Vascular—ophthalmic artery aneurysm, AV malformation
- Granuloma—very rarely in sarcoidosis or pseudotumor.

Local Defect

Roof

- Adjacent neoplasm—meningioma, metastases, and glioma.
- Raised intracranial pressure—due to thinning of floor of anterior cranial fossa.

Medial Wall

- Adjacent neoplasm—carcinoma of ethmoid/sphenoid
- Sphenoid mucocele.

Optic Nerve Glioma

- Occur in children, most often in association with neurofibromatosis-1.
- Slow growing, non-aggressive with a benign course.
- Fusiform enlargement of optic nerve.
- Enhance after contrast administration with variable pattern.

Optic Nerve Sheath Meningioma

- Most common in middle-aged females
- Tubular appearance on CT and MR
- Enhance more than gliomas with "railroad track" appearance
- Calcific within mass/hyperostosis around optic canal may be seen.

Neurofibromatosis-1

- In addition to optic nerve glioma may have orbital flexiform neurofibroma.
- Orbital bone changes of sphenoid, dysplastic egg-shaped enlargement of orbital rim, bony defects in posterior orbit, AP enlargement of middle cranial fossa, enlargement of other cranial foramina.

Retinoblastoma

- Most common intraocular tumor in children
- Presents in first 2 years of life
- High density areas arising from retina
- Calcification common, subretinal fluid on MR.

Arteriovenous Malformation

- Isolated anomalies are rare, usually associated with intracranial AV malformation.
- Usually present with orbital congestion and proptosis.
- Bright enhancement on CECT, serpiginous low, void on MR.

Orbital Pseudotumor

- Nonspecific inflammation of orbital fissures involving predominantly issues behind the globe.
- On CT, seen as area of soft tissue density with poorly-defined margins.
- MR with fat suppression, most sensitive to detect early changes
- If discrete mass—lymphoma must be considered.

Sarcoidosis

- Rarely involves orbit
- May mimic pseudotumor.

BARE ORBIT/HYPOPLASIA OF GREATER WING OF SPHENOID (FIG. 8.20)

Causes

- Meningioma
- Optic glioma
- Relapsing hematoma
- Metastasis
- Aneurysm
- Retinoblastoma
- Idiopathic
- Neurofibromatosis
- Eosinophilic granuloma.

Meningioma

- Most common below 40–60 years of age in females.

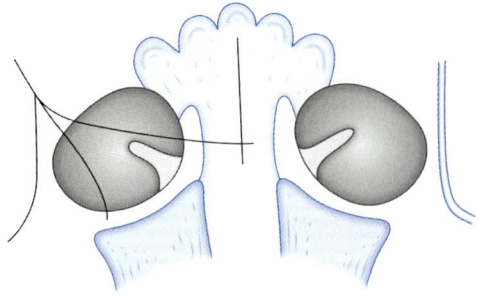

Fig. 8.20: "Bare" orbit.

- Arises from arachnoid granulations. Extra-axial dural-based mass.
- Associated with neurofibromatosis.
- Sites
  - 25% parasagittal.
  - 20% convexity.
  - 15–20% sphenoid ridge.
  - 5–10% olfactory grooves.
- Plain film
  - Hyperostosis
  - Erosion
  - Enlarged vascular channel
  - Tumor calcification
  - Pneumosinus dilatans.

CT: Enhancing hyperdense mass with areas of calcification and cystic areas with peritumoral edema.

MR: Strongly enhancing typically isointense mass with gray matter.

Optic Glioma

- Usually a tumor of childhood (2–6 years).
- Presents with unilateral loss of vision and rapidly progresses to bilateral blindness and death within or 2 years.
- CT shown homogeneously enhancing well-defined fusiform enlargement of the optic nerve. It shows characteristic kicking and buckling (sinusoid) appearance.

MRI: Enlarged fusiform and kicked optic nerve. T1 weighted and proton weighted images, the optic glioma will appear isointense or slightly hypointense compared to the white matter.

On T2WIs, the lesion may show greater variability in intensity. However, it may appear hyperintense compared to the white matter.

Retinoblastoma

- Most common intraocular tumor of childhood.

CT: Moderate to markedly enhancing mass with calcification within it.

MRI: Slightly or moderately hyperintense in relation to normal vitreous on T1 weighted or proton weighted MR images.

On T2WIs, they appear as areas of markedly to moderately low SOI.

Neurofibromatosis

- Two types:
  1. NF-1/von Recklinghausen's disease/peripheral NF chromosome no. 17.
  2. NF-2/central NF/B/L acoustic schwannoma, chromosome no. 22.
- Autosomal dominant.
- Osseous dysplasia in particular bony orbit is associated with von Recklinghausen's disease.
- Partial or complete absence of the greater or lesser wing of the sphenoid; the body of the sphenoid bone may be involved producing an abnormal and dysplastic sella turcica.
- Herniation of the temporal lobe of the brain of pulsating exophthalmos.
- Associated hypoplasia of frontal and maxillary sinuses as well as of adjacent ethmoid air cells.

Eosinophilic Granuloma

- Children, especially boys below 3 years and 12 years of life are most commonly affected
- The skull, pelvis, and femora are most commonly affected
- There are usually solitary lytic lesions in these areas
- Spine
  - Thoracic spine is usually affected
  - Vertebra plana is usually present.

Metastasis

Lung, breast, kidney, and GIT are usually affected.

Aneurysm

- Large retro-orbital aneurysm can erode the bony structures at the back of the orbit or adjacent to the sella.
- Erosion of the inferolateral margin of the optic foramen is characteristic.
- An anterior clinoid process can also be eroded, as can the bone adjacent to it or sella.

ORBITAL HYPEROSTOSIS

Causes

- Meningioma
- Sclerotic metastasis
- Fibrous dysplasia
- Paget's disease
- Osteopetrosis
- Chronic osteomyelitis
- Lacrimal gland malignancy
- Langerhans' cell histiocytosis
- Radiotherapy
- Hyperostosis frontalis interna.

Meningioma (Optic Nerve)

- Most often seen in middle-aged women
- Visual loss, papilledema, and pallor of optic nerve head.

Plain Film

Calcification (common).
Widening of optic canal.
Hyperostosis of sphenoid wing.

CT: Dense sharply-defined tubular mass surrounding and paralleling the optic nerve with enhancement (tram-track appearance).
- *Metastasis*:
  - Uncommon
  - Neuroblastoma, carcinoid, stomach, and colon.
- *Fibrous dysplasia*:
  - Monostotic or polyostotic (McCune–Albright).
  - Skull shows mixed lucencies and sclerosis mainly on the convexity of the calvarium, floor of anterior cranial fossa, sometimes affecting orbit.
  - Usually involvement of other bones like femur, pelvis, mandible, ribs is seen.

Paget's Disease

- Rare below 40 years old.
- Generalized hyperostosis of skull. Vault becomes widened and thickened. Osteomalacic changes lead to platybasia and basilar impression (geographic skull).
- Orbital involvement may be seen.
- Picture frame vertebral body, ivory vertebrae.
- Widening and coarsened trabeculations of pelvic bones.

Osteopetrosis

- Generalized bone thickening.
- Skull—sclerosis and thickening are more prominent in anterior cranial fossa affecting the orbital roof. Cranial nerve compression.
- Sinuses-underpneumatized.
- Erlenmeyer flask deformity.
- "Bone within bone" appearance.
- Rugger–Jersey spine.

Lacrimal Gland Malignancy

- Middle-aged females
- S-shaped upper lid with eyeball displaced down and in lateral rectus involvement may cause restriction of movement
- Erosion or sclerosis of orbital lateral wall may be seen
- Spread along muscle or nerve is characteristic.

Langerhans' Cell Histiocytosis

- Long bones, pelvis, skull, and flat bones.
- Punched-out lesions in skull with little or no surrounding sclerosis, beveled edges (geographic skull).

- Orbital involvement leading to exophthalmos seen in clinical subgroup (Hand–Schüller–Christian disease).
- Other findings like vertebral plana, rib expansion.
- Hepatomegaly, lymphadenopathy, skin lesions, and pulmonary disease.

Hyperostosis Frontalis Interna

- Postmenopausal females
- Irregular nodular thickening of inner table of skull mainly affecting frontal bones, bilateral
- May sometimes involve orbit.

CEPHALOCELES

- A skull defect in association with herniated intracranial contents is termed as cephalocele.
- If the herniation contains solely leptomeninges and CSF, it is termed as meningocele.
- Cephaloceles, in which the protruding structures consist of leptomeninges, CSF and brain, are termed as meningoencephalocele.
- *Incidence*: Cephaloceles occur approximately 1–3 times in 10,000 live births.
- Occipital cephaloceles predominate in individuals of white Europeans or North American origin.
- Sincipital (frontoethmoidal) lesions are more common in Southeast Asians and aboriginal Australians.
- Basal encephalocele are the rarest form of encephalocele.

Occipital and Parietal Cephaloceles (Fig. 8.21 and Table 8.1)

- Occipital cephaloceles originate between the foramen magnum and lambda.
- Brain within these cephaloceles is usually dysplastic and gliotic cerebellum.
- In severe cases, the midbrain and part of ventricular system may also be contained within these cephaloceles.

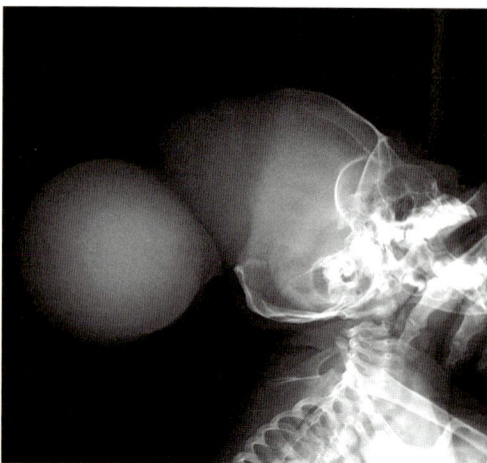

Fig. 8.21: Lateral radiograph of skull shows deficient posterior parietal bones with a large meningo-encephalocele.

Table 8.1: Outline the site and associated anomalies of cephaloceles.

Type	Site	Associated anomalies
Occipital	Between foramen magnum and bregma	Dysplastic and gliotic cerebellum Chiari II and III malformations Dandy-Walker malformation Diastematomyelia Klippel-Feil syndrome
Parietal	Between lambda and bregma	Absent corpus callosum Dandy-Walker malformation Lobar holoprosencephaly Chiari II malformation
Sincipital	Between nasal and ethmoid bones	No association with neural tube defects
Transsphenoidal	Numerous distortion of sellar and parasellar structures and endocrine abnormalities	Callosal agenesis

- Occipital cephaloceles can be associated with neural tube defect such as Chiari II and III malformations, Dandy–Walker malformations, cerebellar dysplasias, diastematomyelia, and Klippel–Feil syndrome.
- Parietal cephaloceles arise from a skull defect between the lambda and bregma.
- They are commonly associated with midline anomalies such as absent corpus callosum, Dandy-Walker malformations, lobar holoprosencephaly, and Chiari II malformations.

Sincipital and Sphenopharyngeal Cephaloceles

- Sincipital (frontoethmoidal) cephaloceles lie between the nasal and ethmoid bones.
- They typically show no association with neural tube defects.
- Transsphenoidal (sphenopharyngeal meningoencephalocele.
- These occur in association with numerous distortions of the sellar and parasellar structures as well as endocrine abnormalities.
- They are frequently associated with callosal agenesis.

Nasal Cephaloceles, Dermoids, and Gliomas

- Nasal cephaloceles as well as nasal dermoids and nasal gliomas occur when a dural diverticulum that traverses the prenasal space and normally connects the superficial ectoderm of the developing nose with the developing brain fails to regress.
- Resulting anomalies range from dermal sinus, dermoid, and epidermoid to nasal cephaloceles and so-called nasal gliomas (which are usually sequestrations of dysplastic or heterotopic glial tissues).
- The crista galli is very important in differential diagnosis of congenital nasal masses. If it is present but split, the mass is typically a dermoid. If it is absent or eroded and the foramen cecum is enlarged, the lesion is a cephalocele.

Atretic Cephaloceles/Meningocele

- They consist of skin-covered subcutaneous lesions that consist of meningeal and ectopic foci of glial or other CNS tissues such as anomalous blood vessels
- They are associated with cerebro-oculo-muscular (Walker–Warburg syndrome).

PATHOLOGICAL INTRACRANIAL CALCIFICATION

Neoplasms

- Glioma
- Craniopharyngiomas
- Meningioma
- Ependymoma
- Papilloma of the choroid plexus
- Pinealoma
- Chordoma
- Dermoid, epidermoid, and teratoma
- Hamartoma
- Lipoma
- Pituitary adenoma (rarely)
- Metastasis (rarely).

Vascular

- Atheroma
- Aneurysm
- Angioma
- Subdural hematoma
- Intracranial hematoma.

Infections

- Toxoplasmosis
- CMV inclusions
- Herpes
- Rubella
- Tuberculosis
- Pyogenic abscess
- Cysticercosis
- Hydatid cyst
- Paragonimus abscesses
- Trichinosis
- Torulosis
- Coccidioides.

Metabolic and Miscellaneous

- Idiopathic basal ganglia calcifications
- Hypoparathyroidism
- Pseudohypoparathyroidism
- Tuberous sclerosis
- Sturge–Weber syndrome
- Neurofibromatosis
- Lissencephaly
- Fahr's syndrome
- Cockayne's syndrome
- X-radiation and methotrexate
- Hemodialysis
- Lead poisoning
- Co-poisoning.

Normal Intracranial Calcification (Fig. 8.22)

- Pineal
- Habenula
- Choroid plexus
- Dura (falx, tentorium, over vault)
- Ligaments (petroclinoid and interclinoid)
- Basal ganglia and dentate nuclei
- Pituitary gland
- Lens.

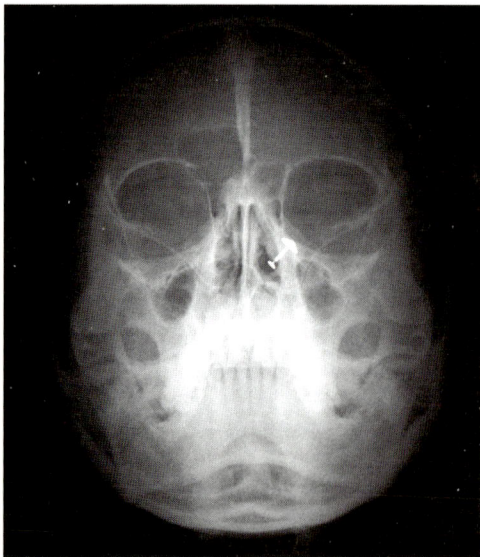

Fig. 8.22: Radiograph of the peripheral nervous system (PNS) region showing calcification in falx cerebri.

Tumors

Gliomas

Most common cerebral tumor
- Calcification is visible on skull films as little as 5%
- Slow growing and less malignant tumor are most likely to calcify
- Oligodendroglioma calcify in 50% of cases
- Posterior fossa gliomas calcify in 20% of cases
- Few punctate dots to a large calcified nodule or linear streaks to large amorphous calcification.

Craniopharyngiomas

- Present mainly in children
- Calcification
  - Midline and just above the sella
  - Few punctate dots to a densely calcified mass
  - Sella is bent forward
  - If the tumor is cystic, curvilinear calcification may be seen.

Meningiomas

- Calcification on plain film in about 10% of cases.
- Calcification is ball-like and amorphous and in a characteristic parasagittal or other typical meningioma sites.
- Other radiological organs include bony hyperostosis where the tumor is involving the vault or sphenoid ridge and increased meningeal vascular markings leading up to the site of attachment.

Dermoids

- Most common in the posterior fossa or near the base of the skull
- Arcs of calcification
- Associated with a characteristic small central defect in the occipital bone.

Epidermoids

- These are much less likely to calcify
- Occasionally show small arc calcifications which can be multiple.

Teratomas

- Found mainly in the pineal and suprasellar regions in children
- They frequently contain calcification and rarely the recognition of a dental element may establish on the plain film.

Pineal Tumors

Calcification in the pineal area, abnormal in extent, particularly in a child.

Ependymomas

- Occur mainly in posterior fossa in children
- In adults occur in supratentorial compartment
- Calcification is unusual but can occur and be quite dense.

Choroid Plexus Papilloma

- Mainly in children
- Show calcification in one of the 4 cases
- Characteristic site is lateral or 4th ventricle.

Lipoma

- Occur in relation to corpus callosum
- Large lesions show a highly characteristic marginal calcification ("bracket sign").

Chordomas

- Irregular calcification in minority of cases
- They grow from the clivus and other radiological features such as a soft tissue mass projecting into the nasopharynx or basal erosion.

VASCULAR LESIONS

Aneurysms

- Characteristic arc-like or circular marginal calcification
- Most occur in the region of the circle of Willis and a linear ring or arc of calcification
- Mostly small (under 1 cm in diameter)
- Occasional calcification is seen in the margins of fusiform carotid siphon or basilar aneurysms.

Angioma

- Consists of scattered flecks of calcium associated with the presence of one or more ring or arc shadows
- The latter arc in the walls of aneurysmal dilatations of vessel on the venous side of the angioma.

Chronic Subdural Hematoma

Calcification in membrane.

Intracerebral Hematoma

Irregular calcification but has no diagnostic features.

Atheromas

- Linear fleck in atheromatous carotid siphons and may be quite extensive
- Atheromatous calcification at the carotid bifurcation in neck.

Infections and Infestations

Tuberculoma

- Calcification on plain film is rare
- Seen in patients successfully treated for tuberculosis and meningitis
- Small nodules in the healed basal exudate at the base of the brain.

Toxoplasmosis

- Most human infestation is derived from cats
- Pregnant carrier can infect the fetus in utero
- Widespread granuloma with calcifications, severe brain atrophy with ventricular dilatation and bilateral choroidoretinitis
- Calcification in congenital toxoplasmosis is characteristic consisting of multiple scattered flecks in the cortex and linear streak in the basal ganglia.

Cytomegalovirus

- There is a severe intrauterine brain infection
- Microcephaly, a characteristic widespread periventricular calcification
- Calcification is stippled, bilateral, and symmetric.

Cysticercosis

- Human autoinfection with the tapeworm *Taenia solium*
- Muscle mass is mainly affected and the calcified cysts present a diagnostic picture
- There is characteristic picture of scattered calcified nodules.

Paragonimus westermani

- This trematode infection is acquired from crabs or crayfish
- Brain lesions are usually in the parietal region and give rise to extensive "roof bubble" calcification in cyst measuring 3–4 cm in diameter.

Metabolic and Miscellaneous

Basal Ganglia Calcification

- Chance of finding in the X-ray of adult skull.
- Bilateral (B/L) and symmetrical and commences in the region of the head of caudate muscles. The globus pallidus, putamen and lateral part of thalamus may be involved. The dentate nuclei in the posterior fossa may be affected with or without supratentorial calcification. The latter is hazy or punctate in type.
- Most cases are primary or idiopathic and the condition is related to age.
- Secondary cases are due to hypoparathyroidism, either spontaneous or following thyroidectomy.

Hyperparathyroidism

- Extensive calcification in falx and tentorium in patients with CRF and on long-term hemodialysis.

Neurofibromatosis

Extensive calcification of the choroid plexus of the 3rd and lateral ventricles.

Tuberous Sclerosis

- Multiple areas of dysplasia in the brain may contain calcifications
- On the plain film, these appear as scattered discrete nodule of varying sizes.

Sturge–Weber Syndrome

- Occipital cortical calcification described as "tram line"
- The parallel lines represent the sulci seen end on since the calcification lies in the atrophic cortex
- Calcification is U/L and occipital region.

Lissencephaly

- Rare anomaly
- Characteristic small (3 mm) calcified nodule in the septum pellucidum and just behind the foramen of Monro.

J-SHAPED SELLA (FIG. 8.23)

Common

- Normal variant
- Mild arrested hydrocephalus
- Optic chiasm glioma.

Less Common

- Achondroplasia
- Congenital hypothyroidism
- Hurler's syndrome
- Neurofibromatosis
- Pituitary tumor
- Intrasellar arachnoid cyst
- Suprasellar tumor.

The normal pituitary fossa in lateral skull radiography can vary considerably in size. A length of 11–16 mm and a depth of 8–12 mm are regarded within the normal limits.

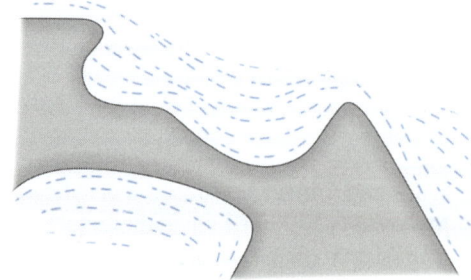

Fig. 8.23: J-shaped sella.

J-shaped sella is an elongated sella with a shallow anterior convexity, which represents an exaggeration of the normal slight impression of sulcus chiasmaticus.

Optic Nerve Glioma

- Appear as fusiform enlargement of optic nerve with secondary involvement of the chiasm or may envelop the chiasm and spread secondary to the optic nerve.
- X-ray—classically, demonstrate a J-shaped sella, optic foramina more than 7 mm or a difference of more than 2 mm.
  CT and MRI—provide the exact localization.
- Usually isodense, and may show enhancement, especially the posterior lesions.
- Calcifications can be seen.
- Eighty-five percent cases seen before 15 years of age.

Hurler's Syndrome

- Caused by deficiency of enzyme alpha-1-iduronidase
- Excess urinary excretion of dermatan sulfate and heparan sulfate
- Macrocephaly, thick vault with ground glass opacity, J-shaped sella
- Chest—wide ribs, wide, short clavicles
- Spine—odontoid hypoplasia, ovoid hook-shaped vertebral bodies, inferior beaking of vertebral bodies
- Pelvis—iliac wings flared with constricted iliac bones, small irregular tumoral capital epiphysis
- Metacarpals—short and wide with proximal coning
- Genu valgum.

Hydrocephalus

- Bulging fontanels, sutural diastasis
- Copper beaten skull
- Usually seen in arrested hydrocephalus, i.e. when the enlargement of ventricles stops due to compensatory mechanisms but they may undergo decompensation.

Hypothyroidism (Cretinism)

- Delayed skeletal maturation
- Fragmented, stippled epiphysis
- Wide sutures, fontanels with delayed closure
- Delayed dentition
- Hypertelorism, wormian bones
- Delayed/decreased pneumatization of sinuses and mastoids
- Calvarial thickening/sclerosis—adulthood
- Hypoplastic phalanges of 5th finger.

Achondroplasia (Autosomal Dominant)

- A skeletal dysplasia with short limbs and a characteristic facial appearance and body habitus.
- Skull—large skull vault, brachycephaly, short skull base, small foramen magnum, and hydrocephalus.
- Spine—platyspondyly, wide disk spaces, narrow spinal canal with lumbar spinal canal stenosis, thoracolumbar kyphosis.
- Square iliac wings, horizontal acetabular roofs.
- Long bone shortening, particularly femur and humerus.
- Trident hand.

Neurofibromatosis

- One or more relatives, primarily with NF
- Optic gliomas (MC CNS tumor in NF-1)
- Typical bone lesions—sphenoid dysplasia or tibial pseudoarthrosis
- Twisted ribbon ribs; splaying of ribs
- Heavy calcification of choroid plexus
- Café-au-lait spots.

Arachnoid Cyst (Leptomeningeal Cyst)

- Benign, congenital, intra-arachnoidal SOL, i.e. filled with clear CSF-like fluid.
- Mainly seen in middle cranial fossa but may involve sella.
- CT—smoothly demarcated, non-calcified extra-axial mass that does not enhance.

Findings on Skull X-ray

- Copper beaten skull – Hydrocephalus bulging fontanel, sutural diastasis

- Optic foramina more than 7 mm or a difference of more than 2 mm — Optic glioma
- Associated sphenoid dysplasia — Neurofibromatosis
- Large skull vault, brachycephaly, short skull base, small foramen magnum — Achondroplasia
- Macrocephaly, thick vault with ground glass opacity, odontoid hypoplasia — Hurler's syndrome
- Wide sutures, fontanels with delayed closure, wormian bones, hypertelorism, calvarial thickening decreased pneumatization of mastoid and sinuses — Hypothyroidism

CEREBELLAR MALFORMATIONS

Differential Diagnosis

- Chiari IV malformations
- Joubert's syndrome
- Rhombencephalosynapsis
- Tectocerebellar dysraphia
- Lhermitte-Duclos disease.

Chiari IV Malformations

- Absent or severely hypoplastic cerebellum
- Small brainstem
- Large posterior fossa, CSF fluid spaces.

Joubert's Syndrome

- Autosomal recessive presents with marked global developmental delay and neonatal breathing abnormalities.
- Dysgenetic vermis that appears split, segmented or disorganized.
- The inferior and superior cerebellar peduncles are often small.
- The 4th ventricle roof appears superiorly convex on sagittal MR scans.
- No hydrocephalus.
- Associated with callosal dysgenesis, congenital retinal dystrophy, oculomotor abnormalities, polydactyly, and cystic kidney.

Rhombencephalosynapsis

- Presentation is with mental retardation and severe ataxia
- Vermian agenesis or hypogenesis
- Midline fusion of cerebellar hemispheres and peduncles
- Apposition or fusion of dentate nuclei
- Variable fusion of colliculi
- Keyhole 4th ventricle
- Associated with ventriculomegaly, absent septum pellucidum, anterior commissure hypoplasia, fused thalami, schizencephaly, and cephalocele.

Tectocerebellar Dysraphia

- Vermian hypoplasia or aplasia
- Occipital cephalocele
- Dorsal traction of brainstem
- The hypoplastic cerebellar hemispheres are rotated lying ventrolateral to brainstem.

Lhermitte-Duclos Disease

It is also known as dysplastic gangliocytoma of cerebellum.

- Gross thickening of cerebellar folia with or without mass effect.
- Mimics posterior fossa neoplasms.
- On CT, there are poorly delineated hypo- or isodense posterior fossa lesions that do not enhance.
- Mass effect and displacement of 4th ventricle may occur.
- Calcification and hydrocephalus may be present.
- On MR decreased signal non-enhancing mass is seen on T1 weighted images and a very characteristic laminated folial pattern of increased signal intensity is seen on T2WIs.
- Usually an isolated abnormality.

Miscellaneous

Dandy-Walker Complex

- Failure of development of anterior medullary velum (roof of 4th ventricle) or atresia of foramina of Luschka and Magendie
- Large posterior fossa
- High tentorial insertion
- High transverse sinus
- The 4th ventricle communicates with a posterior fossa cyst
- Hydrocephalus
- Vermian or cerebellar hemispheric hypoplasia
- Anterolaterally winged cerebellar hemispheres in front of the cyst
- Brainstem may be hypoplastic and compressed
- Heterotopias and cerebellar dysplasias are common
- Associated with corpus callosum agenesis.

Dandy-Walker Variant

- Mild vermian hypoplasia
- Communication of 4th ventricle to cisterna magna with enlargement of 4th ventricle
- Posterior fossa size is normal.

DEMYELINATING DISORDERS

- *Two main categories*:
  1. Dysmyelinating disorders—primary abnormality of formation of myelin.
  2. Demyelinating—result of myelin loss after its normal formation.
- *General imaging features*:
  - Hypodense on CT
  - Hypointense on T1WI
  - Hyperintense on T2WI
  - Acute lesions may show focal contrast uptake.

Demyelination

- Multiple sclerosis
- Acute disseminated encephalomyelitis (ADEM)
- *Infections*:
  - Congenital or perinatal
  - CMV
  - Rubella
  - HSV
- *Acute encephalitis*:
  - HSV
  - Mumps
  - Rubella
  - Measles, chicken pox
  - AIDS encephalitis
  - PML
  - Subacute sclerosing panencephalitis (SSPE)
  - CJD
- *Toxic/metabolic*:
  - Osmotic demyelination
  - Wernicke's
  - Marchiafava-Bignami syndrome
- *Vascular*:
  - Subcortical arteriosclerostic encephalopathy
  - HIE.

Radiation and Chemotherapy

Dysmyelination

- Metachromatic leukodystrophy
- Krabbe's disease.

Paroxysmal/Peroxisomal Disorders

- ALD
- Zellweger's syndrome.

Amino Acid Metabolism

- Canavan's disease.

Mitochondrial Dysfunction

- Leigh's disease
- MELAS syndrome
- MERRF syndrome
- Kearns–Sayre syndrome.

Unknown

- Alexander's disease
- Pelizaeus–Merzbacher disease.

DEMYELINATION

- Multiple sclerosis
- Unknown etiology—autoimmune mediated demyelination

- Most common demyelinating disorder, except for age-related vascular demyelination
- 20–40 years F > M, 1.7–2:1
- *Location*: Ovoid periventricular lesions, oriented parallel to long axis of the brain and lateral ventricles
  Demyelination around subependymal and deep white matter medullary veins.
    – Calloso-septal interface.
- *Infratentorial with 10% in adults*:
    – Posterior fossa—more commonly involved in children and adolescents.
- *C/F*:
    – Prolonged relapsing-remitting disease.

Imaging

- *CT*;
    – May be normal
    – Iso- to hypodense lesions on NCCT
    – Variable contrast enhancement—both nodular and rim-like.
- *MRI*, iso- to hypointense on T1WI, lesion within lesion appearance (beveled appearance).
    – Hyperintense on T2WI.
- *Criteria*:
    – Presence of three or more discrete lesions, more than 5 mm in size, characteristic location with compatible clinical H/O.
    – Oblong lesions at callososeptal interface are typical with characteristic periventricular extension into adjacent white matter, called Dawson's finger.
    – Variable and transient CE, only during active demyelinating stage.

Acute Disseminated Encephalomyelitis

- Immune mediated response to a preceding viral infection or vaccination
- Any age, mostly children and young adults
- Abrupt onset, with monophasic course, neurological symptoms characteristically develop 1–3 weeks after infection
- Multifocal subcortical hyperintense foci on T2WI
- Deep white matter, brainstem and cerebellum can be affected
- Occasionally basal ganglia involvement occurs
- Typically bilateral, but asymmetric
- Usually nonhemorrhagic
- Some but not all lesions enhance, often contrast enhancement.

INFECTIOUS

Congenital and Perinatal Viral Infections

Cytomegalovirus

- Most common cause of congenital infections
- More than 60% of infected fetuses have multisystem involvement
- Most common intracranial abnormalities 70%
- Cardiac abnormalities and hepatosplenomegaly (HCM)—one-third cases
- *C/F*:
    – Prematurity, hepatosplenomegaly, jaundice, thrombocytopenia, chorioretinitis, during newborn period
    – Seizures, mental retardation, optic atrophy, sensorineural hearing loss
    – Hydrocephalus—later manifestations.
- *Imaging*:
    – X-ray—microcephaly with egg-shell like periventricular calcification, due to widespread periventricular tissue necrosis with subsequent dystrophic calcification.
- *USG*:
    – Ventriculomegaly with periventricular calcification.
- *CT*:
    – Hydrocephalus, atrophy, and periventricular calcification.
- *MRI*:
    – Migrational anomalies, encephalomalacia, ventriculomegaly, delayed myelination, subependymal periventricular cysts, and calcification.
- *Rubella*:
    – Interferes with multiplication of cells located in germinal matrix—microcephaly, delayed myelination, vasculopathy with perivascular necrosis in basal ganglia, periventricular region, and cerebral white matter.
- Parenchymal calcification.

- *Other*:
  - Cataract, glaucoma chorioretinitis, microphthalmia cardiac malformations
  - Deafness.

Herpes Simplex Encephalitis

Most common viral encephalitis
- Neonatal herpes simplex encephalitis (HSE) is caused by HSV-2
- In older children and adults, HSV-1
- HSV causes fulminant hemorrhagic necrotizing meningoencephalitis
- Neonatal HSV-2 infection is a diffuse non-focal infection
  HSV-1—limbic system predilection.
  - Temporal lobe, insular cortex, subfrontal area, the cingulate gyrus
  - "Sequential bilaterality".
- *CF*:
  - Altered mental states, seizures, fever, and headache.
- *CT*:
  - Normal or low density lesion in temporal lobe with mild mass effect
  - Hemorrhage—if present highly s/o HSE—usually seen later in the course of disease.
- *CECT*:
  - Ill-defined patchy or gyriform contrast enhancement.
- Neonatal HSE-2:
  Strikingly increased density of cortical gray matter, and diffuse low attenuation in the white matter.
- *MR*:
  - Decrease—T1WI
  - Increase—T2WI
    - In limbic system, with sequential bilaterality with variable contrast enhancement and subacute hemorrhage
- Encephalomalacia, atrophy, and dystrophic calcification late sequelae.

HUMAN IMMUNODEFICIENCY VIRUS ENCEPHALOPATHY

Progressive subcortical dementia-subacute encephalitis
- Develops in 60% of AIDS patients.

- *CT*:
  - Most common finding—atrophy
  - Multifocal hypodense areas in deep white matter.
- *MR-T2WI*:
  - Ill-defined diffuse or confluent patches of increased signal intensity in the deep white matter
  - Most common site—frontal lobes, often—B/L and symmetric
  - Gray matter—typically spared
  - No contrast enhancement.
- *PML*:
  Group B human papovavirus (JC virus)
  - Infects and destroys oligodendroglia—demyelination
  - Adults immunocompromised patients, extremely rare in children
  - Periphery to central progression, subcortical areas first to be affected
  - Typically bilateral and asymmetric
  - Posterior centrum semiovale—most common site
  - Rarely, unilateral, thalamic, and basal ganglia lesions.
- *SSPE*:
  - Rare progressive encephalitis (subacute sclerosing panencephalitis) that develops several years after measles infection
  - Affects children and young adults.
- *CF*:
  - Behavioral abnormalities, myoclonus, tremors and seizures.
  - NCCT—hypodense lesion in subcortical and periventricular white matter basal ganglia.
  - Generalized atrophy.
- *T2W MRI*: Multifocal, hyperintensities in cerebral white matter and basal ganglia.

Osmotic Demyelination

- Alcoholics
- Malnourished or chronic debilitated adults
- Rapid correction of hyponatremia
- Hypernatremia

- Myelinolysis with selective neuron sparing
- MC site—central pons (CP myelinolysis)
- Extrapontine sites: Putaminal, caudate, midbrain, thalami, and subcortical white matter
- NCCT—hypodense, hypointense on T1WI, hyper on T2WI
- CE—most lesions do not enhance, some show variable CE
- Transverse pontine fibers are most severely affected with sparing of corticospinal tracts.

Marchiafava–Bignami Disease

- Chronic alcoholism.
- Corpus callosum demyelination and necrosis, with or without—cerebral hemispheric white matter and other commissural fibers may be affected.
- Wernicke's encephalopathy—nutritional thiamine deficiency—chronic alcoholics.
- TRIAD—ophthalmoplegia, ataxia, confusion.
- Involves both gray and white matter.
- Characteristic topographic distribution. Periventricular regions, mammillary bodies.
- Periaqueductal gray, midbrain reticular formation and tectal plate.
- Postcontrast enhancement—may or may not be present.
  Radiation and chemotherapy—cyclosporine A, methotrexate, cytarabine, 5-FU.
- Small and medium-sized vessel injury.
- Predominant involvement of deep white matter with relative sparing of the cortex and underlying subcortical arcuate fibers.
- Widespread perivascular calcification condition known as mineralizing angiopathy (MA), typically occur in children receiving irradiation and chemotherapy for acute leukemia.
- MC site—basal ganglia and junction of the cortex with subcortical white matter.

Vascular Lesions

HIE: Premature infants—periventricular leukomalacia (PVL) ischemic infarction.
- Isolated PVL reflects second or early third-trimester injury.
- CF—spastic diplegia, non-progressive but permanent.
- MR—peritrigonal hyperintensities focal ventricular enlargement with irregular ventricular contour, atrophy of posterior corpus callosum.
- Bilateral (B/L), and asymmetric.
- *Term infants*: Predominant involvement of cortex and subcortical white matter, with common involvement of deep gray matter nuclei.
- *Children and adults*: Watershed infarction, with B/L selective neuronal necrosis in basal ganglia, thalami, hippocampus, parahippocampal gyrus, cerebellum, and brainstem.

Subcortical Arteriosclerotic Encephalopathy: Binswanger's Disease

- Patients with chronic hypertension
- Dementia, spasticity, seizures, gait apraxia, and incontinence
- Multifocal white matter lesions in periventricular and deep white matter, extending peripherally with increasing severity
- Associated with lacunar infarcts in central gray matter and atrophy.

DYSMYELINATION (LEUKODYSTROPHIES)

- Disorders of children
- Present with variable mental retardation.

Metachromatic Leukodystrophy

Most common hereditary (AR) leukodystrophy.
- Lysosomal disorder, deficiency of arylsulfatase-A, AR
  – Symmetric demyelination with subcortical U-fiber sparing
  – Cerebellum—often atrophic.
- Anterior white matter is most severely affected.
- CT:
  – Moderate ventricular enlargement
  – Hypodensity in white matter, progressing anterior to posterior with no contrast enhancement.

- MR:
  - Increased T2, with arcuate fiber sparing initially
  - Increased intensity in cerebellar white matter
  - Thalamic hypointensity, mild to extreme.

Krabbe's Disease (Globoid Cell Leukodystrophy)

- Deficiency of galactocerebroside β-galactosidase, AR.
- Cerebral atrophy with small brain, extensive symmetric demyelination of the centrum semiovale and corona radiata with subcortical arcuate fiber sparing.
- Cerebellar white matter is affected to a lesser degree.
- Parieto-occipital lobes may be selectively involved early in disease
- NCCT:
  - Periventricular white matter hypodensity
  - Thalami and basal ganglia-hyperdense
  - Corona radiata, cerebellum—also are hyperdense
- MR:
  - Periventricular white matter hyperintensity on T2WI
  - Late onset disease may show changes limited to posterior hemispheric white matter.
- Cerebral atrophy.

Adrenoleukodystrophy

Single peroxisomal enzyme deficiency—acetyl coenzyme-A synthetase
- X-linked recessive
- Three types:
  1. Adrenoleukodystrophy (ALD)
  Rare neonatal form
  2. Adrenomyeloneuropathy (AMN)
  Neonatal ALD-AR
  3. Adrenoleukomyeloneuropathy (ALMN)
- Multiple enzyme deficiency
- Ventricular enlargement, cerebral atrophy.
  - First involvement of occipital lobes and splenium-B/L
  - Centrifugal and anterior extension symmetrical.
- ALD–3 months–1 year of age
  - Sparing of subcortical white matter early in disease.
- AMN–20–30 years
  - Auditory pathway involvement common
  - Typically three zones.
- Innermost central and posterior zone with necrosis, gliosis, and sometimes calcification.
- Intermediate zone of active demyelination and inflammatory change.
- Peripheral zone of demyelination with inflammatory change.

CT

Large symmetric hypodensity in parieto-occipital region ± calcification (peritrigonal).
- After contrast enhancement, in advancing rim with more peripheral non-enhancing edematous zone.

MR

- Central necrosis, zone of decreased intensity on T1WI and increased intensity on T2WI
- Intermediate zone shows contrast enhancement
- Peripheral zone of decreased T1 and increased T2 signal intensity
- Abnormal signal in lateral geniculate bodies, auditory pathways, corpus callosum splenium, and corticospinal tracts.

AMN

Symmetric hyperintensity in posterior limb of internal capsule.

Zellweger's (cerebrohepatorenal syndrome)—autosomal recessive and multiple peroxisomal enzyme deficiency.
- Neuronal migration disorders with heterotopic gray matter pachygyria, polymicrogyria, with white matter hypomyelination.

Leigh's disease: Subacute necrotizing encephalopathy.
- Multiple mitochondrial enzyme deficiencies, automatic recessive.

- Involvement of both gray and white matter.
- CF—hypotonia, seizure, vomiting, loss of head control, and respiratory failure.
- CT—hypodensity in caudate and putamen, no contrast enhancement.
- MR—symmetric hyperintensity in globus pallidus putamen, caudate, periventricular white matter, and periaqueductal gray.

MELAS SYNDROME

- Cerebral infarcts—occipital lobes most common site
- Focal cortical and brainstem white matter changes with basal ganglia calcification with or without cerebral and cerebellar atrophy.

MERRF SYNDROME

- Kearns-Sayre syndrome
- Childhood/adolescence AD
- Progressive external ophthalmoplegia
- Pigmentary retinal degeneration
- Heart block/increased CSF protein/cerebellar dysfunction
- White matter disease with cortical and/or cerebellar atrophy, and calcification in basal ganglia or deep white matter.

LEUKODYSTROPHIES: DISTINCTIVE FEATURES

- Complete/near complete lack of myelination
    - Canavan's disease
    - Pelizaeus–Merzbacher disease
- Frontal white matter most involved—Alexander's disease
- Occipital white matter most involved—ALD
- Macrocephaly
    - Alexander's disease
    - Canavan's disease
- High density basal ganglia—Krabbe's disease
- Enhancement following contrast enhancement
    - Alexander's disease
    - ALD
- *Stroke*:
    - Leigh's syndrome
    - MELAS syndrome
    - MERRF syndrome.

PREVERTEBRAL SOFT TISSUE THICKENING

(Cervical Region)

Normal Values of Prevertebral Soft Tissue

Level	Thickness (in mm)
C1	10
C2	5
C3	7
C4	7
C5	20
C6	20
C7	20

- Weight and age variation
- Flexion and extension less than 1 mm variation.

Fascial Spaces in Prevertebral Region

- Retropharyngeal space between buccopharyngeal fascia anteriorly and alar fascia posteriorly.
- Laterally—cloison sagittale.
- *Retroesophageal space*: Continuation of the above space in mid and lower neck surrounds the esophagus.
- *Danger space*:
    - Ventrally: Alar fascia
    - Dorsally: Prevertebral fascia.
- From skull base down to posterior mediastinum.
- Prevertebral space between prevertebral fascia and vertebrae from skull base to coccyx.

Causes of Prevertebral Soft Tissue (Cervical Region)

- *Retropharyngeal space*:
    - Lymphadenopathy
    - Abscess
    - Cellulitis
    - Edema
    - Hematoma
    - Lipoma
    - Hemangioma
    - Tortuous carotid artery
    - Extension of goiter.
- *Prevertebral space*:
    - Abscess

- Phrenic nerve—schwannomas
- Mesenchymal tumors of muscles.
- Extension of tumors like nasopharyngeal or esophageal carcinoma or lymphoma.

Retropharyngeal Lymph Adenopathy

- Lateral group is involved more than median group
- Reactive, suppurative, metastatic, lymphoma—4 main categories: (1) Metastasis nasopharynx, (2) oropharynx, (3) nasal cavity, and (4) hypopharynx (unresectability of primary tumor).
  CT—inflamed lymphoid tissue enhances homogeneously or heterogeneously or may appear edematous with decreased attenuation and mild delayed peripheral enhancement, nodal edema or suppuration.

Retropharyngeal Cellulitis and Abscess

- Retropharyngeal infections result from suppurative lymphadenitis, associated tonsillitis, pharyngitis, sinonasal infection, otitis media, etc.
- Fever, sore throat, swelling, stridor, odynophagia, and trismus.
- *Plain film*:
  - Widening of retropharyngeal soft tissue
  - Loss of cervical lordosis
  - Occasionally air in retropharyngeal soft tissue.
  CT is used to differentiate adenitis, abscess, and cellulitis.
- Like lymphadenopathy, abscess is also characterized by low attenuation and ring enhancement but the margins no longer confine to nodal morphology (skull base to T4).
- So CT gives invaluable information but it is not entirely accurate.
- US:
  - Differentiate between abscess and adenitis
  - Guidance for intraoperative aspiration and drainage.
- Diagnosis of cellulitis on CT is made when edema of soft tissues and obliteration of fat planes without rim enhancement.
- *Necrotizing cellulitis*: Extensive stranding of subcutaneous fat planes.
- *Complications*:
  - Airway obstruction
  - Displacement and compression of internal carotid artery
  - Internal jugular vein-compression/thrombophlebitis.

Retropharyngeal Edema

- Usually seen following radiation therapy in patients with head and neck cancer
- May also follow trauma or infection of oropharynx or vertebral column.

Hemangioma

These are vascular nests subdivided in three types:
1. Capillary
2. Cavernous
3. Mixed type.

On CT and MRI

- Intensively enhance after contrast injection
- Phleboliths.

Lipoma

- Predominantly found in posterior cervical space but may occur in RPS
- Seen as fat density, well-defined encapsulated on CT and MR
- Lipomas tend to enlarge with weight gain but do not decrease with weight loss.

Tortuous Carotid Artery

- A tortuous common or internal carotid artery may present submucosal mass displacing the posterior pharyngeal wall
- Palpation may not be feasible, pulsation overlooked
- CT diagnosis is straightforward.

Extension of Thyroid Masses

Pretracheal space communicating with retropharyngeal space between levels of thyroid cartilage and inferior thyroid artery can extend through this space.

Prevertebral Abscess
- Abscess in prevertebral space is usually from osteomyelitis of vertebral bodies
- Displaces RPS anteriorly and carotid sheath laterally.

Tumors
- Masses arising from prevertebral muscles are mesenchymal in origin
- Erosion of vertebral body—malignant
- Rhabdomyosarcoma—mostly from pharyngeal mass
- In children—rhabdomyosarcoma and neuroblastoma
- Nasopharyngeal lymphoma or minor salivary gland malignancy may directly invade.

NASOPHARYNGEAL MASSES

Nasopharynx is a space situated posterior to the posterior nares and bounded superiorly by the floor of the middle cranial fossa and posteriorly by the base of skull and laterally by the pharyngeal musculature, the mandible and the parotid.

Methods of Investigations

Plain X-ray soft tissue neck: This is now only sometimes used as a lateral projection of the pharynx. The film is placed against the shoulder and the central ray is centered at the angle of the mandible.

Computed Tomography

Computed tomography is now the optimum method of imaging; it shows not only the outlines of the nasopharynx but also the soft tissue structures of the infratemporal fossa and parapharyngeal space. The scan can be done in axial views and sagittal and coronal reconstructions can be done or direct coronal scanning can be done. Both pre- and postcontrast scans should be undertaken. The role of CT for lesions in this region may be defined as follows:
- Used as a complement to direct examination.
- To assess the size, situation and relations of a well-defined mass for prospective surgical removal, or the extent of local and deep infiltration for radiotherapy planning.
- To assess the relationship of the mass with great vessels and the parotid gland on postcontrast scans.

Magnetic Resonance Imaging

Now the imaging investigation is of choice, but careful selection of cases is necessary. It shows the major vessels of neck without contrast enhancement and clearly depicts the soft tissue anatomy in multiplanar projections. T1-weighted sequences have the best spatial resolution and give a strong signal from fat in the tissue planes. However, T2-weighted protocols are most useful for showing muscle invasion by carcinomas. A standard head coil is all that is used for the assessment of nasopharynx.

Differential Diagnosis of Nasopharyngeal Masses
- Meningoceles
- Adenoid hyperplasia (Fig. 8.24)
- Antrochoanal polyps
- Infections
- Juvenile angiofibroma
- Chordomas
- Carcinomas
- Lymphoma
- Extension of neoplasms (sphenoid/ethmoid carcinoma, parotid tumor).

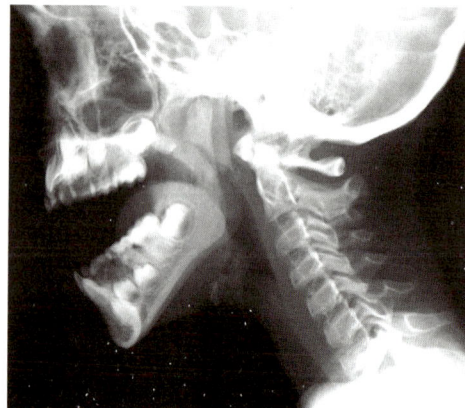

Fig. 8.24: Radiograph of nasopharynx showing adenoid hypertrophy.

Meningoceles

These present as a smooth well-defined mass in an infant or a young child posterior to and projecting into the nasopharynx. These are rare manifestations and are usually associated with a defect in the skull base. These masses may show fluid or CSF density of intracranial contents. These are best shown by coronal CT or MRI, which will differentiate meningocele from an encephalocele.

Adenoid Hyperplasia

- Presents in younger age group with nasal blockage and recurrent attacks of rhinitis.
- There is a verrucoid polypoidal mass in the nasopharynx with no evidence of bone involvement or mucosal invasion.
- CT and MRI best delineate the size, volume, and extent of the lesion.

Antrochoanal Polyp

- These are antral polyps, which outgrow from the antrum and present in the nasopharynx.
- They are smoothly outlined pear-shaped masses in the nasopharynx.
- They are associated with partial or complete opacification of the antrum but with no evidence of bone destruction or erosion. However, thinning of bones, secondary to the expansile nature of the mass, may be seen.
- On CT they present as hypodense soft tissue masses. On MR they have high homogeneous signal on T2-weighted sequences. CT and MR can elegantly define the origin of mass from the maxillary antrum and will also define the extent of the mass.

Infections

- Abscess in the parapharyngeal spaces may present in the nasopharynx posterior to the mucosal lining presenting clinically as masses in the nasopharynx with or without associated changes of inflammation on the overlying mucosa and the patient may show signs of toxemia.
- The abscesses are usually secondary to infection extending either from the parotid glands, the sinuses and hematogenous spread from a distant location.
- On CT, they are seen as well-defined walls of necrotic masses with enhancement of walls on CECT. Associated changes may be seen in the nearby structures from which the abscess has originated.

Juvenile Angiofibroma

- Most common benign tumor in pubescent males presents classically with epistaxis and nasal obstruction and a dark red or ulcerated mass in the nasal cavities and postnasal space.
- CT and MR clearly define the extent and origin of the lesion.
- The mass arises at or close to the base of the pterygoid lamina, thus bone erosion at this site is probably a pathognomonic feature.
- The tumor not only spreads into the nose and PNS but has a special tendency to spread laterally through the pterygomaxillary fissure and anterior bowing of the posterior wall of the antrum, an important differentiating feature. It causes destruction of the adjacent bones.
- Neglected cases may also show extension into the orbit, sphenoid sinus and the cranial cavity.
- There is considerable contrast enhancement on CECT and MR may show presence of flow voids as well as marked enhancement after gadolinium, which is characteristic to the tumor.

Chordomas

- These are midline tumors arising from commonly the clivus, but may also arise from basisphenoid and present as postnasal mass.
- They are usually found in patients of older age group.
- They present on CT as a large soft tissue mass in the postnasal space associated with destruction of the basisphenoid and flecks of calcifications. There is usually an associated intracranial mass.

Carcinomas
- Eighty percent of the carcinomas are squamous cell type. When they are large and exophytic, they present as a mass in the postnasal space. Usually, however, they infiltrate into the base of skull so that the patient presents with a cranial nerve lesion or with enlarged neck glands. Serous otitis media due to blockage of Eustachian tubes may be another presenting complaint.
- There is erosion of the floor of middle cranial fossa.
- There is obliteration of the lateral pharyngeal recess (fossa of Rosenmüller).
- CT and MR may also show the obliteration of soft tissue planes suggestive of invasion.
- Extension in the cranial cavity and evaluation of neck glands by CT and MR help in staging the tumor. In cases of adenoid cystic carcinoma, MR may also show perineural spread, which is characteristic to the tumor.

Lymphomas
- In the postnasal space, these tumors tend to grow in a bulky circumferential pattern without early invasion of the parapharyngeal spaces.
- CT and MR show bulky masses in the postnasal space with homogeneous attenuation or intensity.

Extension from Nearby Structures

This is usually due to the spread of pathological process in the nearby structures like in cases of sphenoid or ethmoid carcinoma or parotid masses. CT and MR will show the presence of primary pathology elsewhere and its extension in the postnasal space.

LARYNGEAL MASSES

Causes

Malignant	Benign
Carcinoma	Papillomas/polyps
Chondrosarcomas	Laryngocele/mucocele
Salivary gland tumors	Hemangioma
Metastases	Cartilage tumors
Miscellaneous	Salivary gland tumors

Malignant Lesions

- *Carcinoma*: Masses in the larynx are usually malignant, and virtually all are squamous cell carcinomas.
  - M:F is 5:1, almost always associated with tobacco and alcohol.
  - Peak incidence is 7th decade.
  - Divided into the supraglottic, glottic, and subglottic (infraglottic) types.
  - Role of radiologist is to describe the deep extension, the relationship of the mass to the surrounding structures, and lymphadenopathy. Pay particular attention to: laryngeal cartilage invasion, transglottic extension, extension into adjacent fascial spaces, especially parapharyngeal space and carotid space, regional lymph nodes including internal jugular chain of nodes and the midline Delphian node. Be observant for possible lung metastasis or secondary lung primary. Needle biopsy of suspicious deep masses may be necessary under imaging guidance.
  - Pitfalls of CT include the inability to reliably differentiate inflammation and edema from tumor, to accurately identify the subsite involvement in the presence of anatomic distortion from large tumors, and to clearly define margins in the absence of well-developed fat planes.
  - MRI has an advantage of multiplanar display especially in determining subglottic extension and in identifying the pre-epiglottic spread. MRI also has difficulty in differentiating edema from tumor but is superior to CT in detecting cartilage invasion.
- *Chondrosarcomas* are slowly growing neoplasms
  - Present usually in the 6th and 7th decades
  - Cricoid cartilage is usually involved (80%) followed by thyroid cartilage
  - Lesions in virtually all patients demonstrate coarse or stippled calcifications

- Features differentiating from carcinomas include older age at diagnosis, absence of smoking history, and predominately calcified tumor matrix.
- Minor salivary gland tumors as adenocystic carcinomas have been reported. They are indistinguishable from the laryngeal carcinomas but should be considered in patients with laryngeal mass and no history of smoking or drinking.
- Metastases to the larynx usually occur in the terminal stages of the disseminated malignancy. Primary tumors include melanoma (30%), renal cell carcinoma (15%). Site of deposit include supraglottic (40%), subglottic (20%), glottic (5%), and multifocal (35%).
- Rare tumors include fibrosarcomas, liposarcomas, and lymphomas.

Benign Lesions

- *Papillomas* constitute 80% of the benign mucosal tumors and are the most common pediatric laryngeal tumors. These appear as multiple nodular excrescences on the false and true cords producing contour abnormalities of the mucosal surfaces.
- Small cystic lesions can arise in the vallecula or epiglottic surface secondary to the obstruction of minor salivary gland.
- *Vocal cord polyps* can arise secondary to vocal abuse.
- *Laryngoceles* are the air-filled diverticulae arising from the saccule of the laryngeal ventricle. They are common in musicians who play wind instruments. They are associated with airway obstruction, pyoceles, and vocal cord paralysis. 25% are bilateral. These are of three types:
  1. *Internal*: When confined within thyroid lamina
  2. *External*: Lesions that pierce the thyroid membrane
  3. *Mixed*: Combination of the internal and external.
- *Laryngeal mucocele* is a fluid-filled laryngocele that arises secondary to a small ventricular cancer obstructing the saccule.
- *Subglottic hemangioma* is the most common laryngeal and upper tracheal neoplasm in the newborn and the young infant. It appears as a well-defined mass in the posterior or lateral portion of the subglottic airway.
- *Chondromas* arise from the hyaline or elastic cartilages of the larynx.
- *Chondrometaplasia* is a condition in which nodules of cartilage arise in the soft tissues of the larynx. Lesions arising in the close vicinity of the laryngeal cartilages may be difficult to differentiate from chondromas or chondrosarcomas on imaging.
- *Schwannomas* typically involve the sensory nerves such as the internal branch of the superior laryngeal nerve and usually arise in the 4th–6th decades as a palpable mass.
- *Minor salivary gland* tumors as pleomorphic adenomas have been reported.
- Rare tumors include paragangliomas, atypical carcinoid tumor, amyloidosis, etc.

ORBITAL MASSES

The pediatric patient with an orbital tumor differs substantially from the adult patient with a much greater incidence of congenital lesions, higher frequency of infection, and unique benign and malignant tumors involving the orbit.

Pediatric Orbital Tumors

- Most common orbital masses are cystic lesions of the orbit, mainly dermoids.
- Vasculogenic lesions are the second most common.
- Others include inflammatory lesions, fat-containing lesions, lacrimal gland masses, lymphoid tumors and leukemia, optic nerve and meningeal tumors, osseous and fibro-osseous masses, rhabdomyosarcoma, and metastatic lesions.
- Common malignant processes include rhabdomyosarcoma, metastatic disease, lymphomas, and leukemia.
- Most orbital tumors in children are benign.

Cystic Lesions

Dermoid Cysts

- Arise from trapped embryonic ectoderm in the suture lines between the orbital bones.
- Classified into juxtasutural, sutural, and soft-tissue types.
- Most common type—juxtasutural in the superotemporal and superonasal quadrants.
- Presents as painless mass in superotemporal area at the lateral portion of the eyebrow.
- Usually unattached to overlying skin, mobile, smooth, and non-tender.
- CT scan reveals a well-circumscribed lesion with a low-density lumen.

Teratomas

- Congenital germ-cell tumors arise from primordial germ cells with ectodermal, mesodermal, and endodermal components.
- Typically present at birth, with no bone invasion, often cause orbital enlargement.
- Large intraconal masses cause massive proptosis.

Vasculogenic Lesions

Capillary Hemangioma

- One-third are diagnosed at birth, and over 90% are visible by 6 months of age.
- Most common presentation—superficial involvement appearing as tumor and telangiectatic vessels in the skin that with time develops the typical strawberry-like appearance.
- Deeper lesions may appear as raised soft, purplish nodules.
- Deep orbital involvement may present solely with proptosis and no skin changes.
- Orbital hemangiomas frequently produce proptosis, globe displacement and enlarge with Valsalva maneuvers or crying.
- The typical course is—normal appearance at birth, lesion first noticed at one month, enlarging till 1–2 years followed by a stabilization and spontaneous involution by age 4–8 years of age.
- Best evaluated with CT or MRI—a diffusely infiltrating non-encapsulated mass, conforming to the surrounding orbital structures. No bony erosion, although expansion of the orbit is possible.
- Ultrasonography is also a valuable non-invasive test.

Lymphangiomas

- Benign congenital malformation—may affect the conjunctiva, eyelids or deep orbit.
- Classically, viewed as separate from the vascular system, although some overlap has been noted.
- Typically, the tumor is identified within the first two decades of life.
- Present as slow enlargement with increasing proptosis over many years, or one of sudden proptosis from intralesional hemorrhage (chocolate cyst).
- The classic lesion is a smooth, pink-orange mass (Salmon patch) under an intact conjunctiva.
- CT scan shows a homogeneous mass with well-defined borders that does not destroy surrounding structures or bone.
- Most lesions are extraconal and in the superior orbit.

Orbital Meningiomas and Schwannomas

- Most common during the 4th–7th decade of life.
  Primary orbital meningiomas arise from the optic nerve, 70% invade the orbit from the cranium infiltrative, and enhancing. The classic "railroad track" describes calcifications of the tumor along the optic nerve in the subarachnoid space.
- MRI is used to evaluate intracranial extension, showing a hyperintense tumor after contrast administration.
  Schwannoma or *neurilemmoma* is a benign, noninvasive, peripheral nerve tumor.
- They are relatively rare; usually occur in adults from age 20–70 years.
- CT shows well-circumscribed, homogeneous, elongated ovoid mass displacing the surrounding structures.

- MRI—the tumor is hypointense on T1WI and hyperintense on T2WI.
- The tumor is extraconal when associated with the 4th cranial nerve, but is more commonly intraconal.

CAVERNOUS HEMANGIOMA (ENCAPSULATED VENOUS MALFORMATION)

- Most common vascular and the most common primary intraconal orbital lesion in adults.
- Average age of onset is around 40 years.
- More common in women (70%) than men (30%) and is generally unilateral.
- Present with a slowly progressive painless proptosis over several years.
- These do not enlarge with Valsalva.
- CT or MRI reveals a well-defined mass with an oval shape.
- Most are intraconal, but occasionally extraconal.
- On CT they are homogeneous with increased density.
- On MRI they are homogeneous and iso-intense to muscle, on T1WI and hyperintense on T2WI.
- Following contrast addition, the lesions enhance inhomogeneously.

METASTATIC TUMORS

- Breast carcinoma is most common metastatic tumor in women followed by lung carcinoma.
- In men, the most common are lung and prostate.
- The average age at presentation is the 7th decade, most being female (due to the higher incidence of breast metastasis).
- On CT, the most common finding is a well-defined, contrast enhancing, intraconal mass.
- The orbital bony walls are also a common site for metastasis, especially with prostate cancers.
- These tumors may show expansion during an acute upper respiratory infection.
- Superficial lesions are more common and have a better prognosis for vision than deeper lesions. No enlargement of the tumor with Valsalva maneuvers.
- Imaging studies include CT and MRI, which both show the multicompartmental nature of the venous-lymphatic malformations.
- MR imaging is preferred over CT because it delineates the internal structure of the cysts.

MISCELLANEOUS

Rhabdomyosarcoma

- Most common orbital malignant tumor found in children.
- Presents early in the 1st decade with rapid unilateral proptosis and displacement of the globe.
- CT scan shows an irregular tumor with moderately well-defined margins, soft tissue attenuation, and often evidence of bony destruction (50%).
- MR imaging demonstrates a signal similar to muscle on T1 and higher than muscle on T2Ws.

Optic Nerve Gliomas

- Often associated with neurofibromatosis type I (18–50% of cases), often bilateral.
- Mean age of presentation is about 8 years.
- Typical presentation is proptosis and visual loss or visual field changes.
- Appear as fusiform enlargement of the optic nerve which is isodense to brain on CT.
- Intracranial extension into the optic canal and chiasm is best evaluated with MRI.

Fibrous Dysplasia

- Most frequent fibro-osseous tumor seen exclusively in children in the first two decades of life.
- Replacement of normal bone with collagen, fibroblasts, osteoid, and giant cells.
- *Two types of fibrous dysplasia*: (1) Polyostotic (Albright's syndrome) and (2) monostotic.
- Polyostotic fibrous dysplasia involves multiple bones, not generally the orbit, abnormal skin pigmentation and precocious puberty.
- Monostotic fibrous dysplasia occurs most often in the bones of the face.

- The orbital roof is the most common site of orbital involvement.
- Usual presentation—adolescent child with proptosis, globes, and orbit displacement and facial asymmetry.
- The CT shows thickened abnormal bone with sclerotic lesions with a "ground-glass" appearance.
- Biopsy is usually necessary to confirm the diagnosis and to rule out more aggressive lesions.

Metastatic Tumors

- Neuroblastoma is the most frequent metastatic orbital disease in children.
- Others include Ewing's sarcoma, leukemia, and lymphoma.
- Neuroblastoma is common in children, majority occurring before age 5 (median 22 months).

Adult Orbital Tumors

In the adult population, the more common types of orbital tumors vary significantly from children. The most common tumor includes carcinomas (paranasal sinus, secondary, and metastatic), inflammatory masses (pseudotumor), lacrimal gland tumors, cysts, lymphomas, meningiomas, and vascular tumors (cavernous hemangiomas). Secondary tumors commonly invade the orbit and include mucoceles, squamous cell carcinoma, meningioma, vascular malformations, and basal cell carcinoma.

Paranasal Sinus Masses

Mass in the paranasal sinuses has the potential to extend into the orbit. The most common mass lesion of the orbit originating in the sinus is the *mucocele*.

Mucocele results from obstruction of a sinus ostium leading to an enlarging fluid-filled sinus, which eventually may erode through the orbital bony wall.
- The median age of presentation is around 50 years.
- Most arise from the ethmoid and frontal sinus
- Patients will present with unilateral proptosis with globe displacement away from the mass, lid swelling, and sometimes a palpable mass.
- CT scan reveals a well-defined homogeneous mass extending into the orbit through a bony defect associated with an opacified sinus cavity.

Neoplasms of the Paranasal Sinuses

- Benign tumors push the periorbital structures aside, while malignant lesions invade the periosteum.
- Most common malignancy is squamous cell carcinoma.
- Disease is usually advanced at presentation with orbital invasion in almost two-thirds of the patients.
- Adenocarcinoma arising from the ethmoid sinuses is frequently associated with wood workers.
- Adenoid cystic carcinomas show perineural spread via the infraorbital nerve.
- Locally invasive neoplasms as esthesioneuroblastoma and benign paranasal neoplasm as inverted papilloma may also extend into the orbit.
- Evaluation best done radiologically with CT scan, because of the ability to detect early bony destruction with either orbital or intracranial extension.
- MRI scans are useful in detecting intracranial extension and distinguishing certain neoplastic diseases from one another.

ORBITAL PSEUDOTUMOR (IDIOPATHIC ORBITAL INFLAMMATION)

- An inflammatory condition of the orbit of unknown etiology.
- Common cause of proptosis from the 2nd to 7th decade of life.
- Multifocal involvement is common and any orbital structure may be involved.
- Onset of symptoms is acute; however, subacute or chronic forms have been described.
- The typical symptom is dull orbital pain, which is worse with eye movement.
- Proptosis is the most common finding.

- CT findings show hazy enlargement of affected structures with enhancement after intravenous contrast injection.
- MR T1WIs show lesions with similar signal to muscles that enhance with contrast. T2WIs have increased signal similar to or greater than fat.

Lacrimal Gland Tumors

- About half are epithelial neoplasms, while the other half are in lymphoproliferative disorder.
- Lymphoid lesions include benign lymphoid hyperplasia, malignant lymphoma, and leukemias. Lymphoid lesions appear as smooth enlargement of the gland on CT scans.
- Epithelial neoplasms appear irregular on CT and include pleomorphic adenomas (benign), adenocystic carcinoma, adenocarcinoma, mucoepidermoid carcinomas, and undifferentiated carcinomas.
- The most common of epithelial lesions is the pleomorphic adenoma (benign mixed tumor) which occurs primarily between the ages of 20 and 50 years.
- Most common malignant epithelial neoplasm is adenoid cystic carcinoma.
- CT scans will often show bony destruction and infiltration of the lacrimal mass.

Lymphoid Tumors

- Orbital lymphomas may be primary or associated with systemic disease.
- Most orbital lymphomas are localized to the orbit but many patients develop systemic lymphoma over time.
- Orbital lymphoma is an adult disease usually presenting between the ages of 50 years and 70 years.
- Usually an anterior mass, enlarges slowly, causing progressive painless proptosis over months.

OCULAR MASSES

Melanoma

- Arise from choroid in elderly.
- Most common malignancy in adults.
- Highly invasive with extraocular spread as well.
- Ultrasound typically shows raised echogenic focus along post wall of vitreous chamber (collar button).
- On MRI, melanotic type shows increased T1W and decreased T2W while amelanotic type is isointense to soft tissue.
- Trans-scleral spread and perineural spread are common.

Retinoblastoma

- Most common malignancy in childhood.
- One-third are bilateral with autosomal dominant inheritance.
- Trilateral retinoblastoma when B/L tumor associated with pineal tumor.
- Highly malignant and aggressive with trans-scleral and hematogenous spread.
- Ultrasound shows highly echogenic mass with DAS.
- CT is modality of choice and shows dense calcification in a retinal based soft tissue mass.
- Any calcification within the globe on CT scans in pediatric patient should be considered retinoblastoma unless proved otherwise.
- MRI is superior to CT in evaluation of trans-scleral or perineural spread or in evaluation of pineal region for additional masses.

INTRAORBITAL CALCIFICATION

Causes

- Cataract
- Retinoblastoma
- Parasitic infection:
  - Hydatid cyst
  - Cellulose cysticercosis
- Phleboliths:
  - Hemangioma
  - Arteriovenous malformation
  - Venous varix
- Orbital meningioma
- Others:
  - Adenocarcinoma and cystic carcinoma of lacrimal gland
  - Neurofibroma
  - Rhabdomyosarcoma.

Cataract

- Immature cataract—scattered opacities are separated by clear zones.
- Mature cataract—totally opaque cortex is noted on ultrasound.

Retinoblastoma

- Most frequent intraocular tumor of childhood.
- 85% are less than 3 years; 20–40% have B/L tumors.

Classified as:
Grade 1: Solitary or multiple, less than 4 disk dram in size at or behind equator
Grade 2: Solitary or multiple; 4–10 disk dram
Grade 3: Anterior to equator or solitary more than 10 disk dram
Grade 4: Tumors that are multiple and extend up to or a serrata
Grade 5: Tumors that involve half of the retina or presence of vitreous seeds.

Most children present with leukokoria or white pupillary reflex.
RF: Irregular intraocular mass, 90% cases show calcification on CT.

Endophytic extension:
- Projects into vitreous.

Exophytic extension:
- Subretinal space—radiopaque density
- Contrast enhancement is variable.
  Orbital and intracranial extension.

Orbital Meningioma

Primary: Optic nerve sheath.

Secondary: Originates from greater wing of sphenoid with temporal and orbital extension.

Optic Nerve Meningioma

Adults: 3rd–5th decades.
R/F:
- Tubular or fusiform thickening of optic nerve
- Homogeneous contrast enhancement
- Tram track sign: Hyperdense mass surrounding hypodense optic nerve
- Calcification +ve
- Optic canal widened by mass or narrowed by hyperostosis
- Intracranial extension ±.

Hemangioma

Capillary Hemangioma

- Tumor of early childhood; involutes spontaneously by 6–7th year.
- Forms a soft bluish mass which may involve any part of orbit.
  - US—well-defined anterior soft lesion with small irregular echoes.
  - Calcification ±.
  - Color Doppler flow imaging (CDFI)—high flow within immature vessels.

Cavernous Hemangioma

- Most common benign retrobulbar tumor; 3rd to 4th decade.
- Usually, it lies within the muscles' core and displacing the optic nerve.
- RF: Honeycomb pattern of altered strong and weak signals on ultrasound.
- CT: Homogeneous mass (hyperdense) with smooth margin showing uniform contrast enhancement.
- Phleboliths +.
- Expansion of the orbital wall +.

Arteriovenous Fistula (Carotid Cavernous Fistula)

- Post-traumatic/postsurgical
- Spontaneous:
  - Atherosclerosis, osteogenesis imperfecta, Ehlers-Danlos syndrome, pseudoxanthoma elasticum
  - Clinically patient presents with pulsatile exophthalmos
  - RF: Dilated superior ophthalmic vein which cannot be compressed
  - Reverse flow in the superior ophthalmic vein which is arterialized
  - Increased size of extraocular muscles
  - Angiography required for endovascular treatment
  - Phleboliths ±.

Orbital Varices

Varix becomes prominent on prone position, compression of jugular veins, and Valsalva's maneuver.
- Ultrasound shows soft echo-free lesion with pheboliths.
- CDFI may demonstrate movements of blood flow as malformation fills with blood or empties.
- Orbit may be expanded.
- CT shows nodular or serpiginous mass, containing phleboliths, with marked contrast enhancement.
- MRI—vase stream with signal void or flow-related enhancement or echo rephasing due to slow flow.
- Permanent signal may indicate a clot.

Rhabdomyosarcoma

- Highly malignant tumor; most frequent in childhood.
- RF—seen as a well-defined mass in a muscle or adjacent to it.
  - Mass may include the lacrimal gland with osseous and extraorbital invasion
  - Calcifications are frequently seen after radiotherapy.
- *Adenocystic carcinoma of lacrimal gland*:
  - Most common malignant lacrimal gland tumor.
  - RF—enlarged gland with irregular serrated bodies, bony erosion of orbital roof.
  - Presence of calcific deposit.
- *Hydatid cyst*:
  - It can be seen in the retrobulbar region.
  - RF—spherical or oval mass of low reflectivity or low density.
  - *Enhancement of walls +ve*
  - *Calcification +ve*
  - *Cellulosae cyst.*
- Intraocular (vitreous or subretinal space).
- *Extraocular (EOMS, eyelid, lacrimal gland, and optic nerve)*:
  - RF—cystic lesion with an eccentrically placed hyperdense scolex showing ring enhancement.
  - In the later stages, nodular calcification is seen.

INNER EAR MASSES

- *The temporal bone*:
  - Petrous part 1
  - Squamous part 2
  - Tympanic part 3
  - Mastoid part 4
  - Styloid process 5
  - Zygomatic process 6
- Houses the structures of middle and inner ears (Fig. 8.25):
  - Cochlear apparatus (for hearing)
  - Vestibular apparatus (for equilibrium)
- The bony case is known as otic capsule or bony labyrinth while the functioning inner organ system is known as membranous labyrinth (Fig. 8.26).

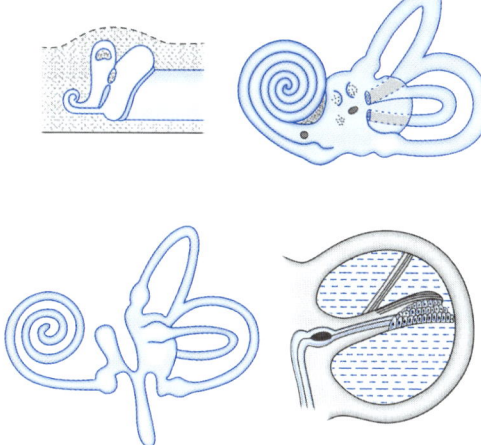

Fig. 8.25: Structures of middle and inner ears.

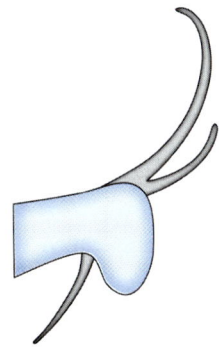

Fig. 8.26: Bony labyrinth.

METHODS OF IMAGING
- Plain X-ray, e.g. Stenvers' view
- Tomography of temporal bone
- CT scan:
  - Axial—especially bony
  - Coronal—labyrinth
- MRI:
  - Axial—especially membranous
  - Coronal—labyrinth.

Masses

Inflammatory:
- Granulomatous labyrinthitis
- Labyrinthitis ossificans
- Sarcoid granuloma:
  - Cholesteatoma or cholesterol granuloma.

Neoplastic
- Schwannoma
- Lipoma
- Arachnoid cyst
- Epidermoid cyst
- Arteriovenous malformation (AVM)
- Hemangioma
- Meningioma
- Lymphoma
- Metastasis
- Temporal bone tumors.

Miscellaneous
- Intralabyrinthine hemorrhage
- Vestibular aqueduct syndrome (VAS).

Salient Features

Inflammatory
- Labyrinthitis is a term used to describe inflammation of inner ear.
- Viral, bacterial, and autoimmune.
- Tympanogenic, meningogenic, hematogenic, post-traumatic; iatrogenic, may be associated with cholesteatoma.
- Bilateral >> unilateral: A cholesteatoma may occur here per se.
- On CT and especially MR, membranous labyrinth shows faint and segmental enhancement (as compared to schwannoma which shows complete and well-defined enhancement)—acute and subacute.
- Associated enhancing granuloma and facial nerve enhancement may be seen.
- In late stages when treatment failure occurs, a fibrous and very late bony labyrinth, also known as labyrinthitis ossificans, is seen. The imaging pattern corresponds accordingly, i.e.:
  - Fibrous:
    - Hypointense on T1WI; minimal or no enhancement
  - Hypointense on T2 WI and T2 gradient-echo.
    - Isodense on CT.
  - Calcified:
    - Hypointense on T1WI, T2 WI with no enhancement.
    - Hyperdense on CT.

Intralabyrinthine Bleed
- Coagulopathy, trauma, and tumor
- Rare
- Hyper on CT and T1.

Vestibular Aqueduct Syndrome
- Most common cause of congenital sensorineural hearing loss diagnosed by imaging.
- On imaging, a large endolymphatic duct and sac are seen. Associated deformity of cochlear modiolus is also present.

Schwannoma
- Of 8th cranial nerve known as acoustic neuromas is usually combined intra- and extracanalicular (i.e. CP angle) but may sometimes be purely intracanalicular.
- Sometimes purely intralabyrinthine schwannomas may be seen.
- Slow-growing noncalcifying masses, larger in females.
- When small, they are uniformly isodense (CT), isointense (T1 and T2) while enhance uniformly but as the size increases, areas of necrosis and cyst formation may also be seen.

Other neoplasia: But these are not stressed as they are not primary inner ear conditions.
- The appearances are general with the epicenter of lesion being the only feature helping in predicting an inner ear origin, e.g.:
  - *Lipoma:* Hyperintense on T1, T2WI hyper, while hypodense on CT, no enhancement
  - *Arachnoid cyst:* Follows fluid signal
  - *Epidermoid:* Follows with specific changes
  - *Bone tumors:* Bony changes
  - *Vascular tumors:* Extreme vascularity.

MIDDLE EAR MASSES (TABLE 8.2)

Congenital

- *Aberrant internal carotid artery*:
  - Vascular tympanic membrane
  - Pulsatile tinnitus
  - Imaging reveals a tubular soft tissue mass entering middle ear cavity posterolateral to cochlea, crossing mesotympanum along cochlear promontory, extending anteromedially to become continuous with horizontal portion of carotid canal.

Table 8.2: Middle ear masses.

Tumor	Location	Imaging	Comments
Aberrant internal carotid artery	Posterolateral to cochlea crossing mesotympanum along cochlear promontory	Enhancing mass on postcontrast images and continuous with carotid canal	Protrusion in middle ear cavity without a bony margin
Dehiscent jugular bulb	Posteroinferior middle ear	Enhancing mass contiguous with jugular bulb	Absence of bony plate between jugular bulb and middle ear
Cholesteatoma	Usually in the epitympanic recess	Hypointense on T1WI and hyperintense on T2WI	Erosion of the epitympanic wall, especially the scutum and ossicles
Cholesterol granuloma	Nonspecific	Hyperintense on T1WI and T2WI	Associated with CSOM
Granulation tissue	Nonspecific	Linear stranding of middle ear cavity with enhancement on postcontrast images	No bony erosive changes
Glomus tympanicum	Cochlear promontory	Enhancing mass on postcontrast images with erosion and displacement of ossicles	Inferior wall of middle ear cavity remains intact
Glomus jugulare	At the jugular foramen	Enhancing mass on postcontrast images with destruction of ossicles and posteromedial surface of petrous bone	Destruction of inferior wall of middle ear cavity, roof of jugular fossa and bony spur separating vein from carotid artery
Meningioma	Nonspecific	Enhancing mass with remodeling of bone	Sclerosis of adjacent bone
Malignant masses as squamous cell carcinoma rhabdomyosarcoma	Nonspecific	Enhancing mass on postcontrast images with destruction of ossicles and other adjacent bones	Histopathology is confirmative

(T1WI: T1-weighted image; CSOM: Chronic suppurative otitis media)

- Protrusion into middle ear without bony margin.
- *Dehiscent jugular bulb*:
  - Vascular tympanic membrane
  - Pulsatile tinnitus
  - Imaging reveals a soft tissue mass contiguous with jugular foramen and there is absence of a bony plate separating jugular bulb from posteroinferior middle ear.

Inflammatory

- *Cholesteatoma*:
  - Tumor-like mass of exfoliated keratin within a sac of stratified squamous epithelium.
  - Cholesteatoma is usually an acquired disease (secondary cholesteatoma) but can be congenital (primary cholesteatoma).
  - Acquired cholesteatoma results from in-growth of squamous epithelium through marginal tympanic membrane perforations, from retraction pockets or from in-growth into the middle ear of the basal layer of the tympanic membrane and is usually related to chronic otitis media.
  - High resolution CT is an excellent technique for showing the location and extent of the lesion prior to surgery.
  - On CT images, cholesteatoma usually presents as a more or less rounded soft tissue mass, often centered within the epitympanic recess and lesions are commonly associated with erosion of the lateral epitympanic wall (more specifically the scutum) and the ossicular chain.
  - Associated findings are thickening of the tympanic membrane and inflammatory polyps in the medial part of the external auditory canal (EAC).
  - MRI may provide additional information, as the signal characteristics and/or enhancement pattern of cholesteatoma are characteristic being low-signal intensity on T1WI and a high-signal intensity on T2WI.

- *Cholesterol granuloma*:
  - Expansile lesion arising from a pneumatized cavity which becomes closed; the subsequent decrease in air pressure causes edema, fluid accumulation, and intralesional bleeding; that promotes granulomatous reaction leading to neovascularity and continuing hemorrhage.
  - In the middle ear cavity, they usually arise in the context of chronic otitis media; on otoscopy, this may give rise to a blue tympanic membrane, suggesting the presence of a vascular mass lesion.
  - On CT images, a well-demarcated expansile lesion is seen, indistinguishable from cholesteatoma.
  - MR characteristics of cholesterol granulomas are hyperintensity on both T1WI and T2WI (this being due to their hemorrhagic components).

- *Granulation tissue*:
  - Vascular reparative tissue, commonly seen in the middle ear and mastoid, in conjunction with other diseases (such as cholesteatoma) or in isolation.
  - It may produce a bluish discoloration of the tympanic membrane, causing clinical doubt as to the presence of a true hypervascular lesion.
  - On CT, granulation tissue causes opacification (linear stranding) of the middle ear and mastoid without erosive changes.
  - On MRI, pronounced enhancement is seen after injection of gadolinium.
  - In rare cases, granulation tissue itself may behave aggressively and cause bone erosion.

Neoplastic

Benign Tumor

- *Glomus tumor/chemodectomas/nonchromaffin paragangliomas/glomerulocytomas* (slow growing vascular lesion arising from glomus body).
  - *Glomus tympanicum* at the cochlear promontory.

- Appears as a globular soft tissue mass with intense postcontrast enhancement.
- It may cause erosion and displacement of the ossicles; however, the inferior wall of the middle ear cavity is left intact.
  - Glomus jugulare at the jugular foramen
- It causes invasion of the middle ear from below and destroys the bony roof of the jugular fossa and bony spur separating vein from the carotid artery.
- There is intense postcontrast enhancement, destruction of ossicles (usually incus), otic capsule, and posteromedial surface of the petrous bone.
- MR imaging shows *"salt and pepper appearance"* due to multiple small tumor vessels.
- Angiography is also diagnostic.
- Malignant transformation with metastases to regional nodes is seen in 2–4% cases.
- *Facial neuroma*:
  - It appears as a tubular mass in enlarged or scalloped facial canal.
- *Choristoma*:
  - Ectopic mature salivary tissue.
- *Meningioma*:
  - Extracranial meningiomas are rare.
  - Extracranial meningiomas are formed by direct extension outside the skull of a primary intracranial meningioma, by metastasis from a malignant intracranial meningioma, or from extracranial arachnoid cell clusters, which accompany certain cranial nerves outside the cranium.
  - The imaging characteristics are similar to those of intracranial meningioma. An enhancing mass lesion with remodeling of the bone is seen; the neighboring bone may appear very sclerotic.

Malignant Tumor
- *Squamous cell carcinoma*:
  - It appears as a soft tissue mass with variable enhancement on postcontrast images.
  - Destruction and displacement of ossicular chain and adjacent bones.

- *Metastases*
- *Rhabdomyosarcoma*:
  - The most common soft tissue tumor in children.
  - This appears as a bulky soft tissue mass with uniform postcontrast enhancement producing bony destruction as well.
  - MR is the imaging modality of choice with the tumor being intermediate in signal intensity on T1WIs and hyperintense on T2Ws.
- Adenocarcinoma (rare), adenocystic carcinoma.

EXTERNAL ACOUSTIC MASSES
Causes
- Keratosis obturans
- External auditory canal cholesteatoma
- Malignant external otitis
- Benign tumors:
  - Exostosis
  - Osteomas
  - Epidermoid or primary congenital
  - Cholesteatoma.
- Malignant tumors:
  - Squamous cell carcinoma
  - Basal cell carcinoma
  - Ceruminoma
  - Rare
  - Metastasis, myeloma
  - Osteosarcoma, chondrosarcoma.
- Histiocytosis
- Some middle ear masses may also extend.

Keratosis Obturans
- Usually occurs in individuals below 40 years.
- History of sinusitis or bronchiectasis (results in reflux sympathetic stimulation of ceruminous gland of EAC).
- Keratin plugs occlude the medial portion of EAC and the adjacent bony canal is diffusely widened (reflux hyperemia).

External Auditory Canal Cholesteatoma (0.1% to 0.5% in EAC)
- Usually occurs in individuals above 40 years.
- Unilateral, chronic, associated with otorrhea.

- Localized erosion of the canal wall with elevation of epidermis by cholesteatoma embedded in the bony wall.
- Formation of sequestrum and sinus tracts may be present.
- Most common site is along the posteroinferior wall of EAC but lateral to temporomandibular joint.
- Exact cause—unknown; periostitis of the bony canal.

Malignant External Otitis

- Disease of elderly who are diabetic or immunocompromised.
- Causative agent is usually *Pseudomonas*, *Staphylococcus* and *Aspergillus*.
- Often begins in an insidious fashion at the osseocartilaginous junction as a focal area of ulceration and osteitis of EAC. Tympanic membrane (TM) is resistant to the infectious process.
- Infection may spread—parotid gland, temporomandibular joint, soft tissue of neck, skull base or involvement of mastoid, petrous apex, and middle ear may also occur.
- Intracranial extension can occur through the petro-occipital synchondrosis.
    - *CT*: Bone destruction and sequestrum, soft tissue edema. Abscess in parapharyngeal spaces and intracranial invasion.
    - *MRI*: Superior to CT for detection of marrow invasion and soft tissue changes.
    - Indium-111 white blood cell and technetium-99m single photon emission computed tomography—best imaging approach to assess the post-therapeutic response.

Exostosis

- Most common benign tumor of EAC.
- Arises in the medial aspect of the osseous portion of the EAC near tympanic annulus.
- Seen in patients with prolonged exposure to cold sea water, swimming pool water.
- Seen as sessile multinodular bony masses. Unilateral or bilateral.

Osteomas

- Less common than exostosis.
- Mastoid is the most common extracanalicular site.
- Seen as solitary, U/L pedunculated growths of mature bone located in the outer portion of the EAC.

Squamous Cell Carcinoma

- Most common malignant tumor of the ear.
- History of chronic external otitis is usually positive.
- Tumor destroys the adjacent bone in the EAC and middle ear and invades the surrounding tissue.
- The most important CT finding suspected of carcinoma is erosion of the walls of EAC or middle ear by a soft tissue mass in a patient who does not have a history of cholesteatoma.
- Predictor of poor outcome:
    - Extensive tumor, 8th nerve involvement, cervical or periparotid lymph nodes.

Ceruminomas

Apocrine glands within the EAC are known as ceruminous glands. Tumors arising from ceruminous glands:
- Ceruminous adenoma:
    - Rare-5th to 6th decade
- Pleomorphic adenoma:
    CT: Soft tissue mass without bony destruction.
- Adenoid cystic carcinoma
- Mucoepidermoid carcinoma
- Ceruminous adenocarcinoma
- Most common.

Computed tomography findings are similar to squamous cell carcinoma except that metastases to regional lymph nodes are more common.

Metastasis

- *Hematogenous*: Breast, prostate, lung, kidney, and thyroid.
- *Direct spread*: Skin, parotid, nasopharynx, brain, and meninges.

- *Systemic involvement:* Leukemia, lymphoma, and myeloma.
- These lesions present as diffuse or focal osteolytic destructive pattern.

Epidermoidomas (Primary Congenital Cholesteatoma)
- Consists of masses of ectodermal rests (different from true cholesteatomas whose formation is a reaction to inflammation and trapped squamous epithelium).
- Seen as a soft tissue mass with widening of EAC.

Histiocytosis
- Primarily affects the pediatric age group.
- In the temporal bone, EAC and mastoids are commonly involved.
- Patients present with otalgia and draining ear.
- Cases are diagnosed only after treatment with antibiotic first to cure a suspected middle or external ear infection.
- Early imaging findings mimic inflammatory diseases beveled. Bony destruction pattern is usually geographical with edge. Enhancement of soft tissue may be homogeneous or peripheral.

INTRAMEDULLARY LESIONS (FIG. 8.27)
- Intramedullary lesions are lesions of spinal cord.
- Tumors:
  - Most are malignant
  - 90–95%.
- Gliomas:
  - More than 95%.
- Ependymomas:
  - Low-grade astrocytomas
  - Oligodendroglioma.
- Less common:
  - Hemangioblastomas
  - Paragangliomas
  - Lipoma
  - Epidermoid—rare
  - Gangliocytoma.
  - Metastasis.
- Non-neoplastic cystic lesions:
  - Hydrosyringomyelia
  - Hematomyelia.

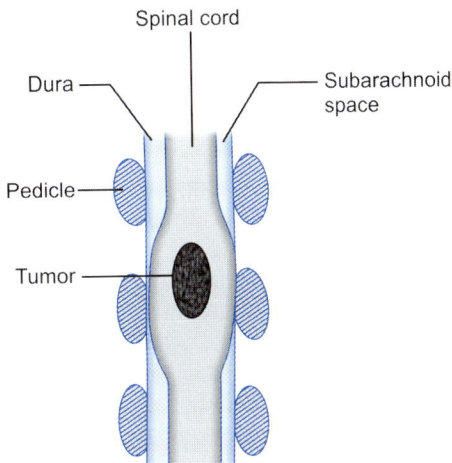

Fig. 8.27: Intramedullary lesions.

- Inflammatory diseases:
  - Multiple sclerosis
  - Transverse myelitis
  - Tuberculoma is rare
  - Cysticercosis
  - Intramedullary abscess
  - Sarcoidosis.
- Infarct.

Ependymoma
- Most common spinal cord tumor overall.
- Most common intramedullary tumor in adults.
- Arise from ependymal cells.

Intramedullary
Most common—cellular type—circumscribed, sharply.
- Most common site—cervical cord
- Mean age 43 years:
  - Cystic degeneration.
- Female > Male:
  - Hemorrhage.
- Typically—symmetric cord expansion
- *Myxopapillary type* exclusively in conus and filum terminale
- Mean age 28 years:
  - Slow growing, filling and expanding lumbosacral spinal cord
  - Male > Female hemorrhage and cystic degeneration—common.

- Cystic fibrosis (CF)—back or neck pain, leg or sacral pain.
- X-ray: Widened canal or bone destruction in 20%.
- Myelography:
  - Nonspecific cord widening
  - Multisegmental lesion
  - Small conus medullaris or filum terminale lesions
  - Well-delineated intradural mass with contrast meniscus.
- CT:
  - Nonspecific canal widening
  - Posterior scalloping
  - Neural foraminale enlargement.
- MRI:
  - Isointense on T1 and hyperintense on T2
  - Hypointensity at tumor margin on T2WI
  - Cyst formation, hemorrhage, and necrosis
  - Enhance strongly following contrast administration.

Astrocytomas

- Second most common spinal cord tumor overall.
- Most common cord tumor in children.
- Usually low grade-fibrillary astrocytomas.
- Anaplastic astrocytomas and glioblastoma multiforme.
- Mean age at presentation –21 years (9 years–70 years).
- Male = Female.
- Most common site—cervical cord and thoracic cord:
  - Multisegmental involvement.
- Most common clinical feature—pain.
- Sign and symptom of neurological dysfunction, often absent early in disease.

X-ray

- X-ray may be normal
- Widened interpedicular distance.

Myelography

- Nonspecific cord enlargement

- Canal widening:
  - MRI—isointense to hypointense on T1, hyperintense on T2, enhance after contrast
- Intratumoral cyst formation and associated syrinx are common.

Hemangioblastoma

- 1–5% of cord: Tumors 75% intramedullary
- Fourth decade: 10–15% combined intra- and extramedullary (intradural)
- Most common site (50%): Thoracic cord, cervical cord (40%)
- Highly vascular nodule with an extensive cyst that diffusely enlarges the cord with prominent leptomeningeal vessels.

Cystic Fibrosis

- Sensory changes—typically impaired proprioception.
- One-third—associated with Von Hipped-Lindau (VHL) disease.
- Myelocord expansion with prominent dilated tortuous vessels seen in 50% patients.
- Angiography—highly vascular mass with dense prolonged tumor blush with prominent vessels.
  MR-cord expansion with high signal intensity on T2WI with strong CE with prominent foci of high velocity signal loss.
- Cyst formation and syrinx—50–70%.

Oligodendroglioma

- Nonglial neoplasms:
  - Ganglioglioma
  - Schwannoma—rare.

Lipoma

- Rare
- May be associated with dysraphism
- CT—fat density
- MR—high signal intensity on T1WI.

Epidermoid

- Rare
- Congenital or iatrogenic
- Usually oval-shaped lesions with variable signal intensity depending upon contents.

Syringohydromyelia

- Fluid-filled cavity usually centered on the central canal + extending into dorsal column through the white commissure.
- Cylindrical—involve most of the cord. May enlarge the cord.
- Fusiform—usually segmental.
  - 80% associated with Chiari-I malformation
  - Most of the rest are idiopathic.
    * Post-traumatic.
    * Postarachnoiditis
    * Above and below intramedullary tumors especially hemangioblastoma.
- Well shown by MRI—signal characteristics similar to cerebrospinal fluid (CSF).
- Intravenous (IV) gadolinium may be necessary to exclude tumor in idiopathic cases.
- Plain CT—may or may not reveal dilatation of central canal.
- CT myelo early and delayed imaging after contrast administration (6 or 10 hours)—helps in diagnosis.

Hematomyelia

May or may not be associated with subarachnoid hemorrhage.
- Trauma
- SVM:
  - Spinal cord AVM most common course of nontraumatic spinal hemorrhage
- Anticoagulant therapy
- Hemorrhage into cord tumor, syrinx, or hemorrhagic area may be associated with inflammatory myelitis.
  MRI—aside from intramedullary hematoma and their primary causative lesions, may show superficial hemosiderosis, seen as a coat of marked hypointensity on T2WI.

Intramedullary Abscesses

- Very rare.
- Usually associated with dermal sinuses.
- Enhancement of the meninges after IV gadolinium contrast can be helpful to indicate inflammation in some of the rare conditions.

- Enhancement is not seen with multiple sclerosis or acute transverse myelitis.
- Metastatic disease to the cord:
  - Rare
  - Variable incidence—0.9% to 8.5%
  - Most common primary lung 40–85% of total metastatic lesions.
- Breast carcinoma, melanoma, lymphoma, colonic Ca, and kidney Ca.
- Thoracic cord > cervical > lumbar.
  CF pain, weakness, paresthesias, bowel, and bladder dysfunction.
- Rapid clinical progression as compared to primary cord tumors.
- Plain X-ray and myelography—usually normal.
- Vertebral metastasis may or may not be associated.
- MR—hypointense on T1 and hyperintense on T2—with or without cord widening.
- Usually central—hypointensity, on T1 which may be confused with syrinx
- Contrast enhancement is present.
  Note: Size of metastasis is disproportionately small compared to the amount of the edema.

Infarction

- Usually involves long segment of the cord.
- Shown only by MRI.
- Usually intensified centrally.
- Particular clinical setting.
- Most common—after:
  - Thoracoabdominal aortic aneurysm repair
  - Thrombosis of dural arteriovenous fistulas and their draining veins.

INTRADURAL EXTRAMEDULLARY MASSES (FIG. 8.28)

Intradural extramedullary masses arise inside the dura but outside the spinal cord. Nerve sheath tumors and meningiomas account for 80–90% of such masses. Other tumors are uncommon and include paraganglioma, epidermoid, dermoid, arachnoid cysts and meningoceles, lipoma, sarcoma, metastases, and non-Hodgkin's lymphoma.

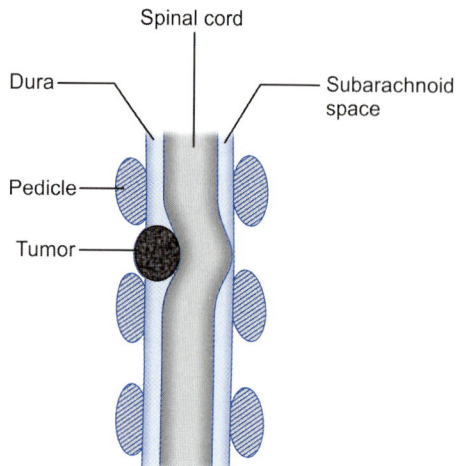

Fig. 8.28: Intradural extramedullary masses.

From a *radiological point of view*, the classical myelographic criteria are:
- Widening of the subarachnoid space on the side of the mass
- Contralateral displacement of the cord and nerve roots away from the mass
- Delineation of the mass by a sharp meniscus of contrast abutting the lesion.

Nowadays, MRI is the modality of choice and clearly shows not only the signs of cord displacement and CSF space widening but also the lesion itself. Plain films may show bony changes when the tumor has enlarged the spinal canal, erosion of the pedicle with widening of the neural foramen, and scalloping of the vertebral body.

Nerve Sheath Tumors

Nerve sheath tumors usually arise from dorsal roots, rarely are entirely intramedullary, presumably from aberrant nerve roots. They include schwannomas, neurofibromas, and rare ganglioneuromas and neurofibrosarcoma.

Clinical symptoms are often similar to those of a disk herniation, with pain and radiculopathy. When they compress the spinal cord, myelopathic signs may be present.
- *Nerve sheath tumors* are the most common intradural extramedullary mass (25–30%) and are primarily seen in middle-aged adults between the ages of 20 years and 50 years, with no predilection for either sex.
- *Schwannomas* (synonyms—neurinoma or neurilemmoma) are typically lobulated, encapsulated masses; nerve fibers do not course through them. They are slightly more common than neurofibromas.
- Neurofibromas are unencapsulated, typically fusiform and less well-defined lesions. Nerve fibers course through them.
- Nerve sheath tumors are variable in location: 70% are intradural extramedullary, 15% are "dumb-bell" shaped tumors, and 15% are extradural.
- These lesions typically enlarge the adjacent neural foramen; calcification within them is rare.
- They are typically (75%) isointense on T1WI and the vast majority is hyperintense on T2WI; virtually all exhibit marked and homogeneous enhancement with gadolinium.
- Other nerve sheath tumors such as ganglioneuroma or neurofibrosarcoma are rare.
- Multiple intraspinal neurofibromas and schwannomas are pathognomonic of NF1 and NF2, respectively. Malignant degeneration of neurofibromas and rarely schwannomas may occur in NF.

Meningiomas

Meningiomas arise from arachnoid cluster cells located at exit zones of nerve roots or entry zones of arteries. Slowly progressive myelopathy is the most common clinical presentation with motor and sensory deficits, sphincter dysfunction, and pain.
- Meningiomas are second to nerve sheath tumors, in frequency, accounting for 25% of all spinal tumors. They are, however, much less common than intracranial meningiomas, the ratio being 1:8.
- Peak incidence is in the 5th and 6th decades. More than 80% occur in women.
- The thoracic spine is the most common site (80%) followed by the cervical spine (15%). The lumbar spine is an uncommon location.
- Meningiomas may rarely calcify and can be seen also on plain films and at CT.

- On MRI, they are isointense on both T1WI- and T2WI and enhance markedly.
- Most spinal meningiomas are benign and slow-growing neoplasm. Ninety percent of spinal meningiomas are intradural, whereas 5% each are "dumb-bell" shaped or extradural lesions.
- Plain films are usually normal. Bone erosion is uncommon (15%). Calcification is rare (1–5%).
- MR scans may demonstrate broad-based dural attachment; a "dural tail" sign in some cases. Occasionally, densely calcified meningiomas are markedly hypointense on MR and show only minimal contrast enhancement.
- A rare variant of spinal meningioma is meningiomatosis characterized by diffuse involvement of the meninges by the tumor. MR imaging demonstrates thick or nodular enhancement, but is nonspecific. This variant carries a dismal prognosis.
- Another rare type of meningioma is angioblastic meningioma, a significantly more aggressive type that carries the potential for extraneural metastases and possibly subarachnoid seeding. These contain a dense capillary bed and varied cellular element including xanthomatous features with intracellular fat. This results in varied signal intensity on T1WI, depending on the amount of fat present, and generally increased signal on T2WI because of the rich capillary bed.

Embryonal Tumors

Embryonal tumors are a less common group, with the exception of lipomas, which are probably the most common. Lipomas, dermoids, and epidermoids may present as primary intramedullary mass lesions at the level of the spine. They are most frequently recognized as intradural intramedullary lesions at or near the conus medullaris in conjunction with dysraphic complexes.
- *Lipomas*:
  - These are characterized by the high-signal intensity on T1WI which is less intense with more T2-weighting.
- *Epidermoid cysts*:
  - These are lined only by superficial epidermal contents of the skin and are filled with keratinized debris and cholesterol.
  - They are congenital or may be acquired as a result of subarachnoid implantation of epidermal elements following lumbar puncture or spinal surgeries.
  - They are found in thoracic spine.
  - They have signal characteristics that follow CSF on T1- and T2WI and are detected on proton density and fluid attenuated inversion recovery images on the basis of their "cottage cheese" appearance.
- *Dermoid cysts*:
  - These are lined by simple or stratified squamous epithelium containing hair follicles, sweat glands, and sebaceous cysts that secrete fatty material into the cyst.
  - Approximately 80% are isolated masses and the rest are associated with dorsal dermal sinuses.
  - They display a variety of noncharacteristic signal intensity patterns with MR not only among different lesions but also within the same tumor. This may be related to the physical state (solid vs. liquid) and lipid content (cholesterol vs. fatty acid) of the cyst.

Paragangliomas

- Usually found in the cauda equina and filum terminale.
- They are usually isointense to spinal cord on T1WI and hyperintense on T2WI. MRI may show a "salt-and-pepper" appearance because of multiple areas of flow voids secondary to hypervascularity.

Arachnoid Cysts

- These are common in mid and lower thoracic region, most commonly located posterolaterally, displacing the cord anteriorly and compressing it.

They are believed to result from the proliferation of arachnoid adhesions caused by trauma, hemorrhage, inflammation or congenital abnormalities. They are accurately characterized noninvasively by MRI.

Metastases

- May be in the form of single or multiple nodules or diffuse subarachnoid seeding.
- Medulloblastoma in pediatric age group and ependymomas and glioblastoma in adults are the most common intracranial tumors producing CSF seeding followed by pineoblastoma, germinoma, retinoblastoma, and choroid plexus carcinoma. Extracranial tumors seeding the meninges include the carcinoma of the lung and breast, leukemia, lymphoma, and melanoma.
- The overall sensitivity of unenhanced and enhanced MRI in detecting intradural extramedullary metastases is only 19% and 36%, respectively in patients with CSF cytological findings positive for neoplasia. So, the CSF examination remains the gold standard (despite the fact that the single CSF specimen is only 50% sensitive to drop metastases).

Cysticercosis

- A parasitic infestation that can result in cysts within the subarachnoid space.
- Most cases are associated with extraspinal involvement.
- These are most commonly seen in the thoracic region.
- MRI reveals lesion with typical cyst-like intensity.
- In addition, nonspecific cord changes resulting from arachnoiditis can be seen characterized by an enlarged cord with irregular margins on T1WI and focal increased signal on T2WI.

Lateral Thoracic Meningoceles

- Seen in association with NF-1 and Marfan's syndrome
- They represent CSF outpouchings that extend into and enlarge the neural foramina, containing both the dura and arachnoid, and follow CSF signal intensity on MRI. No enhancement is seen on postcontrast images.

Spinal Subdural Empyema

- Collection of pus in the subdural space.
- It is a very rare event.
- Different factors including the absence of veins, the filter action of the epidural spinal space, and the centripetal direction of spinal blood flow have been suggested to explain the rarity of this event as compared to spinal epidural empyemas on the one hand and to intracranial subdural empyemas on the other.

EXTRADURAL EXTRAMEDULLARY LESION (FIG. 8.29)

Epidural Space

- Space between dura mater and bone
- Contains epidural venous plexus, lymphatic channels connective tissue and fat.
- Classic myelographic feature is displacement of the thecal sac away from bony walls of the spinal canal with extrinsic compression.
- If block-interface between lesion and contrast column is poorly defined with "feathered" appearance of level of obstruction.

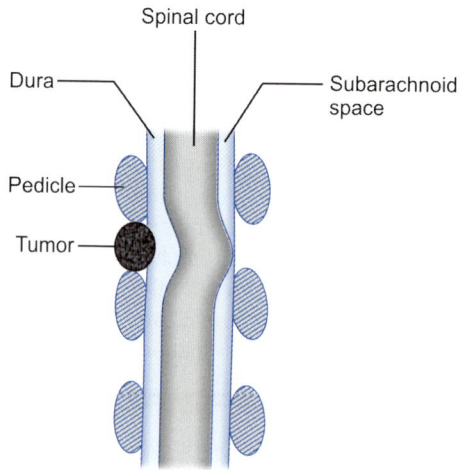

Fig. 8.29: Extradural extramedullary lesions.

- MR scan clearly shows the dura draped over the mass.
- Crescent of epidural fat can be seen capping the lesion.

Differential Diagnoses

- Disk disease:
  - Bulging disk
  - Disk protrusion
  - Herniated nucleus pulposus
  - Sequestrated nucleus pulposus.
- Inflammation:
  - Epidural abscess.
- Hematoma:
  - Post-traumatic
  - Spontaneous.
- Tumors:
  - Benign
    - *Nerve sheath tumor*
    - Meningioma
    - Hemangioma
    - Epidural lipomatosis
    - Angiolipoma
    - Cysts:
      - Arachnoid cysts
      - Synovial cysts
  - Malignant
    - Metastasis:
      - Adult:
        Breast
        Lung
        Prostate
    - Lymphoma:
      - Children:
        Ewing's sarcoma
    - Neuroblastoma.

Disk Bulge

- Loss of turgor of nucleus pulposus and loss of elasticity of annulus fibrosis → disk bulges.
- Decreased height of intervertebral disk space.

X-ray

- Vacuum sign
- Endplate sclerosis or osteophyte.

Nonenhanceed Computed Temography/Magnetic Resonance

- Loss of (normal) posterior disk concavity
- Diffuse, nonfocal protrusion of disk material beyond the adjacent vertebral endplate.

Disk protrusion → Focal incomplete extension of contents of nucleus pulposus through an incomplete tear of annulus fibrosis.

Disk herniation → Herniation of nucleus pulposus through an annular defect causes focal protrusion of disk material beyond the adjacent endplate.

Free disk or sequestrated disk → Disk material migrates inferiorly, superiorly, medially or laterally.

Epidural Abscess

- Hematogenous dissemination → *Staphylococcus aureus*
  - Phlegmonous stage: Thickened inflamed tissue with granulomatous material and embedded microabscesses.
  - Frank abscess—with collection of liquid pus.
- *Clinical features* → Fever and local tenderness
  - Predisposing condition → diabetes, IV drug abuse.
- Imaging → X-ray →
  - Osteomyelitis
  - Disk space narrowing
- CT/MR/Myelo/CT myelo → extradural soft tissue mass with extradural block
- Contrast enhance (CE) → diffuse homogeneous or slightly heterogeneous → 70% →
- In phlegmonous stage.
  - Thick or thin rim enhancement, 30% frank necrotic abscess.

Epidural Hematoma

- Most common cause:
  - Trauma
- Spontaneous →
  - Anticoagulation
  - Vigorous exercise
  - Hypertension

- Vascular malformation
- Postsurgical
- Collagen vascular disorders.

- Most common site → upper thoracic region, in dorsolateral aspect of spinal canal.
- CT → high density lentiform collection located adjustment to neural arch.
- MRI → investigation of choice.

Hemangioma

- Slow growing benign neoplasm, 4th to 6th decades
- Most common site—vertebral body, 10–15% → posterior elements
- Most epidural → secondary to expansion of intraosseous lesion
- 1% → completely extraosseous.

Cystic fibrosis

- Most → Asymptomatic
- Pain → Due to pathological fracture
- Epidural mass.

X-ray → Lytic lesion with honeycomb trabeculations or thick vertical striation.

NCCT → Lytic lesion with typical Polka-dot densities in medullary space.

Myelo/CT myelo → Epidural mass.

MR → Hyperintensity on T1WI and T2WI with foci of very low SI, suggestive of thickened vertical trabeculae. It shows contrast enhancement.

Epidural Lipomatosis

- Excessive deposition of unencapsulated fat in epidural space.
- Part of—morbid obesity:
  - Associated with central or truncal lipomatosis.
- Male >> Female.
- 60% thoracic spine, 40% in lumbar spine.

Clinical Features

- Weakness and back pain
- Radicular pain and numbness
  - Myelo → (Normal) to extradural blocks
  - CT/MR → Increased extradural fat with diminished subarachnoid space.

Spinal Angiolipoma

It is very rare—mature adipose tissue with blood vessels.

- Fifth decade, Female > Male
- Most common → Thoracic spine
- Dorsal or dorsolateral to cord.

Myelo → Extradural mass or block.

CT → Low to intermediate density, epidural mass showing contrast enhancement.

MR → Isointense to hyperintense on T1 and hyperintense on T2.

- Diffuse homogeneous contrast enhancement → Typical.

Cysts

Extradural arachnoid cysts → CSF filled-out pouching of arachnoid that protrude through dural defect.

- Two-thirds → Mid to low thoracic level
- 20% → Lumbosacral region.
- Imaging studies show → long segment CSF equivalent extradural mass that causes spinal cord.

Compression or myelographic block:

- Secondary bony changes → Widened interpedicular distance
- Scalloping of vertebral bodies
- Pedicle thinning or erosion
- Synovial (juxta-articular) cysts—Rare.
  - Associated with facet degeneration.

Malignant Lesions

Metastasis:

- In adults from → Breast
  - Lung → 50%
  - Prostate.
- Other from → Lymphoma, melanoma, renal cancer, sarcoma, and multiple myeloma.
- In children:
  - Ewing's sarcoma
  - Neuroblastoma
  - Pediatric tumors → invade via neural foramen causing a circumferential cord compression
  - Adult → initial site is in vertebral body with secondary involvement of epidural space
  - Lower thoracic and lumbar spine.

X-ray

- Pedicle destruction
- Multifocal lytic vertebral body lesion
- Sclerotic lesion → breast or prostate
- Indistinct posterior vertebral body margin
- Paraspinal soft tissue mass
- Myelography—extradural blocks
- Bone scintigraphy →sensitive
- NCCT →lytic or blastic lesion, with epidural soft tissue mass
- Intrathecal contrast required to delineate precise extent of lesion
- MR → exquisitely delineates epidural and paraspinal soft tissue involvement
- Low signal on T1 and high signal on T2.

Lymphoma—NHL →85%

- HL → less common
- 40–60 years, Male >> Female
- Spinal extradural mass with nonspecific imaging findings
- NHL→ can cause bone destruction and hyperostosis
- Epidural extension best delineated on MRI
- Ewing's sarcoma → Children second decade Male > Female
- Nonspecific findings
- Eroded vertebral body with paraspinal soft tissue mass
- Hypointense to isointense T1WI and hyperintense on T2WI.

DIFFERENTIAL DIAGNOSIS OF FLOATING TOOTH

Definition

The term "floating tooth" applies to a state where there is no supporting bone or periodontal structures, the tooth, however, maintaining its normal position.

Causes

- Infective pathology:
  - Chronic osteomyelitis
  - Acute osteomyelitis
- Osteonecrosis
- Malignant pathology:
  - Osteosarcoma
  - Local extension of malignancy in nearby structures
  - Burkitt's lymphoma
  - Histiocytosis
  - Metastasis especially from lung, breast, and kidney
  - Multiple myeloma.
- Others:
  - Fibrous dysplasia
  - Cementoma and cemento-ossifying dysplasia
  - Ossifying fibroma
  - Hyperparathyroidism
  - Severe periodontal disease.

Salient Features

- *Acute osteomyelitis*:
  - Iatrogenic, traumatic, extension of pulpal infection or acute exacerbation of chronic process.
  - Various forms may be seen as acute periapical abscess, subacute abscess or Gum boil or chronic apical infection.
  - On imaging: Earliest feature seen is widened periodontal space (but this is nonspecific).
  - After 7–14 days, definitive features like blurring of trabecular pattern, loss of lamina dura, and finally a periapical abscess are seen. Associated sequestra and periosteal reaction may be seen. MR shows marrow changes early or in association to bony changes.
- *Chronic osteomyelitis*:
  - A persistent low-grade infection or an untreated or inadequately treated infection
  - It is usually the chronic suppurative osteomyelitis that leads to "floating tooth"
  - This is simply a more protracted form of the above disease process and shows similar features.
- *Osteonecrosis*:
  - Irradiation of developing tooth leads to hypoplasia of both primary and

secondary dentition. Also it leads to an associated mandibular hypoplasia.
- It further leads to reduction in salivary gland function and more acidic, dry environment leading to increased chances of dental infection.
- Direct cell death caused by radiation leads to osteoporosis, bone resorption, pathological fracture, and associated infection in a devitalized bone.

- *Osteosarcomas and other primary bone malignancies*:
  - Osteosarcomas of jaw are rare lesions but have a very similar appearance to that seen elsewhere. The age of occurrence is 30–40 years and the prognosis is much better.
  - Ewing's sarcoma has an epidemiology and appearance similar to that at other sites.

- *Metastasis*:
  - Four times more common in mandible (posterior especially) than maxilla.
  - Breast, kidney, lung, colon, prostate, and thyroid.
    * Localized lucent lesion
    * Moth-eaten lesion
    * Permeative lesion.

- *Direct invasion*:
  - Squamous cell carcinomas. Salivary gland tumors and lymphomas can invade the dental sockets by direct invasion.

- *Multiple myeloma*:
  - Seen more commonly in mandible than metastasis
  - 30% of all cases involve the mandible
  - Skull >> mandible
  - Appearance is similar.

- *Burkitt's lymphoma*:
  - A condition occurring in maxillary bone or jaws of children in equatorial Africa.
  - Probably Epstein-Barr virus.
  - Leads to large soft tissue mass with involvement of all adjacent structures.
  - New bone formation may be seen.

- *Langerhans' cell histiocytosis*:
  - Multifocal resorptions of periapical bone and may be also the tooth root.
  - Children below 5 years, most common.
  - Above 50% of cases have jaw or dental involvement.
  - Hand-Schüller-Christian disease is the condition most commonly forming such an appearance.
  - Geographic skull and vertebra plana are other associated findings.

- *Hyperparathyroidism*:
  - Subperiosteal bone resorption (Lamina dura being one such bone area) is a pathognomonic sign of hyperparathyroidism.
  - Loss of lamina dura is always associated with changes in hand and feet, Brown's tumor, etc.
  - These, though specific, are poorly sensitive indicators of disease.
  - Now seen rarely due to early diagnosis and treatment.

- *Fibrous dysplasia*:
  - A homogeneous, hyperdense, enhancing, and greatly expansile lesion totally replacing the normal bone.
  - Both polyostotic and mono-ostotic forms involve mandible and maxilla but mono-ostotic form involves maxilla slightly more.
  - Craniofacial fibrous dysplasia is a specific form involving more than 1 bone on one side.
  - Cherubism is a familial form of fibrous dysplasia involving predominantly the mandible but also the maxillary tuberosity.

- *Ossifying fibroma*:
  - Mandibular molar or premolar region of women in 3rd or 4th decade.
  - Well-defined, well-circumscribed, expansile.
  - Initially lucent but later may become opaque
  - If a lot of cementum is present, then may be known as cemento-ossifying fibroma.

- *Cementoma-cemento-ossifying dysplasia*:
  - It is periapical lucent lesion that may lead to floating teeth.
  - Cementoma is due to benign fibrous proliferation of periodontal membrane that later becomes ossified.

CYSTS OF JAW

Classified into (Fig. 8.30):
- *Cysts of dental origin*:
  - Developmental:
    - Odontogenic keratocyst (primordial cyst)
    - Dentigerous cyst (follicular cyst).
  - Postinflammatory:
    - Radicular (apical) cyst.
- *Nondental or developmental or fissural cyst*:
  - Medial mandibular
  - Medial maxillary
  - Nasopalatine
  - Globulomaxillary.
- *Nonepithelialized bone cyst*:
  - Simple bone cyst
  - Aneurysmal bone cyst.

Odontogenic Keratocyst

- Follow cystic degeneration, enamel arises before the tooth is formed, so cyst replaces the tooth.
- More common in young men but seen in all ages.
- Cortex is thinned and axial view shows expansion in buccal-lingual plane.
- Most common in posterior mandible and usually monolocular.
- Usually keratinized and may react unless removed completely.

Dentigerous Cyst

- Cystic degeneration of enamel after formation but before eruption of tooth.
- Cyst related to crown of an unerupted tooth.
- Seen in adolescents and young adults.

- Permanent mandibular third molar and maxillary canine are affected.
- Usually unilocular.
- If multiple, may be associated with Gorlin's syndrome.

Radicular (Apical) Cyst

- Most common jaw cyst.
- Lies directly upon the apex of a tooth.
- Follow inflammation of bulb and apical bone.
- Unilocular cyst with dense opaque margin continuous with lamina dura or at periphery of cyst. Within the cyst, lamina dura is destroyed.
- Usually less than 1.5 cm and associated with carious teeth.
- It persists after dental extraction—residual cyst.

Medial Mandibular

Medial Maxillary

It is similar in appearance to radicular cyst but with normal teeth.

Nasopalatine

It is usually seen due to failure of obliteration of nasopalatine ducts behind the central incisors.

Globulomaxillary

These look like inverted pear and lie lateral of upper lateral incisor and canine, the roots of which are diverged.

Simple Bone Cyst

- Usually follows trauma and is known as traumatic cyst.
- In young patients, in posterior aspect of body of mandible.
- Diagnosis is usually histologic.

Aneurysmal Bone Cyst

- Not common in jaws.
- Diagnosis is histologic.

Differential Diagnosis

Location

- Lateral: More common

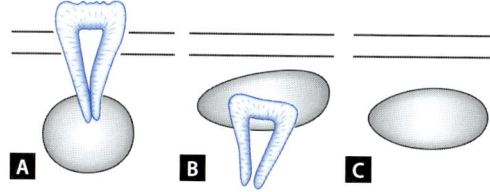

Figs. 8.30 A to C: Types of cysts. (A) Radicular cyst at apex of carious tooth; (B) Dentigerous cyst related to crown of unerupted tooth; (C) Primordial cyst replacing the tooth.

- Medial or midline:
  - Fissural or developmental
  - Usually rare.

Cystic Lesions of the Jaw

It includes benign, dental origin, developmental, odontogenic keratocyst (primordial cyst).
- Monolocular cyst that forms from cystic degeneration of tooth enamel before tooth is formed.
- Cyst replaces the tooth.
- Common in young men and in posterior mandible.
- Cyst demonstrates expansion with cortical thinning.

Dentigerous Cyst (Follicular Cyst)

- Monolocular cyst related to the crown of unerupted tooth.
- Common in adolescents or young adults and the permanent mandibular third molar and maxillary canine are commonly affected.
- Multiple such cysts are associated with Gorlin's syndrome.

Postinflammatory

- *Radicular cysts (apical)*:
  - Unilocular cystic lesion associated with apex of a diseased tooth
  - Dense sclerotic margins of the cyst are continuous peripherally with lamina dura but, within the cyst, lamina dura is destroyed.
- *Nondental or developmental/fissural cysts*:
  - These occur at sites of fusion of embryonic processes and include:
    - Medial mandibular
    - Medial maxillary
    - Nasopalatine duct cyst.
  - Seen in 4th to 6th decades
  - Asymptomatic cyst near anterior palatine papilla:
    - Globulomaxillary cyst
  - Seen between the lateral incisor and canine
    - Nasolabial cyst arises in the soft tissues between the nose and upper lip with resorption of adjacent maxilla.

- Nonepithelialized bone cysts
- Simple bone cyst
- *Traumatic cyst*:
  - Seen in young patient following trauma
  - Common in posterior part of body of mandible
  - Is vaguely spherical but well-defined with thin sclerotic margin
  - May extend upward displacing the vital teeth.
- *Aneurysmal bone cyst*:
  - Well-defined multilocular expansile cystic lesion uncommonly seen in jaws
  - May be secondary to fibrous dysplasia.
- *Brown tumors*:
  - Seen in hyperparathyroidism
  - Commonly involves mandible
  - Arises as a cystic lesion unrelated to tooth
  - Associated loss of lamina dura.
- *Giant cell reparative granuloma of Jaffe*:
  - Soft tissue mass appearing like cyst with well-defined margin
  - Common between 7th year and early 20s.
- *Malignant*:
  - Ameloblastoma (Figs. 8.31A and B)
  - Common in middle-aged males in molar region of mandible
  - Lesions are cystic, multilocular, expansile with thinning of cortex with peripheral satellite defects.
- *Giant cell tumor*:
  - Multilocular cystic lesion with expansion
  - Rare in the jaws.
- *Burkitt's lymphoma*:
  - Jaws are frequently affected with deformed face
  - Multilocular cystic destruction beginning around the roots of the tooth
  - A "sun ray" type periosteal reaction may be associated
  - It is seen in childhood.

LOSS OF LAMINA DURA OF TEETH

Lamina dura is a layer of compact bone that lines the tooth socket and provides anchorage for the fibers of the periodontal membrane.

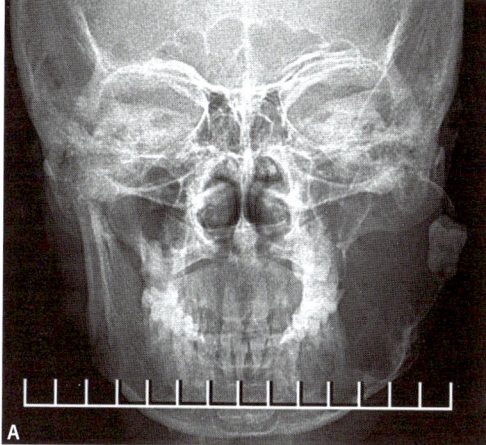

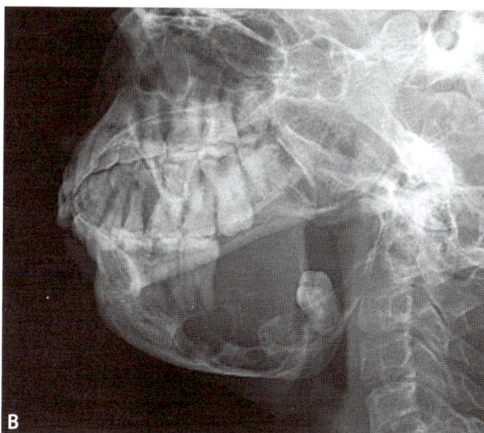

Figs. 8.31A and B: Posteroanterior and lateral radiographs of mandible showing ameloblastoma with floating tooth appearance.

Causes

Generalized:
- Endocrine or metabolic
  - Osteoporosis
  - Hyperparathyroidism
  - Cushing's syndrome
  - Osteomalacia
- Paget's disease
- Scleroderma.

Localized:
- Infection
- Neoplasms:
  - Leukemia
  - Multiple myeloma
  - Metastases
  - Burkitt's lymphoma
  - Langerhans' cell histiocytosis.

Osteoporosis

- There is reduced bone mass of normal composition secondary to either osteoclastic (85%) or osteolytic (15%) resorption.
- Incidence is 7% of all women between 35 and 40 years of age and 1 in 3 women of greater than 65 years of age.

Hyperparathyroidism

- Loss of the lamina dura surrounding the roots of the teeth is an early manifestation of hyperparathyroidism, with alterations in the jaw trabecular pattern characteristically developing next. Not all teeth are affected.
- There is a decrease in trabecular density, and blurring of the normal pattern produces a "ground glass" appearance on the radiograph.
- With persistent disease, other osseous lesions develop, such as the so-called "Brown tumor" of hyperparathyroidism. The name of this lesion is derived from the color of the gross tissue specimen, which is usually dark reddish-brown due to the abundant hemorrhage and hemosiderin deposition within the tumor.
- Radiographically, brown tumors are unilocular or multilocular well-demarcated radiolucencies, which commonly affect the mandible, clavicle, ribs, and pelvis. They may be solitary, but more often are multiple. The long-standing lesions may produce significant cortical expansion.
- The value of loss of lamina dura as a radiodiagnostic sign is poor.
- All patients have hand changes, i.e. subperiosteal bone resorption.

Cushing's Syndrome or Hypercortisolism

- It results from a sustained increase in blood glucocorticoid levels. This can be due to either corticosteroid therapy or endogenous

overproduction from the adrenal gland. Excess adrenocorticotropic hormone from a pituitary tumor also causes hypercortisolism and Cushing's disease.
- Associated osteoporosis is seen in the jaws. Pathological fractures of the mandible, maxilla or alveolar bone may occur.
- Lamina dura may be poorly visualized or absent.

Osteomalacia
- There is accumulation of excessive amounts of uncalcified osteoid with bone softening and insufficient mineralization of osteoid.
- There is poor visualization of the lamina dura.

Paget's Disease
- In the jaw, bone enlargement and sclerosis are usually seen.
- Irregular dense sclerotic patches may form on teeth.
- Mandible usually remains normal, either jaw can become very large indeed.
- Infection is the most common complication and may be the presenting lesion, especially in the mandible.

Scleroderma
- Also called progressive systemic sclerosis, it is a generalized disorder of connective tissue of unknown cause.
- Many of the diverse clinical manifestations in this disease are represented on radiographs as atrophy and calcification of soft tissue and bone resorption. Frequently the abnormalities predominate in the phalanges of the hand, although diffuse subcutaneous calcification, widespread peri-articular calcification, and bone resorption are encountered at other sites, such as the mandible, the ribs and the clavicles. Joint alterations include erosive arthritis and intra-articular calcific collections.
- On radiographs, hand alterations include soft tissue resorption of the fingertips, subcutaneous calcification and bone destruction. Erosion of the phalangeal tufts leads to penciling, sometimes with destruction of much or the entire distal phalanx.
- Thickening of the periodontal membrane and mandibular resorption may result in loss of the lamina dura and loosening of the teeth.
- Erosions may also occur on the superior aspect of multiple ribs. In the spine, paraspinal calcification may be evident.
- Joint involvement may be seen in the proximal interphalangeal (PIP) and distal interphalangeal (DIP) joints, the first carpometacarpal (CMC) joints, the elbow, the inferior radioulnar joints of the wrist, metacarpophalangeal (MCP) and metatarsophalangeal (MTP) joints, knee and hip.
- Incidence is lower than in the axial skeleton.

Burkitt's Lymphoma
- It occurs throughout the world but especially in equatorial Africa, where it accounts for 50% of all childhood malignancies
- Jaws are frequently affected which deforms the face
- Lesions are multifocal
- Destruction of bone begins around the roots of teeth, which are then exfoliated
- New bone formation in these lesions gives a coarse, spiculated, sun ray appearance.

Langerhans' Sun Ray Histiocytosis
- Langerhans' cell histiocytosis (LCH) represents a spectrum of clinical disorders ranging from a highly aggressive and frequently fatal leukemia-like disease, affecting infants to a solitary lesion of bone.
- The presence of alveolar bone loss in young children with precocious exfoliation of primary teeth should suggest the possibility of LCH. LCH can also occur in adolescents and adults.
- Of the bones of the jaw, the mandible is the most frequently involved. The presenting signs usually include pain, swelling, ulceration, and loose teeth.

- Radiographically, the teeth often appear to be floating in air surrounded by large radiolucent regions. This is due to rapid alveolar bone loss.
- The term "eosinophilic granuloma of bone" is used when solitary lesion is found, but multiple lesions may develop later.
- Forming tooth-buds may be destroyed.

Infection
- Apical tooth abscess is the most common cause of loss of lamina dura
- Hyperemia and trabecular destruction are responsible.

Neoplasms
Leukemia
- Diffuse osteopenia is the most common pattern, which is responsible for the poor visualization of lamina dura
- Leukemic lines, which are the transverse radiolucent metaphyseal bands can be seen in the long bones
- Associated periostitis of long bones infrequently encountered.

Multiple Myeloma
- The incidence of jaw involvement in multiple myeloma averages about 15% and involvement of the mandible is more common than in metastases.
- These lesions cause swelling of the jaws, pain, numbness, mobility of teeth, and pathologic fracture.
- Punched-out lesions of the skull and jaw are characteristic radiographic findings.
- This malignancy is associated with diffuse osteoporosis, which also contributes to the loss of lamina dura.

Metastases
- Overall, the most common primary site for metastases to the jaw is the breast. In men, the lung is the most common primary site for jaw metastases. The molar region of the mandible is the most common bony site for metastasis.

OPAQUE MAXILLARY ANTRUM
Causes and associated features of opaque maxillary antrum has been shown in Table 8.3.

Sinusitis
- Acute sinusitis produces an air-fluid level
- Chronic sinusitis can be due to aspergillosis, mucormycosis, tuberculosis and syphilis. Fungal sinusitis is commonly seen in diabetes mellitus. These produce hyperdense sinus secretions as seen on CT usually with bone destruction.

Cysts in Antrum
Mucous Retention Cyst
- Common complication of chronic sinusitis
- Maxillary sinus is the most common site
- Often arises in the floor
- More common than polyp but cannot be differentiated from it on imaging.

Table 8.3: Causes and associated features of opaque maxillary antrum.

Traumatic	Inflammatory/ Infective	Neoplastic	Miscellaneous
Fracture	Sinusitis	Carcinoma	Fibrous dysplasia
Overlying Soft tissue swelling	Allergy	Lymphoma	Cysts
Postoperative (Caldwell-Luc)	Pyocele (rare)	Mucosal polyp	Wegener's granulomatosis
Epistaxis			Technical (over-tilted view)
Barotrauma			Anatomical (aplasia, sloping antral wall)

Dentigerous Cyst
- It is related to the crown of the unerupted tooth
- Expands into the floor of the antrum
- Involved tooth may be displaced into the antrum.

Neoplasms
Polyps (Fig. 8.32)
- Complication of chronic sinusitis
- May extend up to the posterior choanae (antrochoanal polyp)
- CT shows soft-tissue dense, minimally to mildly enhancing masses
- MRI reveals hyperintense masses on T2WI.

Carcinoma
- Associated bony destruction is seen
- Soft-tissue mass extending beyond the limits of the antrum
- Calcification seen in cases of squamous cell carcinoma.

Wegener's Granulomatosis
- Autoimmune disease
- Usually presents at 40–50 years of age
- Early mucosal thickening progresses to a mass with bone destruction.

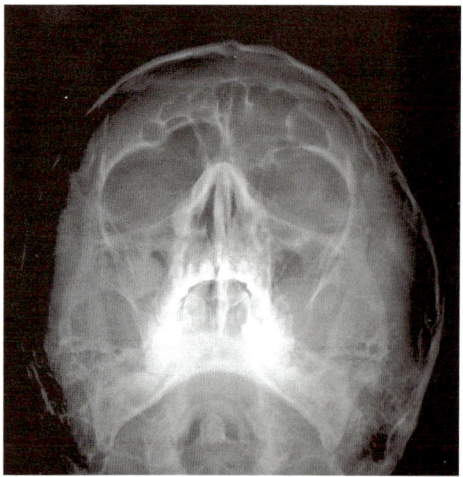

Fig. 8.32: Posteroanterior (PA) radiograph of PNS shows bilateral chronic maxillary sinusitis with antral polyp on the right side.

Fibrous Dysplasia
- There is sclerosis of the facial bones with or without expansion (leontiasis ossea)
- Involvement of the face is usually asymmetrical
- Involvement of the skull may be seen.

THYROID LESIONS
Increased Uptake of Radiotracer
- Grave's disease
- Toxic multinodular goiter
- Toxic solitary nodule
- Dyshormonogenesis
- Hashimoto's thyroiditis
- Following recovery from subacute thyroiditis or antithyroid drug therapy.

Grave's Disease
- It is a very common cause of hyperthyroidism
- The disease tends to occur in a younger age group than does toxic nodular goiter
- The scan findings are quite characteristic. The radioiodine uptake is considerably elevated with 24 hours uptake values considerably in 60–80% range and sometimes higher
- If dynamic range acquisition is performed following intravenous pertechnetate administration, very intense flow to the thyroid will be seen
- The distribution of tracer within the thyroid is typically very homogeneous
- Routine thyroid imaging demonstrates an enlarged gland that is usually rather symmetric. An enlarged pyramidal lobe is frequently present.

Toxic Multinodular Goiter
- Toxic multinodular goiter is a common cause of hyperthyroidism in older individuals with a peak incidence in the 4th and 5th decades, which is later than that of Grave's disease.
- The scan usually demonstrates irregular enlargement of the thyroid without a prominent pyramidal lobe.
- Tracer distribution within the gland is very heterogeneous with varying regions of uptake present.

- Frequently discrete hot and cold regions can be identified even in the presence of hyperfunctioning nodules, the remainder of the thyroid may not be suppressed because of the autonomy present within it.

Hashimoto's Thyroiditis

It is a chronic inflammatory process of the thyroid.
- F > M, may occur at any age, with peak incidence in 4th and 5th decades
- The gland typically is enlarged with patchy traces distribution throughout the gland.

A prominent pyramidal lobe is frequently seen
- Hashimoto's thyroiditis commonly leads to hypothyroidism
- Radioiodine uptake is variable, but is frequently low
- In some instances, Hashimoto's thyroiditis is associated with thyrotoxicosis (called Hashitoxicosis) and they may demonstrate markedly increased radioiodine uptake.

Dyshormonogenesis: In the presence of defective thyroid hormone production.

Increased Thyroid-stimulating Hormone Levels

- Increased thyroid-stimulating hormone (TSH) levels may lead to adenomatous hyperplasia of thyroid, associated with hot thyroid nodule on thyroid scan.
- These TSH dependent lesions will involute following administration of exogenous hormones.

Toxic Solitary Nodule

- It may be TSH dependent (adenomatous hyperplasia) or independent (adenoma)
- Adenomatous hyperplasia if associated with increased TSH levels
- Toxic adenoma is associated with decreased TSH level, with partial or total suppression of remainder of gland
- Rarely malignant thyroid nodule may show increased tracer uptake.

Hot Thyroid Nodule

- A hot nodule concentrates traces more rapidly than does the adjacent normal thyroid
- They are seen in 8% of Tc-99m pertechnetate scans.

Causes
- *Adenoma*
  - Autonomous adenoma
    - Hot nodule
    - TSH independent
    - Associated with decreased/normal TSH level
    - Patient can be hyperthyroid or euthyroid
    - Partial or total suppression of remainder of gland.
  - Adenomatous hyperplasia:
    - Hot nodule
    - TSH dependent
    - Associated with increased TSH level secondary to defective thyroid hormone production.

Note: These nodules can be further evaluated by performing a suppression test. By following administration of exogenous thyroid hormone:
  - An autonomous nodule deep in the lobe will become visible as extranodular uptake is suppressed, and the nodule may be more easily palpable as the gland shrinks.
  - Any TSH-dependent lesion will involute with exogenous hormone administration. Although the nodule may not be visible on scan, its diminution in size, or actual absence on palpation at the time of follow-up may be just as diagnostic. Those nodules that persist following suppression without activity present are treated as cold nodules.
- *Thyroid carcinoma (extremely rare)*
  - Shows discordant uptake.

Note: Any hot nodule on Tc-99m scan must be imaged with I-123 to differentiate between benign or cancerous lesion.

Discordant Nodules

- Most cold nodules lack the ability to either trap or organify iodine. In a small percentage of tumors, however, the organification is blocked, but the trapping function is intact, such a nodule will be hyperfunctioning on Tc-99m pertechnetate scan and

hypofunctioning on I-131 scan, which indicates reduced organification capacity.
- A nodule that is hot on technetium scanning reflecting trapping, but cold on iodine scanning because of absent organification, may represent either a benign or malignant lesion.
- Malignant
  - Follicular/papillary carcinoma.
- Benign
  - Follicular adenoma/adenomatous hyperplasia.

Cystic Lesions of Thyroid

- *Thyroglossal duct cysts*:
  - Appears in the midline along the migratory path of the embryonic thyroid gland anywhere from the foramen cecum at the base of the tongue to the lower neck.
- Characteristically moves with protrusion of tongue and swallowing.
  - Usually cystic, these thyroglossal duct cysts can become infected and develop increased echogenicity but rarely develop thyroid papillary carcinoma.
  - On CT, most cysts are isodense to water. However, they may be hyperdense when there is high protein content.
  - MR imaging—hypointense on T1WI and hyperintense on T2WI. When cyst contents are proteinaceous, the cyst may be hyperintense on T1WI and intermediate to hyperintense on T2WI.
  - Characteristically shows thin peripheral rim enhancement of cyst well. Thick peripheral enhancement is unusual unless cyst is secondarily infected.
- *Simple cyst*:
  - True epithelial cysts are rare (<1% of all thyroid masses)
  - They are smooth-walled anechoic masses with posterior, acoustic enhancement.

Degeneration of Adenomatous Nodules

- Most cystic thyroid masses are degenerating adenomatous nodules.
- These are not true epithelial-lined cysts.
- These may contain bloody fluid, chocolate-colored fluid or xanthochromic fluid, depending on the age of the degeneration of the blood products.
- On USG-anechoic with thin walls and posterior acoustic enhancement.
- The presence of a "comet-tail sign" on USG has been said to be highly specific sign of benign colloid nodule.
- Low density on CT and hyperintense on T2WI and decreased or increased signal intensity on T1WI.
- Increased signal intensity on T1WI is related to the presence of hemorrhage, colloid or increased protein content.

Cystic Papillary Carcinoma

- Any cystic thyroid mass with a solid component must be approached with suspicion for malignancy (especially papillary carcinoma) although a completely cystic nodule with uniformly thin walls is almost always benign.
- Cystic papillary carcinomas show a predominantly liquid content, with one or more solid, irregularly marginated projection in the lumen, each generally containing microcalcifications and central branching blood supply.

Thyroid Abscess

- *Less common*:
  - Clinical features of fever, pain, tenderness.
  - Ultrasound—ill-defined/well-defined hypo- to anechoic lesion with thick irregular shaggy wall with internal debris.

Cold Nodules

- All nodules that cannot be demonstrated to function are considered cold.
- *Causes*:
  - *Benign tumor*:
    - Non-functioning, adenoma
    - Cysts (11–20%)
    - Involuting nodule.

- *Inflammatory mass*:
  - Focal thyroiditis
  - Granuloma
  - Abscess.
- *Malignant tumors*:
  - Carcinoma
  - Lymphoma
  - Metastasis.
- All thyroid carcinomas will be cold, as will be lymphoma and metastatic disease. Many benign nodules, as enlisted above, will also be cold. Because of the relative frequencies of these abnormalities, the vast majority of cold nodules are benign. Although, the specificity of finding a cold nodule on scan is low, it does permit trial of the patient into a diagnostic pathway in which tissue diagnosis is needed to exclude the presence of malignancy. The true incidence of carcinoma in nonfunctioning nodules is difficult to determine, but probably lies somewhere near 6–20% range.
- However, in an attempt to provide more definitive diagnosis, the following feature may be helpful:
  - Ultrasound can easily identify a cystic lesion as a well-defined anechoic lesion, with thin wall showing posterior acoustic enhancement. The presence of a comet-tail sign on ultrasound has been said to be a highly specific sign of a benign colloid nodule.
- There are no specific imaging features to differentiate the varying inflammatory processes that affect the thyroid gland. Acute suppurative thyroiditis is rare, particularly affecting the children. It may be associated with fourth branchial cleft anomaly. The patient will present with painful thyroid swelling and fever. Abscess formation is common and the role of ultrasound is to confirm this, demonstrate its boundaries and its relationship to the major neck vessels.
- *Papillary carcinoma*:
  - F > M, younger age group
  - Slow growth with good prognosis
  - USG characteristics.
- Hypoechoic (90%)
- Microcalcifications (85–90%)
- Hypervascular (90%) with widespread internal flow.
  - Nodal metastasis (50–55%), which can show the same features as the primary lesion
  - Can be echo-free, owing to serous cystic contents.
- *Follicular carcinoma*:
  - F > M, older age group
  - Nonspecific features that suggest follicular carcinoma are irregular tumor margins, a thick, irregular halo, and a tortuous or chaotic arrangement of internal blood vessels on color or power Doppler.
- Sonographic features of medullary carcinoma are similar to that of papillary carcinoma (low reflectivity, irregular margins, microcalcifications, and hypervascularity).
- *Anaplastic carcinomas* are often associated with papillary or follicular carcinomas, and presumably represent a differentiation of the neoplasm. They tend not to spread via lymphatics, but are prone to local aggressive invasion of muscles and vessels. Low reflectivity and signs of invasion or encasement of large blood vessels and neck muscles are the most distinctive sonographic features of anaplastic carcinomas.
  - When they are not adequately imaged and staged with ultrasound, CT or MRI scans are performed to define the extent of the disease.

Lymphoma

- Accounts for about 4% of all thyroid malignancies.
- Mostly of non-Hodgkin's type, affects older female.
- The typical finding is a rapidly growing mass which may cause symptoms of obstruction such as an dyspnea and dysphagia.
- About 70–80% of cases arise from a preexisting chronic thyroiditis (Hashimoto's disease), with subclinical or overt hypothyroidism.

- More commonly present as a solitary mass, but multiple nodules may be seen.
- On USG, lymphoma of thyroid appears as an echo-poor lobulated mass that is nearly avascular. Large areas of cystic necrosis may occur, as well as encasement of adjacent neck vessels.
- Diffuse involvement may cause thyroid enlargement with little detectable abnormality, or a heterogeneous pattern may be seen in the adjacent thyroid parenchyma due to associated chronic thyroiditis.
- There may be associated cervical lymphadenopathy.

Metastasis

- Metastatic disease involving the thyroid is uncommon
- The common primary sites include melanoma, breast and renal cell carcinoma.

DECREASED OR NO UPTAKE OF RADIOTRACER

- *Blocked trapping function*:
  - Iodine load (most common)
  - Exogenous thyroid hormone (replacement therapy)
- *Blocked organification*:
  - Antithyroid medication/goitrogenic substances
- *Diffuse parenchymal destruction*:
  - Subacute/chronic thyroiditis
- *Hypothyroidism*:
  - Congenital hypothyroidism
  - Surgical/radioiodine ablation
  - Thyroid ectopia.

Iodine Load

- Previous administration of iodine-containing medications is the most common extrinsic factor for decreased uptake of radiotracer. Extrinsic iodine administration will depress the thyroid uptake for a variable period, regardless of the thyroid's functional status.
- If thyroid uptake is markedly reduced because of previous iodine exposure, little diagnostic information can be obtained from the scan. Therefore, all the patients should be screened prior to radioisotope administration.

Exogenous Thyroid Hormone

- It is another frequent cause of decreased tracer uptake. In some cases, thyroid suppression scans are intentionally performed in the evaluation of nodules. At other times, however, unintentional thyroid suppression scans are likely to be performed, either because of patients' confusion about discontinuing medication.
- Administration of thyroid hormone (factitious hyperthyroidism).
- Very rarely, functioning ectopic thyroid tissue, such as struma ovarii or functioning metastatic thyroid cancer will cause thyroid suppression.
- Antithyroid drugs—antithyroid drugs, such as propylthiouracil (PTU), or methimazole, block organification and will decrease radioiodine uptake.
  However, pertechnetate uptake will not be affected and useful information can be obtained from Tc-99m scans in selected instances.

Subacute Thyroiditis

- Supposed to be caused by viral infection.
- These patients usually present with a painful, tender and enlarged thyroid, and signs of hyperthyroidism are frequently present secondary to an outpouring of thyroid hormone into the blood from the inflamed thyroid.
- The natural history is variable, but over the subsequent weeks to months, the hyperthyroid phase is succeeded by euthyroid and sometimes hypothyroid stages, before the gland recovers and functioning returns to normal.
- Initially the gland is inflamed and functions poorly with very low radioiodine uptake, as the patient progresses through the hypothyroid and recovery phases, the

radio-iodine uptake gradually increases to the normal range in some patients transiently rising above normal.

Congenital Hypothyroidism
- Scintigraphy is helpful by demonstrating the absence of thyroid tissue, which is the underlying problem in 30–40% of cases.
- Ectopic thyroid tissue may be seen in 40–50% of cases, most commonly seen as a nodule or mass at the base of the tongue.
- In the latter case, increased tracer uptake is present at the foramen cecum of the tongue and there is absence of the normal uptake in the neck.

Ectopic Thyroid
- Ectopic thyroid tissue may lie along the line of thyroglossal duct cyst or adjacent to it.
- The presence of ectopic thyroid tissue decreases tracer uptake in the normal thyroid gland. The ectopic thyroid tissue may coexist with normal thyroid gland, and in some cases, the ectopic tissue may be the only functioning thyroid gland.
- Most commonly ectopic thyroid tissue presents in childhood as nodule or mass at the base of the tongue.

Solid Thyroid Nodule
- *Benign*:
  - Adenomatous hyperplasia (50%)
  - Follicular adenoma (20%)
  - Ectopic parathyroid adenoma
  - *Hemorrhage/hematoma*: Frequently associated with adenomas
  - Abscess.
- *Malignant*:
  - Thyroid carcinoma
  - Lymphoma
  - Metastasis from breast, lung, kidney, and malignant melanoma.
- Hürthle cell tumors.

Adenomatous Hyperplasia
- Most commonly observed pathology of thyroid gland
- May be familial (disorders of hormonogenesis)
  - Iodine deficiency (endemic)
  - Compensatory hypertrophy (secondary to hypoplasia of one lobe or partial thyroidectomy)
- F > M: 3:1
- May be diffuse or nodular
- Diffuse hyperplasia results in enlargement of one on both lobes
- Nodular hyperplasia is usually seen as multiple discrete nodules, varying greatly in number and size, separated by normal parenchyma
- The typical hyperplastic nodule is of the same reflectivity as the normal gland, with a regular and complete peripheral halo, which is probably caused by perinodal blood vessels and mild edema or compression of adjacent normal parenchyma.

Adenoma
- Adenomas represent 5–10% of all nodular diseases of the thyroid.
- F:M = 7:1.
- A minority of adenomas is hyperfunctioning, develops autonomy, and may cause thyrotoxicosis (Plummer's disease)
- Follicular adenomas, which are much more frequently encountered than non-follicular adenomas, are true thyroid neoplasms, characterized by compression of adjacent tissue and fibrous encapsulation.
- Thyroid adenomas may be of low, normal or increased reflectivity usually with a thick and smooth peripheral echo- poor halo, owing to the fibrous capsule and blood vessels.
- Often vessels pass from the periphery to the center of the lesion, creating a "spoke and wheel" appearance. Malignant lesions are discussed with cold thyroid nodules.

Hürthle Cell Tumors
- Very rare
- They have been considered benign lesions in the past but may exhibit malignant characteristics with metastatic spread to lymph nodes and lung. This is seen more

frequently (80%) in lesions measuring greater than 4 cm in diameter
- These lesions are of mixed echogenicity on USG, usually solid and often ill-defined with no calcification
- Currently no single ultrasound criterion can distinguish benign from malignant thyroid nodules with complete reliability.
However, some features almost unique for benign goitrous nodules are:
- A thoroughly cystic appearance
- Moving comet-tail artifact
- Fluid-fluid levels
- Widespread cystic appearance in isoechoic or highly echogenic nodules
- Highly reflective nodules
- A perilesional thin, uniform thickness, echo-poor halo
- Well-defined and regular margins
- Peripheral egg-shell-like or large coarse calcifications
- A perilesional blood flow pattern
- If most of these signs are found in a thyroid nodule, the diagnosis of benign disease is highly reliable
- Conversely the possible ultrasound signs for malignancy are:
  - Low reflectivity
  - Irregular margins
  - Thick irregular halo
  - Intranodular blood flow pattern
  - Microcalcification
  - Hypervascularity
  - Invasion of vessels and adjacent structures
  - Vessel encasement.
- The most reliable of these signs for detecting malignancy are microcalcifications and the infiltration of structures adjacent to the thyroid gland.

Thyroid Calcifications

- Calcifications can be seen in both benign and malignant lesions of thyroid.
- Benign calcifications are seen as stromal calcifications in adenoma or in patients with multinodular goiter.
- Benign calcifications are peripheral or egg-shell-like, usually coarse and scattered throughout the gland, unlike the clustered fine calcifications (microcalcifications) which are more typical of malignant nodules.
- Microcalcifications (<1 mm) occur in 54% of thyroid neoplasms, and are most commonly seen in papillary carcinoma of thyroid. Microcalcifications can also be seen in medullary carcinoma of thyroid.

Chapter 9

Obstetrics and Gynecology

ULTRASOUND CHARACTERISTICS OF ABNORMAL GESTATION SAC

Major

Absence of yolk sac when:
- Mean sac diameter (MSD) more than or equal to 20 mm on transabdominal sonography (TAS).
- MSD more than or equal to 8 mm on transvaginal sonography (TVS).

Absence of embryo when:
- MSD more than or equal to 25 mm on TAS
- MSD more than or equal to 16 mm on TVS
- Distorted sac shape
- Growth of less than 1 mm MSD/day.

Minor

- Irregular sac contour
- Thin decidual reaction less than 2 mm
- Weak decidual echo amplitude
- Absent double decidual sac sign
- Sac positioned low in the uterus.

Causes of Empty Gestational Sac

- Anembryonic pregnancy (blighted ovum)
- Early pregnancy
- Pseudogestational sac with an ectopic pregnancy
- Early molar pregnancy.

DIFFERENTIAL DIAGNOSIS BETWEEN BLIGHTED OVUM AND PSEUDOGESTATION OF ECTOPIC PREGNANCY

Differential diagnosis (D/D) between blighted ovum and pseudogestation of ectopic pregnancy has been shown in Table 9.1 and Figure 9.1.

DIFFERENTIAL DIAGNOSIS BETWEEN ECTOPIC PREGNANCY, ABORTION IN PROGRESS (EARLY GESTATION) AND NABOTHIAN CYSTS

Differential diagnosis between ectopic pregnancy, abortion in progress has been shown in Table 9.2.

Hydropic Degeneration of the Placenta

Hydropic degeneration of the placenta is a phenomenon where numerous cystic spaces are formed within the placenta which is often accompanied by placental enlargement. It can occur in a number of situations which include:
- Simple hydropic degeneration in 1st trimester fetal demise

Table 9.1: Differential diagnosis between blighted ovum and pseudogestation of ectopic pregnancy.

	Anembryonic pregnancy (Blighted ovum)	Pseudogestation of ectopic pregnancy (Fig. 9.1)
Uterine size	Usually normal	May be enlarged
Gestation sac with double decidual sac sign	Present	Absent
Yolk sac	±	Absent
Fetal node	Absent	Absent
Other criteria	Abnormal gestational sac	Adnexal mass
Peritrophoblastic high velocity low impendence blood flow within uterus	Present (PSV more than 21 cm/sec)	Absent (Present around adnexal mass)

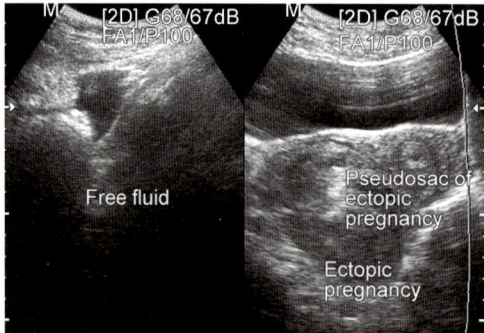

Fig. 9.1: Pseudogestation with free fluid.

- Gestational trophoblastic disease—particularly partial mole
- Triploidy—paternal triploidy
- Beckwith-Wiedemann syndrome.

DIFFERENTIAL DIAGNOSIS BETWEEN PARTIAL MOLE, INTRAUTERINE FETAL DEATH WITH HYDROPIC PLACENTAL DEGENERATION, AND TWIN PREGNANCY (MOLE AND FETUS)

Differential diagnosis between partial mole, intrauterine fetal death (IUFD) with hydropic placental degeneration, twin pregnancy has been described in Table 9.3.

DIFFERENTIAL DIAGNOSIS BETWEEN PELVIC MASSES, EXTRUDED FETAL PARTS WITH UTERINE PERFORATION (FIG. 9.2) AND ECTOPIC PREGNANCY (POSTPARTUM/INTERVENTION)

Differential diagnosis between pelvic masses, extruded fetal parts with uterine perforation and ectopic pregnancy has been shown in Table 9.4.

DIFFERENTIAL DIAGNOSIS OF A PRESACRAL FETAL MASS (TABLE 9.5)

Causes

- Sacrococcygeal germ cell tumors including dermoid cysts.
- Anterior myelomeningocele/meningocele.

Table 9.2: Differential diagnosis between ectopic pregnancy, abortion in progress and Nabothian cyst.

	Ectopic pregnancy	Abortion in progress	Nabothian cysts
Pregnancy test	Positive	Positive	Negative
Uterine size	May be increased	May be increased	Normal; cervix may be bulky
GS/double de-cidual sac sign in uterus	Absent	Present	Absent
Fetal node/Yolk sac	Absent	Present	Absent
Cervical os	Closed	Open	Closed
Adnexal mass	Present	Absent (Except for corpus luteum cyst)	Absent

Table 9.3: Differential diagnosis between partial mole, intrauterine fetal death (IUFD) with hydropic placental degeneration, and twin pregnancy.

	Partial mole	IUFD with hydropic placental degeneration	Twin pregnancy
Uterine size	Often larger for dates	May be smaller for dates	Larger for dates
Placental appearance	Normal tissue with many small cysts (<15 mm)	Normal tissue with few cystic lesions	One normal placenta and one with multiple cystic lesion
Fetus (structurally)	Abnormal either blended/adjacent to placental tissue	Fetus and placenta seen separately	One normal fetus seen/2 fetal poles seen
β-hCG levels	Higher than normal for GA	Lower than expected for GA	Very much higher for GA

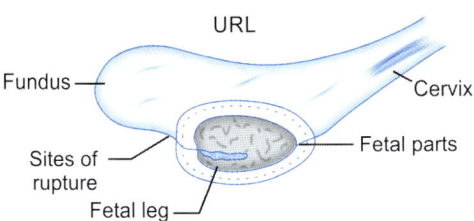

Fig. 9.2: Perforation of lower uterine segment with extension of fetal bones into cul-de-sac (URL: Upper range limit).

- Neurenteric cyst.
- Enteric duplication cysts.
- Retrorectal hamartomas—tailgut cyst.
- Vascular malformation.
- Lymphatic malformation.
- Pelvic abscess.
- *Neurogenic tumors*: Neuroblastoma/peripheral nerve sheath tumors.
- Sarcoma.
- Lipoma.
- Primary bone tumor.
- Lymphoma.

Differentiation between sacrococcygeal teratoma/anterior myelomeningocele and other presacral masses is easily achieved by biochemical tests as amniotic fluid alpha-fetoprotein and acetylcholinesterase levels are increased in the former two.

Table 9.4: Differential diagnosis between pelvic masses, extruded fetal parts with uterine perforation and ectopic pregnancy.

	Pelvic abscess	Extruded fetal parts	Ectopic pregnancy
History of amenorrhea	Usually absent	Present	Present
Uterine size	Normal/enlarged	Small for GA with breach in uterine wall	May be enlarged
USG appearance	Complex echogenic mass	Fetal bones with acoustic shadowing	Heterogeneous adnexal mass
β-hCG level	Normal	Falling titers/normal for GA	Raised
Uterine cavity	Empty/Pus	Fetal parts/only liquor	Pseudosac (Fluid in uterine cavity)

Table 9.5: Differential diagnosis of a presacral fetal mass.

	Sacrococcygeal teratoma	Anterior sacral myelomeningocele
USG appearance	Soft tissue mass with fat and calcifications Mixed and solid (85%) Cystic (15%)	Cystic mass with nerve roots and spinal cord traversing the mass, devoid of any calcifications
Liquor volume	Polyhydramnios (2/3) Oligohydramnios (1/3)	Polyhydramnios
Fetal spine	Normal/destroyed	Defect in spine with widened spinal canal diameter
Location	Type I (~50%)—predominantly external Type II—significant presacral component Type III—both external abdomino-pelvic component Type IV—completely intrapelvic	Presacral
Associated anomalies	NF-I; Marfan's syndrome, partial sacral agenesis' imperforate anus, stenosis, tethered spinal cord, GU tract/colonic placentomegaly, anomalies	Spinal dysraphism, sacral agenesis, dislocation of hip, hydronephrosis, Potter's syndrome imperforate anus, fetal hydrops, curvilinear sacrococcygeal defect.

FETAL NECK MASSES (TABLE 9.6)

Causes

- *Neural tube defects:*
  - Occipital cephalocele
  - Cervical myelomeningocele
- Cystic hygroma—lymphatic malformation (Fig. 9.3)
- Vascular malformation
- Cysts:
  - Midline—thyroglossal cyst
  - Lateral—branchial cleft cyst
  - Lingual cyst
  - Thymic cyst
- Enlarged thyroid (goiter)—congenital hypothyroidism
- Teratoma (Dermoid)
- Rhabdomyosarcoma.

DIFFERENTIAL DIAGNOSIS OF FETAL RENAL CYSTIC DISEASES

Differential diagnosis of fetal renal cystic diseases has been described in Table 9.7.

DIFFERENTIAL DIAGNOSIS OF VARIOUS FETAL ANTERIOR ABDOMINAL WALL DEFECTS

Differential diagnosis of various fetal anterior abdominal wall defects has been described in Table 9.8.

DIFFERENTIAL DIAGNOSIS BETWEEN RENAL CYSTS AND HYDRONEPHROSIS

Differential diagnosis between renal cysts and hydronephrosis has been described in Table 9.9.

DIFFERENTIAL DIAGNOSIS OF CYSTIC ADNEXAL MASSES

- *Ovarian causes:*
  - Physiological ovarian cyst
  - Functional/retention cyst
  - Corpus luteum
  - Theca lutein cyst (in pregnancy)
  - Hemorrhagic cyst
  - Endometrioma
  - Dermoid cyst
  - Serous/mucinous cystadenoma/cystadenocarcinoma

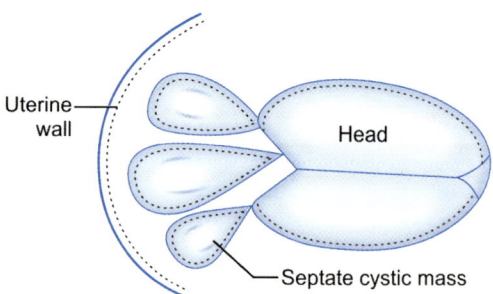

Fig. 9.3: Cystic hygroma.

Table 9.6: Fetal neck masses.

	Neural tube defects	Cystic hygroma	Teratoma
USG-appearance	Predominantly cystic masses	Multiseptate, anechoic mass ± debris	Complex mass containing echo-genic components, some with acoustic shadowing; pre-dominantly solid on 10–31% and purely cystic in 9–15%
Skull and spine defects	Present	Absent	Absent
Other associations	Brain anomalies	Chromosomal defects as trisomy 21; Turner's syndrome, fetal hydrops; may be associated with fetal alcohol syndrome and multiple pterygium syndrome	Associated with thyroid gland

Table 9.7: Differential diagnosis of fetal renal cystic diseases.

	Multicystic dysplastic kidney (MCDK)	Obstructive cystic renal dysplasia	Autosomal recessive polycystic kidney disease (ARPKD)	Autosomal dominant polycystic kidney disease (ADPKD)
Renal size	Usually enlarged	Variable (normal, increased, decreased)	Enlarged	Enlarged
Reniform shape	May be deformed	Usually preserved	Preserved	Preserved
Renal cyst	Multiple of variable size	Multiple in subcapsular region/cortex Usually smaller	May be seen, usually too small to be resolved by ultrasound	Usually presents in adulthood, multiple small to large simple or hemorrhagic cysts
Dilated PC system	Absent	May be present	Absent	Absent
Laterality	Unilateral 80% Bilateral	Usually 20% Bilateral	Bilateral	Bilateral
Normal renal parenchyma	Absent	Usually present around the cyst with thin cortical parenchyma	Present but no CM differentiation	Present but no CM differentiation
Inheritance	Sporadic	NA	Autosomal recessive	Autosomal dominant (so one of the parents is affected)
Association	Contralateral reveal abnormalities as UPJ obstruction, agenesis, hypoplasia, MCDK	Most commonly with urethral obstruction	With hepatic fibrosis, pulmonary hypoplasia, (potters syndrome)	
ADPKD associations—cerebral berry aneurysms, intracranial dolichoectasia, hypertension, colonic diverticulosis, small bowel diverticula, bicuspid aortic valve, mitral valve prolapse, aortic dissection, multiple biliary hamartomas, cysts in other organs including liver, ovaries, spleen, seminal vesicles, prostate, pancreas.				

Table 9.8: Differential diagnosis of various fetal anterior abdominal wall defects.

	Gastroschisis	Omphalocele	Limb body wall complex (aminiotic band syndrome)	Bladder/cloacal exstrophy (OEIS complex)
Location of defect	Right paraumbilical	Midline cord insertion site	Left side lateral defect	Midline, infraumbilical
Size of defect	Small (2–4 cm)	Variable (2–10 cm)	Large	Variable
Covering membrane	Absent	Present	Present, contiguous with placenta, umbilical cord absent	Variable
Contents	Usually small bowel and at times large bowel, stomach and solid viscera	Usually liver but at times with bowel	Evisceration of abdominal viscera especially liver	Bladder wall evisceration with or without bowel
Bowel complication including thickening of wall and dilatation	Present	Absent (usually) present with ruptured membrane	Absent	Absent
Cardiac anomalies	Rare	Common	Common	Uncommon

Differential Diagnosis in Radiology

Table 9.9: Differential diagnosis between renal cysts and hydronephrosis.

	Renal cyst	Hydronephrosis
Size	Variable size	Uniform size
Alignment	Nonspecific	Aligned anatomically
Communication	Absent	Communicate with dilated renal pelvis
Shape	Round to oval	Tapering toward renal pelvis
Reniform contour of kidney	May be distorted	Usually preserved
Renal parenchyma	May be present/absent depending on location	Present peripherally

- Hyperstimulation cysts
- Massive ovarian edema.
- *Tubal causes:*
  - Hydro/Pyosalpinx.
- *Tubo-ovarian:*
  - Abscess
  - Ectopic pregnancy.
- *Miscellaneous:*
  - Peritoneal inclusion cyst
  - Para-ovarian cyst
  - Lymphocele
  - Enteric duplication cyst
  - Appendiceal mucocele
  - Peritoneal carcinoma
  - Malignant mesothelioma.

DIFFERENTIAL DIAGNOSIS OF OVARIAN MASSES (FLOWCHART 9.1)

- Must look for age of the patient
- In middle aged/old always try to differentiate between benign and malignant masses.

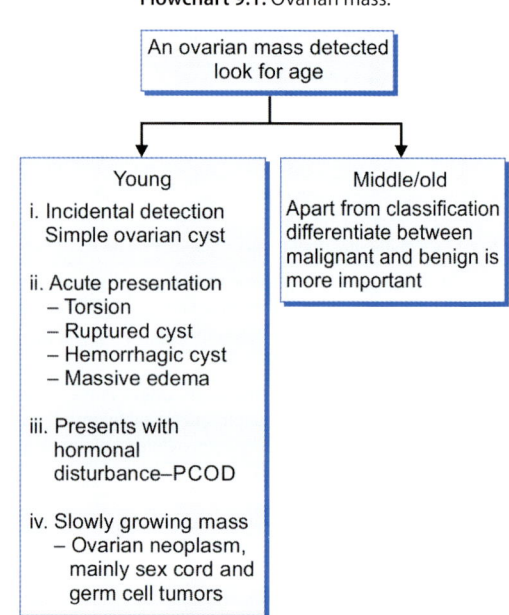

Flowchart 9.1: Ovarian mass.

DIFFERENTIAL DIAGNOSIS OF BENIGN AND MALIGNANT OVARIAN MASSES

Differential diagnosis of benign and malignant ovarian masses has been described in Table 9.10.

DIFFERENTIAL DIAGNOSIS OF CYSTIC ABDOMINAL MASSES

Normal Ovaries

- *Normal tubes:*
  - Peritoneal inclusion cyst
    - USG—multiloculated cystic adnexal mass with intact ovary and mild-septations and fluid.
  - Para-ovarian (Paratubal cyst)
    - USG—cystic
    - Mass frequently located superior to uterine fundus. Ipsilateral ovary seen separately.
- *Abnormal tubes:*
  - Hydro-pyosalpinx
  - USG—cystic tubular mass with incomplete septations and well-defined echogenic wall; anechoic contents in hydrosalpinx and echogenic debris seen in pyosalpinx.

Obstetrics and Gynecology

Table 9.10: Differential diagnosis of benign and malignant ovarian masses.

	Benign	Malignant
Size	Small; less than 5 cm	Large; more than 10 cm
Contour	Well-defined with thin walls	Ill-defined with thick walls
Internal architecture	Cystic with thin septations	Solid/Complex with solid mural or papillary projections with thick septations
Doppler	Absent low or high resist acne flow nodules may be avascular	Vascular nodules with high resistance low
Associated findings		Ascites; peritoneal implants

Abnormal Ovaries

Physiological
- Cysts (Unilocular)
  - Less than 2.5 cm in diameter
  - Sequential changes are most common.

Tubo-ovarian Abscess

Complex multiloculated mass with irregular margins, variable septation with scattered internal echoes and DAS.

Functional Cysts
- (Unilocular), unilateral
- Less than 2.5 cm in diameter
- Changes seen over few next MC
- Low-level reticular echoes may be seen in hemorrhagic cysts
- Theca lutein cysts are bilateral multilocular cysts.

Hemorrhagic Cyst
- Complex multiseptated cystic lesions with fish net appearance
- Intracystic solid clot- with concave margins and absence of internal Doppler signal
- Fluid-fluid level in acute hemorrhage.

Massive Ovarian Edema
- Ovarian edema from partial or intermittent torsion
- Large multicystic adnexal mass is seen on USG.

Endometrioma

Unilocular asymptomatic cystic lesion with homogeneous low-level echoes that rarely show significant changes with menstrual cycles.

Dermoid

Cystic anechoic to echogenic mass with dermoid plug, hair fluid/fat fluid level with foci of calcification.

Cystadenoma/Cystadenocarcinoma

Uni/Multilocular/Bilateral cystic masses with thin/thick septations with mural nodules and low resistance flow in malignant masses with presence of ascites and peritoneal spread.

DIFFERENTIAL DIAGNOSIS OF NON-GYNECOLOGICAL PELVIC LESIONS

These arise most commonly secondary to surgery involving either GIT and urinary tract.
- Appendicular mucocele
- Meckel's diverticulum
- Enteric duplication cysts
- Mesenteric cyst
- Diverticular abscess
- Bladder diverticulum
- Pelvic abscess
- Hematoma
- Lymphocele
- Urinoma
- Seroma.

DIFFERENTIAL DIAGNOSIS OF POSTOPERATIVE PELVIC MASS

Differential diagnosis of postoperative pelvic mass has been described in Table 9.11.

Table 9.11: Differential diagnosis of postoperative pelvic mass.

Abscesses	Hematoma	Lymphoceles/Urinoma/Seroma
Ovoid lesions with thick irregular walls, internal debris, posterior acoustic enhancement with clinical symptomatology	Spectrum of findings from anechoic to echogenic masses with DAS and variable appearance with time	Cystic anechoic collection Fluid cytology helps in diagnosis

DIFFERENTIAL DIAGNOSIS OF OVARIAN ADNEXAL MASS

- Functional cysts
  - Follicular cyst
  - Corpus luteal cyst
  - Hemorrhagic cyst
- Ovarian remnant syndrome
- Paraovarian (Peritubal) cyst
- Peritoneal inclusion cyst
- Endometriosis
- Polycystic ovarian disease (PCOD)
- Massive edema
- Inflammatory T-O mass
- Postoperative lymphocele, seroma, urinoma
- Bowel masses presenting as adnexal.

DIFFERENTIAL DIAGNOSIS OF OVARIAN ADNEXAL MASS OF OVARIAN MASSES

Ovarian Masses are Classified Histologically

- *Epithelial tumors:*
  - Serous
  - Mucinous
  - Mesonephroid (clear cell)
  - Endometrioid
  - Brenner's
  - Mixed
  - Undifferentiated
  - Unclassified.
- *Sex cord (Gonadal stromal) tumors:*
  - Granulosa cell tumor, theca cell tumor
  - Androblastoma (k/a Sertoli-Leydig cell tumor)
  - Gynandroblastoma
  - Unclassified.
- Lipid (Lipoid) cell tumor

- *Germ cell tumors:*
  - Dysgerminoma
  - Endodermal sinus tumor
  - Embryoma
  - Polyembryoma
  - Choriocarcinoma
  - Teratoma
  - Mixed.
- *Gonadoblastoma:*
  - Pure
  - Mixed with dysgerminoma.
- Soft tissue tumors
- Unclassified
- Secondaries
- Tumor-like conditions.

Salient Features

Epithelial Tumors

- Constitute 95% of all malignant neoplasms of ovary
- Most common are serous and mucinous cyst-adenocarcinomas
- Postmenopausal women
- Spreads transcelomically along the direction of ascitic fluid circulation
- Right subphrenic and right paracolic gutters are early sites of spread
- Eighty-five percent have peritoneal deposits at presentation
- Para-aortic and pelvic are the first lymph nodes to be involved One of the few primaries to have splenic secondaries.

On USG:

- First modality used to detect, confirm the presence, and characterize a pelvic mass. Its high sensitivity (97.3%) makes it an ideal screening tool in high-risk groups

- Malignant masses are large, bilateral, complex, with thick walls, thick septa and have mural nodules. Conversely is true for benign.

On Color Doppler:
- Increased abnormal neovascularity
- RI < 0.4; PI < 1 (but these are not highly specific signs).

On CT Scan:
- Mainstay of preoperative assessment.
- The appearance is similar to that seen on USG. The solid components enhance on administration of IV contrast. Solid looking non-enhancing areas have either blood or thick mucin. Calcification is better detected.
- Spread to adjacent—organ is well documented but distant and especially peritoneal spread is difficult to interpret. Conventional scanners detect less than 50% of metastases less than 5 mm.
- Peritoneal deposits may present as small foci of new peritoneal calcification, multiple nodular lesion in omental fat, omental cake, nodules surrounded by bowel loops and thickening along vessels and lymphatics.
- Pseudomyxoma peritonei occurring due to rupture of mucinous tumors present as high density fluid loculi on the serosal surfaces of organ, indenting them.

On MRI:
Basic morphological features are same but it is better in determining the origin, characterization and land masking the spread due to multiplanner capability and better soft tissue contrast.

Germ Cell Tumors
- 5–15% of ovarian malignancies
- Seen in young and adolescent: Peak—16–20 years mostly less than 30 years
- Most common pediatric ovarian tumor
- Most common is dysgerminoma (the counterpart of seminoma)
- U/L, solid, well-defined, large (since aggressive). Dysgerminoma is multiloculated with vascular fibrous septa in between
- Calcification seen in teratoma and dysgerminoma
- Usually extends directly but metastasis to nodes, lung and liver is more common than epithelial tumors.

Stromal/Sex Cord Tumors
- 3–6% of ovarian malignancies
- Most common is granulosa cell tumors
- Almost always malignant
- Hormone (Estrogen) secreting
- Postmenopausal or prepubertal age groups
- Quite variable in appearance.

Metastasis
- 15% of all ovarian malignancies
- Stomach, colon, breast, lung, gallbladder, pancreas
- Krukenberg's tumor is a specific term used to describe a secondary having sarcomatous stroma interspersed between mucin-secreting-Signet ring cells. Usually the primary site is stomach
- Large, B/L, indistinguishable from primary
- Presence of associated deposits in liver, lung are so strong indicators that the ovarian mass is secondary
- Ovary is most common genital organ to receive leukemic deposits
- May be involved in diffuse non-Hodgkin's lymphoma.

Features of Malignancy
- RI less than 0.4
- PI more than 1.0
- Thick septa more than 3 mm
- Mural nodule
- Complex cyst
- Large size more than 10 cm
- Ascites
- Metastasis/peritoneal implants.

SONOGRAPHIC CLASSIFICATION OF ADNEXAL MASSES

Simple Cyst
Always Benign
- Simple ovarian cysts
  - Follicular cyst
  - Corpus luteal cyst

- Hydrosalpinx
- Cystadenoma.
- Non-gynecological
  - Of GI origin
  - Bladder diverticulum.

Solid Masses

Benign
- Pedunculated fibroid.
- Torsion.
- Brenner's tumor.
- Fibroma/thecoma.

Malignant
- Germ cell tumor.
- Endometrioid carcinoma.
- Granulosa cell tumor.
- Metastasis.

Nongynecological
- Lymphadenopathy.
- Bladder tumor.
- GI tumor.

Complex Cyst

Benign
- Cyst with low-level echoes
  - Endometrioma
  - Hemorrhagic cyst
  - Cystadenoma.
- Cyst with hyperechoic component
  - Cystic teratoma.
- Cyst with solid components
  - Tubo-ovarian abscess
  - Cystadenoma
  - Cystic teratoma
  - Fibrothecoma
  - Peritoneal inclusion cyst.

Malignant
- Mucinous/serous cystadenocarcinoma.
- Clear cell carcinoma.
- Endometrioid carcinoma.

- Granulosa cell tumor.
- Cystic teratocarcinoma.
- Metastasis.

Nongynecological
- Abscess
- Hematoma
- Lymphocele.

MRI Classification of Adnexal Masses
- Low T1 + Low T2
  - a. Leiomyoma
  - b. Fibroma/thecoma
- Low T1 + High T2
  - a. Functional cyst
  - b. Peritoneal inclusion cyst
  - c. Cystadenoma
  - d. Hydrosalpinx
- High T1
  - a. Dermoid
  - b. Endometrioma
  - c. Hemorrhagic cyst
  - d. Proteinaceous material
- Heterogeneous
  - a. Malignancies
  - b. Simple cyst with hemorrhage
  - c. Tubo-ovarian abscess
  - d. Ovarian torsion
  - e. Ruptured ectopic pregnancy.

ABSENT INTRAUTERINE PREGNANCY WITH POSITIVE PREGNANCY TEST (FLOWCHART 9.2)

Causes
- Ectopic pregnancy.
- Very early intrauterine pregnancy.
- Recent abortion.
- Molar pregnancy/gestational trophoblastic neoplasia.

Salient Features
- *Ectopic pregnancy:*
  - Specific feature: Live embryo in the adnexa.

Flowchart 9.2: Absent Intrauterine pregnancy with positive pregnancy test.

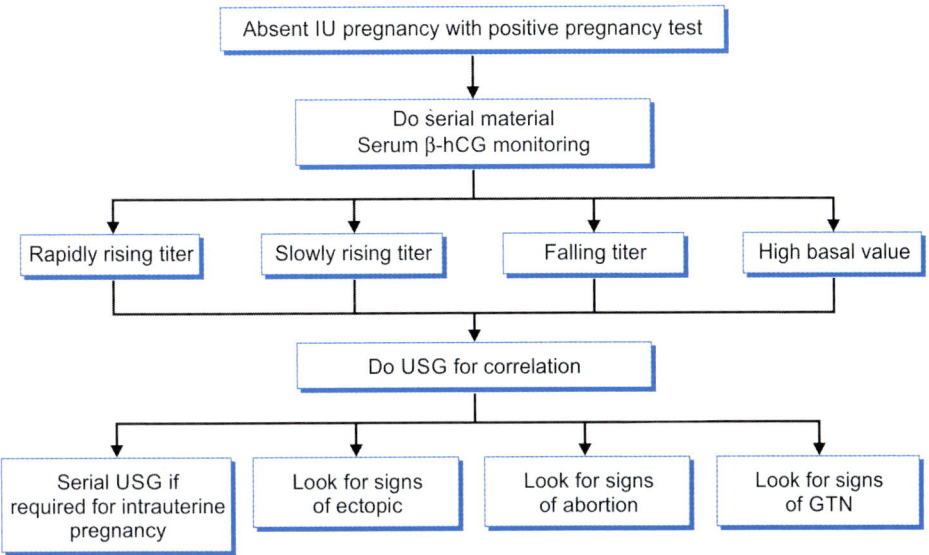

- Nonspecific features (Need β-hCG correlation):
    - Empty uterus
    - Pseudogestational sac in uterus
    - Particulate ascites
    - Adnexal mass
    - Ectopic tubal ring
- Slow rising β-hCG, i.e. doubling time >2 days.
- Nonsupportive features:
    - Live intrauterine pregnancy
    - Peritrophoblastic flow
    - Intradecidual sign/double decidual sac sign
- *Very early intrauterine pregnancy:*
    - Pregnancy test becomes positive at approximately 23 days while the earliest sonographic sign of pregnancy, i.e. intradecidual sign is detected at approximately 25 days. During this window period of 2 days, confusion may occur.
    - It is always wise to screen after 72 hours in case of any confusion.
- *Recent abortion:* In case of positive pregnancy test with USG showing no intrauterine pregnancy serial monitoring of β-hCG should be done. In cases of abortion, a falling titer is seen in maternal serum.
- *Gestational trophoblastic neoplasia:* Uterus is enlarged with cavity filled with multiple small vesicles and soft-tissue nodules. Fetal parts and myometrial invasion may or may not be seen. β-hCG levels are quite high.

DIFFERENTIAL DIAGNOSIS OF THICKENED PLACENTA (FLOWCHART 9.3)

Causes

- Maternal diabetes.
- Rhesus isoimmunization.
- Fetal hydrops.
- Triploidy.
- Intrauterine infections.
- Maternal severe anemia.
- Fetal anemia.
- Fetal hydrops.
- Homozygous alpha thalassemia.
- Placental tumors.
- Retroplacental/Placental bleed.

Differential Diagnosis in Radiology

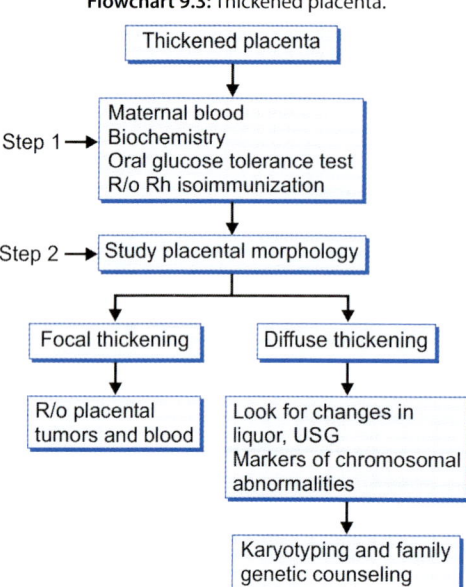

Flowchart 9.3: Thickened placenta.

Salient Features
- Placenta (Figs. 9.4 to 9.6) is called thickened when it measures more than 4 cm in thickness at the cord insertion
- Most of the above causes are better evaluated by microscopic and biochemical evaluation of maternal blood
  - Karyotyping is an essential step in evaluation
  - USG has a corroborative role in evaluating structural abnormalities in above conditions, e.g. fetal hydrops chromosomal abnormalities.

ULTRASOUND SIGNS OF CHROMOSOMAL ABNORMALITY (FLOWCHART 9.4)

Generalized Signs which are Important Even if Isolated
- Borderline ventriculomegaly.
- Posterior fossa abnormality.
- Cystic hygroma.
- Nuchal fold thickness.
- Nuchal translucency.
- Atrioventricular septal defects.
- Double outlet right ventricle.
- Omphalocele.
- Duodenal atresia.
- Echogenic bowel.
- Genitourinary abnormality.
- Nonimmune hydrops.

Important Specific Signs
Trisomy 21
- Cystic hygroma.
- Nonimmune hydrops.
- Nuchal thickening.
- Hydrothorax.

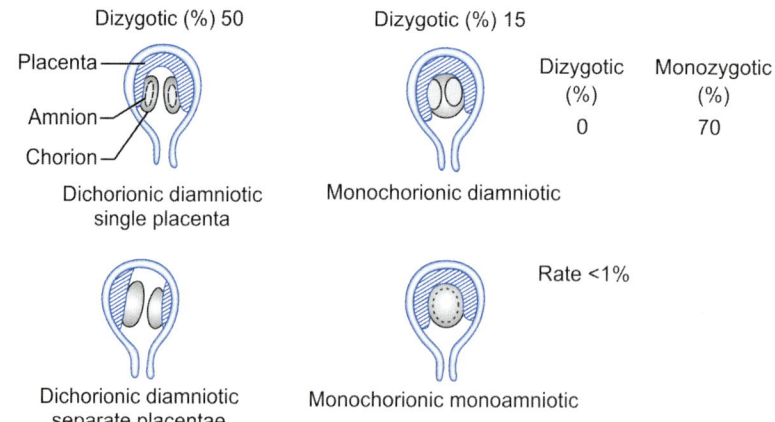

Fig. 9.4: Placenta and membranes in twin pregnancies.

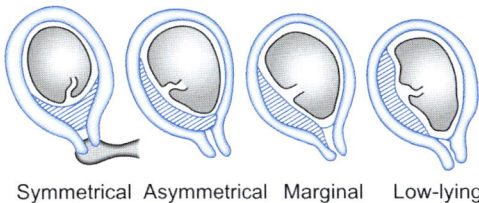

Fig. 9.5: Abnormalities of the placenta.

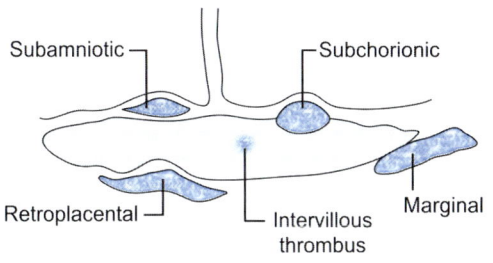

Fig. 9.6: Placental hemorrhage.

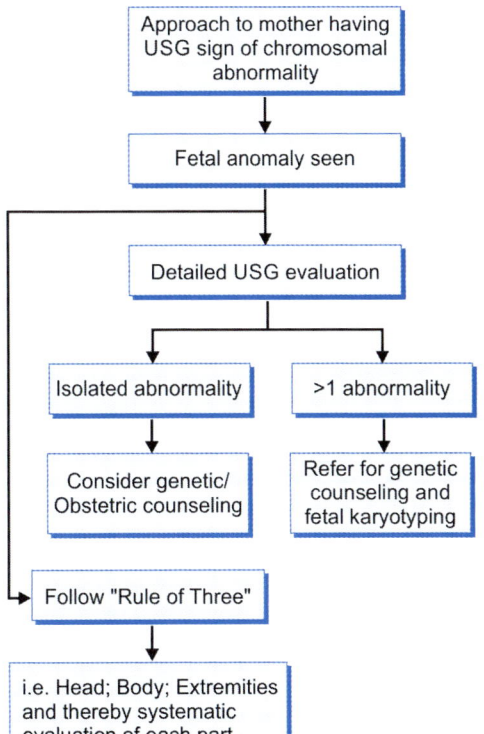

Flowchart 9.4: USG sign of chromosomal abnormality approach.

- Gut atresias.
- Protruding tongue.
- Clinodactyly.
- Increased distance between 1st and 2nd toes.

Trisomy 18

- IUGR.
- Single umbilical artery.
- Cystic hygroma.
- Microcephaly/Dolichocephaly.
- Mega cisterna magna.
- Omphalocele.
- Renal dysplasias.
- Rocker bottom feet.

Trisomy 13

- Cyclopia.
- Anophthalmia.
- Cleft lip/palate
- Low set deformed ear.
- Holoprosencephaly.
- Duplicated kidney.
- Polydactyly.
- Rocker bottom feet.

Triploidy

- Early onset IUGR.
- Myelomeningocele.
- Agenesis of corpus callosum.
- Micrognathia.
- Sloping forehead.
- Postaxial polydactyly/syndactyly.
- Molar placenta.
- Renal cortical cyst.

Turner's Syndrome

- Cystic hygroma.
- Nonimmune hydrops.
- Brachycephaly.
- Small mandible.
- Coarctation of aorta.
- Horse-shoe kidney.
- Cubitus valgus.
- Short stature.

DIFFERENTIAL DIAGNOSIS OF ENLARGED UTERUS (FLOWCHART 9.5)

Causes

- Pregnancy
- Leiomyoma
- Carcinoma endometrium
- Hemato/pyometria
- Gestational trophoblastic
- Puerperal uterus neoplasia
- Ectopic pregnancy
- Soft tissue sarcomas
- Adenomyosis.

Salient Features

- Most common cause of enlarged uterus in childbearing age is pregnant and puerperal uterus, both of which may be evaluated by proper history and signs of pregnancy
- In older females, malignancy is an important consideration
- In young congenitally malformed uterus hemato/pyometria may be seen.

CYSTIC STRUCTURES IN FETAL ABDOMEN (FLOWCHART 9.6)

Causes

- Renal : Multicystic dysplasia and other cystic diseases
  Hydronephrosis
  Megacystis
- GI : Duodenal obstruction
  Jejunal obstruction
- Ovarian : Simple cyst
  Complex cyst associated with torsion
- Mesenteric cyst
- Hepatic cyst
- Pancreatic cyst
- Lymphangioma
- Urachal cyst.

Salient Features

- *Renal:* If multiple cysts with a distorted kidney and absent renal parenchyma are seen, it suggests MCDK. If enlarged echogenic kidneys are seen, it could be either ADPCKD or ARPCKD which are difficult to separate out by USG.
- *GI:* A double bubble sign with polyhydramnios shows duodenal obstruction while multiple air fluid levels indicate jejunal obstruction.
- *Ovarian:* 97% are benign functional cysts due to hormonal stimulation. These are simple cysts located eccentrically in pelvis with a normal GI and urinary system.
- Megacystis is caused by posterior urethral valves; urethral atresia/stricture; prune-belly syndrome; primary megacystis; cloacal malformation; megacystis-microcolon-intestinal-hypoperistalsis syndrome (MMIHS).
- *Meckel-Gruber syndrome:* Polycystic kidney (100%); polydactyly postaxial (55%); occipital cephalocele (60–85%).
- Cystic lesions are usually indeterminate in appearance and correlation to associated features is helpful in final diagnosis.
- Cyst in association with echogenic bowel can be pancreatic cysts in cystic fibrosis.

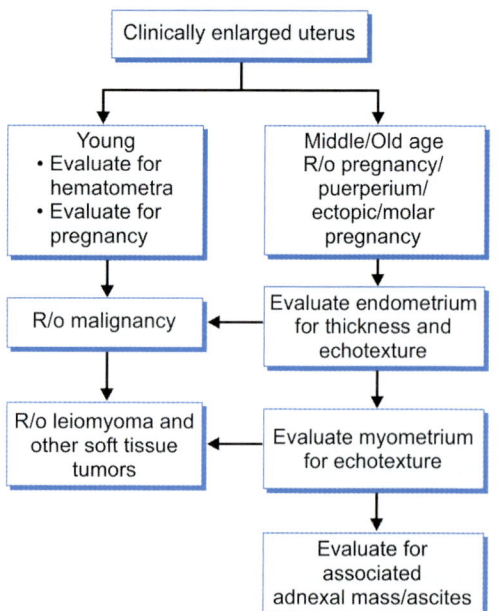

Flowchart 9.5: Enlarged uterus.

Flowchart 9.6: Approach to a cyst lesion in fetal abdomen.

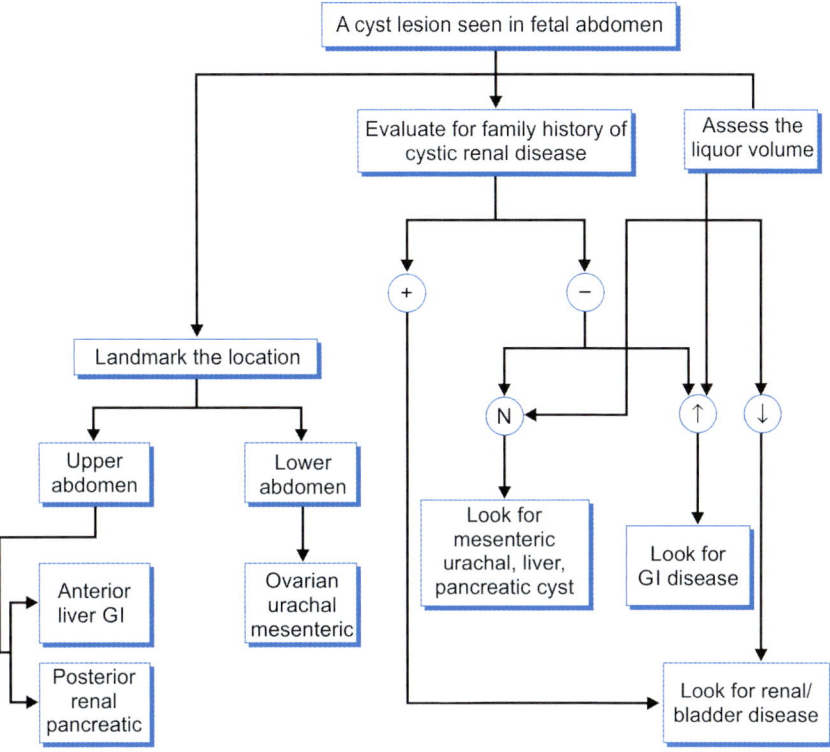

DIFFERENTIAL DIAGNOSIS OF FETAL HYDROPS (FLOWCHART 9.7)

Causes

- *Immune hydrops:*
  - Rh (D) incompatibility.
  - Other blood group antigens incompatibility, e.g. kell.
- *Nonimmune hydrops:*
  - Fetal causes:
    - Idiopathic (15–20%)
    - Infections:
      - CMV; HPVB19; Rubella; Coxsackie; Syphilis; Listeria; Toxoplasma.
    - Cardiovascular:
      - Malformations; arrhythmias; high output failure.
    - Neck/Thorax abnormalities:
      - Cystic hygroma; diaphragmatic hernia; congenital cystic adenomatoid malformation; pulmonary sequestration.
    - Gastrointestinal abnormalities
      - Cirrhosis; hepatitis; atresias; volvulus; meconium peritonitis.
    - Urinary tract abnormalities:
      - Congenital nephrotic syndrome; prune-belly syndrome; polycystic kidney.
    - Anemias:
      - Alpha-thalassemia; HPVB19 infections G-6-P deficiency; Twin-Twin Transfusion syndrome.
    - Chromosomal abnormality:
      - 45,X; Trisomy 13,18,21; Triploidy.
    - Genetic disorders
      - Gaucher's; Hurler's; MPS; sialidosis; achondroplasia; achondrogenesis; thanatophoric dysplasia; Jeune's dystrophy; osteogenesis imperfecta; arthrogryposis multiplex congenita; Pena-Shokeir syndrome; Neu-Laxova syndrome;

Flowchart 9.7: Approach to a cast of fetal hydrops.

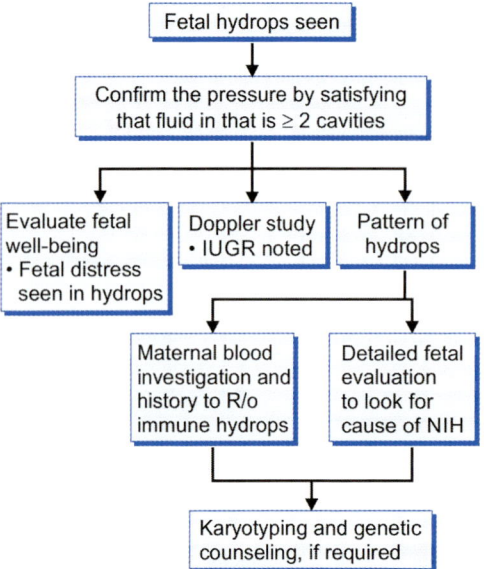

- *Maternal causes:*
  - Severe diabetes.
  - Severe anemia.
  - Severe hypoproteinemia.
- *Placental:*
  - Chorioangioma.
  - Venous thrombosis.
  - Cord torsion, knot, and tumor.

Salient Features

- Hydrops is defined as an abnormal accumulation of serous fluid in at least two body cavities or tissues.
- *Sonographic features:*
  - Ascites.
  - Pleural effusion.
  - Pericardial effusion.
  - Subcutaneous edema.
  - Placental edema.
  - Alteration in arterial/venous Doppler.
  - Alteration in fetal well-being.
- Pseudoascites is a hypoechoic rim seen peripherally in abdomen (<2 mm) due to muscle layer

- Subcutaneous edema is best evaluated over the scalp and head pattern of fluid collection helps in D/D:

Immune hydrops	– Ascites first
Thoracic pathology	– Pleural fluid first
Anemia	– Ascites first
Meconium peritonitis	– Fluctuant ascites with echogenic bowel
Parvovirus infection	– Tense ascites with echogenic bowel

DIFFERENTIAL DIAGNOSIS OF FETAL BRAIN AND HEAD ABNORMALITIES

Causes

- *Abnormalities of dorsal induction:*
  - Anencephaly
  - Encephalocele/iniencephaly
  - Spina bifida/Chiari II malformation
  - Caudal regression.
- *Abnormalities of ventral induction:*
  - Holoprosencephaly
  - Dandy-Walker malformation.
- *Neuronal proliferation/differentiation:*
  - Macrocephaly
  - Microcephaly
  - Vascular malformations/tumors.
- *Abnormalities of migration:*
  - Agenesis of corpus callosum
  - Schizencephaly/lissencephaly
  - Polymicrogyria/pachygyria.
- *Acquired injuries:*
  - Porencephaly
  - Aqueductal stenosis.
- Unclassified.

Salient Features

- Abnormalities are classified according to the time of their origin:

Dorsal induction	– 4th to 7th week.
Ventral induction	– 5th to 10th week.
Neuronal proliferation and differentiation	– 2nd to 3rd month.
Neuronal migration	– 3rd to 5th month.
Acquired injury	– 3rd to 4th month.

- *Anencephaly:*
  - Absence of cranial vault, cerebral hemispheres, diencephalic structures and their replacement by flattened amorphous neurovascular tissue.
  - Mass known as area coxbiovasculosa.
  - Diagnosed earliest by 10 weeks and 100% at 14th week
  - *Acrania*: Absent vault.
  - *Exencephaly*: Brain matter is recognizable.
  - *Cranioschiasis*: Cranial abnormality with spinal dysraphism.
- *Encephalocele:*
  - It is a pouch containing CSF, meninges and brain matter while cranial meningocele has no brain parenchyma.
  - 75% occipital; 13% frontal; 12% parietal.
  - Seen in Meckel-Gruber syndrome.
- *Lemon skull:*
  - Bifrontal indentation is seen in 1% normal fetus, few dwarfism and spina bifida.
- *Strawberry skull:*
  - A skull having reduced OFD, flattened occiput and pointed frontal area. Seen in trisomy 18.
- *Clover leaf skull:*
  - Seen in thanatophoric dwarfism and craniosynostosis.
- *Ventriculomegaly:*
  - Occipital horn more than 10 mm
  - Ventricle to choroid ratio more than 3 mm
  - Anterior horns more than 20 mm (under 24 weeks)
  - VHR—74% at 16th week
  - 35% at 25th week.
- *Banana sign:*
  - Compressed moulded cerebellum about brainstem, seen in spinal dysraphisms.
- *Iniencephaly:*
  - A condition where occiput and cervical spine are involved together in dysraphism. Child is in a "star-gazing" position and spinal segmentation abnormality is present.
- *Holoprosencephaly:*
  - Results from incomplete cleavage and/or diverticulation of forebrain into cerebral hemispheres.
  - May be lobar, semilobar or alobar upon the severity of the disease.
  - Associated with midline facial defects.
- *Dandy-Walker malformation:*
  - A condition where a malformed posterior fossa cyst communicating with fourth ventricle due to vermian agenesis and hydrocephalus is seen.
  - In D-W variant less severe degrees of abnormality is seen.
- Hydranencephaly is the most severe degree of porencephaly or brain destruction where almost the whole of cerebral parenchyma is absent. Mostly due to early and total occlusion of supraclinoid carotids.
- *Schizencephaly:*
  - Characterized by slits lined by gray-matter in brain parenchyma communicating brain surface to ventricles.
- *Lissencephaly (agyria):*
  - Abnormal neuronal migration from germinal matrix to surface leads to absence of convolution formation or formation of broad Gyri (Pachygyria).
- *Corpus callosum agenesis:*
  - Callosal development occurs between 12 and 20 weeks. Any insult leads to total/partial lack of formation of this commissure.
  - Frontal horns are Steer-horn shaped with probst bundles lying medial to them.
  - Colpocephaly and Sun-ray appearance of Gyri radiating to ventricles is seen.

DIFFERENTIAL DIAGNOSIS OF BRAIN AND HEAD ABNORMALITY

- *Anencephaly D/D of amniotic band syndrome:*
  - Amputation of other parts.
  - Membranes in liquor.
  - Asymmetric cranial defects.
  - D/D of large encephaloceles.
- *Encephaloceles:*
  - D/D cystic hygroma.
  - D/D hemangioma.
  - D/D teratoma.
  - D/D scalp edema.
  - D/D branchial cleft cyst.

All the above do not have a cranial defect with protrusion of CSF, brain and meninges.

- *Holoprosencephaly:*
  - D/D severe hydrocephalus.
  - Rim of parenchyma and vessels present.
    - D/D of hydranencephaly-focal brain parenchyma may be seen in the parieto-occipital region. Brain stem and posterior fossa normal.
    Both of the above do not have associated facial defects.
- *Dandy-Walker malformation*
  - D/D variant (Dandy-Walker)
    - Less severe anomaly and hydrocephalus.
  - D/D arachnoid cyst
    - No communication to ventricles.
    - No associated anomaly.
- Hydranencephaly D/D of severe hydrocephalus.
  - D/D alobar holoprosencephaly
  - D/D massive congenital subdural collection.
  - D/D postanoxic/infective encephalopathy.

All the above have thinned or injured brain parenchyma seen to varying degrees.

DIFFERENTIAL DIAGNOSIS OF THICKENED ENDOMETRIUM (FLOWCHART 9.8)

Causes

- Early intrauterine pregnancy/abortions.
- Retained products of conception.
- Ectopic pregnancy.
- Estrogen excess, e.g. polycystic ovary syndrome.
- Endometrial carcinoma/hyperplasia.
- Endometrial polyp.
- Hormonal replacement.
  - Therapy in postmenopausal females.
- Tamoxifen treatment
- Endometritis.

Salient Features

- *Normal thickness*   Phase
  3–5 mm   Proliferative
  Up to 14 mm   Secretory
- *Early intrauterine pregnancy:* With thickened endometrium and increased peritrophoblastic flow look for intradecidual and double decidual sac signs.
- *Ectopic pregnancy:* Pseudogestation sac is an artefact due to minimal uterine collection

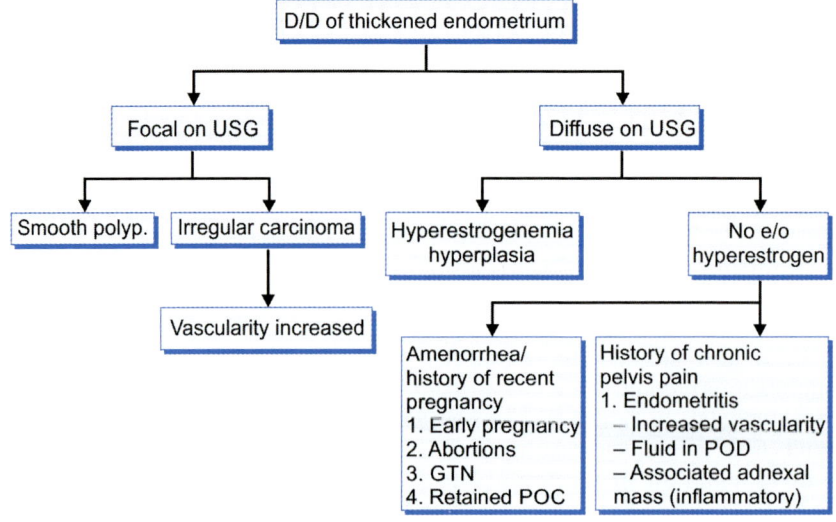

Flowchart 9.8: Thickened endometrium.

with thickened endometrium under hormonal influence seen in these cases.
- *Endometrial carcinoma:*
  - In old ladies
  - Less than 4 cm thickness is normal 4–8 is equivocal and needs histopathological correlation while more than 8 mm is suggestive of malignancy. Associated myometrial invasion is seen in advanced cases.
- Endometrial polyp is a focal thickening seen best by sonohysterography, very minimal if any risk of malignancy is associated.
- Endometrial hyperplasia is said to occur when gland to stroma ratio exceeds that in normal proliferative endometrium. It is divided in hyperplasia with and that without cellular atypia.
  Nearly one-fourth progress to carcinoma if atypia is present. Occurs due to persistent hyperestrogenemia as in estrogen therapy, PCOD, granulosa/theca cell tumors, obesity and persistent anovulatory cycles. Endometrium appears thickened with few cystic areas.

USG SIGNS IN ABORTIONS/MISCARRIAGE (TABLE 9.12)

Abortion

Fetal wastage before viability period.

Induced
- Legal.
- Illegal (Septic).

Spontaneous
- Missed
- Incomplete
- Septic
- Threatened
- Inevitable
- Complete.

Salient Features
- *Missed abortion:* Usually between 8 and 14 weeks.
  - Dead fetus retained inside uterus for more than four weeks.
  - No fetal heartbeat with
    CRL more than 5 mm (TVS)
    CRL more than 9 mm (TAS).
  - Gestational age discordant to menstrual age.
  - Sac more than 25 mm with no evidence of fetus.
  - Distorted sac configuration/shape.
  - Low down location.
  - Internal debris within the sac.
  - Discontinuous/irregular/thin (<2 mm) peritrophoblastic reaction and inadequate flow.
  - Subchorionic collections.

Table 9.12: USG differential diagnosis of abortions/miscarriage.

Points	Missed	Incomplete	Inevitable	Threatened	Septic
Shape of GS	Crumpled non-identifiable	Irregular non-identifiable	Irregular	Well-defined	±
Site of GS	US/LS	US/LS	LS	US	+
Collections around GS	Solid mass forms	±	+	±	+
Peritrophoblastic reaction and vascularity	Not present	Not present	Poor	Present	Not present
Status of fetus	Dead/non-identifiable	Dead/non-identifiable	Dead	Live	Not present
Cervix	Closed	Partially open	Open	Closed	Closed/Open
Abdominopelvic signs of infection	Not present	Not present	Not present	Not present	Present

- *Threatened abortion:*
  - First trimester bleed with a live fetus.
  - Clinical triad of bleeding, cramp, closed cervix.
  - 1/2 progress to spontaneous abortion, 1/2 develop normally.
- *Inevitable abortion:*
  - Gestational sac with fetus having become detached from implantation site and spontaneous abortion likely to occur in the next few hours.
  - Cervix is dilated.
  - Abnormal-shaped sac.
  - Low-lying sac.
  - Collection suggestive of blood seen around the sac.
  - Trophoblastic reaction unsatisfactory.
- *Incomplete abortion:*
  - Consists basically of retained products of conception in the uterus.
  - The product is usually heterogeneous unidentifiable material and/or collection.
  - Associated with bulky uterus and irregular endometrium.
  - May lead to endomyometritis, DIC, septic shock.
- *Septic abortion:*
  - Usually a consequence of illegal abortion.
  - It is very important to look for any foreign body in the uterus/abdomen.
  - Associated uterine perforation, signs of localized/diffuse abdominal sepsis and pelvic sepsis may be seen.

DIFFERENTIAL DIAGNOSIS OF FETAL CAUSES OF ABNORMALITY IN LIQUOR VOLUME

Causes

- *Oligohydramnios (Flowchart 9.9):*
  - Fetal demise/IUD
  - Renal/bladder abnormalities
  - PUV
  - Prune belly syndrome
  - ARPCKD
  - Absent renal artery or renal agenesis
  - IUGR
  - Postdated pregnancy.
- *Polyhydramnios (Flowchart 9.10):*
  - Cardiovascular decompensation
  - Diaphragmatic hernia
  - Anencephaly/other severe cranial anomalies especially ONTD
  - Obstructive malformations of GIT, e.g. TOF, duodenal
  - Stenosis/atresia
  - Bone dysplasias
  - Neuromuscular abnormalities
  - Chromosomal abnormality, e.g. trisomy 18.

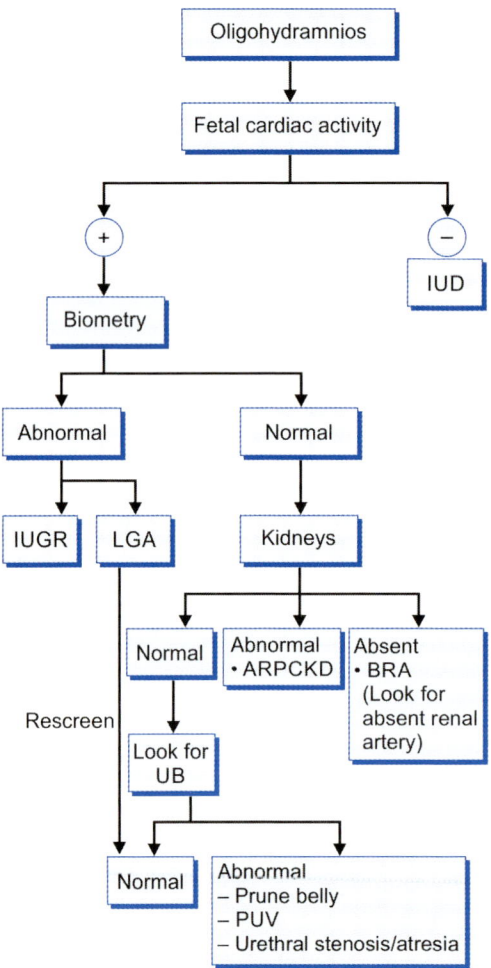

Flowchart 9.9: Approach to a pointing with oligohydramnios.

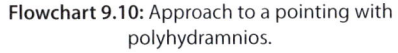

Flowchart 9.10: Approach to a pointing with polyhydramnios.

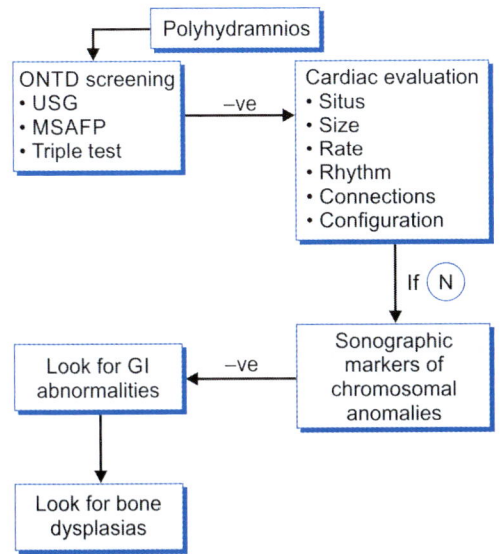

Salient Features

- *Amniotic fluid assessment*

	Single pocket	AFI
Oligohydramnios	<2 cm	<7
Reduced	2–3 cm	7–10
Normal	3–8 cm	10–17
More than average	>8–12 cm	17–25
Polyhydramnios	>12 cm	>25

- *Fetal demise:*
  - Fetal wastage, after the time significant liquor production is seen, leads to slow resorption of liquor.
  - Urine production status at 9 weeks and renal function starts at 11 weeks. At 12 weeks, urine accumulates at the rate of 5 cc per day.
- *Signs of IUD are:*
  - Spalding's sign
    - Overriding of skull bones.
  - Gas in vessels-Robert sign.
  - Fetal maceration.
  - Sometimes associated hydrops.
  - Extended limbs/lost tone.
  - Absent-cardiac activity.
  - Gas in abdomen.
  - Echogenic amniotic fluid.

- *IUGR:*
  - Weight of neonate below 10 percentile of the expected fetal weight for that age.
  - Usually detected after 32–34 weeks, i.e. the age of maximum fetal growth.
  - May be due to uteroplacental insufficiency that leads to asymmetric IUGR.
  - Symmetric IUGR is early onset and leads to concordant reduction of all parameters.
  - Criteria for IUGR:

	Sensitivity	Specificity
Advance placental grade	62%	64%
FL/AC (increased)	34–49%	78–83%
TIUV (decreased)	57–80%	72–76%
Small BPD	24–88%	62–94%
Slow increase in BPD	75%	84%
Low EFW	89%	88%
Decreased AFV	24%	98%
Increased HC/AC	82%	94%
Biophysical profile	<6 = Equivocal <4= Fetal compromise	

  - Doppler indices
  - Uterine artery—S/D >2.3, difference of the two sides >1, RI > 0.6
    - MCA-RI < 0.7
    - Umbilical artery-RI - >0.7
- *Postdated pregnancy/Large for dates:*
  - When weight is more than 90th percentile for the expected fetal weight.
  - Also when weight more than 4000 g.
  - Sonographic criteria.

LGA	Sensitivity	Specificity
AD/BPD (increase)	46%	79%
FL/AC (decrease)	24–75%	44–93%
AFV increase	12–17%	92–98%
Pondrel index increased	13–15%	85–98%
High EFW	20–74%	93–96%
Growth score increased	14%	91%

Macrosomia
- FL increased   24%   96%
- AC increased   53%   94%
- High EFW   11–65%   89–96%
- BPD increased   29%   98%
- *Renal/bladder abnormality*: Any cause of reduction of urine formation as in renal (B/L) agenesis, ARPCKD or of obstruction to outlet of urine as in prune-belly syndrome, urethral atresia/stenosis, posterior urethral valve can lead to oligohydramnios. Look for signs of Megacystitis, i.e. UB more than 8 mm, hydronephrosis, i.e. pelvis more than 6 mm, abnormal renal parenchyma, dilated ureter and urethra.
- Polyhydramnios occurs when either increased production or decreased fetal Gulping of liquor is seen.
- *Cardiovascular decompensation:*
  Bradycardia – <100 BPM of >10 sec
  Tachycardia – >180 BPM
  PSVT – 180–300 BPM with conduction rate 1:1
  Flutter – 300–400 BPM with conduction rate 2:1/4:1
  Fibrillation –>400 BPM
- *Diaphragmatic hernia:* Cystic areas in thorax with small abdomen. Absent fundic bubble, GB with portal vein pointing up.
- Double bubble and triple bubble sign of duodenal and jejunal atresia should be looked for.
- Skeletal dysplasia, chromosomal abnormalities detection has been described elsewhere.

DIFFERENTIAL DIAGNOSIS OF GAS IN THE GENITAL TRACT (FLOWCHART 9.11)

Causes
- Fistula between genital tract and gastrointestinal tract
  - Congenital
  - Postinflammatory, e.g. tuberculosis, Crohn's disease
  - Due to infiltrative malignancies.

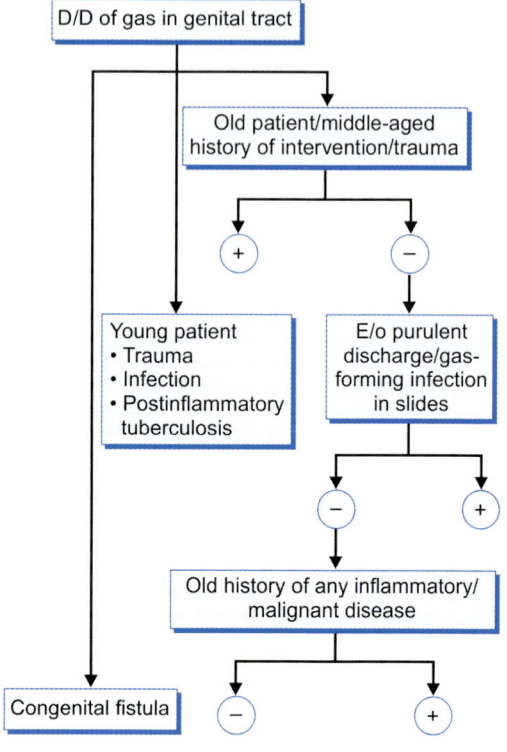

Flowchart 9.11: Gas in genital tract.

- Postintervention
  - Hysterosalpingography
  - Hysteroscopy
  - Pervaginal examination
  - Tubal insulation
  - Laparoscopy.
- Gas-forming infection.
- Post-traumatic.

Salient Features
Fistula between GUT and GIT occurs most commonly due to inflammatory conditions like Crohn's disease and tuberculosis. In such cases, it is usually the small bowel that communicates with uterus.
- Congenital fistulas occur between lower genital tract and terminal GIT leading to rectovaginal and rectouterine fistulas. These occur early during the course of development due to closely associated origin of both the above.

- Malignancies of uterus, cervix, vagina, rectum, rectosigmoid and anal canal lead to fistula formation between them. Feculent material is also seen passing from genital tract.
- Contrast studies from both tracts are good for depiction of site of communication.
- MRI is fast picking up in demonstration of fistula.
- Gas-forming anerobic and gram-negative infections are usually uncommon but occur in cases of immunocompromised, states as diabetes, AIDS, chemotherapy and systemic diseases.
- Trauma to genital tract may be due to vehicle accident, due to obstetric intervention or prolonged labors.

DIFFERENTIAL DIAGNOSIS OF FETAL INTRA-ABDOMINAL CALCIFICATION (FLOWCHART 9.12)

Causes

- *Peritoneal:*
  - Meconium peritonitis.
  - Plastic peritonitis with hydrometrocolpos.
- *Tumors:*
  - Hemangioma.
  - Hemangioendothelioma.
  - Hepatoblastoma.
  - Metastatic neuroblastoma.
  - Teratoma.
- *Infections:*
  - Toxoplasma.
  - Cytomegalovirus.

Salient Features

- *Meconium peritonitis:*
  - Occurs due to meconium exiting from the bowel lumen, due to perforation, causing sterile chemical peritonitis.
  - Perforation occurs due to volvulus, jejunal/ileal atresia, meconium ileus.
  - Immediately ascites occur following which linear streaky or spotty calcification occurs.
  - Pseudocyst formation may also occur.
  - Calcified meconium balls in/out the lumen may also be seen.
- Infections like toxoplasma and CMV lead to calcifications in liver, spleen and also intracranial calcification.
- Hemangiomas may occur at multiple sites in fetal body and may be associated with calcification.
- Hemangioendothelioma and hemangiomas
  - Common fetal hepatic tumors which show areas of specky linear calcification associated with vascular spaces showing high velocity Doppler shifts.
- Hepatoblastoma is the most common hepatic tumor (Primary) in young and

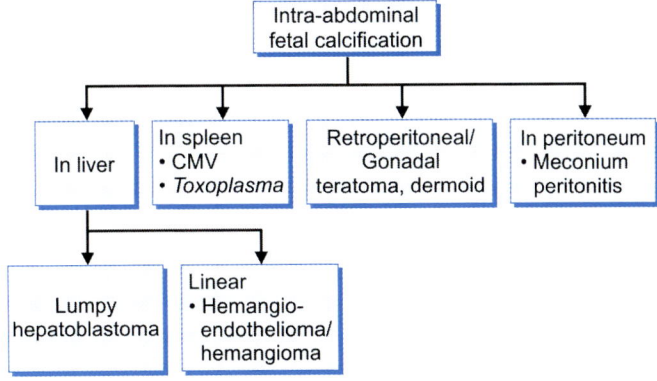

Flowchart 9.12: Intra-abdominal fetal calcification.

nearly all present before the age of five. Associated with hemihypertrophy, 11p13 chromosome and Beckwith-Wiedemann's syndrome. Serum AFP levels are almost always elevated. Shows lumpy calcification.
- Neuroblastoma is the most common neonatal tumor usually occurring in the adrenal gland. It is an echogenic mass, heterogeneous in appearance. It commonly metastasizes to placenta, liver and subcutaneous tissues with the metastasis appearing echogenic calcified. Hydrops may commonly occur.
- Teratomas and dermoids are common fetal tumors occurring in retroperitoneal and gonadal locations most commonly. These show solid and cystic areas with areas of calcification.

DIFFERENTIAL DIAGNOSIS OF FETAL THORACIC ABNORMALITIES (FLOWCHART 9.13)

Causes

- Pleural effusion.
- Congenital diaphragmatic hernias.
- Pulmonary hypoplasia.
- Pulmonary sequestration.
- Pulmonary cystic adenomatoid malformation/CPAM.
- Congenital bronchogenic cyst.
- Esophageal duplication cyst.
- Neuroenteric cysts.
- Bronchial/laryngeal atresia.
- Thymic enlargement.
- Cystic hygroma.
- Teratoma.
- Neuroblastoma.
- Anterior thoracic meningocele.

Salient Features

- *Pleural effusion:*
  - May be isolated or occur as a result of generalized fetal hydrops.
  - Fluid collects as a cresentic rim around lungs forming a 'Bat-Wing-appearance' of lungs floating in fluid.
  - U/L—congenital adenomatoid malformation (CAM), diaphragmatic hernia, sequestration, pulmonary hypoplasia.
  - B/L—infections, CHF, Turner's, Down's, pulmonary lymphangiectasia.
  - Long-lasting larger effusions may lead to pulmonary hypoplasia.
  - May be treated by thoracocentesis.
- *Diaphragmatic hernias:*
  - Bochdalek hernia
    * Posterolateral in location.
    * Left> >right.
    * Small intestine (88%), stomach (60%), colon (56%), liver (51%), spleen (45%).
    * Detected by sonography at 17 weeks.
    * Mediastinal deviation seen by change in position and axis of heart.
    * Hollow viscera may be seen with AC less than 5th percentile and polyhydramnios.
    * Absence of GB in abdomen.
    * Umbilical vein displaced up.
  - Morgagni hernia
    * Anteriorly behind the sternum.
    * Right>>> left.

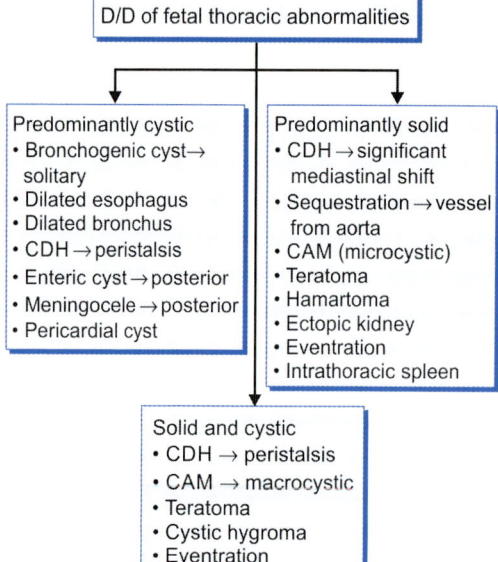

Flowchart 9.13: Fetal thoracic abnormalities.

- Omentum, colon, liver, stomach, small bowel.
- May be covered by peritoneum and pleura or only pleura or none at all. If pericardium is also absent, it lies in direct contact to heart.
  - Eventration of diaphragm
    - Due to absent muscle fibers in the diaphragm.
    - U/L asymptomatic.
    - B/L may cause pulmonary hypoplasia.
    - B/L associated with trisomy 13 and 18, CMV infection, Rubella infection and arthrogryposis multiplex congenital.
- *Pulmonary hypoplasia:*
  - U/L—rare, may be simulated by discordant rate of growth of both lungs. Due to thoracic masses.
  - B/L—commoner, due to restricted chest cage as in thanatophoric dwarfism, Jeune's asphyxiating dystrophy, achondrogenesis and all causes of early onset severe oligohydramnios.

  $$\frac{\text{Chest area} \times \text{heart area}}{\text{Chest area}} \times 100$$

  is accurate (85% sensitive and specific) in diagnosis, as correlated to age.
- *Cystic adenomatoid malformation (CAM):*
  - Are hamartomas in lung divided by Adzich in Macroscopic (cysts >5 mm) and Microscopic (<5 mm).
  - Macroscopic type has better prognosis and is less commonly associated with hydrops.
  - Size of the mass may decrease over time.
  - Has to be D/D from diaphragmatic hernia, bronchial cyst, cystic dilatation of esophagus, pericardial teratoma.
- *Pulmonary sequestration:*
  - Is a segment or part of lung not communicating at the usually bronchovascular tree.
  - Appear as solid echogenic masses inside (Intralobar sequestration) of the lung. Usually in basal parts.
  - Extralobar may occur inside the diaphragm, pericardium, hila, mediastinum.
  - In 50% malformations of sternum and diaphragm are seen but no major anomaly is seen.
  - D/D to diaphragmatic hernia, CAM and lobar emphysema.
  - A supplying vessel from aorta is the most confirmatory sign.
- Up to 27 weeks, the thymus enlarges and appears as echogenic mass (from 14 weeks); after 27 weeks, it becomes hypoechoic
- Cystic hygroma (lymphangiomas) is cystic (predominantly) and solid dumb-bell mass extending in the mediastinum.
- Teratomas usually arise from pericardium and are surrounded by pericardial fluid (diagnostic point). Appearance is the same as in adults.
- Neuroblastomas are echogenic masses with echolucent centers lying in the paravertebral area.
- Enteric cysts lined by GI mucosa are also seen in posterior mediastinum.

Index

Page numbers followed by *f* refer to figure, *fc* refer to flowchart, and *t* refer to table.

A

Abetalipoproteinemia 110
Abortions 383, 384, 384*t*, 401, 401*t*
  incomplete 402
  missed 401
  recent 393
  septic 402
  threatened 402
Abscess 6, 136, 143, 256, 273, 311, 326, 390
  epidural 326, 367
  formation 3
  intramedullary 363
  pancreatic 141
  paracolic 96*f*
  perirenal 253
  prevertebral 346
  prostatic 281
  renal 262
  retropharyngeal 3
  subphrenic 57, 145*f*
  tubo-ovarian 389
Acetabulum, medial wall of 185*f*
Achalasia 10, 99
  cardia 99*f*
  hyperactive 155
Achondrogenesis 175
Achondroplasia 173, 201, 212, 319, 320, 337
  homozygous 175
Acidosis, renal tubular 256
Acoustic masses, external 359
Acoustic neuroma 293
Acrania 399
Acro-osteolysis 204, 205*f*, 226, 296
Acro-osteosclerosis 205
Actinomycosis 125
Adamantinoma 219
Addison's disease 191

Adenocarcinoma 105*t*, 106, 139, 141, 359
  polypoidal intraluminal component 113
Adenoma 28, 135, 136, 260, 377, 381
  adrenal cortical 283
  autonomous 377
  parathyroid 15
  pituitary 305
  simple tubular 126
  tubulovillous 126
Adenomatoid malformation, cystic 35, 407
Adenomyomatosis 131
Adenopathy
  paratracheal 12*f*
  superior
    bilateral 19*f*
    mediastinal 19*f*
Adenosis, sclerosing 71, 75
Adnexal masses, sonographic classification of 391
Adrenal mass
  differential diagnosis of 282
  unilateral 142
Adrenoleukodystrophy 343
Adrenoleukomyeloneuropathy 343
Adrenomyeloneuropathy 343
Agenesis 49, 281
  prostatic 281
  pulmonary 44
Air bronchogram 42
Air trapping 51, 52
Airway 37
Alagille syndrome 134
Albright's syndrome 351
Alexander's disease 344
Alkaptonuria 93, 317

Allergic alveolitis, extrinsic 56
Allergy 375
Alpha fetoprotein 164
Alport's syndrome 235, 257
Alveolar cell carcinoma 27
Alveolitis 56
Ameloblastoma 373*f*
American Joint Committee on Cancer Staging 276
Amino acid metabolism 339
Amniotic band syndrome 387, 399
Ampulla of Vater 165
Amyloidosis 36, 110, 119, 123, 137, 235, 237, 243, 244
Ancylostoma duodenale 112
Anemia 397
  chronic 200
  hemolytic 295
Anencephaly 399
Aneurysm 12, 29, 307, 331, 335
  aortic 9, 319
  myocardial 88
Angiofibroma
  juvenile 300, 346, 347
  nasopharyngeal 314
Angiography 302, 362
  carotid 313
  contrast invasive 238
Angiolipoma, spinal 368
Angioma 180, 335
Angiomyolipoma 259
Angiotensin-converting enzyme inhibitor 254
Ankylosing spondylitis 93, 94*f*, 210, 228, 229*f*, 317, 321
Anorectal malformation 150*f*
Antibiotics 245
Anticonvulsants 245
Antihistaminics 245
Antral gastritis, stenosing 157

Aorta
  aneurysm of arch of 9*f*, 83, 83*f*
  arch of 12
  coarctation of 80
  enlargement 82
  long segment coarctation of 83
  small 83
Aortic arch, right 85, 86
Aortic dissection 387
  emergency situation 13
Apert's syndrome 203
Aplasia 49, 375
Apophyseal joint 229
Apoplexy, pituitary 306
Arachnodactyly 203
Arachnoid cyst 297
  suprasellar 305
Armillifer armillatus 94
Arterial disease, focal 235
Arterial infarction 241
Arterial obstruction 124
Arteriography 254
Arteriosclerosis, generalized 235, 238
Arteriovenography 286
Arteritis 255
Artery 236
  aneurysm, pulmonary 41, 82
  hypertension, pulmonary 82
  inferior pulmonary 79*f*
  pressure, sustained pulmonary 78
  pulmonary 29, 31
  tortuous innominate 10, 14
Arthritides 183, 194
Arthritis 184, 206, 207, 318
  biochemical 206
  degenerative 211*t*
  infective 207
  inflammatory 207, 211*t*
  involving spinal column 228
  juvenile chronic 194, 317
  mutilans 207
  neuropathic 185*f*, 210, 211*t*
  psoriatic 226, 228
  rheumatoid 23, 56, 68, 88, 183, 185*f*, 186*f*, 201, 224, 228, 229, 230*f*, 321
  septic 206
  tubercular 206*f*

Arthropathy 171, 201, 208, 224
  neuropathic 206
  psoriatic 207, 229
Asbestosis 47, 56
Ascending aorta, aneurysm of 15
Ascites 130, 146
Askin tumor 22
Aspergillosis 34
Aspiration 34
Asthma 27, 28
Astrocytoma 304, 327, 362
Atheromas 93, 335
Atherosclerosis 124, 255
Atlantoaxial subluxation 318
Atresia 84
  urethral 268
Atrial septal defect 83, 85
Atrophic kidney, causes of 247
Atrophy
  localized 173
  postinflammatory 235, 237
  postobstructive 235, 236, 250
  reflux 235
Auditory canal cholesteatoma, external 359
Axillary lymphatic obstruction 72
Azygos vein, dilated 20

B

Bacterial overgrowth syndromes 123
Bamboo spine 229*f*
  appearance 210
Banana sign 399
Bare orbit 329, 330*f*
  sign 312
Barium 120, 121, 122
  enema 120*f*, 150*f*, 170
  esophagogram 102*f*
  examination 169, 286
  meal 157
Barotrauma 375
Barrett's esophagitis 98, 100, 153
Basal cell nevus syndrome 203
Basal ganglia calcification 293, 336
Basal pulmonary collapse, bilateral 26
Basilar artery, elongation of 302
Basketwork appearance 192

Battered child syndrome 194
Beckwith-Wiedemann syndrome 384
Behçet's disease 130
Bergman's sign 251
Berylliosis 47
Bicuspid aortic valve 387
Bile ducts
  anatomy of 161
  normal size of 164
  variants 164
Bile-plug syndrome 134
Biliary atresia 134
Biliary tract abnormalities 134
Biliary tree
  dilatation 136
  gas in 131, 143
Bilirubin 163
Binswanger's disease 342
Bird beak appearance 99
Biventricular enlargement 85*f*
Bladder 181
  calculi 269
  carcinoma of 266
  exstrophy 387
  neck stricture, acquired 269
  neuropathic lesions of 270
  outflow obstruction 267
  sphincter dyssynergia 270
  tumors 269
  wall, gas in 252
Blighted ovum 383, 383*t*
Blood
  clot 250, 274
  flow
    pulmonary 50, 51, 89
    volume of 87
  tests 120
Bochdalek's hernia 10, 20, 27, 50
Boerhaave's syndrome 57
Bone 196, 286, 292
  appearance 196
  cancellous 196
  coarse trabecular pattern of 180
  compact 196
  cyst 230
    aneurysmal 182, 182*f*, 189, 221, 221*f*, 234, 234*f*, 371, 372

nonepithelialized 371
simple 182*f*, 184, 218*f*, 232, 371
solitary 219
disease, diffusely infiltrating 192
dysplasias 196
expansion 176
hemangioma of 190*f*
infarcts 217
islands 177, 216
lesion
  benign 182, 184*t*
  common lytic 188
  expansile 218
  malignant 179, 182, 184*t*
  sclerotic 176
  septated 189, 189*t*
  subarticular lytic 183
loss, patterns of 192
malignancies, primary 370
metabolism 191*f*
normal 191*f*
resorption 22
sarcoma, primary 178
scan 221
scintigraphy 279
sclerosis 179
  subchondral 227
sclerotic lesions of 214
spongiosa 191*f*
tumor
  benign 231*f*
  primary 182, 385
tumor 357
Bony ankylosis 199*f*
Bony deformity 230*f*
Bony labyrinth 355*f*
Bowel
  disease, inflammatory 124, 166
  lesions, extrinsic 114
  necrosis 128
  rotation, abnormalities of 150
Brachydactyly 203
Bracket sign 335
Brailsford-Morquio's syndrome 214
Brain and head abnormality, differential diagnosis of 399
Brainstem 327

Breast 181
  abscess 71, 72
  calcification types 72
  carcinoma 38*f*, 72, 75*f*
    spiculated 70*f*
  cysts, simple 68*f*
  edema 72*f*
  edematous 72
  high-resolution sonogram of 69*f*, 70*f*
  mammographic differential diagnosis 66
  masses, spiculated 70
Brodie's abscess 180, 182, 184, 218, 233
Bronchiectasis 28
  cystic 34
Bronchiolitis 29
  obliterans 52
Bronchitis, chronic 28
Bronchus 27
Budd-Chiari syndrome 137
Bull's eye lesions 112*f*
Bulla 52
Bullous costochondral ends 202
Burkitt's lymphoma 370, 372-374
Burns 92
Burr hole 287
Bursitis 161
  iliopsoas 160

C

Caffey's disease 179, 215
Calcification 29, 68, 236, 245
  adrenal 142
  benign 72
  dystrophic 73, 255
  focal 69*f*
  hepatic 132
  intra-abdominal 150
  intraorbital 353
  myocardial 88
  pancreatic 138
  parasitic 94
  parenchymal 256
  pleural 59, 62, 62*fc*
  renal 255
  sheet-like 97, 97*t*
  splenic 138
  types of 73, 74*f*
Calcification, arterial 93*f*

Calcinosis
  generalized 97
  universalis, idiopathic 97
Calcium 190*f*
  pyrophosphate arthropathy 183
Calculi 255
  prostatic 281, 282
Calculus 250, 274
Callus formation, excessive 196
Calyceal diverticulum 261*f*
Calyces 239
  dilated 249, 250
Campomelic dwarfism 175
Canada-Cronkhite syndrome 119, 127
Canavan's disease 344
Candida esophagitis 102
Captopril scintigraphy 238
Carcinoma 10, 27, 33, 70, 76, 104, 105, 106*t*, 111, 113, 115, 124, 125, 127, 156, 346, 348, 375, 376
  adenocystic 359
  adrenal 181
    cortical 283
  advanced 101
  anaplastic 4, 379
  breast 76*f*
  bronchial 39
  bronchoalveolar 40
  bronchogenic 38*f*, 39*f*, 60, 88, 181
  bronchus 29
    exclude 49
  cystic papillary 378
  early esophageal 102
  embryonal 271
  endometrial 401
  esophageal 100, 102*f*
  esophagus 100
  follicular 4, 379
  invasive 70
  medullary 4, 70
  metastatic 115, 117
  mucinous 70
  papillary 4, 70, 379
  primary 65
  prostate 215, 268, 274, 282
  secondary 65
  typical 70*f*

Cardiac failure, congestive 80*f*
Cardiomyopathy, hypertrophic obstructive 83
Cardiophrenic angle mass 63, 63*fc*
Cardiovascular disorders, differential diagnosis of 77
Carney's triad 39
Caroli's disease 134
Carotid artery
  aberrant internal 357
  tortuous 345
Carotid cavernous fistula 354
Carpal fusion 203
Carpenter syndrome 203
Carpets small bowel 126
Cataract 354
Cavernous sinus 298
  lesions 303
Celiac disease 100, 120, 121, 124
Cellulitis
  necrotizing 345
  retropharyngeal 345
Cementoma-cemento-ossifying dysplasia 370
Cephaloceles 332, 332*t*
  atretic 333
  occipital 332
  parietal 332
  sphenopharyngeal 333
Cephalohematoma 292, 293*f*
Cerebellar
  astrocytoma 309
  dysplasias 333
  hemispheres 328
  malformations 338
  vermis 328
Cerebellopontine angle
  anatomy 301*f*
  masses 301
Cerebellum 327
Cerebral
  atrophy 343
  berry aneurysms 387
Cerebrohepatorenal syndrome 198, 343
Cerebrospinal fluid 287, 327
Ceruminomas 360
Cervical
  abscess 3, 6
  nodal calcifications, right 32*f*
  region 344

  rib 2, 6, 7, 21
  spine 2*f*, 229*f*
Cervix 181
Chamberlain's line 294
Chemodectomas 358
Chemotherapy 339
Chest 1, 285
  and upper extremity 296
  radiograph 29
  wall 31
    abnormalities 21, 21*t*
    defects 51
    tumors 22, 23*t*
  X-ray 100
Chiari malformations 338
Chilaiditi's syndrome 144
Choanal atresia 152
Cholangitis, sclerosing 171
Cholecystitis 107
Cholesteatoma 316*f*, 357, 358
  congenital 293
  primary congenital 361
Cholesterol granuloma 293, 357, 358
Cholesterolosis strawberry gallbladder 131
Chondroblastoma 181*f*, 184, 219, 234
Chondrocalcinosis 208
Chondrodysplasia punctata 173, 175, 198, 213
Chondroectodermal dysplasia 173, 175
Chondroid lesions 187
Chondromas 349
Chondrometaplasia 349
Chondromyxoid fibroma 180, 182*f*, 189, 221, 234
Chondrosarcoma 179, 184*f*, 348
Choppy sea appearance 292
Chordoma 300, 308, 335, 346, 347, 359
Choriocarcinoma 271
Choroid plexus papilloma 310, 335
Chromosomal
  aberration 211
  abnormality, ultrasound signs of 394
  disorders 172

Chylothorax 57
Cirrhosis 124, 246
Clavicle 201, 226
  medial end of 201
Clear cell sarcoma 180
Clinodactyly 203
Clivus canal line 294
Cloaca, extroversion of 150
Cloacal exstrophy 387
Clostridium welchii 96
Clover leaf skull 399
Coal miner's pneumoconiosis 46
Coal workers 47
Cobblestone
  appearance 113*f*
  duodenal cap 113, 113*f*
Coccidioidomycosis 182
Codman's triangle 183*f*, 193
Cold nodules 5, 378
Colitis, ischemic 130
Collagen disease 32, 36, 206
Collagen disorders 55
Colloid osmotic pressure 57
Colon 181
  villous adenoma of 124
Comet-tail defect 131
Complex cyst 392
Compression
  atelectasis 25*f*, 61*f*
  extrinsic 114
Computed tomography 3, 5, 64, 100, 102, 168, 170, 221, 242, 247, 248, 250, 251, 253, 254, 256, 259-262, 280, 282, 346
  angiography 238, 254
  contrast-enhanced 116, 310
  criteria 264
  nodule enhancement 39
  scan 277, 286
  urography 286
Congestion
  intramural 108
  pulmonary venous 87
Connective tissue 37
  disorder 57, 202
Contusion 327
Cooley's anemia 289
Copper accumulation 133
Cord
  edema 327
  enlargement, diffuse 326*f*

lesion, suprasacral 270
tumors, stromal 391
Corpus callosum agenesis 399
Corrosive 99, 155
 gastritis 105
Cortex 238
Cortical defect, fibrous 184*f*, 231, 231*f*
Cranial fossa, midline 297
Craniopharyngioma 304, 306, 334
Cranioschiasis 399
Creeping fat appearances 117
Crescent sign 32
Cretinism 212, 320, 337
Crohn's disease 108, 109, 113, 115, 117, 119, 120, 124, 127, 130, 157-159, 168, 169, 228, 230
Crystal deposition disease 208
Cupola sign 145
Curvilinear collapse 144
Cushing's syndrome 190, 223, 373
Cystadenocarcinoma 141, 389
Cystadenoma 141, 389
 carcinoma 141
 mucinous 139
 serous 139
Cystic abdominal masses, differential diagnosis of 388
Cystic adnexal masses, differential diagnosis of 386
Cystic disease
 inherited 257
 localized 261
Cystic duct, duplication of 164
Cystic eye, congenital 312
Cystic kidney disease, acquired 262, 265
Cystic lesions, multiple 231
Cysticercosis 95*f*, 336, 366
Cysticercus cellulosae 94
Cystitis 252
 emphysematous 252
Cystogram 267, 269
Cystosarcoma phylloides 69
Cysts 35, 54, 136, 256, 263, 264, 327, 368, 375, 386, 387
 adnexal 148
 adrenal 284
 apical 371, 372
 arachnoid 298, 307, 328, 337, 357, 365

 atypical 264
 benign 131
 bronchogenic 10, 17, 35, 41
 calyceal 264, 265
 choledochal 134
 cortical 263
 dentigerous 371, 371*f*, 372, 376
 enteric duplication 385
 enterogenous 297, 312, 328
 esophageal duplication 17, 20
 extradural arachnoid 326
 follicular 372
 functional 389
 hemorrhagic 389
 intratesticular 272
 intratumoral 362
 leptomeningeal 287, 337
 medullary 263, 265
 neurenteric 11, 18, 19, 328, 385
 paratubal 388
 pericardial 64
 perinephric 265
 posterior fossa 327
 prostatic 281
 radicular 371, 371*f*, 372
 renal 386, 388, 388*t*
 retention 281
 ruptured 40
 simple 68, 182, 261, 263, 378, 391
 thymic 1, 3, 6
 traumatic 372
 types of 371*f*
 unruptured 40
 wall
  calcification 262
  calcified 138
Cytomegalovirus 109, 335, 340
 congenital 200
 esophagitis 153

D

Dandy-Walker
 complex 339
 malformation 297, 327, 333, 399, 400
 syndrome 297
 variant 328, 339
Danger space 344
Decubitus 26

Demyelination 339
Dental origin, cysts of 371
Dermatomyositis 97
Dermoid 142, 297, 307, 327, 333, 334, 389
 cysts 350, 365
 extra-abdominal 71
 tumor 304
Dextrocardia 89*f*
Diabetes mellitus 246, 273
Dialysis, chronic 107
Diaphragm 25, 31
 elevation of 25
 right dome of 89*f*
 splinting of 26
Diaphragmatic hump 15, 64
 right sided 27
Diaphyseal dysplasia, progressive 316
Diaphysis 189
 proximal tibial 234*f*
Diarthrodial joint 185*f*-187*f*
 osteoarthritis of 186*f*
Diastematomyelia 333
Diastrophic dwarfism 174, 175, 213
Dibroadenoma 69*f*
Digestion, inadequate 121
Digits, abnormal 203
Discordant nodules 377
Disk
 bulge 367
 disease 367
 herniation 367
 protrusion 367
 space 229
Distal phalanges, resorption of 205
Distal ulna, diaphysis of 179*f*
Diverticula, esophageal 152
Diverticulosis, colonic 387
Diverticulum 265
 hypopharyngeal 152
 pharyngoesophageal 152
Dolichoectasia, intracranial 387
Dorsal induction, abnormalities of 398
Down's syndrome 198, 201, 203, 319-321
Dumb-bell tumor 318
Duodenal mucosal fold 107*f*

Duodenal papilla
  major 166
  minor 166
Duodenitis 107, 107f, 121
  erosive 113
Duodenum
  dilated 113
  obstruction of 113
Dwarfism, acromesomelic 213
Dyschondrosteosis 173, 203, 213
Dyshormonogenesis 377
Dysmyelination 339, 342
Dysostosis
  cleidocranial 22, 226
  craniomandibular 227
  multiplex 211, 213
  peripheral 174
Dysphagia, neonatal 152
Dysplasia 127, 212
  acromesomelic 173
  cleidocranial 296
  craniometaphyseal 201
  cystic 272
  fibrous 176, 177, 182, 184, 215, 218, 233, 233f, 288-292, 315, 331, 351, 370, 375, 376
  mesomelic 173
  metaphyseal 201
  multiple epiphyseal 198
  renal 241, 263
  spondyloepiphyseal 174, 198
  urethral 268
Dystrophia myotonica 289
Dystrophy, reflex sympathetic 192

E

Ebstein's anomaly 51
Eccentric expansile 185
Echinococcus 182
  granulosus 40
Echogenicity 236, 237, 239, 241, 242, 246, 262
Ectasia, antral vascular 104
Ectopia, renal 147
Ectopic pregnancy,
  pseudogestation of 383, 383t
Edema 112, 118
  angioneurotic 110
  intestinal 108

  peripheral 91
  pulmonary 42, 43t, 80f, 87
  retropharyngeal 345
  unilateral pulmonary 42
Eggshell calcification 72
Eggshell curvilinear 75
Ehlers-Danlos syndrome 205
Eisenmenger physiology 52
Ejaculatory cyst 281
Ellis-Van creveld syndrome 203, 213
Embolism, pulmonary 52
Embryo, absence of 383
Emphysema 29, 53, 145
  bilateral pulmonary 29f
  compensatory 53
  congenital 51f
Empty gestational sac, causes of 383
Empty sella 306
Empyema 57
  chronic 59
  epidural 311
  subdural 311
Encephalitis, acute 339
Encephalocele 399
Encephalomyelitis, acute
  disseminated 340
Encephalopathy, subcortical
  arteriosclerotic 342
Enchondroma 180, 182f, 184, 219, 232, 232f, 301
Endobronchial metastases 28
Endocrinal disorders 172
Endocrine 222
  disease 211
  disorders 212
Endometrioma 389
Endometriosis 115, 118
Endometrium, thickened 400, 400fc
Endophytic extension 354
Enostosis 177
Enteritis
  eosinophilic 117, 119
  infectious 109
Enthesiopathy 208
Enthesitis 229
Epanutin eptoin therapy 91
Ependymoma 310, 326, 335, 361
Epicardial fat pad 15, 65

Epidermoid 289, 297, 298, 307, 334, 362
  cyst 232, 273, 365
  tumor 302, 304
Epidermoidomas 361
Epiphysis
  irregular 174, 197
  stippled 197
Epithelial neoplasm, papillary 140
Erlenmeyer flask deformity 200
Erosion 201, 227, 229
Erysipelas 72f
Erythrocyte sedimentation rate 115
Escherichia coli 247, 252
Esophageal carcinoma,
  differential diagnosis of 102
Esophageal stricture
  distal 227
  irregular 155
Esophagitis 103, 153, 154
  drug-induced 154
  herpetic 153
  reflux 153
  signs of 153
  tuberculous 154
Esophagus
  abnormal appearance of 98
  dilated 20, 98
  normal appearance of 98
Esophagus, perforation of 27
Esthesioneuroblastoma 299
Ethmoid carcinoma 346
Ewing's sarcoma 22, 179, 179f, 180
Ewing's tumor 181f
Exomphalos 150
Exostosis 189f, 360

F

Facial neuroma 359
Falx cerebri 334f
Fascial spaces 344
Fat 38, 94
  density 6, 63
  deposition 13, 14
  necrosis 71, 75
    idiopathic 72
Fatigue fractures 196
Fatty infiltration, focal 135, 136

Faulty radiologic technique 50, 51, 53
Fecal fat 120
Felson's method 8*f*
Femoral heads, migration of 185*f*
Femoral intercondylar notch, enlarged 208
Femur, osteoid osteoma of 217*f*
Fetal
  abdomen 396, 397*fc*
  alcohol syndrome 198
  bones, extension of 385*f*
  brain, differential diagnosis of 398
  calcification, intra-abdominal 405*fc*
  demise 403
  hydrops
    cast of 398*fc*
    differential diagnosis of 397
  intra-abdominal calcification, differential diagnosis of 405
  mass, presacral 385*t*
  neck masses 386, 386*t*
  node 384
  renal cystic diseases 387*t*
    differential diagnosis of 386
  thoracic abnormalities 406*fc*
    differential diagnosis of 406
  warfarin syndrome 198
Fever, rheumatic 88
Fibroadenolipoma 66
Fibroadenoma 68, 75
  lobulated 68*f*
Fibrogenesis imperfecta ossium 180
Fibroma
  nonossifying 179*f*, 182, 184*f*, 188*f*, 189, 221, 231
  ossifying 289, 290, 370
Fibromatosis 71
  aggressive 4
Fibromuscular dysplasia 255
Fibrosis 44
  cystic 107, 108, 121, 138, 362, 368
Fibrous dysplasia, types of 351
Fishgold's bimastoid line 294
Fissural cysts 371, 372

Fissures
  accessory 163
  bulging 55
  hepatic 162
  transverse 163
Fistula 252
  arteriovenous 354
Flank lines, bulging of 146
Floating tooth
  appearance 373*f*
  differential diagnosis of 369
Fluid accumulation, abnormal 243
Fluoroscopy 116
Fluorosis 93, 94f, 194, 216, 292, 317
Follicle-stimulating hormone 223
Foot, dorsiplantar projection of 185*f*
Football sign 145
Forestier's disease 230
Fracture 197, 375
  depressed 292*f*
  multiple 196
  pathological 217*f*, 218*f*
Frontal sinus, mucocele of 289
Functional segmental liver anatomy 161, 162
Fungal
  ball 269, 274
  disease 12
  sinusitis 300
Fungi 57

G

Galactocele 66, 67
Gallbladder
  agenesis of 164
  anomalies, congenital 164
  ectopia 165
  fissure for 163
  hypoplastic 165
  nonvisualization of 131
  septations of 165
  wall, thickened 136
Ganglion
  cell tumors 20
  intraosseous 233
Ganglioneuroma 142, 283, 326
Gangrene 128

Gardner's syndrome 119, 126
Garré sclerosing osteomyelitis 178
Gas 96
  gangrene 96*f*
  in genital tract, differential diagnosis of 404
Gastric
  abnormality 119
  adenocarcinoma 106*t*, 113
  carcinoma 157, 181
  diverticulum 282
  emphysema, interstitial 113
  folds, thickened 104, 104*fc*, 110
  lymphoma 106*t*, 113*f*
  masses 156
  mucosa, heterotopic 113
  outlet obstruction, mechanical 112
  rugae 113*f*
    hypertrophic 124
  ulcer disease, chronic 157
  volvulus 112
  wall, gas in 113
Gastritis 104
  alcoholic 104
  antral 105
  emphysematous 113
  giant-hypertrophic 105
  hypertrophic 104
  lymphocytic 111
Gastrocolic fistula 124, 159
Gastroenteritis, eosinophilic 110, 115, 119, 122, 157, 158
Gastroenteropathy, allergic 124
Gastrointestinal
  abnormalities 397
  obstruction, congenital 132
  tract system 98
Gastroschisis 150, 387
Gaucher's disease 180
Genetic disorders 397
Genital tract 404*fc*
Germ cell tumors 271, 390, 391
Germinoma 308
Gestational trophoblastic
  disease 384
  neoplasia 393
Giant cell
  reparative granuloma of Jaffe 372

tumor 180, 188f, 189, 220, 220f, 372
Giardiasis 119, 123
Gigantism 322
Gliomas 333, 334
  visual pathway 308
Glomerulocytomas 358
Glomerulonephritis, chronic 235, 238, 257
Glomus
  jugulare 357
  tumor 358
  tympanicum 357
Goiter 386
  intrathoracic 6
  retrosternal 11, 8t, 14
  toxic multinodular 376
Gonadal stroma, tumors of 271
Gonadoblastoma 390
Gout 183, 207, 317
Granular cell myoblastoma 71
Granulation tissue 357, 358
Granulomas 36, 138, 284
  eosinophilic 219, 232, 288, 323, 330, 375
  non-fungal 300
Granulomatous disease 142, 158
Grave's disease 376
Great toe, interphalangeal joint of 185f
Great vessels, transposition of 85
Ground-glass haziness 146
Growth 38
  plate
    abutting 234f
    premature closure of 173
  rate of 40
Guinea worm 94

H

Hair-on-end appearance 295f
Hajdu-Cheney syndrome 226
Hamartomas 28, 66, 156
  multiple 119
    biliary 387
  pulmonary 39
  retrorectal 385
Hand muscle, atrophy of 5
Hashimoto's thyroiditis 377
Haustral loss 167

Heart disease 124
  acyanotic 89
  congenital 78, 194
  cyanotic 89, 296
  ischemic 80
  rheumatic 82f, 85f, 87f
Heart malformations 90
Heel pad
  sign 91
  thickness 91, 91fc, 92f
Helicobacter pylori 105
Hemangioblastoma 327, 362
Hemangioma 1, 2, 7, 15, 180, 189, 225, 287, 296, 317, 322, 323, 325, 345, 354, 368
  capillary 135, 313, 350, 354
  cavernous 351, 354
  neoplastic 289
  subglottic 349
Hematemesis 151
Hematoma 33, 35, 69, 138, 326, 327, 367, 381, 390
  cervicothoracic 5
  chronic subdural 293, 335
  epidural 367
  intracerebral 335
  intramural 114
  perinephric 253
  pulmonary 41
  subperiosteal 191f
Hematomyelia 363
Hematopoietic disorders 199
Hematuria 285
  painless 284
Hemiplegia 26
Hemithoracic volume 48
Hemithorax, opaque 48
Hemochromatosis 139
Hemolytic-uremic syndrome 257
Hemopericardium 77
Hemophilia 110, 183
Hemorrhage 108, 160, 161, 381
  acute 59
  adrenal 284
  intraparenchymal 139
Hemosiderosis 46
Hemothorax 57, 60
Henoch-Schönlein purpura 108
Heparin toxicity 224
Hepatic lesions, hyperechoic 135

Hepatic vein 162
  middle 162
  right 162
Hepatitis, acute 135
Hepatobiliary system 98
Hepatoma 133
Hernia 96
  congenital 65
  diaphragmatic 48, 50, 64, 404, 406
  hiatus 10, 21, 21f, 151f
  paraduodenal 150
Herpes simplex encephalitis 341
Hilar enlargement 29
  bilateral 29, 30t
  unilateral 29, 30t
Hip
  anteroposterior projection of 185f
  avascular necrosis of 199
  joints 185f
  transient osteoporosis of 192
Hirschsprung's disease 150, 150f
Histiocytoma 233
  malignant fibrous 22
Histiocytosis 46, 359, 361
Histoplasma capsulatum 40, 46
Histoplasmoma 40
Histoplasmosis 46
Hodgkin's disease 4, 17, 33
Hodgkin's lymphoma 28, 100, 157, 159
Homocystinuria 198
Honeycomb lung 54, 54t
Honeycomb pattern 55
Horner's syndrome 5
Hot thyroid nodule 377
Human immunodeficiency virus encephalopathy 341
Hunter's syndrome 214
Hurler's syndrome 320, 213, 320, 336, 337
Hürthle cell tumors 381
Hyaline membrane disease 44f
Hydatid 255, 322
  cyst 34, 40, 64, 130, 355
Hydrocalycosis 249
  congenital 250
Hydrocalyx 264
Hydrocephalus 318, 337

Hydrometrocolpos 148
  ruptured 135
Hydronephrosis 147, 386, 388, 388*t*
  grades of 239*f*
Hydropic placental degeneration 384, 384*t*
Hydropneumothorax 31, 61*f*
Hydrops, nonimmune 397
Hydrostatic pressure 57
Hygroma, cystic 14, 16, 18, 386, 386*f*
Hyperalimentation 246
Hypercalcemia 97
  causes of 256
  idiopathic 216
Hypercortisolism 373
Hypergonadism 212
Hyperlucent lung 54
Hyperostosis
  endosteal 316
  frontalis interna 289, 290, 332
  generalized 289
  infantile cortical 179
  orbital 331
Hyperoxaluria, primary 257
Hyperparathyroidism 24, 93, 95, 138, 182, 192, 215, 222, 224, 256, 287, 336, 370, 373
  brown tumor of 220
  secondary 223, 224
Hyperplasia
  adenoid 346, 347
  adenomatous 377, 381
  benign prostatic 267, 282
  thymic 11
Hypertension 387
  pulmonary 85
    arterial 29, 78, 79, 79*f*, 79*fc*
    venous 87, 87*f*
  renovascular 254
  systemic 80, 83
Hyperthyroidism 223
Hypertranslucency, causes of bilateral 53
Hypertrophy
  adenoid 346*f*
  compensatory 242
  diffuse 268
Hypervitaminosis 216
  A 216
  D 216, 257

Hypoalbuminemia 109
Hypochondroplasia 173, 212
Hypogonadism 190, 223
Hypoparathyroidism 198
Hypophosphatasia 175, 200, 201, 212, 296
Hypopituitarism 212, 223
Hypoplasia 49, 281
  congenital 235, 236
  infantile 83
  pulmonary 53, 246, 407
  tubular 83
Hypopseudohypoparathyroidism 215
Hypotension, arterial 235, 238
Hypothalamoneurohypophyseal axis germinoma 304
Hypothyroidism 198, 223, 296, 337, 380
  congenital 381, 386

I

I-cell disease 176
Idiopathic thrombocytopenic purpura 110
Infarction 363
  chronic 235
  end result of 238
  lobar 239
Infections 36, 37, 59, 68, 91, 323, 324, 333, 335, 346, 347, 375
  chronic 273
  congenital 135
  granulomatous 159
  low-grade 225, 317
  prostatic 281
Inflammatory bowel disease, extraintestinal complications of 170
Inflammatory disease 106, 361
Inhalation
  disease 17
  disorder 59
Inner ear masses 355
Interphalangeal joints, ankylosis of 208
Interstitial pneumonitis 56
Interstitial pulmonary disease, bilateral 45*f*
Intestinal bile salt concentration 121

Intestinal obstruction 144*f*, 149
  signs of 150*f*
Intestinal stricture, small 115, 116*fc*
Intrabowel disease 228
Intracranial calcification
  normal 334
  pathological 333
Intradural mass, extramedullary 325*f*
Intrarenal arteries, spectral analysis of 248
Intrauterine
  fetal death 384, 384*t*
  pregnancy
    absent 392, 393*fc*
    early 400
Intrinsic bowel wall lesion 114
Iodine accumulation 133
Iron metabolism 166
Ischemia 118, 121, 125, 235
Ischiopubic rami 191*f*
Islet cell tumor 139, 141
Ivory vertebral body 317

J

Japanese Society of Esophageal Disease 101
Jaundice, neonatal obstructive 134
Jaw
  cystic lesions of 372
  cysts of 371
Jejunal diverticulosis 123
Jejunal obstruction 114, 149
Jeune's disease 174
Joints 172
  distal interphalangeal 374
  metacarpophalangeal 374
  metatarsophalangeal 374
  movements, painful 174
  normal diarthrodial 186*f*
  posterior part of 207*f*
  proximal interphalangeal 23, 374
  vertebrae 230
Joubert's syndrome 338
J-shaped sella 336, 336*f*
Jugular bulb, dehiscent 357, 358
Jugular veins, asymmetric dilatation of 1

K

Kaposi's sarcoma 156
Kearns-Sayre syndrome 339
Keratocyst, odontogenic 371
Keratosis obturans 359
Ketoacidosis, diabetic 27
Kidney 180
  absent 246
  adult 235, 235*t*
  bilateral 237
    large smooth 243
    malrotated 253*f*
  congenital absence of 253
  cystic disease of 262
  ectopic 253
  gas in 252
  large 241
  medullary sponge 256, 265
  multicystic 248
    dysplastic 147, 265, 387
  neonatal 235, 235*t*
  nonvisualization of 246
  normal sectional anatomy of 235*f*
  renal outlined calyces system of 249*f*
  small 235, 235*t*, 237, 239, 254
  smooth 235, 235*t*, 237, 239, 241, 254
  unilateral 235
Kinky hair syndrome 194, 296
Klebsiella pneumoniae 40, 50, 55
Klippel-Feil syndrome 321, 333
Knee joint 96*f*, 184*f*, 188*f*, 207*f*, 208*f*, 228*f*
Kniest syndrome 174, 175
Koch's chest 12*f*, 32, 32*f*, 35*f*, 48, 48*f*
Krabbe's disease 339, 343
Krukenberg tumor 391
Kwashiorkor 138

L

Labyrinthine ossification 316
Lacrimal gland
  adenocystic carcinoma of 355
  malignancy 331
  tumors 353
Lactic dehydrogenase 164
Lactose intolerance 123
Lamina dura of teeth, loss of 372
Langerhans' cell histiocytosis 56, 288, 289, 323, 325, 331, 370, 373
Langerhans' sun ray histiocytosis 374
Laryngoceles 349
Lead 216
Leather bottle stomach 157
Leigh's disease 339, 343
Leigh's syndrome 344
Leiomyoma 10, 99, 103
Leiomyomatosis 63
Leiomyosarcoma 156
Lemon skull 399
Leontiasis ossea 289, 290
Leprosy 93
Léri's disease 180
Léri-Weill disease 213
Léri-Weill syndrome 203
Leukemia 9, 28, 180, 245, 272, 375
Leukocytes 195*f*
Leukodystrophy 342, 344
  globoid cell 343
  metachromatic 339, 342
Lhermitte-Duclos disease 338
Ligamentum teres, fissure for 162
Ligamentum venosum, fissure for 163
Limb
  abnormalities, spinal abnormality besides 174
  body wall complex 387
Linitis plastica 157, 158
Lipoblastoma 4, 6
Lipohemarthrosis 94
Lipomas 4, 6, 15, 16, 60, 65, 66, 94, 283, 335, 345, 357, 362, 365, 385
  infrapatellar 96*f*
Lipomatosis, epidural 368
Liposarcoma 6, 63, 92
Liver 387
  anatomy of 161
  bright 135
  diffusely
    hyperechoic 135
    hypodense 137
    hypoechoic 135
  function tests 163
  hyperperfusion abnormalities of 137
  normal hemodynamics parameters of 163
  normal size of 163
Looser's zone 224, 295
Lumbar
  artery, pseudoaneurysm of 160, 161
  spine, posterior apophyseal joints of 186*f*
Lumbosacral spine 229*f*
Luminal occlusion 114
Lung
  abscess 28, 40, 55
  cyst, traumatic 35
  disease 26
  field
    hypertranslucent 53
    hypertransradiant 50
  lesions 44*t*
  tear 27
  tumors 27
Lupus erythematosus 185*f*
Luschka ducts 164
Lymph node 16, 17, 31, 63, 65, 67
  enlargement 9, 12, 14, 15
  mass, metastatic 7
  mediastinal 100
  metastatic 9*t*
Lymphadenopathy 319
  retropharyngeal 345
  sub-diaphragmatic 102
Lymphangiectasia 110, 121, 124
  intestinal 108, 110, 124
  primary 119
Lymphangioma 1, 2, 14, 63, 350
  cystic 6
Lymphangitis 63
  carcinoma 28
Lymphatic
  malformation 385, 386
  obstruction 124, 147
Lymphoceles 390
Lymphoma 4, 9, 16, 29, 69, 100, 104-106, 106*t*, 110, 111, 113, 114, 119, 124, 125, 127, 130, 141, 156-159, 180, 216, 225, 258, 272, 313, 317, 346, 348, 369, 375, 379, 385

M

Macroadenoma 305
Macrocalcification 75
Macrodystrophia lipomatosa 172*f*
Madelung deformity 202
Magnetic resonance 221, 260
    anatomy 280
    angiography 238, 254, 302
    imaging 2, 170, 219, 248, 264, 278, 286, 346
    urography 286
Malabsorption 119, 120
    signs of 120*f*
Malakoplakia 274
Malformation, arteriovenous 3, 329
Malignancy 68
    features of 391
    primary 64, 115, 117
    secondary 64
Malignant solitary pulmonary nodule 37*t*
Mammogram 66*f*, 75*f*
    craniocaudal 68*f*, 69*f*, 76*f*
    mediolateral 70*f*, 72*f*
Mantoux test 115
Marble bone disease 289
Marchiafava-Bignami disease 342
Marfan's syndrome 24, 203, 209, 319
Maroteaux-Lamy syndrome 214
Masses 131, 356
    abdominal 147, 148
    adnexal 384, 392
    adrenal 142, 282
    cystic 142
    extradural 325, 325*f*
    extrinsic 128
    inflammatory 257, 379
    intramedullary 326, 326*f*
    intraspinal 325
    laryngeal 348
    middle ear 357, 357*t*
    nasopharyngeal 346
    ocular 353
    orbital 349
    pancreatic 139
    pleural 59
    posterior mediastinal 19
    renal 257
    solid 392
    suprasellar 303, 305
    tracheal 13
Massive fibrosis, progressive 34
Mastitis 72
Mastocytosis 119, 124, 179, 216
Mastoiditis, chronic 316, 316*f*
Maxillary antrum, opaque 375, 375*t*
Maxillary sinusitis, bilateral chronic 376*f*
McLeod syndrome 53
Meckel-Gruber syndrome 203, 396
Meconium peritonitis 134, 405
Mediastinal lesion, anterior 14*t*
Mediastinal masses 7, 29
    anterior 7, 14, 15*f*, 16
    posterior 10
    superior 11
Mediastinal thymus, cervical extension of 1, 2
Mediastinitis, fibrosing 87
Mediastinum 7, 19, 19*f*, 88
    posterior compartments of 8*f*
    tumors of 7, 7*t*
Medullary cystic disease 235, 237, 266
Medulloblastoma 309
Mega cisterna magna 297, 328
Megacalyces 250
Meig-Salmon syndrome 57
Melanoma 181, 353
Melas syndrome 339, 344
Melnick-Needles syndrome 201
Melorheostosis 180
Ménétrier's disease 104, 105, 110, 119, 124
Meningioma 289-293, 296, 300, 304, 314, 316, 326, 329, 331, 334, 357, 359, 364
    orbital 350, 354
    primary orbital 350
    suprasellar 307
Meningocele 289, 333, 346, 347
    anterior 20
    lateral thoracic 366
Meningoencephalocele, large 332*f*
Merrf syndrome 339, 344
Mesothelioma 44, 50
    malignant 60, 62

Metabolic disorders 212
Metaphyseal
    band, solitary dense 200
    injury, localized 200
    lines, dense vertical 200
Metaphysis, cupping of 200
Metastasis
    calcifying 28
    hematogenous 101, 314
    osteolytic 220*f*
    osteosclerotic 215
    parenchymal 310
Metastatic lesions, characteristics of 180, 181
Meyer dysplasia 198
Michel's classification 162
Microadenoma 305
Microcalcifications 75, 76
    internal 70*f*
    multiple 75*f*
Microlithiasis, alveolar 46
Middle segment shortening 173, 211
Migration, abnormalities of 398
Milk alkali syndrome 256
Miscarriage 401, 401*t*
Mitchell staging 199, 200*t*
Mitochondrial dysfunction 339
Mitral incompetence 80
Mitral regurgitation 85*f*, 90
Mitral stenosis 81, 83, 85, 85*f*, 87
Mitral valve 88
    prolapse 387
Mitral valvular disease 82
Mixed density lesions 66, 67*fc*
Mole, partial 384, 384*t*
Moniliasis 153
Monoarthritis 205
Morgagni's hernia 8, 16, 27, 63, 64
Morquio's syndrome 198, 319, 320
Moth-eaten bone 189
Moth-eaten nephrogram 274
Moustache sign 145
Mucocele 352
    laryngeal 349
Mucolipidosis 175, 176
Mucopolysaccharidoses 175, 319, 320
Mucous retention cyst 375
Mucoviscidosis 107

Müllerian duct cyst 281
Multilocular cystic lesions,
    nonexpansile 231
Muscle, tumors of 133
Mycobacterium
    avium-intracellulare complex 109
    tuberculosis 311
Myelitis 327
Myelography 362
Myelolipoma 142, 283
Myeloma 216
    multiple 180, 220, 234, 244, 287, 323, 370, 375
Myelosclerosis 216, 318
Myositis ossificans 92
    progressive, congenital 92
Myxedema 91
Myxoma 84

N

Nabothian cysts 383, 384, 384*t*
Nasal cephaloceles 333
Nasogastric tube esophagitis 154
Nasopalatine 371
Nasopharyngeal masses,
    differential diagnosis of 346
Necrosis
    acute cortical 244, 257
    aseptic 198
    avascular 198, 198*f*, 199, 200*t*
    intestinal 132
    papillary 235, 237
Necrotizing disorders 243
Neonatal dysplasia, lethal 175
Neoplasms 35, 37, 59, 114, 292, 313, 333, 375, 376
    cystic 263, 297, 298
    extension of 346
    primary 300, 310
        malignant 156
Neoplastic disease 323, 324
Nephritis
    acute interstitial 245
    hereditary chronic 235
Nephroblastomatosis 261
Nephrocalcinosis 255, 255*f*
    cortical 257
    medullary 256

Nephrogram 236, 239, 241, 242, 245, 246, 262
    abnormal 274
    absent 274
    dense persistent 274
    inhomogeneous arteriographic 274
    persistent
        dense 274
        faint 274
    striated urographic 274
Nephrolithiasis 256
Nephroma
    congenital mesoblastic 260
    mesoblastic 147
    multilocular cystic 261, 263, 265
Nephronophthisis, juvenile 266
Nephropathy, reflux 239
Nephrosclerosis
    benign 235
    malignant 235
Nerve 93
    sheath tumors 20, 300, 313, 364
Neural foramina, enlarged 326*f*
Neural tube defects 386
Neuraminidase deficiency 176
Neurilemmoma 350
Neuroblastoma 5, 6, 142, 148, 180, 181, 260, 283, 326, 385
    metastatic 221, 221*f*
Neurocysticercosis 95*f*
Neuroectodermal tumor,
    primitive 22
Neurofibroma 4, 287, 325, 326*f*
Neurofibromatosis 24, 57, 93, 203, 255, 318, 329, 330, 336, 337
Neuromuscular disease 155
Neuromuscular disorder 152, 320
Neuropathic foot 207*f*
Nipple, retraction of 76*f*
Nodular hyperplasia 267
Nodular lymphoid hyperplasia,
    benign 113
Nodule
    adenomatous 378
    rheumatoid 34, 41
    sand-like 119
    small 119

solitary pulmonary 36, 37, 37*f*, 38
    toxic solitary 377
Non-adenomatous single polyps 126
Nonexpansile unilocular cystic lesions 231
Non-gynecological pelvic lesions,
    differential diagnosis of 389
Non-Hodgkin's disease 17
Non-Hodgkin's lymphoma 28, 157, 187*f*
Nonsteroidal anti-inflammatory
    disorders 245
    drug 198
Non-ulcerative mucosal disease 124
Notched proximal ureter 236
Nutritional
    deficiency 190
    disturbances 222

O

Obesity 91
Obstruction
    complete 251
    ileal 114, 149
    venous 124
Oligodendroglioma 362
Oligohydramnios 402, 402*fc*
Ollier's disease 201
Omphalocele 387
Oncocytoma 260
Optic
    chiasmatic lesions 303
    foramen, enlarged 328
    glioma 330
    nerve 331
        glioma 329, 337, 351
        meningioma 354
Orbital fissure enlargement,
    superior 311
Orbital inflammation, idiopathic 352
Orbital tumors, adult 352
Ormond's disease 159
Ossificans progressiva 97
Osteitis condensans ilii 228

Osteoarthritis 183, 186f, 208f, 228, 228f, 230
Osteoarthropathy, hypertrophic 194, 195
Osteoblastic metastasis 176f, 317
Osteoblastoma 178, 179f, 180, 217
Osteochondrodysplasias 211
Osteochondroma 24, 189f
Osteoclastic activity, disturbance of 22
Osteoclastoma 220, 234
Osteocytes, location of 191f
Osteodysplasty 201
Osteodystrophy, renal 180, 215, 224, 291
Osteogenesis imperfecta 24, 175, 194, 224, 294, 296, 315, 319
Osteoid
  lesions 187
  osteoma 178, 178f, 180, 216, 217f
Osteolytic defects 184
Osteoma 178, 216, 289, 290, 299, 360
Osteomalacia 180, 191, 191f, 222, 224, 295, 374
  causes of 192
Osteomyelitis 179, 190, 194, 217, 300
  acute 369
  chronic 188f, 369
  diabetic 195f
  hematogenous 195f
Osteonecrosis 180, 184, 369
  avascular 198
Osteopathia
  condensans disseminata 177
  striata 178, 200, 316
Osteopenia 190, 222
  causes of diffuse 222
  periarticular 230f
Osteopetrosis 316, 317, 331
Osteopoikilosis 177, 216
Osteoporosis 177f, 180, 190, 222, 222f, 324, 373
  disuse 224
  generalized 222
  juvenile 223
  periarticular 227
  postmenopausal 223
  senile 223

Osteosarcoma 180, 189f, 217, 217f, 370
  multifocal 179
  parosteal 92
  primary 289, 290
Osteosclerosis 94f
  diffuse 94f
  generalized 176
Otitis media, chronic suppurative 316, 357
Otopalatodigital syndrome 296
Oval calcifications, multiple 95f
Ovarian adnexal mass, differential diagnosis of 390
Ovarian edema, massive 389
Ovarian masses 388fc, 390
  benign 388, 389t
  differential diagnosis of 388, 390
  malignant 388, 389t
Ovaries 181, 387
  abnormal 389
  normal 388

P

Pachydermoperiostosis 194, 194f, 296
Paget's disease 176, 177f, 178, 180, 192, 209, 216, 225, 289, 291, 292, 294, 315, 317, 322, 323, 331, 374
  progression of 177f
Pancoast's syndrome 5
Pancoast's tumor 5, 6
Pancreas 165, 387
  anatomy of 161
Pancreatic disease, adjacent 104, 106
Pancreatitis 57, 107
  chronic 138, 159
  focal 139, 141
Papillae 236, 239
Papillary mucinous tumor, intraductal 139
Papillary necrosis
  chronic 238, 239
  grades of 257f
  renal 256
Papilloma 69, 349
  inverted 298
  squamous 102

Paragangliomas 365
  nonchromaffin 358
Paragonimus westermani 336
Paralytic ileus 112
Paranasal sinus
  masses 352
  metastatic 352
  neoplasm of 352
  secondary 352
Para-ovarian cyst 388
Paraplegia 92, 228
Parapneumonic effusion 57
Parasellar chordoma 314
Parasites 57, 121
Parenchymal destruction, diffuse 380
Parenchymal disease, high resolution CT-pattern of 63
Parotid tumor 346
Paroxysmal disorders 339
Pars interarticularis 178f
Patent ductus arteriosus 80, 82
Pectus carinatum 21
Pectus excavatum 21
Pelizaeus-Merzbacher disease 344
Pelken spur 191f
Pelvic
  abscess 96, 385
  kidney 253
  mass 384, 385t
  postoperative 389, 390t
Pelvicalyceal system
  dilated 239, 242
  hypoplastic 239
  hypovolemic 239
Pelvi-infundibulocalyceal system 236, 237
Pelvis 94f, 269, 269f, 296
  calyceal system 237
Pelviureteric junction obstruction 250
Pepper-pot skull 192
Peptic
  disease 159
  stricture 98
  ulcer 145
    disease 104, 107, 124
Periaortic mass 251
Periaortitis, chronic 159
Pericardial calcifications 88

Pericarditis
  constrictive 87, 124
  idiopathic 88
Perihilar cystic bronchiectasis, bilateral 34*f*
Perihilar pneumonia 29
Perinatal viral infections 340
Perineural spread 314
Periosteal reaction 179, 194, 234*f*, 245
  types of 183*f*, 192, 193
Periostitis 206
Peripheral nerve 270
  sheath tumors 385
Peripheral nervous system 91, 334
Periportal hyperechogenicity 135
Peritoneal fistula, pulmonary 145
Peritoneal surface 144
Periurethral glands 280
Peroxisomal disorders 339
Pertechnetate scan 20
Perthes disease 199*f*
Petrous bone, destruction of 293
Peutz-Jeghers syndrome 119, 126, 127
Pharyngocele, lateral 152
Pharyngoesophageal pouch 10, 13, 20
Pheochromocytoma 142, 181, 283
Phleboliths 138
Phosphorus 190*f*
Phrenic nerve palsy 26
Phylloides tumor 69
Pilocystic astrocytoma 303
Pineal tumors 335
Pinpoint opacities, multiple 54
Placenta
  abnormalities of 395*f*
  hydropic degeneration of 383
  thickened 393, 394*fc*
Plantar calcaneal spur 208
Planum sphenoidale 299*fc*
Plasma cell granuloma 39
Plasmacytoma 220, 234, 323
Platybasia 294*f*, 295
Pleural fluid, radiological appearances of 61
Pleuropericardial cyst 8, 15
Plexiform neurofibromas 312
Plummer-Vinson syndrome 100

Pneumatoceles 52
Pneumatosis 110
  coli 145
  cystic 113
  intestinalis 128, 145
Pneumoconiosis 33, 47
Pneumocystis carinii 138
Pneumomediastinum 5, 27, 145
Pneumonectomy 44
Pneumonia 40, 145
  bacterial 40
  lobar 54
Pneumonitis, subsegmental 48
Pneumopericardium 31
Pneumoperitoneum 142, 143, 145, 147*f*
  diffuse 146*f*
Pneumothorax 26, 53, 60, 61, 61*f*
Poland syndrome 22, 203
Poliomyelitis 23
Polyarteritis nodosa 130, 157, 255
Polyarthritis 24
Polycystic kidney
  disease 245, 262-264
    autosomal dominant 264, 387
    autosomal recessive 264, 387
  infantile 147
Polydactyly 174*f*, 203, 203*f*
Polyhydramnios 402, 403*fc*
Polyostotic fibrous dysplasia 219*f*
Polyp 125, 376
  adenomatous 125
  antral 376*f*
  antrochoanal 346, 347
  colonic 125, 126
  hamartomatous 126
  hyperplastic 126
  mucosal 375
  single juvenile 126
Polyposis
  coli, familial 126
  juvenile 126, 127
Polysyndactyly syndrome 203
Popcorn calcification 73
Porcelain gallbladder 133*f*
Porencephalic cysts 298
Portal vein
  gas in 131, 143
  thromboemboli 135

Postburn contracture 204*f*
Postnephrectomy 253
Postpneumonectomy 50
Posturethral valves 268
Pott's spine 6
Potter's syndrome 247
Pregnancy
  ectopic 383, 383*t*, 384, 384*t*, 385*t*, 400
  test 384
    positive 392, 393*fc*
Presacral fetal mass, differential diagnosis of 384
Pressure
  overload 80, 81, 81*t*, 83-85
  ventilation, intermittent positive 145
Prevertebral soft tissue, causes of 344
Proctitis 168
Progeria 226
Proliferative disorders 243
Properitoneal fat lines, normal 146
Prostate 181, 267, 279, 281, 387
  infections of 281
  specific antigen 275, 288
  tumors of 281
  zonal anatomy 279*f*
Prostatitis
  acute 281
  chronic 281
  granulomatous 281
Protein
  deficiency 224
  deposition, abnormal 243
  losing enteropathy 124
Proteus mirabilis 247
Protrusio acetabuli 209, 209*f*
Proximal limb shortening 173, 211
Prune-Belly syndrome 270
Pseudarthrosis 2*f*
Pseudo wall sign 144
Pseudoachondroplasia 174, 212
Pseudoarthrosis 197
Pseudocalcification 73
Pseudochondroplasia 173, 175
Pseudocyst 141
  non-pancreatic 131
  pancreatic 11, 131

Pseudodiverticulosis, intramural 153
Pseudofractures 224
Pseudogestation 384f
Pseudo-kidney sign 117
Pseudolymphoma 104, 105
Pseudomass 71
Pseudomonas 360
Pseudo-obstruction 122
Pseudpneumoperitoneum 144
Pseudopolyp 125
Pseudpseudohypoparathyroidism 215
Pseudotumor 352
  inflammatory 39
  orbital 329, 352
Psuedoachondroplasia 320
Psychiatric disorder 152
Pubic bone, aneurysmal bone cyst of 221f
Punctate calcifications, absence of 184f
Pyelogram 238
  intravenous 253f, 261f
Pyelography, intravenous 286
Pyelonephritis
  acute 242
    focal bacterial 262
  chronic 239
  emphysematous 252
  xanthogranulomatous 242, 247, 256
Pyknodysostosis 215, 226, 291, 296
Pyle's disease 201
Pyloric canal, abrupt narrowing of 113
Pyocele 375
Pyonephrosis 247

R

Radial scar 71
Radiation 339
  enteritis 115, 118, 124
    end-stage 115
  esophagitis 100, 154
  injury 158
  necrosis 311
  neoplasia 235
  nephritis 236, 238
  therapy 72
Radiolucent lesion 66, 67fc
Radionuclide bone scintigraphy 268
Radiotherapy 88, 120
Radiotracer, uptake of 376
Rathke's cleft cyst 305, 307
Raynaud's phenomenon 23
Rectal tumor 130
Rectosigmoid junction, anterior indentation of 130
Rectum 181
Regional migratory osteoporosis 192
Regurgitation
  aortic 82
  pulmonary 82, 85
Reiter's syndrome 185f, 227-229
Renal anomalies, contralateral 247
Renal artery 238
  aneurysm of 256
  occlusion 246
  stenosis 235, 238, 247
    atheromatous 236
    signs of 254
Renal cell carcinoma 181, 248, 256, 258, 286
  cystic 264
Renal cystic disease, unilateral 265
Renal cysts
  classification of 263
  extraparenchymal 263, 265
Renal disease
  atheroembolic 235
  chronic 222
Renal dysplasia, obstructive cystic 387
Renal failure
  acute 244
  chronic 88
Renal infarction
  chronic 236
  end result of 236
Renal vein 241
  thrombosis 147, 241, 248
Rete testes, tubular ectasia of 272
Retinoblastoma 180, 329, 330, 353, 354
Retrocaval ureter 251
Retroesophageal space 344
Retrograde cholangiopancreatography, endoscopic 140
Retroperitoneal
  fibrosis 124, 159, 251
  tumor, primary 159
Retropharyngeal abscess, causes of 3
Rhabdomyosarcoma 180, 270, 351, 355, 357, 359, 386
Rheumatoid arthritis, juvenile 228, 230
Rhombencephalosynapsis 338
Ribs
  abnormal
    density of 202
    shape of 202
    size of 202
  dense 202
  lesions 201
  notching 22, 202
  ribbon 202
Rickets 191f, 194, 198f, 212, 296
Rigler's sign 145
Rim nephrogram 274
Rokitansky-Aschoff sinuses 131
Rubella, congenital 200

S

Sacroiliac joints 210, 228, 228f, 229, 229f, 230
Sacroiliitis 208, 227, 230
  differential diagnosis of 228
Sacrotuberous ligament, bilateral 94f
Salivary gland tumors, minor 349
Salmon patch 350
Salt and pepper appearance 359
Santorini accessory pancreatic duct 165
Sarcoidosis 9, 19, 19f, 29, 35, 46, 56, 68, 157, 158, 206, 227, 257, 329
Sarcoma 28, 115, 385
Scheuermann's disease 324, 324f
Schistosomiasis 251, 274
Schizencephaly 298, 399
Schwannoma 4, 313, 349, 350, 356
Scimitar syndrome 65

Scintigraphy 168
  renal 254
Scleroderma 56, 97, 98, 155, 227, 374
Sclerosis 287, 288, 288*fc*
  progressive systemic 227
  systemic 23, 122
  tuberous 56, 63, 178, 263, 336
Scoliosis 26, 48
  severe progressive 174
Scurvy 191*f*, 194, 224
Sella
  osteoporosis of 305*f*
  turcica 303*f*
Sellar masses 305
Seminal versiculogram 268
Seminal vesicle 387
  calcification 273
  cysts 281
Seminal vesicular invasion 282
Seminoma 271
Septal lines 47
Septations, types of 189
Septic infarct 35
Seroma 390
Sex cord tumor 390, 391
Sexually-transmitted disease 229
Short limb 213
  dysplasias 211
  skeletal dysplasia 173
  spinal abnormality besides 174
Short rib 202
  polydactyly syndrome 203
  syndromes 175
Short spine
  dysplasias 213
  skeletal dysplasia 174
  spinal abnormality besides 174
Short trunk dwarfs 213
Shrunken stomach 113*f*
Sickle cell
  anemia 138, 178, 295, 325
  disease 194
  disorder 318
Silicosis 29, 46, 47, 56, 63
Sinusitis 375
Situs 89
  intermedius 89
  inversus 89, 89*f*
  solitus 89

Skeletal
  abnormalities 226
  hyperostosis, diffuse
    idiopathic 209*f*, 228, 230, 317
  maturation
    abnormal 172
    disorders 172
    system 172
Skeleton
  appendicular 176*f*
  ossification of 175
Skiagram chest, plain 51-53
Skin
  calcifications 73
  edema 72*f*, 76*f*
  squamous cell carcinoma of 181
Skull vault
  density of 292
  thickening of 289
Small bowel folds, thickened 109*fc*, 119
Smooth esophageal strictures, causes of 155
Soft tissue 50, 53, 95*f*, 96*f*, 97
  calcification, periarticular 95*t*, 96
  density
    lesion 68
    mass 16, 46
  infection 195*f*
  lesions 91
    differential diagnosis of 8, 9*t*, 91
  ligamentous calcification 93*f*
  linear calcification of 93
  mass 179*f*
  neck, plain X-ray 346
  nodules 207
  ossification 92
  swelling 375
  thickening, prevertebral 344
Solitary pulmonary nodule
  benign 37*t*
  characteristics of 38
Spectrum 265
  multiple pinpoint opacities 48*t*
Sphenoid 346
  hypoplasia of greater wing of 329
  sinus 303

Spinal anomalies 19
Spinal canal 318
  central 186*f*
Spinal column 228
Spinal cord 325*f*
  mass displaces 325*f*
Spinal fusion 229
Spinal subdural empyema 366
Spine 166, 210, 215, 222, 229, 230, 324*f*
  osteoarthritis of 186*f*
Spleen 387
Splenic lesion, hyperechoic 138
Spondylitis 230
  anykylosing 317
  tubercular 319, 320*f*
  tuberculous 3
Spondyloarthritides, seronegative 210
Spondyloarthropathies, enteropathic 230
Spondylosis, degenerative 316
Sporadic aniridia 260
Squamous cell carcinoma 5, 105*t*, 251, 357, 359, 360
Staghorn calculus 256
Staphylococcus 54, 360
  aureus 34, 55
  pneumoniae 60
Steinberg classification 199
Stenosis
  aortic 80, 82, 88
  pulmonary 77, 85
Sternal mass 15
Stomach 112*f*
  dilatation of 132*f*
  gaseous distension of 26
Storage disorders 201
Strawberry skull 399
Streptococcus
  pneumoniae 54, 55
  pyogenes 55
String sign 117
Strongyloidosis 119
Sturge-Weber syndrome 336
Subclavian artery
  aberrant 1
  anomalous left 86
Subphrenic inflammatory disease 26

Sudeck's atrophy 192
Sunburst periosteal reaction 179*f*
Sunray appearance, divergent spiculated 193
Sunray speculation 133
Superior vena cava syndrome 88
Sylvian fissure, enlarged 297
Symphysis pubis
   fusion of 210
   widening of 210
Syndactyly 203, 203*f*
Synovitis, chronic 230
Syphilis 179, 288
   congenital 194
Syringohydromyelia 363
Systemic lupus erythematosus 24, 57, 77

T

Tailgut cyst 385
Takayasu's arteritis 255
Tectocerebellar dysraphia 338
Temporal bone sclerosis 314
   differential diagnosis of 314
Tendinitis 93
Tenia saginata 112
Tenia solium 112, 336
Tension pneumothorax 60
Teratoma 308, 335, 350, 386
   atypical 308
Testicular tumors
   differential diagnosis of 271
   primary 271
   secondary 271
   spread of 272
Testis 181
   benign lesions of 271
   miscellaneous lesions of 271
Tetralogy of Fallot 51, 77, 85
Thalassemia 295
Thallium 133
Thanatophoric dwarfism 175, 213
Thoracic aortic aneurysm 18
Thoracic dystrophy, asphyxiating 174, 175, 213
Thoracic inlet 1*f*
   anatomy of 1
   lesions of 1, 1*fc*
Thoracic outlet syndrome 6
Thorax abnormalities 397

Thrombosis, subacute 248
Thumb, abnormal 204
Thymoma 15, 16
Thymus, normal 16
Thyroglossal duct cysts 378
Thyroid 16, 180, 181
   abscess 378
   acropachy 194
   calcifications 382
   carcinoma 4, 6, 377
   cystic lesions of 378
   ectopic 381
   enlarged 386
   gland, enlarged 2*f*
   hormone, exogenous 380
   lesions 376
   masses, extension of 345
   nodule, solid 381
   stimulating hormone levels 377
   tumor 7, 14
Thyroiditis, subacute 380
TNM staging 140, 276
Todani's type 134
Tolosa-Hunt syndrome 313
Tophaceous gout, chronic 186*f*, 187*f*
Total anomalous pulmonary venous
   drainage 13
   return 84, 85, 87
Toxoplasmosis 335
Trabecular bone, formation of 92
Trachea 27
Tracheobiliary fistula, congenital 164
Tram tracks calcification 73
Tramline calcification 244
Transitional cell carcinoma 259, 286
Trauma 35, 59, 194, 317, 323, 324
Tricuspid
   atresia 52
   regurgitation 83, 85, 87
   stenosis 77, 84
   valve 89
Tropheryma whipplei 122
Tubercular arthritis
   early phase of 206*f*
   late phase of 206*f*

Tuberculoma 40, 335
Tuberculosis 12, 18, 33, 55, 59, 88, 108, 111, 115, 124, 158, 184, 247, 250, 255, 284, 286, 321
   duodenal 107*f*
   miliary 45, 45*f*
Tuberosity, calcaneal 92*f*
Tubular bone involvement, severe 174
Tumoral calcinosis 92
Tumors 130, 142, 246, 250, 251, 256, 325, 326, 334, 346, 367
   benign 314, 358, 359, 378
   brown 372
   containing adipose 133
   embryonal 365
   epithelial 267, 390
   extracranial 313
   fibrous 64, 65
   head and neck 100
   hepatic 135, 137
   lymphoid 353
   malignant 2, 359, 379
   medullary 283
   mesodermal 267
   metastatic 351, 352
   necrotic 143
   neurogenic 10, 10*t*, 13, 20, 313, 385
   orbital 313
   pediatric orbital 349
   pleural 62
   primary 16, 180, 181*t*
   renal 248, 253
   sacral 130
   stage of 266
   stromal 272, 283
   teratodermoid 8, 15
   testicular 271
   thymic 7
   tracheal 10
   vanishing 59
Tunica albuginea, cysts of 272
Turcot's syndrome 125, 127
Turner's syndrome 203, 212, 263, 395
Twin pregnancy 384, 384*t*, 394*f*
Tympanic membrane 360

U

Ulcerative colitis 124, 127
Ulcers
    aphthous 129
    disease 105, 107
    esophageal 153
Unilateral renal artery stenosis, signs of 254
Urate nephropathy, acute 246
Uremia 107
Ureter 237, 242
    dilated 249
    gas in 252
Ureterocele 274, 251
    ectopic 270
    orthotopic 251
Urethra, posterior 269f
Urethral diverticulum, anterior 268
Urethral valves, congenital 268
Urinary tract 284
    abnormalities 397
    complications 171
    gas in 143, 252
    rupture 268
Urinoma 147, 390
Urogenital system 235
Urography, excretory 160
Urological elements, primary 243
Uropathy, obstructive 242
Uroradiologic elements, secondary 236, 237, 239-241, 243, 259
Uterine
    perforation 384, 385t
    size 384
Uterus 181
    enlarged 396, 396fc

V

Valve
    aortic 88
    calcifications, cardiac 88
    position of 88f
    pulmonary 88
    stenosis, pulmonary 82
Van Buchem's disease 316
van der Hoeve's syndrome 315
Varicoid carcinoma 103
Varicose veins 93
Vascular
    disorders 107
    insufficiency 109, 194
    lesion 17, 304, 335, 342
    malformation 173, 385, 386
    system 147
    tumors 357
Vasculitis 110
Vasculogenic lesions 350
Veins, thrombosed 93
Vena cava
    enlarged superior 87
    thrombosis, inferior 124
Veno-occlusive disease, primary pulmonary 87
Ventral induction, abnormalities of 398
Ventricular septal defect 79, 80f, 85
Vermis 327
Vertebrae
    bullet-shaped 223
    collapse of 222f
    hemangioma of 225f
Vertebral body
    anterior scalloping of 319, 319f
    central beak of 320f
    posterior scalloping of 318, 318f
Vesical calculi 269f
Vesicointestinal fistula 252
Vesicoureteric reflux 249, 251, 270
Vessels, tumors of 133
Vestibular aqueduct syndrome 356
Videocystometrography 270
Villonodular synovitis, pigmented 184
Villous adenoma 124, 126
Viral infection 88
    congenital 340
Vitamin D 192
    deficiency of metabolism of 192
Vocal cord polyps 349
Volume overload 79, 80, 81t, 82, 83, 85
von Hippel-Lindau disease 248
Voorhoeve's disease 178
Voorhoeve's syndrome 316

W

Wachenheim's line 294
Waldenström's macroglobulinemia 119
Wegener's granulomatosis 34, 37, 41, 375, 376
Werner's syndrome 93
Wernicke's encephalopathy 342
Whipple's disease 110, 119, 122, 124, 228, 230
Whipple's triad 139
Wilms' tumor 147, 148, 181, 248, 258, 260
    variant of 180
Wolman's disease 142
Wormian bones 291
    multiple 296
Wounds, penetrating 252

X

Xanthomatosis 110
Xylose breath test 120

Y

Yersinia 124
    colitis 130
    enteritis 130
Yolk sac 384
    absence of 383

Z

Zellweger's syndrome 198, 263, 339, 343
Zenker's diverticulum 13, 20, 152
Zollinger-Ellison syndrome 104, 107, 110, 111, 119, 122